Orthopaedic and Trauma Nursing

Orthopaedic and Trauma Nursing

An Evidence-based Approach
to Musculoskeletal Care

Second Edition

Edited by

Sonya Clarke and Mary Drozd

WILEY Blackwell

Library of Congress Cataloging-in-Publication Data
Names: Clarke, Sonya, editor. | Drozd, Mary, editor.
Title: Orthopaedic and trauma nursing: an evidence-based approach to
    musculoskeletal care / edited by Sonya Clarke and Mary Drozd.
Other titles: Orthopaedic and trauma nursing (Clarke)
Description: Second edition. | Hoboken, NJ: Wiley-Blackwell, 2023. |
    Includes bibliographical references and index.
Identifiers: LCCN 2022029474 (print) | LCCN 2022029475 (ebook) | ISBN
    9781119833383 (paperback) | ISBN 9781119833390 (adobe pdf) | ISBN
    9781119833406 (epub)
Subjects: MESH: Orthopedic Nursing–methods | Trauma Nursing–methods |
    Musculoskeletal System–injuries | Wounds and Injuries–nursing |
    Evidence-Based Nursing
Classification: LCC RD753 (print) | LCC RD753 (ebook) | NLM WY 157.6 |
    DDC 616.7/0231–dc23/eng/20220819
LC record available at https://lccn.loc.gov/2022029474
LC ebook record available at https://lccn.loc.gov/2022029475

Cover Design: Wiley
Cover Image: © SCIEPRO/Getty Images

Set in 9.5/12.5pt STIXTwoText by Straive, Pondicherry, India

Printed in Singapore
M WEP256553 150124

Contents

List of Contributors

Thelma Begley, MSc (Nursing), Bachelor Nursing Studies (Hons), Higher Diploma in Nursing Studies (Children's Nursing) and (Nurse Education), Orthopaedic Nursing Certificate, RGN, RCN, RNT
Assistant Professor in Children's Nursing, School of Nursing and Midwifery, Trinity College Dublin, Dublin, Ireland

Thelma, a nurse for over 30 years, holds qualifications in adult, child and orthopaedic nursing as well as in nurse education. Her clinical experience includes children, young people's medical and surgical nursing, and adult and children's orthopaedic nursing, in particular orthopaedic trauma. She has significant teaching experience in undergraduate and postgraduate nursing programmes, with specialist expertise teaching children's and orthopaedic nursing. She is module leader on undergraduate, postgraduate and MSc children's nursing programmes.

Dr Sonya Clarke (Editor), EdD, MSc, PGCE (Higher Education), PG Cert (Pain Management), BSc (Hons) Specialist Practitioner in Orthopaedic Nursing, RN child, RGN
Senior Lecturer (Education), School of Nursing & Midwifery, Queen's University Belfast, Belfast, UK

Sonya, a nurse for over 30 years, has experience in children's and adult nursing in her nursing career, which commenced in 1988. She qualified as an RGN in 1991, followed by a diploma in Children's Nursing in 1996. Clinical practice was primarily within Northern Ireland's regional elective orthopaedic unit for the adult and child until 2001, with additional nursing experience (bank position) gained as a Marie Currie nurse until 2009. Prior to her teaching position in 2003, she was employed as a Lecturer Practitioner at Queen's University Belfast and Musgrave Park Hospital, Belfast. Current positions within higher education include Professional Lead for a new MSc pre-registration in Children's and Young People's Nursing and established pathway leader within continuing professional for a short course in Orthopaedic and Fracture Trauma

Nursing across the Lifespan. Sonya's teaching, research and scholarly activity reflects both children's nursing (child rights) and her specialist subject area of orthopaedics. Sonya was presented with the Royal College of Nursing (RCN) Award of Merit in 2020, the highest honour for service in recognition of the exceptional contribution she has made to the RCN. She also has an extensive publication history and continues to actively lead, inspire and deliver evidenced-based education that motivates and advances nursing.

Alison Collins, BSc (Hons), RGN, District Nursing Qualification Certificate in Orthopaedic Nursing, Post Grad Dip in Wound Healing and Tissue Repair, MSc
Tissue Viability Nurse, Belfast Health & Social Care Trust, Belfast, UK

Alison is an experienced nurse of more than 25 years. She currently holds a specialist nursing post within the largest health and social care trust within Northern Ireland.

Yvonne Conway, MSc Primary Care, BSc (Hons) Nursing, logy, Adv Dip Ed, RGN, RNT
Department of Nursing, Health Sciences and Integrated Care, Atlantic Technological University (Mayo), Castlebar, Ireland

Yvonne has extensive experience of teaching and curriculum development in both undergraduate and postgraduate general nursing. Her clinical expertise lies principally in emergency nursing, having worked in both UK emergency departments and USA trauma centres before her move into nurse education. She has directed Master's programmes in emergency nursing and acute medicine, and was a Trauma Nursing Core Course instructor. She has presented at conferences nationally and internationally, and been involved in funded research projects covering various topics. Recent publications include a rapid systematic review and qualitative evidence synthesis.

Dr Stefanie Cormack, PhD, MSc, PGCAPHE, FHEA
Senior Lecturer, Faculty of Education, Health and Wellbeing, University of Wolverhampton, UK

Stef is a Senior Lecturer and research lead for paramedic science for the Faculty of Education, Health and Wellbeing at the University of Wolverhampton. She qualified as a paramedic and worked as an operational helicopter emergency medical service (HEMS) critical care paramedic, gaining her Master's degree before moving into paramedic education. She has research interests in out-of-hospital cardiac arrest management, human factors and prehospital trauma/HEMS. Her PhD was a mixed methods approach to designing and evaluating a behavioural marker system for paramedic non-technical skills when managing an out-of-hospital cardiac arrest.

Mrs Julie Craig, MB BCh BAO (Hons.), MSc (Clin. Ed), MRCS MSc (Ortho. Eng.)
Orthopaedic Specialty Doctor, Royal Victoria Hospital, Belfast Health & Social Care Trust, Belfast, UK

Julie Craig is an orthopaedic specialty doctor in the Royal Victoria Hospital, Northern Ireland's regional trauma centre, in the Belfast Health & Social Care Trust (BHSCT). Julie graduated as a doctor from Queen's University Belfast (QUB) and is a member of the Royal College of Surgeons of Edinburgh. She has completed a Master's degree in clinical education at QUB and a Master's degree in orthopaedic engineering at Cardiff University. She is the former undergraduate medical educational lead for fractures in BHSCT, and currently teaches quality improvement and leadership skills to doctors in BHSCT and teaches postgraduate nurses specialising in trauma and orthopaedics. She has a special interest in clinical data analysis, is the specialty improvement lead for the BHSCT trauma database, and is a member of the Royal College of Physician's Falls and Fragility Fracture Audit Programme (FFFAP) board and the National Hip Fracture Database Advisory Group. She has presented her work on the Royal Victoria Hospital's fracture and major trauma patients internationally and has been the recipient of the prizes for best presentations from the British Trauma Society, the Irish Hip Fracture Database Annual Meeting and the British Orthopaedic Association (Bone and Joint Journal Prize).

Peter Davis MBE, Cert.Ed, BEd (Hons), RGN, DN, ONC, MA
Associate Professor (retired), Emeritus Editor International Journal of Orthopaedic and Trauma Nursing

During the late 1980s, Peter held posts in pre- and post-basic nursing education with a specific remit for orthopaedic nurse education. In 1989, he gained a Master's degree in nursing and education. In 1994, his first book, as editor and contributor, was published, *Nursing the Orthopaedic Patient*. From 1992 to 1994, he was chair of the RCN Society of

Orthopaedic and Trauma Nursing, and he has spent several years as a committee member. He was founding editor of the *Journal of Orthopaedic Nursing* and is now Emeritus Editor of the new *International Journal of Orthopaedic & Trauma Nursing*. He has presented numerous papers at national and international conferences. A personal philosophy of practice being primary to theory has kept him close to nursing care throughout his career and ensures an emphasis on research utilisation and evidence-based practice. In 2000, Her Majesty Queen Elizabeth II conferred on him the honour of Member of the Order of the British Empire (MBE) for services to orthopaedic nursing.

Dr Jeannie Donnelly, PhD, Dip. Wound Healing & Tissue Repair, BSc (Hon's) Health Studies incorporating the RCN Nurse Practitioner Professional Award, RN, ONC
Lead Nurse Tissue Viability, Belfast Health & Social Care Trust, Honorary Senior Lecturer, School of Nursing, Queens University Belfast, Belfast, UK

Jeannie qualified as a Registered Nurse in Belfast in 1988 and spent the first 8 years of her career working in the Fracture Trauma Unit of the Royal Victoria Hospital. During her time in this specialty, she became passionately interested in wound healing and tissue repair. In 1996, Jeannie became the first Tissue Viability Nurse on the island of Ireland, and in 2010, the Lead Nurse for Tissue Viability within the Belfast Health & Social Care Trust.

Dr Mary Drozd, Senior Teaching Fellow, Aston Medical School, Aston University, England, UK
Registered Nurse, Doctorate in Health and Wellbeing, MSc Health Sciences, BA (Hons), PGCE (Higher Education), ENB 219, Senior Fellow of the Higher Education Academy

Mary is a Registered Nurse with over 30 years' experience in orthopaedic and trauma nursing. She has worked as a staff nurse, sister, ward manager and advanced nurse practitioner in a variety of orthopaedic and trauma settings prior to joining a Higher Educational Institute in 2004. She has maintained strong clinical links alongside contributing to National Institute for Health and Care Excellence (NICE) guidance as a clinical specialist.

As an elected national steering committee member for the Royal College of Nursing (RCN) Society of Orthopaedic and Trauma Nurses (SOTN) from 2009- 2013 and re-elected in 2013-2017, Mary led the revision and further development of the RCN SOTN national competences for orthopaedic and trauma practitioners in 2012 and more recently was on the working group which published the current national competences in 2019.

Mary successfully completed a Professional Doctorate in Health and Wellbeing in 2019. Her research focused on adults with intellectual disabilities and their experiences of orthopaedic and trauma hospital care. The findings from the study have been disseminated via national and international conferences and papers from her thesis have been published in peer-reviewed and open access journals.

Mary has undertaken the role of Book Review Editor, Assistant Editor and is currently the Social Media Editor and a peer reviewer of manuscripts for the International Journal of Orthopaedic and Trauma Nursing. In 2021, Mary was awarded Senior Fellowship of the Higher Education Academy

Professor Sandra Flynn, PhD, MSc, BA (Hons), PGCE, RN, ONC
Chester Medical School, University of Chester

Professor Flynn qualified at the Chester District School of Nursing, the Robert Jones and Agnes Hunt Orthopaedic Hospital Oswestry and the University of Liverpool in general nursing, orthopaedic and trauma nursing, and education. Sandra started her academic career as a senior lecturer at the University of Chester in 2018 and is responsible for leading on the Doctor of Medicine programme at Chester Medical School. Both her Master's and PhD are orthopaedic based. Sandra worked for the National Health Service (NHS) for 38 years, during which time she advanced her knowledge, skills and expertise in the field of trauma and orthopaedics. She held the title of Consultant Nurse in Orthopaedics at the Countess of Chester NHS Foundation Trust. Introduced in 2008, this was the first consultant nurse post in the country working within this field of practice. Sandra undertook clinical practice at an advanced level and exercised higher levels of judgement, discretion and decision making in clinical care using an advanced practice competency framework. She was one of only two nurses at that time trained to perform hand surgery in the UK. She functioned as an expert resource-providing consultancy both internal and external to the Trust in the field of orthopaedics, monitoring and improving standards of care through clinical audit, dissemination of research, supervision of practice, teaching and provision of support for professional colleagues. Sandra is a former member of the Royal College of Nursing Society of Orthopaedics and Trauma Nursing committee, acting as Nursing Advisor to the Department of Health workforce planning sub-group, 18-week orthopaedic pathway. She has worked as a Specialist Advisor to the Care Quality Commission (CQC), the independent regulator of health and social care in England. Her role with the CQC was to undertake inspections of acute hospital trusts to check the quality of the orthopaedic and trauma services they provide.

Beverley Gray Linnecor, MSc Advanced Practice, BSc (Hons) Nursing Studies, PgCert TLHE, RGN, ONC, Dip CN, Cert in CBT, Cert in Counselling Skills, Professional Cert in Management

Beverley has many years of experience in both trauma and elective orthopaedic nursing. She was formerly the Clinical Nurse Specialist for the Scottish National Brachial Plexus Injury Service and Specialist Lecturer in Orthopaedics at the University of the West of Scotland. Beverley has presented papers internationally and published for books and journals. Beverley is now based in Guernsey, Channel Islands and is currently Clinical Editor with the *International Journal of Orthopaedic and Trauma Nursing*.

Sinead Hahessy, RGN, BA, MA (Soc. Sc.)
Lecturer and Postgraduate Programme Director, School of Nursing & Midwifery, National University of Ireland, Galway, Ireland

Sinead has 20 years' experience as a lecturer in nurse education. Her clinical nursing career includes experience in orthopaedics, gerontology, emergency care and theatre nursing. With a postgraduate background in sociology, she has contributed to the professional and educational development of undergraduate and postgraduate nursing in Ireland through involvement in curriculum design and teaching. Her teaching and research interests are in qualitative research, orthopaedic/theatre nursing, professional development in nursing and academic practice, reflective practice and arts-based pedagogy.

Fiona Heaney, RGN, MHSc (Nursing/Education), PG Diploma (Nursing Studies/Orthopaedics), PG Diploma (Clinical Teaching)
Clinical Nurse Specialist in Bone Health Galway University Hospitals, Galway, Ireland

Fiona started out working in orthopaedic trauma and has been involved in the care of patients following fracture for over 20 years. She worked as Clinical Facilitator/Practice Development Co-ordinator for Orthopaedic Nursing in Galway University Hospitals and later transferred into the role of Clinical Nurse Specialist in Orthopaedic Trauma. During her time working with people following acute fractures she developed an interest in promoting bone health and fracture prevention. She currently works as Clinical Nurse Specialist in Bone Health and is part of the Fracture Liaison Service in Merlin Park Hospital Galway.

Karen Hertz, MSc, BSc, DPSN, RGN, ENB219
Advanced Nurse Practitioner, Royal Stoke University Hospital, University Hospitals of North Midlands, Stoke-on-Trent, UK

Karen is a registered nurse, working in the National Health Service as an advanced nurse practitioner in a trauma and orthopaedic unit. She qualified in 1987 and since then has worked for 35 years in a variety of roles in trauma and orthopaedics, but her passion is for fragility fracture nursing and interdisciplinary care. She has been actively involved in both the Global and National Fragility Fracture Networks (FFNs) since their inception. She is currently leading the

Global Fragility Fracture nurse education team within the FFN. She has co-authored a number of journal articles, book chapters and books on fragility fracture management and allied subjects.

Professor Rebecca Jester, PhD, BSc (Hons)
Head of the School of Nursing, Royal College of Surgeons in Ireland, Medical University, Bahrain

Rebecca is Head of the School of Nursing, RCSI, Medical University, Bahrain. She qualified as a registered nurse in the UK in 1985. Rebecca then worked as a staff nurse, sister and ward manager in several trauma and orthopaedic settings in the UK and Sweden before completing a BSc (Hons) Education Studies in Nursing in 1995 and embarking on a clinical academic career working across the interface of education, research and clinical practice. Rebecca was awarded a PhD in Health Sciences from the University of Birmingham in 2001, supported by a National Smith and Nephew Fellowship. She was awarded a personal chair (professorship) in Orthopaedic Nursing in 2008 by Keele University and has held several senior academic positions, including Head of the School of Nursing and Midwifery, Keele University, Head of the Nursing School Abu Dhabi for Griffith University and Head of Department of Adult Nursing and Midwifery, London South Bank University. She holds several honorary positions internationally, including Emeritus Professor of Nursing, University of Wolverhampton, UK, Honorary Advisor to The Hong Kong College of Orthopaedic Nursing, Associate Editor of the *International Journal of Trauma and Orthopaedic Nursing* and Adjunct Professor of Orthopaedic Nursing Research at the University of Southern Denmark. Rebecca has many years of experience as an advanced nurse practitioner in orthopaedics whilst working in her academic roles and she was awarded Fellow of Nursing by the Hong Kong Academy of Nursing (May 2021) for contribution to excellence in nursing and advancement of nursing practice. Rebecca has a track record of research and associated publications in clinical research related to orthopaedic care.

Julia Judd, MSc, RSCN, RGN, ENB 219
University Hospital Southampton, Child Health. Tremona Rd Southampton, SO16 6YD, UK

Julia is an Advanced Nurse Practitioner in Children's Orthopaedics at the University Hospital Southampton, UK. She qualified as an RSCN and RGN at Queen Mary's Hospital for Children in Carshalton and subsequently gained her orthopaedic qualification and her Master's degree. Julia has a passion for promoting expertise and best practice through the organisation of and presenting at children's orthopaedic conferences. Julia has published extensively, both articles and book contributions, and is a reviewer for the *International Journal of Orthopaedic Trauma Nursing*. She is actively involved with a number of different national and international research projects, specifically focusing on developmental dysplasia of the hip, Perthes disease, clubfoot and the orthopaedic manifestations of vitamin D deficiency. Julia is co-chair of the RCN Society of Orthopaedic and Trauma Nursing.

Dr Carolyn Mackintosh-Franklin, RN, BA (Hons), MSc, PhD, PGDIp HE
Reader, University of Manchester, Manchester, UK

Carolyn is a registered nurse with many years' experience in pain management as a pioneering clinical nurse specialist and educationalist. Her most recent work focuses on educating nurses and other healthcare professionals to develop greater understanding of the nature of pain so that assessment and management can be improved for all pain sufferers. This includes the development of both undergraduate and postgraduate education programmes as well as embedding education around pain assessment and management into pre-registration undergraduate programmes. Carolyn's own area of research focuses on healthcare staff and their attitudes towards people experiencing pain based on existing evidence that demonstrates only slow improvements made in pain management, and the large numbers of people who continue to experience unnecessary and prolonged suffering as a result of poor pain assessment and inadequate management. Healthcare staff, personal attitudes and limited knowledge about pain are likely to be significant factors underpinning this failure to improve care and proactive educational programmes may support future practice improvements, as well as reduce unnecessary suffering.

Rosemary Masterson, RGN, ONC (ENB 219), BNS, MSc in Nursing
National Orthopaedic Hospital, Cappagh, Dublin, Ireland

Rosemary undertook her general training in the northwest of Ireland before completing the ENB 219 certificate in Orthopaedic Nursing at the Royal National Orthopaedic Hospital in Stanmore, London. She has worked in both orthopaedic elective and trauma settings in Ireland and London. She has undertaken the role of book review editor for the *International Journal of Orthopaedic and Trauma Nursing* in the past and contributes to international and national orthopaedic nursing conferences. Rosemary currently acts as treasurer of the Irish Orthopaedic Interest Group. She undertook her Bachelor of Nursing Studies degree at University College Dublin and in conjunction with the Royal College of Nursing and the University of Manchester completed a Master's degree in Nursing. She currently works as a nurse tutor and part of this role involves delivering the specialist modules on a Postgraduate

Diploma Orthopaedic Programme run in conjunction with the Royal College of Surgeons in Ireland.

Paul McLiesh, RN, BN, GDip Orth, MNSc, PhD candidate
University of Adelaide, Australia

Paul is a senior lecturer; he completed his initial training as a registered nurse at the Royal Adelaide Hospital in 1989 and has worked in a number of roles over the subsequent 23 years. He has been lecturing in the Adelaide Nursing School at the University of Adelaide since 2010 and is an education specialist through the Adelaide Education Academy. He is the Education Officer for the Centre for Evidence-based Practice South Australia, an affiliated centre of the Joanna Briggs Institute, and was president of the Australian and New Zealand Orthopaedic Nurses Association (2013–2015) and the South Australian Orthopaedic Nurses Association (2014–2016). He is a deputy editor of the *International Journal of Orthopaedic and Trauma Nursing* and a PhD candidate focusing on the use of structure nursing assessment tools and their value for use by nurses with varying levels of expertise teaching.

Pamela Moore, PgCert Specialist Practitioner in Orthopaedic Nursing, BSc (Hons), RGN
Nursing Development Lead, Belfast Health & Social Care Trust, Belfast, UK

Pamela has many years of experience in both managerial and 'hands on' roles within a busy dedicated fracture clinic/unit and as a development lead for orthopaedic and fracture trauma practice. Pamela is passionate about orthopaedic and fracture trauma care and values ongoing nurse education. Pamela is a frequent specialist lecturer on the orthopaedic and fracture trauma programmes and Objective Structured Clinical Examination examiner at Queen's University Belfast.

Mr Martyn Neil, FRCS, DipSEM (GB&I), MSc
Clinical Director – Orthopaedic Surgery, Consultant Trauma and Orthopaedic Surgeon, Belfast Health & Social Care Trust, Belfast, UK

Martyn has worked in the Royal Victoria Hospital and Musgrave Park Hospital Royal from 2013. He has held the appointment of Clinical Director – Orthopaedic Surgery since 2021.

Lynne Newton-Triggs, MA, RGN, Pre-Assessment Sister
Bedford Hospital NHS Trust, Bedford, UK

Lynne currently works as a pre-assessment nurse manager at a district general hospital with her main focus being the orthopaedic specialty. She qualified as an RGN in 1984 and has since worked in both elective and trauma environments as a ward sister and specialist nurse. She completed the English National Board 219 at the Robert Jones and Agnes Hunt Orthopaedic Hospital in 1987 and has since

completed a BA (Hons) degree in Nursing Studies and an MA in Healthcare Ethics.

Jean Rogers, RGN, BSc (Hons), MSc, ONC, Cert. Ed (Fe)
Practice Education Facilitator for the Open University

Jean qualified as an RGN in 1988 from Salford NHS Foundation Trust. She has worked in a number of areas, including elective orthopaedics, acute trauma and ENT, rheumatology and endocrinology, acute medicine and acute rehabilitation. She undertook the orthopaedic course at the Robert Jones and Agnes Hunt Orthopaedic Hospital in 1991 where she was in the last group to undertake the 12-month course and in her spare time completed a Certificate in Higher Education. Following this Jean held the posts of senior staff nurse, junior sister and lecturer/practitioner, and completed a BSc (Hons) in Nursing Practice and an MSc in Professional Development. She is co-author of the Oxford University Press book *Handbook of Orthopaedic and Trauma Nursing* as well as numerous articles. Her main interests lie in orthopaedics, nurse education and the politics of nursing, and she takes an active role in these areas, being a member of the orthopaedic forum, the practice educator's special interest group and the RCN Education Forum. Jean's current post is as academic assessor and practice tutor for the Open University, where she believes that she has the best of both worlds educating and supporting the nurses of the future in the practice setting.

Dr Julie Santy-Tomlinson (Co-editor of the first edition), PhD, RGN, RNT, MSc, BSc (Hons)

Julie has been Editor of the *International Journal of Orthopaedic and Trauma Nursing* since 2007. She has a clinical background in orthopaedic and trauma nursing with a focus on trauma care, older people, fragility fracture, tissue viability and wound care. She has published numerous articles and chapters related to many aspects of orthopaedic and trauma nursing. She has worked in nursing education since 1995.

Helen Stradling, MSc, BA (Hons), ENB 931, M01750, ENB 237
Sarcoma Specialist Nurse and Support Line Manager, Sarcoma UK, London, UK

Helen qualified from the University of Birmingham in 1998. From there she took up the post of staff nurse at the Nuffield Orthopaedic Centre in Oxford. It was here she was able to mix her passion for orthopaedics and oncology as the sarcoma patients were nursed on the ward. During the first few years on the ward, Helen began to increase her knowledge relating to sarcoma and undertook study in both oncology and orthopaedics. In 2004, the Nuffield Orthopaedic Centre became one of five national centres for the care of bone and soft sarcoma, and it was at this point that Helen was successful in her application for the role of Macmillan Specialist Nurse for musculoskeletal oncology. During the 12 years in that post, Helen grew the sarcoma nursing service in Oxford and introduced nurse-led follow-up for all sarcoma patients. Helen was awarded the Nursing Times Cancer Nurse Leader of the Year award in 2010 in recognition of all the work she had put into improving the pathway for sarcoma patients and their families in Oxford. Helen became the first Chair of the National Sarcoma Forum in September 2011. She also became a Trustee of the charity Sarcoma UK in 2013, and in 2016 she decided to leave the team in Oxford and join the Sarcoma UK staff team as a sarcoma specialist nurse and support line manager. Helen was also able to use her sarcoma knowledge to take forward the charity's strategic plan to continue raising awareness, improving the timeliness of diagnosis and undertaking research to bring about new treatments for all those affected by sarcoma.

Anna Timms, RGN, BSc Psychology, ONC
Limb Reconstruction Clinical Nurse Specialist, Royal National Orthopaedic Hospital, Stanmore

Anna qualified from the Queen Elizabeth School of Nursing, Birmingham in 1994. Since then she has specialised within the fields of rheumatology and orthopaedics. Working within the trauma environment at the Royal London Hospital, she became a limb reconstruction nurse specialist in 2005, leaving to become a member of the team at the Royal National Orthopaedic Hospital in 2012. She has authored articles and presented both nationally and internationally in the field of limb reconstruction.

Elizabeth Wright, RGN, RSCN, MSc Advanced Clinical Practice
Advanced Nurse Practitioner, University Hospital, Southampton, UK

Since qualifying at the Hammersmith Hospital, London, Liz gained experience in general paediatric and neonatal intensive care nursing and then entered the specialist field of orthopaedic paediatric nursing in 1990. She was sister of a paediatric orthopaedic ward for 6 years, then a nurse specialist until she commenced her current post of advanced nurse practitioner, completing her MSc in Advanced Nurse Practice in 2004. She has jointly convened and chaired several national paediatric orthopaedic conferences, established and chaired the Royal College of Nursing (RCN) Children and Young Peoples Orthopaedic and Trauma Group in 1998, participates in the RCN Society of Orthopaedic and Trauma Nursing (SOTN), and has been a member of various SOTN work panels and the SOTN Scientific Committee. She has published and presented several times on the subject of paediatric orthopaedics. More recently, Liz has been a core member of the James Lind Priority Setting Partnership, setting priorities for research, and the British Society Children's Orthopaedic Surgery Consensus Group for Congenital Talipes Equinus Varus.

Elaine Wylie, RGN BSc (Hons) PGDip, Specialist Practice Registration: Rheumatology
Nurse Specialist, Southern Health and Social Care Trust, Northern Ireland, UK

Elaine has worked in rheumatology for 31 years and for the last 21 years has been a nurse specialist. She was appointed to the role of Rheumatology Biologics Manager/ Lead Nurse Specialist in 2019. She is currently based at Craigavon Area Hospital, where her clinical responsibilities include nurse-led biologic therapy clinics, review clinics, telephone review clinics and helpline services. She also manages the biologics service and a team of nurse specialists. She is involved in service development locally and regionally, and has mentored rheumatology nurses in Italy to extend their role and service. Her specific interests in rheumatology are inflammatory arthritis patient and family education and support, along with staff training and development. Elaine teaches on the orthopaedic specialist course at Queen's University Belfast and has presented at meetings locally, nationally and internationally.

Sian Rodger, Spinal Cord Injury Educator (clinical), MSc, BSc (Hons), RN (adult), Royal National Orthopaedic Hospital NHS Trust

Sian is a patient education and health coaching clinical nurse specialist at the London Spinal Cord Injury Centre. A product of project 2000 (1996) Sian has gone on to achieve her BSc Hons in professional nursing practice (spinal cord injury) and a Masters in Clinical Research (2020). Sian has had peer reviewed article s published in Nursing Times and British Journal of Nursing and writes a regular on-line blog for the Nursing Times. She also organises the nurses' online journal club at the RNOH. Sian has worked within the field of spinal cord injury nursing for most of her nursing career- 25 years! She continues to work clinically with patients and staff to educate them in spinal cord injury.

Foreword

Welcome to the second edition of *Orthopaedic and Trauma Nursing: An Evidence-Based Approach to Musculoskeletal Care*. Since the publication of the first edition the world has faced one of its most serious challenges to health with the COVID-19 pandemic, which has impacted on so many of us individually and as healthcare professionals. Orthopaedic and trauma care has been significantly impacted, with many elective procedures being cancelled, patient consultations being delivered remotely using telemedicine and staff being deployed outside of the speciality. It is important to take a moment to reflect and remember family, friends and colleagues who have been affected by COVID-19.

The first edition of this book received a tremendous amount of positive feedback from students, practitioners and educators globally regarding how it influenced patient care and contributed to practitioners' knowledge and competence. I am delighted to say that the second edition builds on this solid platform, providing essential updates and including contributions from a wide range of practitioners, educators and researchers with many years of expertise in orthopaedic and trauma care from many parts of the globe. I have had the privilege to work with many of the contributors through my role as Deputy Editor of the *International Journal of Orthopaedic and Trauma Nursing* and being a member of the guideline development group for the Royal College of Nursing Society of Trauma and Orthopaedic Nursing competency document, and can attest to their expertise and passion for orthopaedic and trauma care.

Every chapter has been reviewed and updated to include the latest evidence-based practice, policy and guidelines. Changes to practice since the first edition include the global implementation of enhanced recovery pathways aiming to shorten hospital length of stay and ensure safe and effective discharge and rehabilitation. Enhanced recovery pathways are based on interdisciplinary teams working in partnership with patients and their families, and embrace shared decision making between practitioners and patients. Rehabilitation has also become embedded in many enhanced recovery pathways to optimise patients' health status prior to elective surgery. Increasingly, patients are spending less time in the inpatient setting with more shared models of care with primary and community services.

Technology continues to provide opportunities to work in new ways, including patient consultations for follow-up assessment being carried out remotely using tele-medicine, which has enabled patients to continue to receive expert care when face-to-face consultations were not possible due to COVID-19. This has required practitioners to develop new skills in assessment and consultation when not having the patient in the same room and has also required patients to engage with practitioners in a different way. Technology is also supporting patients with rapid and easier access to information and monitoring. Many orthopaedic and trauma teams have developed apps that patients can access to gain information about their condition, treatment and care, and can also be used to support patients with their rehabilitation and exercise regimens.

Specialist and advanced practice roles continue to develop within the speciality globally, making a significant impact on services such as fragility fracture and osteoporosis treatment and care, and there is a growing realisation of the need to increase health promotion and prevention in orthopaedic conditions and to address the issue of rising rates of obesity and its detrimental impact on the musculoskeletal system.

My vision for this text is that it will find its way onto wards and departments where staff and students can dip into it to check best practice, and ultimately that it influences the quality of patient care and safety. I also hope that the book becomes a core text on the reading lists of specialist orthopaedic programmes globally and a useful resource for undergraduate nursing and therapy students. I am fortunate to have networks in orthopaedics in the UK, Hong Kong, Denmark and the Middle East, and can attest to this book having relevance and value to practice and education globally. I will certainly be using the book on a regular basis and if you are looking for an orthopaedic and trauma text to support evidence-based contemporary practice this is a must-read.

Rebecca Jester
Head of the School of Nursing, Royal College
of Surgeons in Ireland, Medical University
Deputy Editor, *International Journal of
Orthopaedic and Trauma Nursing*

Preface

Welcome to the second edition of this book. Orthopaedic and trauma care remains a highly specialised aspect of healthcare focused on the person with musculoskeletal problems or injury and following orthopaedic surgery. Such care is delivered across the lifespan, i.e. birth to death, in a wide range of community and hospital settings. The skills required for effective, evidence-based practice must be developed through a regard for the knowledge and evidence base for practice coupled with development of competence and expertise. This area of healthcare shares generic skills but encompasses specialist skills like no other. The aim of this 25-chapter edition is to provide practitioners working in orthopaedic and musculoskeletal trauma settings with the evidence, guidance and knowledge required to develop their skills and underpin effective practice.

This book continues to reflect the focus on the practice of musculoskeletal care as well as putting a specific focus on the evidence base for that practice. It builds on the first edition and differs with a larger focus on fragility fractures across two chapters, 18 and 19. All other chapters have been updated and modified by either their original author(s) or new co-authors from clinical practice and/or higher education. For example, we are delighted to welcome Mrs Julie Craig (Chapters 17 and 20) and Mr Martyn Neil (Chapter 20) from the Trauma and Orthopaedic Department, Royal Victoria Hospital, Belfast, as well as paramedic Dr Stefanie Cormack (Chapter 16) and Paul McLiesh, an Education Officer for the Centre for Evidence-based Practice in South Australia, who has revamped Chapter 2. The editors and contributors have again tried to not achieve the impossible in providing information about all of the available knowledge on a given topic, but offer a pedagogical approach to teaching and learning or, more simply, building blocks for extending knowledge and understanding the issues that drive safe, effective practice. The book once more provides relevant information about key theory and summaries of the evidence base underpinning all the main aspects of orthopaedic and trauma practice. This approach will enable the practitioner to easily gain an understanding of the existing evidence base for their practice. This will ensure that the book is relevant for those studying for a degree as well as those clinicians practicing in developing and advanced orthopaedic and trauma practitioner roles. Evidence is rarely out of date, but it is sometimes superseded. One danger with this approach in this book, therefore, is that the evidence base is likely to move on as time progresses, so it is important that the practitioner is also encouraged to seek more up-to-date evidence through knowledge of how to access and appraise it.

Because the focus of this text is on evidence-based practice, summaries, or digests, of the available evidence as well as reference to relevant and seminal research support each chapter. This will enable the practitioner to focus on the evidence essential for modern practice. The book is not only mindful of the person's lifespan but also of equality, diversity and inclusion, for example of those with a learning disability. Whilst much is on the care of the adult, a proportionate amount of content is transferable and purposely includes sections focusing specifically on the infant, child and young person and on older people with orthopaedic conditions following surgical intervention and after injury.

Although the title of the book reflects a focus on nursing care of the orthopaedic and trauma patient, it also aims to provide a wealth of useful and thought-provoking information for other practitioners working in the orthopaedic and trauma setting. Equally, the book is aimed at practitioners outside the United Kingdom (UK), where the editors are based.

Part I of this edition again provides an overview of the key issues that relate to orthopaedic and trauma nursing practice. It considers the theory underpinning orthopaedic care and places it in context with the history and development of practice in the musculoskeletal care environment. An important aspect of this is a discussion of how the evidence base for orthopaedic trauma practice has developed, and how the reader might develop skills in seeking out and evaluating evidence. There is also an overview of how professional and practice development, based on theoretical knowledge and evidence, can lead to ensuring and developing competence and effective practice. Integral to this introductory section is an overview of the musculoskeletal system that will enable the practitioner to further develop their knowledge of anatomy and physiology, which can then be applied to the other sections of the book. Rehabilitation begins at the patient's very first contact with healthcare services and the central concepts within, and practice of, rehabilitative care are also considered.

Part II focuses on six specific aspects of practice, which although generic, take on a specific specialist focus in the musculoskeletal care setting. Consideration of general and specialist assessment of the patient, casting, traction and external fixation, prevention and management of complications and patient safety, nutrition and hydration, pain assessment and management, and wound management and tissue viability are considered specifically within the context of orthopaedic and trauma care. These aspects of care, along with the key principles discussed in the previous part, need to be applied to the practice advice provided in the remainder of the book.

Part III considers the care of the patient with musculoskeletal conditions not attributed to trauma, but to degeneration of the bones, joints and soft tissue, with a specific focus on arthropathies such as osteoarthritis. The section considers the management of these conditions with a specific focus on elective surgery, which constitutes much of the need for orthopaedic care in the non-emergency setting.

Part IV provides an overview of the principles and practice of care of the patient following musculoskeletal trauma and injury. It begins with a discussion of the principles of trauma care, providing the practitioner with important knowledge to underpin safe and effective trauma care practice in both the emergency situation and subsequent care. This is followed by specific consideration of the principles of fracture management and care and then by specific consideration of fractures in the older person with a focus on fragility fractures of the hip. This is followed by an overview of the care of the person with spinal cord injury aimed specifically at practitioners who provide that care in the general hospital setting. Finally, there is a brief overview of the knowledge required to care for the patient with soft tissue and nerve injury, including brachial plexus injuries.

Part V refers to the first part of the lifespan; it provides an overview of key concepts and fundamental issues that relate to the neonate, infant, child and young person. The material is specific to this client group and values the expertise of children's nursing relating to skeletal growth and development, person- and family-centred care, safeguarding/non-accidental injury, and pain management. This is followed by key information relating to the assessment and management of common children's musculoskeletal conditions that the practitioner may come across in everyday practice. A review of fracture healing, diagnosis and classification then follows before the complexities of diagnosing and treating children's fractures, considering the immature and developing skeleton, are discussed along with the principles of conservative and surgical treatment.

We hope that the readers of this book will use the text as a general reference source for maintaining and developing their knowledge, but that they will also extend that knowledge by accessing the further reading and seeking new material that is relevant to their own learning needs through online and traditional sources of information. We hope that this will help to ensure orthopaedic and trauma practice will remain safe, effective and evidence-based.

Finally, we would like to thank Dr Julie Santy Tomlinson, co-editor of the first edition, for her continued support and contribution to the second edition, especially around the co-development of fragility fracture in the older person.

Sonya Clarke and Mary Drozd
Belfast and Birmingham

Part I

Key Issues in Orthopaedic and Musculoskeletal Trauma Nursing

1

An Introduction to Orthopaedic and Trauma Care

Julie Santy-Tomlinson[1], Sonya Clarke[2], and Mary Drozd[3]

[1] *International Journal of Orthopaedic and Trauma Nursing*
[2] *Queen's University Belfast, Belfast, UK*
[3] *Aston University, Birmingham, UK*

Introduction

Orthopaedic and trauma nursing is a discrete but diverse specialty focused on the care of the patient with musculoskeletal problems. The aim of this chapter is to provide the reader with an overview of today's orthopaedic nursing by exploring the essence of orthopaedic care, patient care needs, and the nature and development of orthopaedic nursing as a specific nursing specialty. It is important to understand what is special about orthopaedic nursing to excel in its delivery and to ensure its continued existence.

The Changing Nature of Orthopaedic Practice over Time

History provides important perspectives for contemporary practice. The history of orthopaedic nursing provides the lens through which we can understand today's experiences and perspectives. Orthopaedic nursing as a specific entity has only existed since the early decades of the twentieth century. Prior to this, nursing care for patients with musculoskeletal conditions and injuries had been provided by nurses and others with generic skills and limited, if any, healthcare education.

Many musculoskeletal diseases such as tuberculosis and poliomyelitis that were common in the eighteenth and nineteenth centuries were eradicated in higher income countries during the twentieth century. This was largely because of improvement in living conditions, public health and healthcare, and resulted in important and far-reaching change in priorities for orthopaedic and trauma care. Even so, this history remains pertinent to the way in which care is provided today.

Orthopaedic care has been provided for as long as the musculoskeletal system has been prone to disease and injury, although this previously took place under the auspices of bone setters, barber surgeons and other 'informal' carers. Trauma nursing is most often evident in nursing stories from war, such as those surrounding the Crimean War and the role played by both Florence Nightingale and Mary Seacole. The care of patients sustaining musculoskeletal trauma has often made strides forward during times of conflict, war, great societal change and disaster. Much of the knowledge and skills in musculoskeletal trauma nursing derives from the part that nurses have played, and still play, in war. It could be argued, for example, that the likes of Florence Nightingale and Mary Seacole would have provided musculoskeletal trauma care to those injured during the Crimean war and could, therefore, be seen as the forerunners of today's trauma nurses. Before that, when nursing was not an organised profession, care on or near the battlefield would have been provided by military personnel engaged in field care or by wives who travelled to war with their soldier husbands.

Orthopaedic nurses have always worked closely with orthopaedic surgeons, although their development has not always been parallel. The formalisation of medical specialties began in the late nineteenth century once medical knowledge began to expand and there was an increasing need to organise and manage the growth of medical care (Weisz 2003). In the late 1800s doctors began to organise themselves into groups of specialists according to specific organs of the body or categories of diseases. The management of patients with musculoskeletal disease and injury, however, was largely conducted by general surgeons until the twentieth century.

The term 'orthopaedic' is credited to Nicholas Andry, an eighteenth century French professor of medicine who published an introduction to orthopaedics in 1741, the first time the word orthopaedic was written. The word derives from two Greek words, *orthos* meaning 'straight and free from deformity' and *paidios* meaning 'child', with a collective meaning of 'straight child'. This reflects the roots of orthopaedic care of children with deformities of bones and joints from congenital conditions and childhood disease affecting the musculoskeletal system (Swarup and O'Donnell 2016). Later, this theme was continued with the philanthropism of the nineteenth century, which was often focused on what were perceived at the time as 'crippled' children from poor backgrounds whose families could not care for them.

Orthopaedic nursing has been entwined with the development of orthopaedic and trauma surgery. The efforts of pioneering surgeons such as Hugh Owen Thomas and Robert Jones led to the inception of orthopaedic surgery in the 1940s as part of the development of the National Health Service (NHS) in the United Kingdom as well as the development of orthopaedic and trauma services around the world.

The early development of orthopaedic nursing is widely attributed to Dame Agnes Hunt in Shropshire, England in the early twentieth century. She initially set up a small rural care facility for children with chronic musculoskeletal conditions from nearby industrial cities such as Liverpool. Her approach involved a focus on rest, fresh air and good nutrition, with the aim of ensuring the proper development and recovery of diseased, injured and deformed bone, joints and soft tissue. She enlisted the help of Sir Robert Jones as a consulting surgeon and together they set up a specialist orthopaedic hospital at Gobowen, not far from the initial site of the home. This became the Robert Jones and Agnes Hunt Orthopaedic Hospital, one of several specialist hospitals set up around the UK around that time to provide expert care to patients with musculoskeletal disease. Some of these hospitals still exist today with a focus on expert specialised diagnosis, treatment, surgery, care and rehabilitation for those with complex musculoskeletal health problems.

The development of orthopaedic surgery has been driven by a desire to improve lives by, for example, facilitating healing and preventing disability following trauma and ameliorating the pain and disability of osteoarthritis and other chronic conditions. Elective orthopaedic surgery, and the subsequent need for specialised nursing to care for patients undergoing such procedures, only fully developed following the advent of successful surgical orthopaedic implants from the 1960s onwards. Both hip and knee arthroplasties were initially developed in the 1960s and gradual improvements in implants, surgical procedures and aftercare have resulted in great success in treating patients with severe joint arthropathies such as osteoarthritis and rheumatoid arthritis. Until then orthopaedic nursing would have been largely focused on musculoskeletal trauma, often relating to war, and on diseases of bones, joints and muscles.

In an early textbook, Mary Powell (1951) wrote of the general principles of orthopaedic nursing, which embodied the principles of rest balanced with movement and exercise, treatment of the patient as a whole, optimum positioning for joints using splinting and traction, relief of pain and the provision of the best conditions for recovery and healing. This encompassed pre-operative and post-surgical care, trauma care and rehabilitation. With a focus on the nurse–patient relationship and teamwork, many parallels can be drawn with orthopaedic and trauma nursing today.

Musculoskeletal care previously involved the enforcement of many weeks and months of rest, while the current focus is on early mobilisation and avoiding inactivity. Although much is very different in the twenty-first century, there are some principles of early twentieth century care that remain relevant, in particular the need for what Mary Powell (1951) would have called an 'orthopaedic conscience' (which she later renamed the 'orthopaedic eye'), a special sense or consciousness of how movement, position, posture and comfort are central to both the assessment and care of the orthopaedic patient in modern healthcare. Orthopaedic practitioners develop this intuition through experience of working with patients affected by musculoskeletal problems. Skilled and experienced orthopaedic and trauma practitioners are able, for example, to recognise patient care needs by instinctively observing posture and the way in which people move. Skilled orthopaedic practitioners understand how gentle and minimal repositioning of a limb or supporting it with a pillow can improve comfort and support healing and recovery. Such observation and subsequent intervention are not as simple as they sound, rooted in insight and skill, and demonstrate how nurses make judgements about the needs of patients and formulate decisions about care based on clinical information derived from a variety of sources including, but not exclusively, evidence (Thompson and Dowding 2002).

As mentioned earlier, at the beginning of the twentieth century several specialist orthopaedic hospitals sprang up in the UK. This led to the rapid creation of a network of centres, often in rural or suburban locations, focused on the specialist care of patients and the education of practitioners in the principles and specifics of musculoskeletal care. These organisations also became early developers of the evidence base for orthopaedic care. As services have become more centralised, several of these centres closed and were integrated into acute urban hospital centres. Those remaining specialist hospitals continue to develop the specialist knowledge and research evidence for musculoskeletal care alongside emergency departments and acute, outpatient and community units.

Modern Orthopaedic Care

During the twentieth century, musculoskeletal care began to evolve into two related entities: elective care and musculoskeletal trauma care. Elective orthopaedic surgery involves procedures that are planned and usually aim to improve known conditions that are causing pain and/or disability. This often includes surgery for arthropathies such as osteoarthritis and rheumatoid arthritis, and might also involve surgery to further manage the effects of trauma once initial recovery and healing has taken place. This might include, for example, surgery to correct deformity or the removal of metal work inserted electively or following injury. Patients with rheumatoid arthritis and other rheumatological conditions are often cared for in specialist centres where the focus is on medical management and rehabilitation rather than on surgery. They might, however, be referred for elective surgery when this is of potential benefit.

Trauma care, conversely, is unplanned and involves the care and rehabilitation of patients who have sustained injury following an unexpected event such as a fall, road traffic accident or sporting injury. All structures of the human body are prone to injury and trauma care can therefore take place in a variety of settings, including the emergency department, intensive care unit and neurosurgical setting as well as the orthopaedic trauma unit. Orthopaedic trauma care is focused specifically on trauma to the musculoskeletal system while considering the need to include other aspects of trauma management as necessary. The focus in this book is specifically on those aspects of trauma care which involve the musculoskeletal system. Often orthopaedic nurses are specialists in one or the other of elective or trauma orthopaedics, but many have skills in both areas and work in units where the two are combined.

The Nature of Orthopaedic and Musculoskeletal Trauma Nursing

The orthopaedic practitioner has a unique role, with associated skills and knowledge. Nursing theory applied to orthopaedic and musculoskeletal trauma nursing comes both from general sources relating to nursing and healthcare (such as surgical and medical nursing), and from specialist sources relating specifically to the orthopaedic and trauma specialty. The theory which underpins orthopaedic nursing practice is based on an in-depth knowledge of the anatomy and physiology of the musculoskeletal system and of those physical and psychosocial factors which affect musculoskeletal health and wellbeing as well as recovery from injury and surgery.

Specialisation in nursing has been moving back towards generic nursing for a few decades largely because of nursing resource shortages and the erosion of specialist nursing education. Despite this, orthopaedic nursing remains very much a discrete entity, different from all other nursing specialisms. The exact nature of orthopaedic nursing has been a matter of some discussion over many years. Work has focused on its status as a discrete specialty and the specific nursing actions which make it distinct from other nursing specialisms and from generic nursing. This debate has highlighted the importance of specialist skills and the need for specific education for orthopaedic and trauma nursing. One example of this is the assessment skills needed to recognise a very specific set of potential complications of orthopaedic surgery, conditions and injuries (see Chapter 9 for further detail) that are not part of the generic skills required of nurses and other practitioners. See Box 1.1 for further detail of the present state of inquiry into the specialist nature of orthopaedic nursing.

Within orthopaedic nursing itself, there are several additional areas of specialisation. These focus, for example, on either specific conditions or regions of the musculoskeletal system such as the spine, osteoporosis, hand injuries, skeletal oncology etc. The focus may also be on specific age groups across the person's life span. For example, children's orthopaedic care involves the provision of healthcare to the neonate, infant, child and young person. Caring for this population is highly specialised and requires specially trained and educated nurses who are able to combine skills in the care of the person from birth to 18 years and (sometimes beyond) with musculoskeletal problems (see Chapters 13 and 22–25). Children's nursing, although allied to mental health and learning disability nursing because of the child-specific stage of human development, remains different to adult nursing (Clarke 2019). Therefore, many countries continue to educate a dedicated group of children's nurses to provide nursing care to a diverse population, who are both a service user and rights holder, in partnership with their family (Clarke 2017). Many orthopaedic patients are older and have conditions that are a result of primary (normal ageing) or secondary (changes caused by illness or disease) ageing. A more recently recognised subspeciality of orthopaedic nursing is orthogeriatric

---

Box 1.1   Evidence Digest: The Nature of Orthopaedic Nursing

An early study by Love (1995) attempted to clarify and discriminate between orthopaedic and general nursing using a questionnaire survey of orthopaedic nurses that asked which nursing activities were highly orthopaedic nursing functions and which were not. There was a range of activities deemed to be unique to orthopaedic nursing, including 'elevation of limbs to prevent swelling' and 'removal of splintage if ischaemia is threatening safety of a limb'.

More recently a number of researchers (Santy 2001; Drozd et al. 2007) have used qualitative approaches to research, such as grounded theory, to explore the nature of orthopaedic and trauma nursing, and examine the detail of what specific interventions practitioners undertake with orthopaedic patients. Work by Judd (2010) has undertaken similar inquiry into issues related to working with children with orthopaedic problems.

This work is a foundation on which theory, education and practice frameworks can be developed to ensure that

musculoskeletal care can be increasingly effective in the future and enable practitioners to articulate their specialist role and value. The studies collectively demonstrate that there are many specialist interventions which focus on supporting mobility, managing and caring for the patient with orthopaedic devices such as splints, traction, casts and external fixators, and caring for the patient following specific surgical procedures and injuries as well as preventing and recognising the complications of those interventions. The studies also highlight how specialist skills are developed and used alongside the generic interventions and actions considered to be fundamental aspects of nursing as a whole. The studies can be used as evidence to help ensure that the skills, knowledge and attitudes required for effective orthopaedic and trauma nursing practice are maintained. The findings therefore ensure that the specialty of orthopaedic care is protected from erosion and that patients are cared for by practitioners who are competent in providing that care in all its forms.

---

nursing, where practitioners have specific skills in providing expert care to older people sustaining fragility fractures (see Chapters 18 and 19).

Even so, orthopaedic nursing has tended to continue to use generic nursing models applied to the care of the adult or child. Nursing models ideally aim to illustrate the theory of nursing practice to enable the practitioner to organise and prioritise effective and safe patient care. The nursing process, developed by Orlando (1961), provides a logical, structured approach that directs the practitioner's critical thinking in a dynamic manner. It encourages the nurse to balance scientific evidence, personal interpretation and judgement when delivering patient/family-centred care. This is supported by models of nursing and philosophies of care that help to define the care role and guide practice (Corkin et al. 2012). Currently, service users (patients) have become active partners in their care, being holistic, and person-centred.

Mobility and Function

Mobility, movement and function are concepts that have long been argued to be central to orthopaedic nursing (Balcombe et al. 1991; Davis 1994; Love 1995). The concept of mobility itself has been difficult to define. Ouellet and Rush (1992, 1996, 1998) and Rush and Ouellet (1998) began to highlight the complex and essential nature of mobility and its link with immobility as well as the care needs generated from mobility problems. Davis (1994) also

emphasised the centrality of mobility for patients with musculoskeletal problems within the physical, psychological and social domains of care. Key to this discussion is an acknowledgement that movement is an essential aspect of human health and wellbeing. It also acknowledges that both musculoskeletal problems and the associated nursing interventions can lead to immobility and that such immobility or restricted mobility leads to consequences, including serious complications.

The centrality of mobility in orthopaedic and trauma nursing practice has led to one proposed model for orthopaedic nursing (Balcombe et al. 1991; Davis 1994) which holds mobility at its core. The work of Ouellet and Rush in the 1990s has done much to illuminate the centrality of mobility in caring for patients with musculoskeletal problems. Even though the work has largely been conducted in older people's care settings, the findings have direct relevance to orthopaedic and trauma nursing.

Ouellet and Rush (1998) proposed a conceptual model of mobility which is broken down into six components: mobility capacity, forces, perceptions, actuation in all dimensions, patterns and consequences. These components can have direct relevance to the role of the orthopaedic practitioner in directing assessment and interventions that assess and improve mobility capacity. This takes account of the forces involved in mobilisation for patients with specific conditions, allowing for the patient and carer perceptions of their own mobility, how people actually mobilise, and the results of both mobilisation and the care provided.

Public Health and Musculoskeletal Conditions and Injury

Public health focuses on the health and wellbeing of individuals from a societal perspective. It is synonymous with the prevention of disease and ill-health through public action. The public health agenda applied to orthopaedic and trauma care is complex. It is mainly focused on skeletal health but this, in itself, is a multifaceted issue and necessarily involves consideration of numerous factors which affect musculoskeletal health, such as:

- bone development in the child and young adult
- bone health, including, specifically, vitamin D deficiency, osteoporosis, rickets and osteomalacia
- exercise and musculoskeletal fitness
- diet, nutrition and obesity
- lifestyle factors and risk-taking behaviours
- accidental injury and its prevention, e.g. road traffic, work place and sports injuries
- ageing.

Musculoskeletal conditions and injuries can affect any member of society and there are few personal, social and cultural boundaries. Human anatomy evolves slowly, but injury can be a result of immediate changes in the weather and other natural conditions as well as societal variations such as diverse and migrating cultures amongst countries. Other issues include changes in population dynamics, with an increasingly ageing population leading to an upsurge in fragility fractures (see Chapters 18 and 19). For the young person and young adult there is a heightened rate of injury due to risk-taking behaviour. The epidemiology of orthopaedic-related conditions alters as the pathophysiology of disease processes and the treatment options continue to evolve due to emerging technology, research evidence and the ongoing drive for safe, cost-effective care.

Concerns about vitamin D deficiency illustrate the changing nature of the public health agenda and musculoskeletal care. Deficiency is associated with rickets, fractures and musculoskeletal symptoms, and studies suggest a worrying link with deformity and generalised bone and muscle pain (Judd 2013). Such deficiency is attributed to an increasingly multiethnic population, poor diet and lifestyle choices made by families. Previously a condition linked with poverty, the recent recurrence of rickets in the UK, for example, is linked to changes in the lifestyle of children, which has resulted in them spending less time playing out of doors, reducing their exposure to the sunlight that is important for vitamin D and calcium synthesis.

The Diverse Orthopaedic Patient

Contemporary orthopaedic nursing is an advocate of equality, diversity and inclusion (EDI) because it ensures fair treatment and opportunity for all people, thus eradicating prejudice and discrimination on the basis of an individual or group of individuals' protected characteristics, i.e. age, gender, disability, etc. Veselinova (2014), for example, highlights the importance of person-centred care in the context of people with dementia (often cared for by orthopaedic nurses following fracture), and how workers care can ensure that rather than being marginalised, these service users are actively included in all aspects of their lives. EDI is an ethos that must be embedded by all healthcare providers, healthcare settings and care givers. Within the context of EDI, this chapter presents a valuable insight into people with intellectual/learning disabilities who present with orthopaedic-related conditions. The vast age range of the orthopaedic trauma patient means that there are a number of conditions and injuries that are more common in different age groups. Age groups carry different risk factors for musculoskeletal problems; these are outlined in Table 1.1. Changes occur as the musculoskeletal system develops, grows and deteriorates, and as humans age. Many orthopaedic conditions and fracture trauma injuries are related to changing musculoskeletal structure. Normal and abnormal changes occur in utero, at birth, in childhood, in adulthood and from old age to death. Intrinsic factors affecting this include abnormal musculoskeletal development such as developmental dysplasia of the hip, scoliosis and osteogenseis imperfecta, for which there are considerable variations in treatment and outcome. Other conditions are often age-related, such as osteoporosis and osteoarthritis, which are associated with intrinsic factors such as increasing age. Such variations can hopefully be reduced as a result of national guidance and globally relevant initiatives such as those published by the World Health Organization (WHO). Extrinsic factors include the risk-taking of the young person/adolescent leading to road traffic trauma alongside accidental and non-accidental injury in vulnerable children and adults. In spite of political and economic development in most parts of the world, social status and environmental conditions continue to impact on musculoskeletal health problems due to issues such as low income and poor education leading to poor diet.

A diverse society which focuses on the health and wellbeing of individuals includes people with intellectual disabilities (IDs) (referred to as 'learning disabilities' in England). The Royal College of Nursing (2017) defines 'intellectual disability' as 'a lifelong condition, resulting in a reduced intellectual ability and thus difficulty with

Table 1.1 Age groups in relation to orthopaedic problems

Age group	Examples often specific to age group
Familial/hereditary	Paget's
	Osteogenesis imperfecta
Congenital/developmental	Developmental dysplasia of the hip
	Talipes
Post-natal and pre-walking	Birth injuries
Early childhood	Rickets and osteomalacia
	Non-accidental injury
	Accidental injury
Mid to late childhood	Juvenile idiopathic arthritis
	Perthes' disease
Young person/adolescence	Slipped upper femoral epiphysis
	Osgood–Schlatter disease
Early adulthood	Injuries resulting from high-energy trauma
	Sports injuries
	Rheumatoid arthritis
	Ankylosing spondylitis
Middle and late adulthood	Work-related injury
	Back pain
Later life/older age	Injuries resulting from low-energy trauma
	Fragility fractures
	Osteoporosis
	Degenerative joint conditions

everyday tasks'. An ID affects the way a person understands information and includes a lifelong difficulty with learning new skills and understanding information (NHS England 2017). People with IDs are at increased risk of poor bone health but, despite this, assessment of bone health is often not undertaken (Michael 2008), with evidence of an underutilisation of the preventative services related to musculoskeletal conditions and injuries amongst people with IDs (Srikanth et al. 2011). Burke et al. (2019) demonstrated that the prevalence of poor bone health in people with IDs is substantial, implying an increased risk of fracture due to reduced skeletal integrity.

Lifestyle factors are contributors to poor bone health in people with IDs, such as poor dietary habits, constipation, poor mobility, low levels of exercise, low levels of vitamin D and obesity (McCarron et al. 2011). Finlayson (2011) and Finlayson et al. (2010, 2014) reported that people with ID sustain more injuries, falls and accidents than the general population. Eye disease is associated with falls risk and is highly prevalent among older people with IDs (McCarron et al. 2013). Fractures may occur from a low impact injury if a person has osteoporosis and this places people with IDs at an increased risk of injury following a fall (Cox et al. 2010).

A large, population-based cross-sectional study was undertaken in Scotland, UK and concluded that the most prevalent physical health conditions affecting people with IDs included osteoporosis, bone deformity and musculoskeletal pain (Kinnear et al. 2018). A staggering 48% of people with IDs in this study with 1023 participants had musculoskeletal conditions. Although this study was undertaken in one region of Scotland it highlights the prevalence of these conditions as well as the complexity related to multimorbidity for people with IDs.

The Context of Hospital Experiences of People with an ID

Mainstream health services have difficulty in providing an equitable service for people with IDs compared with the general population (Box 1.2) (Mencap 2007; Emerson and Baines 2011; Heslop et al. 2013; Iacono et al. 2014). The hospital can be a high-pressure environment for staff with challenging targets to achieve, such as seeing and treating people quickly as well as reducing the length of stay of patients in hospitals. Blair (2017) affirmed that there were challenges for people with IDs receiving hospital care as hospitals can be very frightening environments for a person with IDs; they are often unfamiliar places and the person with an ID may have had previous negative experiences. Alongside this, Blair (2017) contended that healthcare professionals may have limited knowledge about people with IDs as they may not have been prepared, trained or educated to adequately care for them. This can result in healthcare professionals lacking in understanding of the fundamental needs and abilities of people with IDs. People with IDs require equity in the form of the provision of reasonable adjustments to achieve effective clinical outcomes (Equality Act 2010).

Health professionals need to see the 'person' with an ID and not just the 'disability'. 'Diagnostic overshadowing' occurs when a health professional makes the assumption that the behaviour of a person with IDs is related to their disability without exploring other factors such as illness (Blair 2017). Furthermore, a person with IDs may be unable to communicate their symptoms to healthcare professionals and therefore be at risk of symptoms being missed, which can lead to clinical deterioration and premature death (Heslop et al. 2013).

Box 1.2 Evidence Digest: The Voices of Adults with an ID about their Orthopaedic and Trauma Hospital Care in the UK

People with IDs have a greater prevalence of musculo-skeletal conditions and injuries than the general population and this has significant impacts on wellbeing. Despite this, orthopaedic and trauma hospital care had not been investigated with this group, who seldom have their voices heard or their experiences valued and interpreted. This study contributes to the existing evidence base by exploring the experiences of people with IDs who have received orthopaedic and trauma hospital care.

Aim: To understand the orthopaedic and trauma hospital experiences from the perspective of adults with an ID.

Methods: A qualitative approach, focusing on peoples' lived experiences, was utilised. A purposive sample of five participants was recruited and one-to-one, semi-structured interviews were undertaken. Analysis of the interviews employed an interpretative phenomenological analytical framework.

Findings: The findings from each participant in the study were discussed in relation to their orthopaedic and trauma hospital care. A cross-case comparison was then undertaken and the themes below represent common experiences across participants:

- communication challenges
- lack of person-centred care
- issues related to pain management
- lack of confidence in hospital care
- valuable support and expertise of carers
- incompetence of hospital staff
- isolation and loneliness.

Discussion and conclusions: This study contributes to the evidence base by being the first to specifically focus on and provide experiential findings pertaining to the orthopaedic or trauma hospital experiences of adults with IDs. There were significant shortcomings in the orthopaedic and trauma hospital experiences of adults with IDs, who perceived they were unsupported and received poor care in orthopaedic and trauma hospital settings.

Recommendations and implications for practice: Person-centred care for adults with IDs in orthopaedic and trauma hospital settings is needed along with specific education and training, including close liaison with the experts by experience, people with IDs and their carers as well as the specialists in IDs (Drozd 2019).

The Care Journey in Different Settings

In many of the chapters in this book we see that the care journey takes place against a background of changing health services and political priorities as well as individual needs. During the COVID-19 pandemic, this has been even more evident as services have had to change and develop very rapidly. There is no reason to believe that the enormous change and development of healthcare services seen in the later decades of the twentieth century and at the beginning of the twenty-first century is likely to slow down. The practitioner, therefore, needs to ensure they have a dynamic understanding of how this affects the care of the orthopaedic and trauma patient, especially in relation to the setting in which care takes place.

Ambulatory care is increasingly providing opportunities for patients to be offered treatment and care without a stay in hospital or, at most, a very short stay. This is driven by the need to reduce the costs of healthcare as well as an acknowledgement that an acute hospital is not always the best place for the patient to be. In the orthopaedic and trauma setting, this has increasingly been the case for major orthopaedic surgery such as hip and knee arthroplasty. Fast-track, rapid recovery and enhanced recovery will be discussed often in this book as they are now embedded features of orthopaedic care everywhere. It is important to bear in mind, however, that non-admission to, or early discharge from, hospital is not always in the patient's best interests and can be anxiety provoking and painful for patients and their families. Thus, there is a need to provide support that ensures that specialist orthopaedic advice and services are accessible remotely from the hospital. In particular, services need to ensure that patients recovering at a distance from an acute hospital setting in their own homes are afforded support and a care package which includes fundamental elements such as effective pain relief, good nutrition, support for rehabilitation, access to advice and support, and all of the things the patient needs to reach both their recovery and rehabilitation potential as well as maintain their safety. Such services can be complex and difficult to coordinate. One of the difficulties in providing adequate support in the patient's home can be funding and purchasing mismatches between the acute hospital and community services, which may be quite separate entities depending on the structure and funding of the healthcare system. Family support for care in the home is also becoming increasingly challenging as the role and employment of family members changes and increasing pressure is placed on families to provide complex care.

For more than a quarter of a century there has been a strong focus on reducing lengths of hospital stay and moving from hospital-based to community-based care. This focus is driven by the need to stretch limited resources while maintaining the quality of care. While this shift has long been an important aim for healthcare managers and policy makers, the reality has been more problematic, and this change is taking place slowly. Musculoskeletal conditions, injuries and surgery are problems which take time to resolve and may leave the individual of any age with varying degrees of temporary or permanent disability that require careful support and rehabilitation. Within this drive is a danger that patients are being discharged from hospital with residual nursing needs and there is a consequent need to develop care practice at the boundaries of the care settings. The development of technology is offering new opportunities for monitoring and supporting patients in their homes, especially in rural and remote settings, but in many areas this has yet to be applied to the orthopaedic patient. Meanwhile orthopaedic and trauma practitioners need to develop skills in providing care and support from a distance, and the use of communication technology is likely to increase as this aim becomes more relevant in the future.

Ethical and Legal Aspects of Orthopaedic and Trauma Care

Practitioners are increasingly required to consider the complex nature of ethical issues which affect the orthopaedic and trauma patient. As with all other branches of nursing, there are both specialised and general issues that affect the specific patient group, and the orthopaedic practitioner needs a deep working understanding of these.

Much of the discussion about ethical issues in all aspects of nursing is related to the nature and quality of care. Nursing care is often seen as being synonymous with holistic patient-centred approaches, which are non-judgmental and include the demonstration of attitudes and behaviours that are sensitive to the needs of patients and carers, and respect individuality and choice (McSherry et al. 2012). This is especially important when orthopaedic and trauma care takes place in highly pressurised environments in which it is possible to lose sight of patient-centred priorities. Effective education of orthopaedic practitioners, insightful and transformational leadership, and the development of a strong patient priority-centred evidence base

are central to this. Within this is the need to develop practitioners not only with the right knowledge, skills and attitudes but with a passion for working with patients with very specific and significant needs related to their musculoskeletal problem.

The provision of quality care within a framework that values and respects dignity is a constant source of discussion in all healthcare settings. This is particularly important in maintaining the practitioner's own safety when the patient is a vulnerable child or older adult or other individual with impairment. As people with learning disabilities live longer they are more likely to require care in orthopaedic settings. Mental health problems such as debilitating depression frequently affect care and recovery. There remains a need for the practitioner to develop the skills to care for orthopaedic patients with a wide variety of needs that make them vulnerable. The safeguarding from harm of both children and vulnerable adults is becoming an increasing priority and must be central to all care provided.

In any healthcare setting, informed consent for all procedures and activities is an important part of care along with consideration of the mental capacity of the patient. Orthopaedic interventions carry with them significant risks. Understanding how to assess the capacity of an individual to make decisions about their care is an important part of informed consent, as is the ability to ensure that patients, carers and families understand the risks of the decisions they are being asked to make. Practitioners must adhere to Acts of Parliament in their own country, which provide a statutory framework to empower and protect people of all ages who may lack capacity to make their own decisions.

There is a danger that orthopaedic practitioners assume that 'do not resuscitate' orders and living wills do not relate to the orthopaedic/trauma patient group except in the oncology setting. This can perhaps be traced to the specialty's focus on healing and recovery. However, as caring develops in the coming decades it is likely that there will be a greater focus on end of life issues and practitioners must be aware of the national guidance and legislation that requires them to be aware of best practice in both decision making and communication. One example of this is in the discussion regarding the need to consider palliative care for frail older patients with major orthopaedic injuries. Research increasingly shows that some conditions are life-limiting. One example is hip fracture, which often occurs in very frail elderly patients and may need to instigate a sensitive discussion about the need to implement end-of-life care (Murray et al. 2012). Decisions and discussions about such matters may not have been, but will need to be, part of the orthopaedic practitioner's skills set as the quality of end-of-life care reaches a more prominent place in all settings.

Summary

This chapter has examined the nature of orthopaedic and trauma nursing, and the main issues which drive its development, including public health, political, practical, and legal and ethical agendas. It has highlighted the diverse needs of the orthopaedic patient along the entire age continuum and in the variety of settings in which care takes place. It acknowledges that modern healthcare is complicated and has many drivers, and that this leads to numerous complex ethical issues with which the practitioner must engage. It is hoped that these principles can be successfully applied to the material contained within the remainder of this book.

Further Reading

Judd, J. (2010). Defining expertise in paediatric orthopaedic nursing. *International Journal of Orthopaedic and Trauma Nursing* 14 (3): 159–168.

McSherry, W., McSherry, R., and Watson, R. (2012). *Care in Nursing: Principles, Values and Skills*. Oxford: Oxford University Press.

Santy, J. (2001). An investigation of the reality of nursing work with orthopaedic patients. *Journal of Orthopaedic Nursing* 5 (1): 22–29.

Santy Tomlinson, J. and Mackintosh-Franklin, C. (2020). *How to be a Great Nurse: The Heart of Nursing*. M&K.

Sellman, D. (2011). *What Makes a Good Nurse?* London: Jessica Kingsley.

References

Balcombe, K., Davis, P., and Lim, E. (1991). A nursing model for orthopaedics. *Nursing Standard* 5 (49): 26–28.

Blair, J. (2017). Diagnostic overshadowing: see beyond the diagnosis. *British Journal of Family Medicine* 37–41. http://www.intellectualdisability.info/changing-values/diagnostic-overshadowing-see-beyond-the-diagnosis (accessed 17 August 2021).

Burke, E., Carroll, R., O'Dwyer, M. et al. (2019). Quantitative examination of the bone health status of older adults with intellectual and developmental disability in Ireland: a cross-sectional nationwide study. *British Medical Journal Open* 9: e026939. https://doi.org/10.1136/bmjopen-2018-026939.

Clarke, S. (2017). The history of children's nursing and its direction within the United Kingdom. *Comprehensive Child and Adolescent Nursing* 40: 3. https://doi.org/10.1080/24694193.2017.1316790.

Clarke, S. (2019) *An exploration of the child's experience of staying in hospital from the perspectives of children and children's nurses using child-centered methodology*. EdD thesis, Queen's University Belfast.

Corkin, D., Clarke, S., and Liggett, L. (ed.) (2012). *Care Planning in Children and Young People's Nursing*. Oxford: Wiley-Blackwell.

Cox, C.R., Clemson, L., Stancliffe, R.J. et al. (2010). Incidence of and risk factors for falls among adults with an intellectual disability. *Journal of Intellectual Disability Research* 54 (12): 1045–1057.

Davis, P.S. (1994). *Nursing the Orthopaedic Patient*. Edinburgh: Churchill Livingstone.

Drozd, M. (2019). *The Voices of Adults with a Learning Disability and a Carer on their Orthopaedic and Trauma Hospital Care in the UK*. Unpublished thesis, University of Wolverhampton for the degree of Professional Doctorate in Health and Wellbeing.

Drozd, M., Jester, R., and Santy, J. (2007). The inherent components of the orthopaedic nursing role: an exploratory study. *Journal of Orthopaedic Nursing* 11 (1): 43–52.

Drozd, M., Chadwick, D., and Jester, R. (2020a). An integrative review of the hospital experiences of people with an intellectual disability: lack of orthopaedic and trauma perspectives. *International Journal of Orthopaedic and Trauma Nursing* 39: https://doi.org/10.1016/j.ijotn.2020.100795.

Drozd, M., Chadwick, D., and Jester, R. (2020b). A cross-case comparison of the trauma and orthopaedic hospital experiences of adults with intellectual disabilities using interpretative phenomenological analysis. *Nursing Open* https://doi.org/10.1002/nop2.693.

Drozd, M., Chadwick, D., and Jester, R. (2021). The voices of people with an intellectual disability and a carer about orthopaedic and trauma hospital care in the UK: an interpretative phenomenological study. *International Journal of Orthopaedic and Trauma Nursing*. https://doi.org/10.1016/j.ijotn.2020.100831.

Emerson, E. and Baines, S. (2011). Health inequalities and people with learning disabilities in the UK. *Tizard Learning Disability Review* 16: 42–48.

Equality Act (2010) www.legislation.gov.uk/ukpga/2010/15/pdfs/ukpga_20100015_en.pdf (accessed 17 August 2021).

Finlayson, J. (2011). *Injuries, Accidents and Falls in Adults with Learning Disabilities and Their Carers: A Prospective Cohort Study*. Ph.D. thesis, University of Glasgow.

Finlayson, J., Morrison, J., Jackson, A. et al. (2010). Injuries, falls and accidents among adults with intellectual disabilities. Prospective cohort study. *Journal of Intellectual Disability Research* 54 (11): 966–980. 319. https://doi.org/10.1111/j.1365-2788.2010.01319.x.

Finlayson, J., Morrison, J., Skelton, D.A. et al. (2014). The circumstances and impact of injuries on adults with learning disabilities. *The British Journal of Occupational Therapy* 77 (8): 400–409.

Heslop, P., Blair, P., Fleming, M., et al. (2013). *Confidential Inquiry into premature deaths of people with learning disabilities (CIPOLD)*. University of Bristol, Bristol. www.bris.ac.uk/cipold/reports/index.html (accessed 17 August 2021).

Iacono, T., Bigby, C., Unsworth, C. et al. (2014). A systematic review of hospital experiences of people with intellectual disability. *Biomedical Central (BMC) Health Services Research* 14: 505. http://www.biomedcentral.com/1472-6963/14/505 (accessed 17 August 2021).

Judd, J. (2010). Defining expertise in paediatric orthopaedic nursing. *International Journal of Orthopaedic and Trauma Nursing* 14 (3): 159–168.

Judd, J. (2013). Rickets in the 21st-century: a review of low vitamin D and its management. *International Journal of Orthopaedic and Trauma Nursing* 17 (4): 199–208.

Kinnear, D., Morrison, J., Allan, L. et al. (2018). Prevalence of physical conditions and multimorbidity in a cohort of adults with intellectual disabilities with and without down syndrome: cross sectional study. *British Medical Journal Open* 8: e018292. https://doi.org/10.1136/BMJ open-2017-018292.

Love, C. (1995). Orthopaedic nursing: a study of its specialty status. *Nursing Standard* 9 (44): 36–40.

McCarron, M., Swinburne, J., Burke, E., et al. (2011). *Growing older with an intellectual disability in Ireland 2011: First results from the Intellectual Disability Supplement to the Irish Longitudinal Study on Ageing (IDSTILDA)*. Dublin: School of Nursing and Midwifery, Trinity College.

McCarron, M., Swinburne, J., Burke, E. et al. (2013). Patterns of multimorbidity in an older population of persons with an intellectual disability: results from the intellectual disability supplement to the Irish longitudinal study on aging (IDS-TILDA). *Research in Developmental Disabilities* 34: 521–527.

McSherry, W., McSherry, R., and Watson, R. (2012). *Care in Nursing. Principles, Values and Skills*. Oxford: Oxford University Press.

Mencap (2007). *Death by Indifference*. London: Mencap.

Michael, J. (2008). *Healthcare for all: report of the independent inquiry into access to healthcare for people with learning disabilities*. London. http://webarchive.nationalarchives.gov.uk/20130107105354/http:/www.dh.gov.uk/prod_consum_dh/groups/dh_digitalassets/@dh/@en/documents/digitalasset/dh_106126.pdf (accessed 17 August 2021).

Murray, I.R., Biant, L.C., Clement, N.C., and Murray, S.A. (2012). Should a hip fracture in a frail older person be a trigger for assessment of palliative care needs? *Supportive and Palliative Care* 1 (1): 3–4.

NHS England (2017). *Helping people with a learning disability to give feedback*. London: NHS England. https://www.england.nhs.uk/wp-content/uploads/2017/04/bitesize-guide-learning-disability.pdf (accessed 17 August 2021).

Orlando, I.J. (1961). *The Dynamic Nurse-Patient Relationship: Function, Process and Principles*. New York: G.P. Putnam's Sons.

Ouellet, L.L. and Rush, K.L. (1992). A synthesis of selected literature on mobility: a basis for studying impaired mobility. *International Journal of Nursing Knowledge* 3 (2): 72–80.

Ouellet, L.L. and Rush, K.L. (1996). A study of nurses' perceptions of client mobility. *Western Journal of Nursing Research* 18 (5): 565–579.

Ouellet, L.L. and Rush, K.L. (1998). Conceptual module of client mobility. *Journal of Orthopaedic Nursing* 2 (3): 132–135.

Powell, M. (1951). *Orthopaedic Nursing*. Edinburgh: E&S Livingstone.

Royal College of Nursing (2017). *The Needs of People with learning disabilities. What pre-registration students should know?* Royal College of Nursing, London.

Rush, K.L. and Ouellet, L.L. (1998). An analysis of elderly clients' views of mobility. *Western Journal of Nursing Research* 20 (3): 295–311.

Santy, J. (2001). An investigation of the reality of nursing work with orthopaedic patients. *Journal of Orthopaedic Nursing* 5 (1): 22–29.

Srikanth, R., Cassidy, G., Joiner, C., and Teeluckdharry, S. (2011). Osteoporosis in people with intellectual disabilities: a review and a brief study of risk factors for osteoporosis in a community sample of people with intellectual disabilities. *Journal of Intellectual Disability Research* 55: 53–62.

Swarup, I. and O'Donnell, J.F. (2016). An overview of the history of orthopedic surgery. *The American Journal of Orthopedics* 45 (7): E434–E438.

Thompson, C. and Dowding, D. (ed.) (2002). *Clinical Decision Making and Judgement in Nursing*. Edinburgh: Churchill Livingstone.

Veselinova, C. (2014). Understanding equality, diversity and inclusion in dementia care. *Nursing and Residential Care* 16 (7): https://doi.org/10.12968/nrec.2014. 16.7.406.

Weisz, G. (2003). The emergence of medical specialization in the nineteenth century. *Bulletin of the History of Medicine* 77 (3): 536–574. https://doi.org/10.1353/bhm. 2003.0150.

2

Evidence and Refining Practice

Paul McLiesh

Adelaide Nursing School, University of Adelaide, Adelaide, Australia

Introduction

The aim of this chapter is to consider how individual nurses and healthcare systems can use evidence to strengthen practice and improve the outcomes and experiences for patients.

As orthopaedic nurses we aim to continually reflect on our practice and refine our knowledge, skills and application of nursing care, with the aim of ensuring that the care we deliver is effective, timely, suitable and appropriate for the needs of our patients. While over time, individual nurses will gradually refine their ability to accurately judge the value of the care they deliver, there is a risk that what guides their practice will be solely based on what they have seen and learnt locally, and may not necessarily incorporate evidence from a broader range of sources. Traditionally, nursing practice has been based on knowledge passed from nurse to nurse and while this is a useful practice and a key part of learning, it can lack rigour of certainty and lacks a contribution from a broader range of sources. While in contemporary healthcare settings nursing practice is more likely to be guided by a range of sources and evidence than in the past, there are still significant challenges in identifying suitable evidence to guide practice, getting that evidence incorporated into practice and dealing with large amounts of evidence, some of which may be contradictory.

Evidence-based practice (EBP) is a broad term that refers to knowledge and practice that has been developed over time with the purpose of 'generating knowledge and evidence to effectively and appropriately deliver healthcare in ways that are effective, feasible, and meaningful to specific populations, cultures, and settings' (Pearson et al. 2012).

To better understand contemporary practice and evidence utilisation, it is helpful to understand the historical journey of how orthopaedic nursing practice has developed over time. Hunt (1938) gives a very insightful view of her experience in developing orthopaedic nursing and the impact of the social and political factors she had to face. Since this publication there have been many books written to help both student and qualified orthopaedic practitioners (Powell 1986; Footner 1987; Davis 1994; Maher et al. 2002; Kneale and Davis 2005) along with journals and individual papers. Much of the early literature published in relation to orthopaedic nursing practice discussed the practicalities of specific skills to guide delivery of care. However, there were also those leaders who sought to not only influence the way nurses' practice, but how they learnt, how they developed the specialty and how they prepared other nurses to deliver better care over time. Dame Agnes Hunt was one of those early leaders in the UK and she identified that there were gaps in the care needs of 'crippled' children and was able to influence the leaders of the time to change healthcare systems to better meet the needs of this patient population (McLiesh and Wiechula 2013).

There have been a number of influences on the development of nursing knowledge. The Briggs report in 1972 (Committee on Nursing) suggested that nursing should become a research-based profession and there has been much written about how and why this is necessary, the impact it has on patient care and the view of nursing by other professions. Care up to this point had often been based on what had traditionally been delivered under the authority of senior staff. Whilst this may have been based on years of experience there was no real assurance that the care delivered was the best possible or was even effective. Policies and education began to respond to this, but over subsequent decades it was noted that the uptake of research by nurses was sporadic and sometimes limited. Hunt (1981) identified that research was still not really finding its way into practice a decade after the report was published. Another decade later Close and Cheater (1994) felt that research had started to permeate the culture of nursing, although they did not think it was a clearly embedded concept. Even in the late 1990s Batteson (1999) felt that many practices were still based on local circumstance rather than research. Even in today's contemporary practice there are significant reasons why good-quality evidence does not find its way into the daily practice of orthopaedic nurses around the world. The reasons for this and the barriers that prevent this 'translation' into practice are key considerations here and have been the subject of a significant body of research (Kitson 2011; Harvey et al. 2016).

Clarke (1999) considered care in terms of efficiency and effectiveness in clinical decision making, and Gerrish and Clayton (1998) add the concern for quality improvement and cost consciousness. Particular attention was paid to effectiveness by the NHS executive (1998) as they began to ask that clinical decisions should be based on the best possible evidence. This approach, guided by consideration of effectiveness, is useful and is valuable in the generation and application of clinical guidelines. But effectiveness is not the only criteria by which to judge new knowledge and evidence: feasibility, appropriateness and meaningfulness, particularly for the patient, are also important. The Joanna Briggs Institute uses this approach as the basis for their Model of Evidence-Based Healthcare:

'The best available evidence, the context in which care is delivered, the individual patient and the professional judgement and expertise of the health professional inform this process' (Joanna Briggs Institute 2021a).

Hicks and Hennessy (1997) discussed the notion of accountability as care cannot be delivered based solely on opinion and/or authority; it needs some form of justification. So while recognising the importance of the individual nurse's knowledge, there is value in creating systems to appraise new knowledge (evidence) through ever-expanding research activity. As the sheer scale of the amount of evidence that is being generated through research expands, it becomes difficult for the individual orthopaedic nurse to be able to assess and apply this knowledge. This need led to the formation of a number of organisations such as Cochrane, the Joanna Briggs Institute (2021a) and the National Institute for Health and Care Excellence (NICE) where processes were developed to appraise and summarise evidence for both practice and teaching purposes.

There was also the encouragement of research utilisation, and Horsley et al. (1978) examined the complex organisational functions that range from problem identification to the implementation of an innovation. Many research texts were then published looking at how to undertake and critique research, including chapters on change management. However, research can be used in more than one way and may not just be about innovation and change in practice. Estabrooks (1998) identified that it can be used as action research when directly applied to practice, with change and evaluation taking place as part of the research. It can also be used conceptually to enlighten understanding and persuasively to change the views of others. The function of systematic reviews grew from a sense that there was a lack of ability to critique research-generated evidence and be able to combine the evidence from a number of primary research projects to provide a summary for clinicians and researchers. A range of individuals were responsible for the development of this approach, including people such as Archie Cochrane (https://www.cochrane.org/about-us/difference-we-make).

Evidence-based Practice

This term and what it means, how it is applied and who it is relevant to has been transformed over time. Even the term itself has a number of iterations for different groups, for example evidence-based medicine, evidence-based learning and evidence-based care. Ingersoll et al.'s (2000) definition brings in the nursing context and notes that it is more about theory-derived research-based information, about care delivery to groups and individuals, and, most importantly, is considerate of individual needs and preferences. This definition does not imply that primary research is the only form of evidence and it includes the patient in decisions reflecting the increased levels of health-related knowledge of patients and the view that 'medicine knows best' is quickly being eroded by the 'expert' patient.

Nurses must embrace this issue from their own professional perspective as well as differentiate their professional roles and responsibilities. EBP is a broad term and its focus is on using evidence to influence or change/confirm practice, the notion being that using existing evidence will ensure that care is delivered in a manner that is best suited for the patients' needs at that time and place. Evidence such as this has been generated out of research or observation, synthesised and/or critiqued (such as in systematic reviews), and used to inform guidelines and policies which then, ideally, inform and direct practice. While this is a sound approach, there is much to get in the way of ensuring that evidence is used to inform those guidelines/practice and ensuring that the knowledge is used by nurses who are delivering care. This is where the notion of knowledge translation (KT) arises, which focusses on the argument that successful implementation of evidence into practice requires consideration of a range of factors such as the evidence itself, the context of where and when it is being implemented and how the integration is facilitated (Kitson et al. 2008). Just because evidence exists in regard to a particular topic does not mean it will be adopted and implemented by those who would benefit the most from using it. This notion of KT is key to individual nurses, as well as healthcare systems, in designing ways that high-quality evidence can be disseminated to individuals delivering care and influence their practices (Harvey and Kitson 2016).

There are two main considerations for EBP, however. The first is the assumption that research has been conducted and strong evidence exists on the particular clinical issue or problem of interest. This may not always be the case. For example, if a search is conducted for evidence to support the premise that early mobilisation in orthopaedic patients is beneficial, very little original research may be found. The second assumption is that all published research is of good quality. Just because research is published, even in a peer-reviewed source such as a quality journal, does not necessarily mean the evidence is strong and should be adopted without questioning its quality or applicability. Poorly designed, implemented and presented research can still be found in peer-reviewed journals and should be subjected to continual critical appraisal. The appraisal process often shows research to be poorly constructed and conducted, and therefore must be measured in its implementation. Santy and Temple (2004) identify in their critical review of skeletal pin site care that only two pieces of evidence were found that were of sufficient quality to be trusted and used to direct nursing care. It is challenging then for the individual nurse to spend time critiquing individual research to determine what is high-quality evidence. This is where processes such as systematic reviews (Joanna Briggs Institute 2021c), where the evidence is sought, critiqued, combined and knowledge synthesised to produce a higher level of evidence, can be used to guide policies and practice. There are organisations whose main purpose is to conducted these reviews and use the synthesised knowledge to create guidelines, etc. that are based on high-quality evidence. Examples of these are the Joanna Briggs Institute, Cochrane and the University of York Centre for Reviews and Dissemination. As identified earlier in this chapter, evidence should incorporate elements of the following:

> *Feasibility*: The extent to which an intervention is practical or viable in a specific context.
> *Appropriateness*: The extent to which an intervention fits within the context of a specific situation.
> *Meaningfulness*: How the intervention is experienced by individuals or groups.
> *Effectiveness*: The extent to which an intervention achieves the intended result
> (Jordan et al. 2019)

It is essential that any evidence that is adopted is first assessed and appraised for quality. This can be a formal or informal process but should involve critique of elements such as consideration of research design and methodological approach, rigour in research design, methods of data collection and analysis, statistical methods used, and congruency between research design, conduct of the research and presentation of the findings. Finally, the evidence should be applied to the context in which it is relevant. An example of the entire process, from setting the question to implementing findings, is provided in a review of preoperative exercise in knee replacement surgery (Lucas 2004).

Hierarchies (and Quality) of Evidence

There is a good deal of debate about what is best evidence and nurses need to be able to navigate this complex, evolving web of information. When deciding what evidence is best, a number of authors have made some attempt to apply categories to help clarify what may be the most rigorous. Bircumshaw (1990) suggests a fairly simplistic hierarchy to help the reader understand the relationship between research and practice, tying the availability of research into the responsibility of the nurse. This model places the emphasis on the primacy of empirical research. This should not be seen as too much of a problem as different research designs may be regarded as more valid and reliable than others, although this may vary depending on who is asked the question and what is their background. However, other models are much more encompassing than this and encapsulate a broader range of evidence types ranging from personal and peer experience to meta-analyses and systematic reviews. A basic overview of these is:

- quantitative research
- qualitative research
- expert opinion
- personal experience.

Historically the hierarchy of evidence, and even the inclusion of various philosophical approaches to research, has evolved significantly. Empirical research appears to have great pre-eminence in these early hierarchies and Griffiths (2002) feels that this may be because questions about issues such as effectiveness and efficiency are best addressed by such methods, particularly the randomised controlled trial (RCT). Quantitative research may not, however, be able to solve all problems and the integration and acceptance of qualitative methodologies gradually became more accepted as a way of creating evidence and informing practice. Munhall (2012) points out that there are 'untidy' aspects of caring that need to be examined, such as emotion and feeling. Decision making around these may not be best served by purely quantitative approaches such as RCTs. McCormack (2004) suggests that qualitative research is an important element of practice but, because of perceived problems relating to reliability and validity, it may be placed lower in the hierarchy. Howard and Davis (2002) describe and explain the relatively weak position of qualitative research in orthopaedics and suggest a new approach they label 'diagnostic research'. More contemporary research approaches, using qualitative methodologies, are now more commonplace and more widely accepted (McLiesh and Rasmussen 2017; Rasmussen and McLiesh 2019).

More and more, it is accepted that to better understand the complex nature of healthcare both qualitative and quantitative research is valuable in creating evidence that can be used to inform practice, maintain patient safety and improve experience.

Various research organisations around the world will produce guidelines regarding hierarchy of evidence, such as the National Health and Medical Research Council Levels of Evidence and Grades for Recommendations in Australia (Levels of Evidence and Grades for Recommendations for Developers of Guidelines 2009).

Mantzoukas (2007) suggests we abandon the hierarchy altogether as this often serves to impede the implementation of EBP. An alternative offered is reflection on practice to make decisions relating to care. To do this, a good deal of clinical experience is required and at the same time as there is a growing body of evidence in nursing, there is also a growing body of experience that has been gained by individual practitioners. So the knowledge of experienced and expert individual orthopaedics nurses should not be dismissed on face value, as that knowledge is valuable and will be highly contextualised and can serve as a valuable resource for other nurses developing their practice. Intuition and experience in expert practice are important as the development of quality services cannot be delayed by lack of research findings (Ellis 2000) and intuition uses the untapped resource of tacit knowledge (Meerabeau 1992). This complicates matters: on the one hand EBP tends to underemphasise intuition and experiential knowledge and stresses the examination of clinical research, whilst on the other hand it can never replace individual expertise (Rolfe 1999). What is likely absent from this evidence, from individual experience and practice, is a formalised critique of that knowledge. The expert orthopaedic nurse will develop that practice over time in response to a wide range of clinical scenarios and experiences. That nurse's expertise may develop at an almost subconscious level and they may not spend time formally reviewing or considering the way they have learnt to practice in that manner and the evidence on which they base their care interventions. A balance of

formal review processes and evidence generation, translation and implementation when combined with expert knowledge and practice is likely to ensure the best outcomes for all, especially patients.

Finding Evidence

The general clinical orthopaedic nurse may be unlikely to have a strong sense of individual research methodologies and what makes good-quality research design, as this has not been a focus of traditional nursing training. Developing a better level of research literacy across the broad orthopaedic nursing workforce will likely have a range of beneficial effects, as it teaches individuals how to approach problems identified in practice, plan ways of measuring what is occurring, critically reviewing the results and then implementing changes to improve the situation. For existing evidence, practitioners have to be able to extract evidence/ data that is relevant and be able to recognise the different range of approaches that can inform practice. Accessing this evidence can be difficult and time-consuming for the individual. Most large healthcare organisations will provide access to online databases of resources such as journals, health databases and evidence synthesis organisations, but knowing how to search these effectively and spend time looking through the results can be challenging. Other smaller organisations or those in lower income countries may not have access to that information, which makes this even more difficult. Using evidence that has already been subjected to the critique and synthesis processes, such as systematic reviews or evidence summaries, can be a useful way to consider change to practice. Approaching known issues as a group or organisation is also effective and may be far more likely to have the intended outcome of improving practice.

Finally, it is essential that a well-developed plan, and appropriate skills and resources are allocated to create a suitable culture for EBP to work effectively (Munhall 2012).

Using Evidence in Practice: An Example

Having looked at some of the issues around research and evidence, we now must look at how you can start to develop your own knowledge base relevant to orthopaedic or trauma practice. The ability to think critically in solving a healthcare problem is of essence to the process of EBP because each context is unique and just knowing the evidence is not sufficient to ensure that a certain practice is adopted and integrated without identifying barriers, strategies and appropriateness. Jones-Devitt and Smith (2007, p. 7) define critical thinking as:

> Making sense of the world through a process of questioning the questions, challenging assumptions, recognising that bodies of knowledge can be chaotic and evolving; ultimately with the aim of continually improving thinking.

Sometimes we respond to a problem quickly and may not consider the specific nuances of that situation, especially if our practice is not well developed and the situation is demanding, complex or if we are under time pressure to make quick decisions. For example, with respect to surgical wound care, the orthopaedic nurse may consider the best type of dressing to use for a particular patient and search for evidence to support or make that choice. However, maybe other elements should be considered first: does the wound need a dressing, what is the history of the wound, what has been tried before for this wound, what worked and what did not work for this person, what specific patient factors may influence healing (such as compliance, smoking) or are there other disease processes that may impact healing such as unstable diabetes? Once these questions are considered, and answered, the choice of dressing type can then be addressed utilising a range of evidence that best meets the context of this situation.

Below is a step-by-step process which you can use to consider this type of approach to the care you deliver. It does not have to lead to a full research project and be undertaken for educational purposes, you can do it just to improve patient care, but it demonstrates a good way to approach care questions and reflection on practice using evidence.

- Choose a subject area or set a question and discuss this with your managers and colleagues (nurses and other disciplines). Think about an area of practice that you want to consolidate or develop. Maybe there is something in your clinical area that makes you and others just stop and question why? Or could this be done in a better way? Is there something that just does not seem to work well? A sense of curiosity, as a nurse, is one of the most essential characteristics needed for development of expert practice. This first stage is probably the most important, as without a clear search question the end result will be weak, inconclusive or unusable.
- Start to look for information and identify resources that pertain to your chosen area. Make notes of:
  - the databases that you searched
  - the key words that you used for your search and how you refined them

  - if you undertook any incremental searching (looking at the reference list at the back of published articles)
  - conversations with others who have a particular specialist interest in the area you have chosen
- Spend time learning how to search each database specifically.
- Look for evidence summaries or systematic reviews from organisations identified in the EBP section above.

All the above are ways of accessing existing sources of knowledge, but each will have its own issues for consideration:

- Databases may be selective in the information that they hold or may contain so much information that it is difficult to decide what is important. Don't limit your search to primary research only, as evidence/knowledge is much wider than this, but do try to make sure the information you collect is peer-reviewed from reputable journals to ensure its credibility. Key words can be difficult to determine and define so it is important to ensure that you have been very specific in the choice of subject. Again, it is useful to discuss this with managers, peers or others with experience in research or development of search strategies to ensure that you have the correct terms for the correct focus.
- Incremental searching (looking at the reference lists on articles that you already have) is useful, particularly when the databases do not appear to be yielding very much.
- Asking specialist/advanced nurses for information is also useful and may yield some articles that you had not thought of or may be finding difficult to obtain. However, because of their specialist focus, you may find that the article selection may be narrowed.

While each method may have its limitations, if you identify material from a wide range of sources it is likely that you will end up with a pertinent dataset for use in the development of your knowledge base.

- Once you have collected all the resources, read through them and identify the ones that you will select for consideration. While you are reading each paper, consider the authors and their experience, think about the type of journal and the date of the publication. Some databases will allow you to see how many others have cited that publication, which may potentially indicate the quality of the information.
- Spend time re-reading each paper. Get a feel for the area, write down notes as you read. Identify the papers that are primary research and those that are literature reviews, editorials, professional opinion, etc.

Table 2.1 Research summary

Reference	Make a note of the full reference here so that you have a lasting record of it
Themes/key words	Under what theme/key word can the work be summarised?
Principal findings	What are the main findings of the research?
Ethics	Is there evidence that the research project was subject to ethical scrutiny? Are there any obvious problems to note?
Sample	Has the population under study been described?
	What type of sample was drawn from the population? Is the sample representative of the population?
	Are the characteristics of the different participant populations similar (i.e. the control versus intervention groups)
	How many were selected for the study and what was the response rate?
	How many dropped out of the study/what was the attrition rate?
	How might the above affect the generalisability (external validity) of the study?
	Does the method of the research (qualitative) match the research methodology?
Design	*Quantitative* *Qualitative*
	RCT Grounded theory
	Experiment Phenomenology
	Quasi-experiment Ethnography
	Correlational
	Cohort
	Survey
	Try to ascertain if the study is retrospective or prospective
	In terms of hierarchies of evidence is the design used trustworthy?
Data collection	Were the groups being compared (quantitative) treated the same except for the intervention being considered?
	Identify the ways data have been collected. Were those involved as participants or as researchers blinded (quantitative) to which group received what interventions? Were outcomes measured correctly and consistently?
	Some studies may use more than one method
	Was data collected in a suitable way? (Some examples are interviews, observations, care records, clinical data, scales, questionnaires)
	How valid/reliable is the method utilised?
Data analysis	*Quantitative* *Qualitative*
	What is/are the name(s) of the test(s) used? How have the data been dealt with?
	Are these parametric or nonparametric? How trustworthy do you feel this is?
	Do the authors represent the participants' 'voice' in their findings/analysis?
	What is the level of significance?
Clinical significance	Have the researchers looked at the clinical as opposed to the statistical significance of the findings?
	Have they identified the implication (and recommendations) for practice and future research?

- Start to summarise the research articles using research evidence summaries (see Table 2.1) and the other articles using literature evidence summaries (see Table 2.2). You may want to design your own format if you find these too restrictive.
- Once you have completed all the summaries, have a look through and see if you can identify any themes. For

example, if you are looking at pre-operative fasting you may find that some of the articles are about fasting times whilst others may look at the outcomes associated with fasting times. Separate these and then put each of the articles on a matrix for each theme. Matrices for the research articles and other literature can be found in Tables 2.3 and 2.4, respectively.

Table 2.2 Literature summary

Reference	Make a note of the full reference here so that you have a lasting record of it. You can export these citations into a citation reference manager program such as EndNote
Summary	What are the main points being made by the author(s)?
Themes/key words	Under what theme/key word can the work be summarised?
Article type	Is the article type any of the following: opinion, editorial, group consensus, conference proceedings, review?
	In terms of hierarchies of evidence what is the position of this material relative to research?
Clinical relevance	Of what clinical relevance is the article?

- Once you have identified all the different approaches taken in the research articles and inserted them into the matrix start reading around the research methods that have been utilised by the authors. Justham (2007) suggests a simple checklist of questions that will get you started. The Critical Appraisal Skills Programme (2021) and Joanna Briggs Institute (2021b) websites provide more in-depth appraisal tools. Access research methods texts from the library to help you to understand the methods discussed in the papers.
- For the other articles it is useful to identify what type of evidence they represent (professional opinion, group consensus, etc.) and their position relative to research in a hierarchy of evidence.

Developing confidence in critiquing research and evidence will be more effective based on your understanding of different research methods and methodologies. Developing a higher level of research literacy will not only assist you in critiquing research but also being able to apply that evidence in your practice. Reading methods and methodology papers can assist in strengthening this knowledge (McLiesh 2019; McLiesh et al. 2018; Rasmussen and McLiesh 2019).

Table 2.4 Literature matrix template

Author/date/source	Article type	Summary of points for comment	Clinical reflections

Translation of Evidence

Having gone some way to develop your knowledge base, what do you do with it now? It is helpful to have a way of summarising the evidence and identifying key elements of the evidence, especially in relation to your specific practice context. Using a tool such as that shown in Table 2.4 will go some way to help that process.

Taking evidence and translating that into refinement of practice is likely one of the most underestimated elements of practice change in healthcare. It may stem from the thought that once evidence is made obvious, then it will naturally be adopted by those in practice and find its way into care delivery. But this thought process seriously underestimates the difficult nature of practice change and the complexity and amount of information competing for nurses' attention.

There are a number of frameworks or literature that consider this step in the process of evidence utilisation. Kitson et al. (2018, p. 231) identify that some of the existing models for evidence translation are not well designed to match the complex world of healthcare:

> Most are linear or cyclical and very few come close to reflecting the dense and intricate relationships, systems and politics of organizations and the processes required to enact sustainable improvements. We illustrate how using complexity and network concepts can better inform KT and argue that changing the way we think and talk about KT could enhance the creation and movement of knowledge throughout those systems needing to develop and utilise it.

Table 2.3 Research matrix template

Author/date/source	Summary of findings	Ethics	Sample type/size	Design	Data collection	Tests/analysis	Discussion/clinical relevance

They suggest that using elements of a theoretical framework that identify the complexity of healthcare systems and the way we practice can enhance the creation and movement of knowledge throughout those systems. They suggest five subnetworks of key processes be considered, (i) problem identification, (ii) knowledge creation, (iii) knowledge synthesis, (iv) implementation and (v) evaluation (Kitson et al. 2018), with the understanding that these will vary depending on the location, setting, context and differences in times. Spending time allowing for all these elements is likely to achieve more effective implementation of evidence and change of practice. Other considerations regarding the willingness for the individuals and/or organisation to change, how the change is facilitated, and organisational culture and leadership are also key factors. This was presented as a framework of translation of knowledge into practice by Harvey et al. (2016).

Context, collaboration and culture may be particularly important in the field of orthopaedics and trauma because of the multiprofessional nature of the speciality. Field (1987) identifies the different roles of the professionals:

- doctor = curative
- physiotherapist = restorative
- nurse = evaluative.

Each member of the team will have a different role but will need common knowledge to function effectively, therefore it makes sense to make sure that all are involved if there is to be any development in EBP as this may involve multiple adoption decisions.

In the UK, advanced practice roles have been developed and Health Education England (2017) have published a framework, 'Multiprofessional framework for advanced clinical practice in England', which builds on previous frameworks that were used in Wales and Scotland. It sets out an agreed definition for advanced clinical practice for all health and care professionals and articulates what it means for individual practitioners to practise at a higher level from that achieved on initial registration. The framework lists the capabilities expected of practitioners working at an advanced level across four pillars: clinical practice, leadership and management, education and research. Thompson and McNamara (2021) acknowledge that the role of the advanced nurse practitioner (ANP) is relatively new to the Irish healthcare system and it has undergone significant transformation since its inception, transcending both nursing and medical domains. See Chapter 7 for further information about advanced practice in orthopaedic and trauma nursing.

Given the various frameworks presented above, it is possible to adopt these, which have been designed for system change, to your individual practice as well. You can start with an issue or problem that needs solving (something that is not working well) and then consider the evidence, the strength of that evidence, how it could be applied to your local context/practice, the likelihood of whether that would be effective (or not), the reasons why, the culture of willingness to change (for those key people in your setting), the timing, the way it is/will be implemented or facilitated, and how those who will be affected are prepared (or not). This all takes time and effort to plan and implement but the more time that is spent in preparation, the more likely positive outcomes are later on, with benefits for patient care/experience.

In summary, an approach that develops knowledge and understanding to use in an EBP approach has six elements:

- search for evidence
- critique of evidence
- summarise evidence
- plan the implementation
- translate into practice
- evaluate the impact.

At its simplest, EBP is about good practice and improving the quality of healthcare (Baker 2010). Practitioners must continue to strive to generate and identify new knowledge for practice and apply it only after casting a critical orthopaedic nursing eye over it. We must listen to patient stories or narratives as they can be powerful and enlightening directors of decisions about care (Davis 2007). We must also listen to our own hearts and instincts, and utilise evidence in a caring and empathetic manner.

Further Reading

Aveyard, H. (2010). *Doing a Literature Review in Health and Social Care*, 3e. Maidenhead: Open University Press.

Aveyard, H. and Sharp, P. (2013). *A Beginner's Guide to Evidence Based Practice in Health and Social Care*, 2e. Maidenhead: Open University Press.

Gerrish, K., Lathlean, J., and Cormack, D. (2015). *The Research Process in Nursing*. Wiley.

Jones-Devitt, S. and Smith, L. (2007). *Critical Thinking in Health and Social Care*. London: Sage.

Harvey, G. and Kitson, A. (2015). *Implementing Evidence-Based Practice in Healthcare: A Facilitation Guide*. Taylor & Francis.

References

Australian Government (2009). *NHMRC additional lvels of evidence and grades for recommendations for developers of guidelines.* www.mja.com.au/sites/default/files/NHMRC. levels.of.evidence.2008-09.pdf.

Baker, J. (2010). *Evidence-Based Practice for Nurses.* London: Sage.

Batteson, L. (1999). Health visiting and clinical benchmarking. *Primary Health Care* 9 (9): 10, 12, 14.

Bircumshaw, D. (1990). The utilization of research findings in clinical nursing practice. *Journal of Advanced Nursing* 15: 1272–1280.

Clarke, J. (1999). Evidence-based practice: a retrograde step? The importance of pluralism in evidence generation for the practice of health care. *Journal of Clinical Nursing* 8: 89–94.

Closs, S. and Cheater, F. (1994). Utilization of nursing research: culture, interest and support. *Journal of Advanced Nursing* 19: 762–773.

Committee on Nursing (1972) *Report of the Committee of Nursing*, Briggs Report, Cmnd 5115. HMSO, London.

Critical Appraisal Skills Programme (2021) https://casp-uk. net (accessed 5 September 2021).

Davis, P.S. (1994). *Nursing the Orthopaedic Patient.* Edinburgh: Churchill-Livingstone.

Davis, P. (2007). Listening to patient stories. *Journal of Orthopaedic Nursing* 11 (1): 1.

Ellis, J. (2000). Sharing the evidence: clinical practice benchmarking to improve continuously the quality of care. *Journal of Advanced Nursing* 21 (1): 215–225.

Estabrooks, C.A. (1998). Will evidence-based nursing practice make practice perfect? *Canadian Journal of Nursing Research* 30 (1): 15–36.

Field, P.A. (1987). The impact of nursing theory on the clinical decision making process. *Journal of Advanced Nursing* 12: 563–571.

Footner, A. (1987). *Orthopaedic Nursing.* London: Balliere-Tindall.

Gerrish, K. and Clayton, J. (1998). Improving clinical effectiveness through an evidence-based approach: Meeting the challenge for nursing in the United Kingdom. *Nursing Administration Quarterly* 22 (4): 55–65.

Griffiths, P. (2002). Evidence informing practice: introducing the mini review. *British Journal of Community Nursing* 7 (1): 38–40.

Harvey, G. and Kitson, A. (2016). PARIHS revisited: from heuristic to integrated framework for the successful implementation of knowledge into practice. *Implementation Science* 11 (1): 33.

Harvey, G., Marshall, R.J., Jordan, Z., and Kitson, A.L. (2016). Exploring the hidden barriers in knowledge translation. *Qualitative Health Research* 25 (11): 1506–1517.

Health Education England (2017). *Multi-Professional Framework for Advanced Clinical Practice in England.* London: Health Education England.

Hicks, C. and Hennessy, D. (1997). Mixed messages in nursing research: their contribution to the persisting hiatus between evidence and practice. *Journal of Advanced Nursing* 25: 595–601.

Horsley, J.A., Crane, J., and Bingle, J.D. (1978). Research utilization as an organizational process. *Journal of Nursing Administration* July: 4–6.

Howard, D. and Davis, P. (2002). The use of qualitative research methodology in orthopaedics – tell it as it is. *Journal of Orthopaedic Nursing* 6: 135–139.

Hunt, A. (1938). *This Is My Life.* London: Blackie.

Hunt, J. (1981). Indicators for nursing practice: the use of research findings. *Journal of Advanced Nursing* 6: 189–194.

Ingersoll, G., McIntosh, E., and Williams, M. (2000). Nurse-sensitive outcomes of advanced practice. *Journal of Advanced Nursing* 32 (5): 1272–1281.

Joanna Briggs Institute. (2021a) *JBI Approach to Evidence Based Healthcare.* https://jbi.global/jbi-approach-to-EBHC (accessed 29 August 2021).

Joanna Briggs Institute. (2021b) *Critical Appraisal Tools.* http://joannabriggs.org/research/critical-appraisal-tools. html (accessed 11 May 2017).

Joanna Briggs Institute. (2021c) *Database of Systematic Reviews.* https://journals.lww.com/jbisrir/Pages/default. aspx (accessed 15 January 2021).

Jones-Devitt, S. and Smith, L. (2007). *Critical Thinking in Health and Social Care.* London: Sage.

Jordan, Z., Lockwood, C., Munn, Z., and Aromataris, E. (2019). The updated Joanna Briggs Institute model of evidence-based healthcare. *JBI Evidence Implementation* 17 (1): 58–71.

Justham, D. (2007). Finding and evaluating an article. *Journal of Orthopaedic Nursing* 11: 60–65.

Kitson, A. (2011). Mechanics of knowledge translation. *International Journal of Evidence-Based Healthcare* 9 (2): 79–80.

Kitson, A., Rycroft-Malone, J., Harvey, G. et al. (2008). Evaluating the successful implementation of evidence into practice using the PARiHS framework: theoretical and practical challenges. *Implementation Science* 3 (1) 2008/01/07: 1.

Kitson, A., Brook, A., Harvey, G. et al. (2018). Using complexity and network concepts to inform healthcare knowledge translation. *International Journal of Health Policy and Management* 7 (3): 231–243.

Kneale, J.D. and Davis, P.S. (2005). *Orthopaedic and Trauma Nursing.* Edinburgh: Churchill Livingstone.

Lucas, B. (2004). Does a pre-operative exercise programme improve mobility and function post total knee replacement: a mini-review. *Journal of Orthopaedic Nursing* 8: 25–33.

Maher, A.B., Salmond, S.W., and Pellino, T. (2002). *Orthopaedic Nursing*. Philadelphia: Saunders.

Mantzoukas, S. (2007). The evidence-based practice ideologies. *Nursing Philosophy* 8 (4): 244–255.

McCormack, B. (2004). Commentary on fortuitous phenomena: on complexity, pragmatic randomised controlled trials, and knowledge for evidence-based practice by Carl Thompson. *Worldviews on Evidence-Based Practice (First Quarter)* 18–19.

McLiesh, P. (2019). Understanding research: systematic reviews for orthopaedic and trauma nursing. *International Journal of Orthopaedic and Trauma Nursing* 34: 48–51.

McLiesh, P. and Rasmussen, P. (2017). An overview of research in orthopaedic and trauma nursing. *International Journal of Orthopaedic and Trauma Nursing* https://doi.org/10.1016/ j.ijotn.2017.04.001.

McLiesh, P. and Wiechula, R. (2013). Orthopaedic nursing in the 2010s: a critical ethnography. Master of Nursing Science thesis, University of Adelaide, Adelaide Research & Scholarship. http://digital.library.adelaide.edu.au/dspace/handle/2440/76546.

McLiesh, P., Rasmussen, P., and Schultz, T. (2018). Quantitative research in orthopaedic and trauma nursing. *International Journal of Orthopaedic and Trauma Nursing* 30: 39–43.

Meerabeau, L. (1992). Tacit nursing knowledge: an untapped resource or a methodological headache? *Journal of Advanced Nursing* 17 (1): 108–112.

Munhall, P. (2012). *Nursing Research*. Jones & Bartlett Learning.

NHS Executive (1998). *Information for Health: An Information Strategy for the Modern NHS 1998–2005*. London: Department of Health.

Pearson, A., Jordan, Z., and Munn, Z. (2012). Translational science and evidence-based healthcare: a clarification and reconceptualization of how knowledge is generated and used in healthcare. *Nursing Research and Practice* 2012: 792519.

Powell, M. (1986). *Orthopaedic Nursing and Rehabilitation*. Edinburgh: Churchill Livingstone.

Rasmussen, P. and McLiesh, P. (2019). Understanding research: qualitative research in orthopaedic and trauma nursing. *International Journal of Orthopaedic and Trauma Nursing* 32: 41–47.

Rolfe, G. (1999). Insufficient evidence: the problems of evidence-based nursing. *Nurse Education Today* 19: 433–442.

Santy, J. and Temple, J. (2004). A critical review of two research papers on skeletal pin site care. *Journal of Orthopaedic Nursing* 8: 132–135.

Thompson, W. and McNamara, M. (2021). Constructing the advanced nurse practitioner identity in the healthcare system: a discourse analysis. *Journal of Advanced Nursing* https://doi.org/10.1111/jan.15068 (accessed 11 October 2021).

3

Professional Development, Competence and Education

Mary Drozd[1] and Sinead Hahessy[2]

[1] Aston University, Birmingham, UK
[2] National University of Ireland, Galway, Ireland

Introduction

The aim of this chapter is to discuss ongoing or continuing professional development (CPD) for orthopaedic and trauma nurses. Nursing is a constantly changing profession and engaging in CPD is a compulsory part of being a professional. Keeping up to date with research, and evidence-based or best practice, and acquiring new skills helps to facilitate an effective and safe contribution to patient care. Patients have a right to expect, at the very least, a practitioner who is competent in their sphere of practice. One existing competency framework (*Royal College of Nursing, Society of Orthopaedic and Trauma Nurses* 2019) will be discussed along with specialist orthopaedic and trauma nurse education, mentorship in orthopaedic and trauma nursing practice, social media and the role of reflection in CPD.

Continuing Professional Development

Literature detailing the relevance of CPD emerged in the 1980s and is mainly UK orientated (e.g. Charles 1982; Brown 1988). It focused on philosophical debates, underpinning frameworks, the relevance of continuing education and the challenges associated with implementation. Barribal et al. (1992) noted a lack of empirical data analysing nurses' perceptions of their continuing education needs. Further debates focused on what constituted an effective continuing professional education (CPE) system (Nolan et al. 1995) or the tensions between the 'luxury' or 'necessity' of the endeavour (Perry 1995). Nonetheless, CPE has developed at an accelerated pace. The pioneers of

educational change embraced the pursuit of 'new' knowledge through various curricular and pedagogical approaches. Concepts central to the professionalisation debate, such as pursuing the accumulation of a distinct body of knowledge through research activity and reflective practice, have emerged and remain as central tenets in nurse education. CPE in orthopaedic and trauma nursing strives to promote the specialist nature of knowledge and the majority of postgraduate/post-qualifying programmes are designed to address this. The 'artistic' forms of nursing knowledge such as intuition and experience are increasingly being accepted as valid forms of knowledge.

Continuing professional development (CPD) can be defined as 'the systematic maintenance, improvement and broadening of knowledge and skills, and the development of personal qualities necessary for the execution of professional, managerial and technical duties throughout one's working life' (Tomlinson 1993, p. 231). The broad-based function of CPD in healthcare is to ultimately improve patient outcomes (Cervero and Gaines 2015) but should also endeavour to sustain personal motivation, job satisfaction and commitment to the overall professional development of nursing (Hariyatia and Safril 2018). Activities to promote professional development can take the form of both informal and formal activity, and can help the practitioner to move beyond prescribed parameters of practice and develop expertise to further the body of knowledge in nursing.

Professional regulation is the hallmark of professions and ensures that standards are adhered to and that practice is maintained and developed (Munro 2008). Internationally, regulatory bodies require practitioners to meet specific standards for both practice and education. The purpose is to link professional development and the maintenance of competence to protect the public through safe practice. Nurses have a specific professional responsibility to engage with CPD (O'Shea 2008; Nursing and Midwifery Council 2019a) and employers need to recognise that their most valuable resource is their staff. Carlisle et al. (2011) have highlighted the organisational benefits of providing effective and tailored CPD which can directly benefit issues with staff turnover. The current landscape of increasing nursing vacancies and problems with staff retention in the UK National Health Service (NHS) has long been a subject of discussion where an emphasis has been placed on an urgent focus on productivity and investment in the workforce as a means of retaining and investing in staff (Buchan et al. 2019).

However, it is often learning and development opportunities that are sacrificed in financially constrained healthcare environments and continue to be affected by a lack of funding. Detailing staffing trends, Buchan et al. (2019, p. 6) have noted there has been a continued lack of investment in CPD for NHS staff in the UK. Extraneous barriers also exist and have been identified in the literature to include financial issues, workload demands, work schedules, anxiety, the learning climate, support for learning and lack of job satisfaction (Cooley 2008). These factors continue to impede engagement in CPD. In a meta-synthesis Mlambo et al. (2021) thematically present the complex nature of engagement in CPD that offers a detailed representation of the concept. They argue that organisational culture and commitment need to be supportive of staff, that organisations need to focus on incremental and constant development of practice, and that flexibility regarding work schedules to facilitate staff to participate in CPD are important (Mlambo et al. 2021, p. 8). The rapid growth in online CPD in nursing may help to alleviate some of the challenges identified regarding restraints, but it is partly dependant on the information technology competence of staff to be successful.

The employer has an important role in facilitating and encouraging CPD, and in investing in staff to ensure that professional learning occurs in the workplace alongside development of the organisation (Gopee 2002). There is an expectation that individuals will contribute to their own learning and that of others because of the perceived benefit to the individual and the team's professional growth, future employability and ability to perform their current role effectively. Modernisation agendas for health services include the development of a culture of learning that enables staff to progress and develop. CPD is often an obligatory element of this that values evidence of personal development and this is achieved in various ways.

The focus of CPD has moved towards evaluating the impact of post-registration programmes from the perspectives of the student and the impact learning has on clinical practice and patient outcomes, although there is a paucity of research in relation to the latter. A review of the CPD literature (Hegarty et al. 2008) concludes that patient outcomes are neglected in 61 studies and they advise that future research endeavours should aim to include patient outcomes. Gijbels et al.'s (2010) systematic review focused on the student perspective and concluded that nurses welcomed the effects that CPD has on professional and career trajectories. There is little research that has addressed the impact of orthopaedic and trauma CPD from either the student perspective or as measurement of patient outcomes as a consequence of CPD (see Box 3.1 for factors that optimise the impact of CPD in nursing).

Mentors

Literature from a wide range of disciplines refers to the use of mentoring to assist career development. This is practiced differently in particular locations, settings and healthcare professions. Mentors are crucial in facilitating the development of other practitioners as they assist the next generation in developing skills and accumulating knowledge. In the UK, the Nursing and Midwifery Council (2018a,b) introduced new standards of proficiency for nurses and midwives and replaced the term 'mentor' with 'practice assessor' and 'practice supervisor' (Nursing and Midwifery Council 2018a,b; Feeney and Everett 2020).

Mentorship roles are aligned to the context of clinical leadership, which as a concept has evolved as a central focus of ensuring the professional development of nursing (Stanley 2012; Daly et al. 2014). The importance of the clinical leadership aspect of the mentor's role is identified by nursing students as being a valuable mechanism for bridging the theory practice gap (Démeh and Rosengren 2015). To this end a mentor must have a sound evidence-based knowledge and skill base along with an understanding of how individuals learn and grow professionally to be able to nurture practitioner development (Gopee 2018). Mlambo et al. (2021) have highlighted the importance of emphasising the connection of CPD initiatives to patient care and that staff are more likely to engage with CPD where this is apparent. This is important in the context of the role of mentorship. At the point of socialisation to the orthopaedic and trauma environment the mentor can help to instil values associated with life-long learning and professional development in the specialty by relating a sense of partnership (Ali and Panther 2008) and professional identity in which the student or practitioner feels assimilated into the clinical setting.

Box 3.1   Evidence Digest: Factors that Optimise the Impact of Continuing Professional Development in Nursing: A Rapid Evidence Review (King et al. 2021)

Continuing professional development is essential for healthcare professionals to maintain and acquire the necessary knowledge and skills to provide person-centred, safe and effective care. This is particularly important in the rapidly changing healthcare context of the Covid-19 pandemic. Despite recognition of its importance in the UK, minimum required hours for re-registration and related investment have been small compared to other countries. The aim of this review is to understand the factors that optimise CPD impact for learning, development and improvement in the workplace.

Design

A rapid evidence review was undertaken using Arksey and O'Malley's (2005) framework: identifying a research question, developing a search strategy, extracting, collating and summarising the findings.

Review Methods

In addressing the question 'What are the factors that enable or optimise CPD impact for learning, development and improvement in the workplace at the individual, team, organisation and system level?', the British Nursing Index, the Cochrane Library, the Cumulative Index to Nursing and Allied Health Literature, the Health Technology Assessment database, the King's Fund Library and Medline databases were searched for key terms. A total of 3790 papers were retrieved and 39 were included.

Results

Key factors to optimise the impact of nursing and inter-professional continuing development are self-motivation, relevance to practice, preference for workplace learning, strong enabling leadership and a positive workplace culture. The findings reveal the interdependence of these important factors in optimising the impact of CPD on person-centred care and outcomes.

Conclusion

In the current, rapidly changing healthcare context it is important for educators and managers to understand the factors that enhance the impact of CPD. It is crucial that attention is given to addressing all of the optimising factors in this review to enhance impact.

Mentors provide a spectrum of learning and supportive behaviours such as challenging and being a critical friend, being a role model, helping to build networks and develop resourcefulness, simply being there to listen, helping people work out what they want to achieve and planning how they will bring change about (Clutterbuck 2004). Price (2004) suggests that a mentor will be in a position to shape other nurses' understanding of practice and practice wisdom for years to come. The specialist knowledge and skills, such as post-operative orthopaedic care, the prevention and recognition of complications or the application of traction, are best learned in the practice setting. Great responsibility for this is placed on mentors even though resources are finite and mentors must juggle the delivery of care with their teaching and supportive roles (Price 2004). No other role in nursing has such power to shape other nurses' practice and knowledge, and nothing can be more important than passing on clinical skills and knowledge to others while caring for patients and their families (Price 2004). A system of mentorship is essential in enabling the less experienced practitioner to be supported in specialist knowledge and skill development, and such a mentor should aim to provide leadership in developing learning (Gopee 2018).

Competence

Competence has become a defining feature of practice-based professions (Bradshaw 2000). Axley (2008, p. 217) argued that 'there is no officially agreed upon theoretical or operational definition of competency among nurses, educators, employers, regulating bodies, government and patients' and that the attributes of 'competency' are multi-faceted and context-dependent, which can lead to confusion. Pijl-Zieber et al. (2014, p. 677) have discussed the complexity of understanding that exists amongst key stakeholders (i.e. educators, practitioners and students) regarding competency in nursing. They argue that student nurses may feel underprepared to enter the clinical environment if competence in clinical skills is not adequately addressed in their educational programmes, and they question the emphasis placed on the development of generic skills in nurse education at the expense of clinical competency. Pijl-Zieber et al. (2014) call for a consistent approach to competency assessment in nurse education.

The aspects of competence most frequently cited are:

a) knowledge (information, teaching, training)
b) actions (ability, skill)

c) professional standards (criteria, requirements, qualification)
d) internal regulation (accountability, attitude, autonomy)
e) dynamic state (ongoing change, consistent improvement).

Competence is not fixed or static but part of the development of expertise and an intrinsic aspect of professional practice (Eraut 1994). It is concerned not only with skill acquisition and application but also with the development of knowledge to support assessment and decision making (Proctor-Childs 2011). Other professional qualities such as attitude, motives, personal insight, interpretative ability, maturity and self-assessment should be included (Axley 2008).

It is essential that clinical decision making is examined (Hagbaghery et al. 2004) and understood by orthopaedic and trauma nurses to ensure critical analysis is applied to the decision-making process, as this enhances competency development. There are two broad philosophical approaches that support clinical decision making as identified by Krishnan (2018). These are the analytical model (sometimes referred to as the systematic-positivist model) and the intuitive model (sometimes referred to as the intuitive-humanist model). Orthopaedic and trauma nurses employ components of these approaches to clinical decision making concurrently in respective patient encounters. The analytical model refers to the process of, for example, collecting patient data in the form of vital signs or completing a fall risk assessment tool and is based solely on an objective mindset to the task in hand. Conversely, in the intuitive model the driving force is the individual (the nurse) and the experience they bring to the situation (Benner 1984) and this approach encompasses the subjective view of the patient. This means, for example, when making a decision about care the nurse would take into consideration the holistic human and cultural context of the individual patient and how these elements would influence the care trajectory. As Krishnan (2018, p. 75) notes 'when the nurse becomes experienced, he or she observes the patterns and themes and can quickly differentiate between relevant and irrelevant information'.

Patients with orthopaedic conditions or traumatic injuries require specialist knowledge and skills which develop over time and via various strategies that will be discussed later. Benner (1984) highlights that a nurse who was expert in coronary care found it difficult to perform even at the competent level on an intermediate care surgical unit supporting clinical specialisation and a structure of clinical preceptors or mentors to teach the beginning nurse or the experienced nurse who transfers to a new unit.

Orthopaedic and Trauma Practitioner Competences

Contemporary healthcare requires efficiency and competence. The Royal College of Nursing (RCN) Society of Orthopaedic and Trauma Nurses (SOTN) in the UK has provided an example of specialist competences for orthopaedic and trauma practitioners (RCN Society of Orthopaedic and Trauma Nurses 2019). The benefit of a competency framework is that it provides a foundation on which to develop and evaluate safe and effective practitioners. The framework aims to provide a solid foundation to optimise evidence-based practice and provide safe and competent care.

Orthopaedic and trauma practitioner competences highlight the specialist nature of orthopaedic and trauma practice, and provide clarity for organisations regarding what they can expect from orthopaedic and trauma practitioners. They can also be used as benchmarks for organisations to use in recruitment, selection, development, appraisal and individual performance management as well as to contribute to the CPD of practitioners. The specialist orthopaedic and trauma practitioner domains within the RCN framework include those described in the following sections (RCN Society of Orthopaedic and Trauma Nurses 2019).

Partner/Guide

The unique partnership between the patient and the healthcare professional encompasses the importance of guiding the patient on their journey within orthopaedic and trauma healthcare. Supporting the patient and ensuring they are at the centre of their care is essential, as is working in partnership with the patient's family/informal carers along with liaison and collaboration with all members of the multiprofessional team (MPT) to ensure seamless, holistic care.

Comfort Enhancer

Comfort is a concept which is fundamental to the care of the orthopaedic/trauma patient. It is a complex human experience that can be interpreted in different ways. It is closely related to the experience of pain, especially for patients who have received an assault to musculoskeletal tissue (Cohen 2009). The comfort of orthopaedic/trauma patients is central to good healthcare outcomes. This aspect of care may become more complex for the patient depending on the nature of their condition, injury or surgery. Musculoskeletal instability and movement can result in significant pain and discomfort. Competence in providing essential care within this context is therefore central to high-quality care and highlights the need for that care to be provided in a specialist setting where practitioners possess the requisite specialist competence (Santy et al. 2005; Drozd et al. 2007).

Risk Manager

One of the central aspects of orthopaedic and trauma practice is the fact that orthopaedic and trauma surgery and injuries may carry with them a high risk of complications. The range of complications varies from those which are common to all situations where there is immobility and/or an assault to body tissues. However, there are a number of complications which are specific to trauma and orthopaedic patients such as compartment syndrome, fat embolism, osteomyelitis, neurovascular impairment, venous thrombo-embolism and complex regional pain syndrome. The nature of these complications requires highly specialised care.

Technician

The highly technical aspects of orthopaedic and trauma practice require knowledge, understanding and skill in managing, for example, specialised devices and equipment which are used to either treat orthopaedic conditions and injuries or to protect patients from complications. The practitioner needs to be competent in managing such treatment modalities, which are highly specialised and carry their own risk of complications (linked to the risk management domain). Some practitioners develop enhanced expertise in specific aspects. For example, while many practitioners care for patients with casts, additional expertise is required for the application of casts. In turn, these highly skilled and educated practitioners require focused, in-depth training and education. Appropriate education, training and development of practitioners is essential in ensuring that the right level of practitioner, with the requisite knowledge, understanding and skills is caring for orthopaedic and trauma patients. Maintaining the currency of such specialist skills is imperative for safe and effective care. For example, traction is now used less extensively for adults and such competences may require regular updating.

Although these domains relate directly to UK practice, there is scope for transferability internationally.

There are various strategies for achieving ongoing professional development within orthopaedic and trauma nursing, such as:

- self-study by engaging with current evidence-based material (see Chapter 2)
- seeking learning opportunities in the workplace

- supervised practice by experienced mentors/practice supervisors and practice assessors
- coaching/mentoring others
- case studies
- viva voce
- objective structured clinical examinations
- oral and/or written reflections about care
- critical incident analysis
- reflecting on practice
- self and peer assessments
- undertaking clinical audit
- formal appraisals with line managers
- in-house courses and study programmes
- accredited university programmes
- learning through electronic means such as online applications and other mobile media with instant access to evidence-based information
- professional portfolios containing evidence of learning and development.

Learning can also occur through personal experience, for example from personal family experiences that can be transferred to the work context (Munro 2008). There should be a forum for discussion of clinical practice in which nursing knowledge is coherently charted and explored (Benner 1984). Careful record keeping and sharing of paradigm cases are important strategies for documenting the significance of nursing practice. Teaching rounds/master classes by expert nurses open vistas to other nurses while recognising the value of expertise and its importance in transmitting wisdom and judgement.

Social Media

Social media describes the online and mobile tools that people use to share opinions, information, experiences, images and video or audio clips, and includes websites and applications used for social networking (International Council of Nurses 2015). Common sources of social media include social networking sites such as Facebook and LinkedIn, blogs and microblogs such as Twitter, content-sharing websites such as YouTube and Instagram as well as discussion forums and message boards.

The use of social media by nurses can help them to stay abreast of recent healthcare developments, enrich practice and provide a dialogue with the professional community and the public (International Council of Nurses 2015). However, it is important that nurses understand their professional responsibilities regarding its use (Barry and Hardiker 2012; Nursing and Midwifery Council 2018c, 2019b). Nurses must understand the benefits and risks of using social media both inside and outside the workplace. The professional, ethical, regulatory and legal issues associated with the use of social media have to be considered and addressed by nurses, healthcare provider organisations, educational institutions, professional associations and regulators. The Nursing and Midwifery Council (2019b) has produced guidance related to the use of social media, which is underpinned by The Code (Nursing and Midwifery Council 2018c) and covers the need to use social media and social networking sites responsibly.

Reflection

An essential aspect of professional development is to undertake structured, facilitated reflection as a central component of CPD (Bolton and Delderfield 2018) to explore practice and competence, although CPD does not guarantee competence. Lillyman (2011) believes that reflection is a strategy that helps the practitioner to link evidence-based theory with current practice. Alongside this, reflective learning involves actively thinking about and learning from experience. Moloney and Hahessy (2006, p. 50) state that:

> for educational development to happen the reflective nurse must see knowledge attainment as part of a developmental cycle where new knowledge is mixed with existing knowledge and practice, in order for a change in practice to occur

This is in accordance with Schon's (1987) notion of integrating formal and espoused theory to develop personal knowledge.

The majority of reflective models suggest three main stages: awareness, critical analysis and the development of new perspectives (Freshwater et al. 2008). Effective reflection requires a supportive and reflective culture, and is a process that all individuals can use to develop professionally and maintain professional accreditation as part of their involvement in daily care delivery (Lillyman 2011). Learning can change attitudes as well as challenge habitual or outdated practices and is often stimulating and rewarding, but can also be associated with a degree of discomfort as existing knowledge is tested and attitudes challenged (Pross 2005).

Dubé and Ducharme (2015) suggest a combination of verbal and written practice as the most beneficial approach for capturing learning in reflection. However, verbal reflective practice is viewed as less onerous. This has implications for reflective practice in the complex and busy orthopaedic and trauma environment. The importance of the mentor's role in the clinical setting is emphasised here, where a continuous and consistent awareness of the potential for reflective learning can be reinforced in all nurse/patient encounters.

Education

Pre-registration nurse education and training programmes may cover limited aspects of orthopaedic and trauma nursing, and aspects of orthopaedic and trauma nursing may be wrongly subsumed under the surgical nursing specialty without the recognition of this as a separate specialism. Orthopaedic and trauma practitioners require specific, specialist knowledge and skills at different levels of practice (Clarke 2003; Santy et al. 2005; Royal College of Nursing 2005; Lucas 2006; Flynn and Whitehead 2006; Drozd et al. 2007; RCN Society of Orthopaedic and Trauma Nurses 2019). An assumption is often made that post-qualifying/graduate nurses who undertake further academic courses relating to orthopaedic and trauma nursing will have an appreciation of the basic anatomy and physiology of the musculoskeletal system. This is often unsubstantiated and basic anatomy and physiology need to be revisited early in post-qualifying orthopaedic and trauma nursing courses to build on this underpinning basic knowledge.

One way that nurses can achieve personal and professional growth is by learning through formal defined education programmes (Munro 2008) at postgraduate level, but learning can also be nonaccredited workplace learning. It is vital that the evidence of this ongoing learning and development is documented by practitioners. This can be done by keeping a CPD portfolio to provide evidence of competency development and as Farrell (2008 cited in Timmins 2008, p. 24) argues can function to move beyond the parameters of professional development to incorporate the personal dimension, thus linking professional and personal growth. Further education can lead to opportunities for advancing role development, but there is a lack of standardisation of orthopaedic and trauma nursing education in many countries.

Summary

It is essential that practitioners are enabled to provide the highest quality effective orthopaedic and trauma patient care, and professional development should be an ongoing and integrated activity. Practitioners must recognise and seize opportunities for professional development. Ongoing learning and role development are essential for the dramatic changes practitioners experience, but educators also have a significant responsibility to maintain links with the clinical environment to ensure that they remain cognisant of clinical developments along with appropriate pedagogical approaches. Meskell et al. (2009, p. 789) have argued that:

> lecturers must demonstrate a value for the practice component of the role and the maintenance of clinical credibility appears to be crucial in order to address the theory-practice divide and preserve the right to continue teaching nurses

Various strategies for accessing ongoing professional development have been discussed along with active engagement in reflection and the consistent support and challenge from current mentors in practice. Excellence in orthopaedic and trauma nursing practice is the aim of CPD. Registered nurses have a code of conduct and statutory requirements for maintaining registration that necessitate CPD. Other practitioners in orthopaedic and trauma settings must also keep updated and continue to develop both personally and professionally.

Orthopaedic and trauma nursing will continue to evolve and encouragement is needed to pursue lines of inquiry and raise research questions from clinical knowledge and practice for the benefit of patients. It is clear that further research is required into the effects and outcomes of CPD on patient care in clinical practice.

Further Reading

Bolton, G. and Delderfield, R. (2018). *Reflective Practice: Writing and Professional Development*, 5e. London: Sage.

Lobo, C., Paul, R., and Crozier, K. (2021). *Collaborative Learning in Practice. Coaching to Support Student Learners in Healthcare*. Oxford: Wiley Blackwell.

Lawson, S. and Hearle, D. (2020). *A Strategic Guide to Continuing Professional Development for Health and Care Professionals: The TRAMm Model*, 2e. Cumbria: M&K Publishing.

McIntosh, A., Gidman, J., and Mason-Whitehead, E. (ed.) (2011). *Key Concepts in Healthcare Education*. London: Sage.

Royal College of Nursing, Society of Orthopaedic and Trauma Nurses (2019) *A Competence Framework for Orthopaedic and Trauma Practitioners*. Royal College of Nursing, London.

Royal College of Nursing (2018) *Improving Continuing Professional Development: How reps can make a difference in the workplace*. Royal College of Nursing, London.

Royal College of Nursing (2018). *Investing in a Safe and Effective Workforce. Continuing professional development for nurses in the UK*. Royal College of Nursing, London.

References

Ali, P.A. and Panther, W. (2008). Professional development and the role of mentorship. *Nursing Standard* 22 (42): 35–39.

Arksey, H. and O'Malley, L. (2005). Scoping studies: towards a methodological framework. *International Journal of Social Research Methodology* 8 (1): 19–32.

Axley, L. (2008). Competency: a concept analysis. *Nursing Forum* 43 (4): 214–222.

Barribal, K.L., While, A.E., and Norman, I.J. (1992). Continuing professional education for registered nurses: a review of the literature. *Journal of Advanced Nursing* 17: 1129–1140.

Barry, J. and Hardiker, N. (2012). Advancing nursing practice through social media: a global perspective. *The Online Journal of Issues in Nursing* 17 (3): Manuscript 5.

Benner, P. (1984). *From Novice to Expert. Excellence and Power in Clinical Nursing Practice*. New Jersey: Prentice Hall.

Bolton, G. and Delderfield, R. (2018). *Reflective Practice: Writing and Professional Development*, 5e. London: Sage.

Bradshaw, A. (2000). Competence and British nursing: a view from history. *Journal of Clinical Nursing* 9: 321–329.

Brown, L.A. (1988). Maintaining professional practice: Is continuing education a cure or merely a tonic? *Nurse Education Today* 8: 251–257.

Buchan, J., Charlesworth, A., Gershlick, B. and Seccombe, I. (2019) A critical moment: NHS staffing trends, retention and attrition. Health Foundation. www.health.org.uk. (accessed 19 May 2021).

Carlisle, J., Bhanugopan, R., and Fish, A. (2011). Training needs of nurses in public hospitals in Australia review of current practices and future research agenda. *Journal of European Industrial Training* 35 (7): 687–701. https://doi.org/10.1108/03090591111160797 (accessed 19 May 2021).

Cervero, R. and Gaines, J. (2015). The impact of CME on physician performance and patient health outcomes: an updated synthesis of systematic reviews. *Journal of Continuing Education in the Health Professions* 35 (2): 131–138. https://doi.org/10.1002/chp.21290 (accessed 19 May 2021).

Charles, M. (1982). Continuing education in nursing: whose responsibility? *Nurse Education Today* 2: 5–11.

Clarke, S. (2003). A definitional analysis of specialist practice in orthopaedic nursing. *Journal of Orthopaedic Nursing* 7 (2): 82–86.

Clutterbuck, D. (2004). *Everyone Needs a Mentor*. London: Chartered Institute of Personnel and Development.

Cohen, S. (2009). Orthopaedic patient's perceptions of using a bed pan. *Journal of Orthopaedic Nursing* 13 (2): 78–84.

Cooley, M.C. (2008). Nurses' motivations for studying third level post-registration programmes and the effects of studying on their personal and work lives. *Nurse Education Today* 28 (5): 588–594.

Daly, J., Jackson, D., Mannix, J. et al. (2014). The importance of clinical leadership in the hospital setting. *Journal of Healthcare Leadership* https://www.dovepress.com/getfile.php?fileID=22523 (accessed 20 May 2021).

Démeh, W. and Rosengren, K. (2015). The visualisation of clinical leadership in the content of nursing education – a qualitative study of nursing students' experiences. *Nurse Education Today* 35: 888–893.

Drozd, M., Jester, R., and Santy, J. (2007). The inherent components of the orthopaedic nursing role: an exploratory study. *Journal of Orthopaedic Nursing* 11 (1): 43–52.

Dubé, V. and Ducharme, F. (2015). Nursing reflective practice: An empirical literature review. *Journal of Nursing Education and Practice* 5 (7): 91–99.

Eraut, M. (1994). *Developing Professional Knowledge and Competence*. London: The Falmer Press.

Farrell, M. (2008). The Purpose of Portfolios, Chapter 2. In: *Making Sense of Portfolios: A Guide for Nursing Students* (ed. F. Timmins). Berkshire: McGraw Hill/Open University Press.

Feeney, A. and Everett, S. (2020). *Understanding Supervision and Assessment in Nursing*. London: Sage Publications.

Flynn, S. and Whitehead, E. (2006). An exploration of issues related to nurse led clinics. *Journal of Orthopaedic Nursing* 10 (2): 86–94.

Freshwater, D., Taylor, B.J., and Sherwood, G. (2008). *International Textbook of Reflective Practice in Nursing*. Oxford: Wiley Blackwell.

Gijbels, H., O'Connell, R., Dalton-O'Connor, C., and O'Donovan, M. (2010). A systematic review evaluating the impact of post registration nursing and midwifery education on practice. *Nurse Education in Practice* 10 (1): 64–69.

Gopee, N. (2002). Human and social capital as facilitators of lifelong learning in nursing. *Nurse Education Today* 22 (8): 608–616.

Gopee, N. (2018). *Supervision and Mentoring in Healthcare*, 4e. London: Sage.

Hagbaghery, M.A., Salsali, M., and Ahmadi, F. (2004). The factors facilitating and inhibiting effective clinical decision making in nursing: a qualitative study. *Biomed Central Open Access* http://www.biomedcentral.com/1472-6955/3/2 (accessed 4 October 2021).

Hariyatia, R.T.S. and Safril, S. (2018). The relationship between nurses' job satisfaction and continuing professional development. *Enfermería Clínica* 28 (Suppl. 1 Part A): 144–148. https://doi.org/10.1016/s1130-8621(18)30055-x (accessed 19 May 2021).

Hegarty, J., Mc Carthy, G., O'Sullivan, D., and Lehane, B. (2008). A review of nursing and midwifery education research in the Republic of Ireland. *Nurse Education Today* 28: 720–736.

International Council of Nurses (2015) *Nurses and Social Media*. ICN Postion paper. Adopted in 2015.

King, R., Taylor, B., Talpur, A. et al. (2021). Factors that optimise the impact of continuing professional development in nursing: a rapid evidence review. *Nurse Education Today* 98: https://doi.org/10.1016/j.nedt.2020.104652.

Krishnan, P. (2018). A philosophical analysis of clinical decision making in nursing. *Journal of Nursing Education* 57 (2): 73–78.

Lillyman, S. (2011). Reflection. In: *Key Concepts in Healthcare Education* (ed. A. McIntosh, J. Gidman and E. Mason-Whitehead), 156–161. London: Sage.

Lucas, B. (2006). Judgment and decision making in advanced orthopaedic nursing practice in relation to chronic knee pain. *Journal of Orthopaedic Nursing* 10 (4): 206–216.

Meskell, P., Murphy, K., and Shaw, D. (2009). The clinical role of lecturers in nursing in Ireland: perceptions from key stake-holder groups in nurse education on the role. *Nurse Education Today* 29: 784–790.

Mlambo, M., Silé, C., and McGrath, C. (2021). Lifelong learning and nurses' continuing professional development, a metasynthesis of the literature. *BMC Nursing* 20: 62.

Moloney, J. and Hahessy, S. (2006). Using reflection in everyday orthopaedic nursing practice. *Journal of Orthopaedic Nursing* 10: 49–55.

Munro, K.M. (2008). Continuing professional development and the charity paradigm: interrelated individual, collective and organisational issues about professional development. *Nurse Education Today* 28 (8): 953–961.

Nolan, M., Owens, R.G., and Nolan, J. (1995). Continuing professional education: identifying the characteristics of an effective system. *Journal of Advanced Nursing* 21: 551–560.

Nursing and Midwifery Council (2018a). *Standards Framework for Nursing and Midwifery Education*. London: Nursing and Midwifery Council.

Nursing and Midwifery Council (2018b). *Standards for Student Supervision and Assessment*. London: Nursing and Midwifery Council.

Nursing and Midwifery Council (2018c). *The Code. Professional Standards of Practice and Behaviour for Nurses, Midwives and Nursing Associates*. London: Nursing and Midwifery Council.

Nursing and Midwifery Council (2019a) *Revalidation. How to revalidate with the NMC. Requirements for renewing your registration.* how-to-revalidate-booklet.pdf, http://nmc.org.uk (accessed 1 October 2021).

Nursing and Midwifery Council (2019b). *Guidance on Using Social Media Responsibly*. London: Nursing and Midwifery Council.

O'Shea, Y. (2008). *Nursing and Midwifery in Ireland. A Strategy for Professional Development in a Changing Health Service*. Dublin: Blackhall Publishing.

Perry, L. (1995). Continuing professional education: luxury or necessity? *Journal of Advanced Nursing* 21: 766–771.

Pijl-Zieber, E.M., Barton, S., Konkin, J. et al. (2014). Competence and competency-based nursing education: finding our way through the issues. *Nurse Education Today* 34: 676–678.

Price, B. (2004). Mentoring: the key to clinical learning. *Nursing Standard* 18 (52): suppl.1–suppl.2.

Proctor-Childs, T. (2011). Clinical competence. In: *Key Concepts in Healthcare Education* (ed. A. McIntosh, J. Gidman and E. Mason-Whitehead), 17–22. London: Sage.

Pross, E. (2005). International nursing students: a phenomenological perspective. *Nurse Education Today* 25: 627–633.

Royal College of Nursing (2005). *Competencies: An Integrated Career and Competency Framework for Orthopaedic and Trauma Nursing*. London: Royal College of Nursing.

(2019). Royal College of Nursing, Society of Orthopaedic and Trauma Nurses. In: *A Competence Framework for Orthopaedic and Trauma Practitioners*. London: Royal College of Nursing.

Santy, J., Rogers, J., Davis, P. et al. (2005). A competency framework for orthopaedic and trauma nursing. *Journal of Orthopaedic Nursing* 9 (2): 81–86.

Schon, D.A. (1987). *Educating the Reflective Practitioner*. London: Temple Smith.

Stanley, D.J. (2012). Clinical leadership and innovation. *Journal of Nursing Education and Practice* 2 (2): 119–126.

Timmins, F. (2008). *Making Sense of Portfolios: A guide for nursing students*. Berkshire: McGraw Hill, Open University Press.

Tomlinson, H. (1993). Developing professionals. *Education* 182 (13): 231.

4

The Musculoskeletal System and Human Movement

Lynne Newton-Triggs[1] and Jean Rogers[2]

[1] *Bedford Hospital, Bedford, UK*
[2] *Open University, Milton Keynes, UK*

Introduction

The aim of this chapter is to provide an overview of musculoskeletal structure and function in relation to human movement. Structure and function are linked and it is impossible to discuss one without the other. It is essential that orthopaedic and trauma practitioners know and understand the terms used to describe anatomical positions and the structures involved in musculoskeletal conditions, injuries and surgery to facilitate safe, high-quality effective care. It is also essential to provide a common language that is effective in interdisciplinary communication as this ensures practitioners can explain specific conditions, injuries, surgery and treatment to other staff, patients and relatives to enable them to engage in their care.

Anatomical Positioning

The human body is described as being in anatomical position when the body is upright with the head facing forward, hands at the side facing forward with the thumbs pointing away from the body and the feet hip-width apart with the feet and toes pointing forward (Figure 4.1). This is a universally known position. When referring to the right and left of the body, this is the right and left of the person who is the subject of discussion (e.g. the patient) not the left and right of the observer.

The skeleton has two distinct sections: the axial skeleton consists of the skull bones, inner ear, ribs, vertebrae and sternum. It provides structural support, attachment points for ligaments and muscles, and protection for the brain, spinal cord and major organs of the chest. The appendicular skeleton consists of the pectoral girdle and the upper limbs, pelvic girdle and lower limbs that make movement possible and protect the organs of the pelvis.

Human movement is described in three dimensions (or planes) which divide the human body (Figure 4.2):

- The sagittal (vertical/median) plane lies vertically through the body dividing it into left and right parts.
- The coronal (frontal) plane lies vertically through the body dividing it into anterior and posterior parts.
- The transverse (horizontal) plane lies horizontally through the body dividing it into superior and inferior parts.

Anatomical Terminology and Movement

Anatomical directions and terminology assist practitioners to use a systematic approach to describing and orientating the human body. Box 4.1 gives the most commonly used terms.

Movement can be described in a variety of ways depending on where and how the movement occurs. Types of movement are often given in pairs describing opposite movements (see Box 4.2).

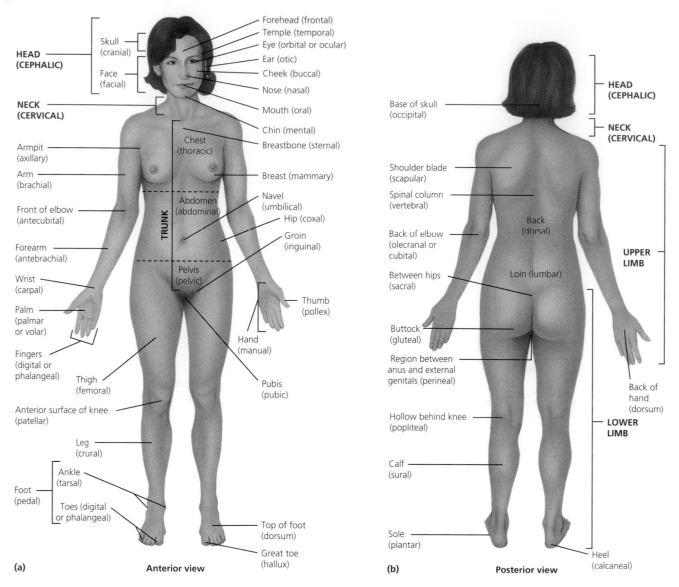

Figure 4.1 Anatomical position. *Source:* Tortora, G.J. and Derrickson, B.H., *Essentials of Anatomy and Physiology*, 2018, Wiley. Reproduced with permission of John Wiley & Sons.

The Skeleton

The skeleton is made of bone, cartilage and ligaments, which work in unison to allow movement. The skeleton is strong, light and flexible, representing about 20% of the total body weight, half of which is water. At birth, there are over 300 bones, some of which fuse later. Adults have approximately 206, varying slightly between individuals depending on small bone fusion during growth.

Bones are classified in many ways, with their shape and structure being governed by genetic, metabolic and mechanical factors (see Table 4.1).

Bone Physiology

Bone is a highly vascular tissue containing an intercellular substance surrounding widely separated cells. This dynamic tissue is continuously remodelled and features four characteristic types of cells (see Table 4.2).

Bone is made up mainly of collagen and mineral salts, principally calcium phosphate and some calcium carbonate with small amounts of magnesium hydroxide, fluoride and sulphate. These salts are deposited in a framework of collagen fibres which then calcify. Bone is not completely solid; it has some spaces between its hard components, providing channels for blood vessels and a lighter

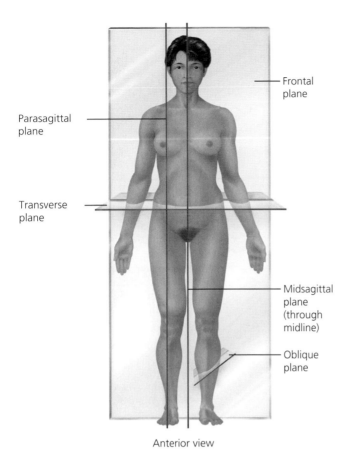

Parasagittal plane

Frontal plane

Transverse plane

Midsagittal plane (through midline)

Oblique plane

Anterior view

Figure 4.2 Planes of the body. *Source:* Tortora, G.J. and Derrickson, B.H., *Essentials of Anatomy and Physiology*, 2018, Wiley. Reproduced with permission of John Wiley & Sons.

Box 4.1   Common Anatomical Terms

- Anterior/ventral: towards the front of the body
- Deep: away from the surface of the body
- Distal: away from the body
- Inferior/caudal: away from the head or towards the lower part of the body
- Lateral: away from the midline of the body
- Medial: towards the midline of the body
- Midline: the centre line of the body when it is in the anatomical position
- Posterior/dorsal: towards the back of the body
- Proximal: closer to the trunk
- Superficial: close to the surface of the body
- Superior/cranial/cephalic: towards the head or upper part of the body
- Valgus: deviated away from the midline
- Varus: deviated towards the midline

Box 4.2   Terminology for Describing Movement

- Flexion: bending movement, the angle of the joint is decreased
- Extension: straightening movement, the angle of the joint is increased
- Pronation: rotation of the arm, the hand faces away from the anatomical position to face backwards
- Supination: rotation of the arm so the hand faces forwards
- Abduction: movement of the limb away from the midline
- Adduction: movement of the limb towards the midline
- Inversion: movement of the foot and ankle, leaving the sole of the foot facing towards the midline
- Eversion: movement of the foot and ankle, leaving the sole of the foot facing away from the midline
- Plantar flexion: the toes are pushed down away from the body
- Dorsiflexion: the toes are pushed up towards the body
- Rotation: rotation of a joint along the horizontal axis of the bone laterally or medially
- Protraction: movement forward in the transverse plane, e.g. biting the upper lip with the lower teeth
- Retraction: movement backwards in the transverse plane, e.g. moving the teeth back into position
- Elevation: motion of the limb upwards, e.g. shrugging the shoulders
- Depression: motion of the limb downwards, e.g. opening the jaw
  One term does not relate to a pair and is unique to the movement of the thumb:
- Opposition: moving of the thumb to the fingers or the palm for grasping objects

---

structure. Bone tissue can be categorised into compact or cancellous (spongy) depending on the size and distribution of the spaces.

Compact bone surrounds cancellous bone and is thicker in the diaphysis (shaft) than the epiphyses (ends). It provides support and protection, and helps long bones resist the stress of weight bearing. Adult compact bone has a concentric ring structure, with blood vessels and nerves traversing it from the periosteum through Volkmann's canals that connect with the blood vessels and nerves of the medullary cavity and the central Haversian canals. The Haversian canals run longitudinally through the bone and are surrounded by rings of hard calcified bone, concentric lamellae, between which are spaces called lacunae that contain osteocytes. Canaliculi radiate in all directions from the lacunae, forming an intricate network

---

Box 4.3   Functions of The Skeleton

- Support: framework for support of the body and maintaining its shape
- Movement: muscles, bones and joints provide the principal mechanics for movement, all coordinated by the nervous system
- Protection: encases and protects vital organs
- Blood cell production: haematopoietic stem cells (HSCs) in the medulla of the bone (bone marrow) give rise to all of the different mature blood cell types and tissues; this is a vital process in the body
- Storage: the matrix of bone stores calcium and the bone marrow stores iron
- Endocrine regulation: bone cells release the hormone osteocalcin, which contributes to the regulation of blood sugar and fat deposition

---

Table 4.1 Bone classifications.

Bone	Examples	Features
Long bones	Femur, tibia, humerus	Tubular in shape with a central shaft (diaphysis) which contains bone marrow
		Two extremities (epiphyses)
		Completely covered (except for joint surfaces) in periosteum
		The epiphyses contain epiphyseal cartilage/plates near each end of the bone which are active in growth and ossify when growth is completed in early adulthood
Short bones	Found in the wrist and ankle (carpals and tarsals)	Cuboid in shape
		No shaft
		Hard outer shell of compact bone
		Spongy (cancellous) bone in the centre
Flat bones	Cranium, scapula, pelvis, ribs	Hard compact bone outer casing with a soft cancellous bone centre
		Usually curved
Irregular bones	Bones of the face, vertebrae	Do not fit in other categories
Sesamoid bones	Patella, distal portion of first and second metacarpals, pisiform, first metatarsal	Embedded in tendons

Table 4.2 Bone tissue cell types.

Osteoprogenitor (osteogenic) cells	• Unspecialised cells derived from mesenchyme • With mitotic potential and the ability to differentiate into osteoblasts • Within the periosteum, endosteum, Haversian and Volkman's canals
Osteoblasts	• Have no mitotic potential • Involved in bone formation by secreting organic compounds and mineral salts • Found on the surface of bone
Osteocytes	• Maintain the daily cellular activities of bone • Have no mitotic potential and are osteoblasts that have become trapped within the bony intercellular substance that they have laid down
Osteoclasts	• Develop from circulating monocytes • Found around the surfaces of bone • Function is the resorption of bone which is important in the development, growth, maintenance and repair of bone

providing numerous routes for nutrients to reach the osteocytes and also for the removal of waste. Each central canal with the surrounding lamellae, lacunae, osteocytes and canaliculi is known as a Haversian system or osteon (see Figure 4.3).

Cancellous (spongy) bone consists of an irregular latticework of thin plates of bone called trabeculae within which lie lacunae containing osteocytes. The spaces between the trabeculae of some bones are filled with red marrow (responsible for red cell production). Blood vessels from the periosteum penetrate through to the cancellous bone.

Bone Growth and Development

The process of bone formation, ossification, begins in the embryo. The skeleton at this time is composed of fibrous membranes and hyaline cartilage shaped like bones and providing the medium for ossification. Ossification occurs in two ways:

- *Intramembranous ossification*: Osteoblasts cluster in a fibrous membrane, forming a centre of ossification, and secrete intercellular substances partly composed of collagenous fibres, forming a framework around which calcium salts are deposited (calcification). When the

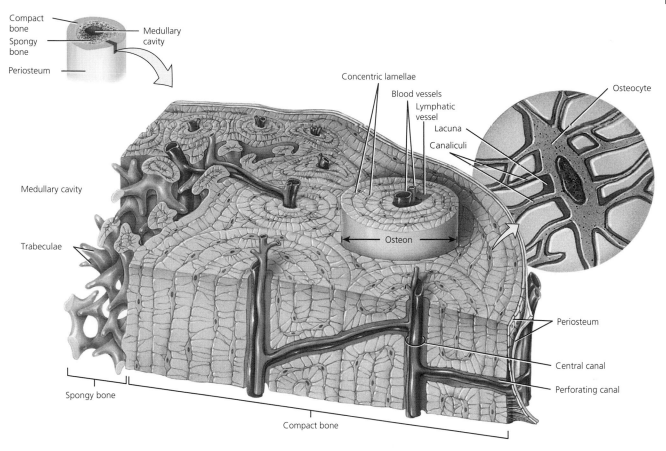

Figure 4.3 Haversian system (osteon). *Source:* Tortora, G.J. and Derrickson, B.H., *Essentials of Anatomy and Physiology*, 2018, Wiley. Reproduced with permission of John Wiley & Sons.

cluster of osteoblasts is completely surrounded by the calcified matrix, it is called a trabecula (plural trabeculae). Trabeculae radiate out from each centre of ossification into a framework. The original connective tissue becomes the periosteum and the ossified area becomes cancellous (spongy) bone with a covering of compact bone. Bone is continuously destroyed and reformed until it reaches its final adult size and shape.

- *Endochondral ossification* (the replacement of cartilage by bone): Most bones of the body are formed by this process. Early on in embryonic development a cartilage template of the future bone is laid down and covered by a membrane, the perichondrium. Midway along the shaft a blood vessel penetrates the perichondrium, stimulating osteoprogenitor cells within the perichondrium to enlarge and become osteoblasts. These cells then form osteocytes, which form a periosteal collar of compact bone around the middle of the diaphysis of the cartilage model. This then forms the membranous covering of bone known as the periosteum. At the primary centre of ossification, chondrocytes hypertrophy and the matrix becomes mineralised and spaces in the

shaft of the bone join together, forming the medullary cavity which then fills with bone marrow. Secondary centres of ossification form at the extremities of long bones in the epiphyses and lay down spongy bone. One secondary ossification centre develops in the proximal epiphysis soon after birth and the other centre develops in the distal epiphysis during a child's second year. After the two secondary ossification centres have formed, bone tissue completely replaces the cartilage except in these two regions: cartilage continues to cover the articular surfaces of the epiphyses as articular cartilage as well as in the region between the epiphysis and diaphysis (the epiphyseal plate), where lengthwise growth of bone continues into early adulthood.

Bones continue to grow in length and width following birth. Appositional growth is the growth in diameter of bone by the formation of new bone on the surface of existing bone. This occurs at the same time as growth in the length of bone. Bone lining the marrow cavity is destroyed by osteoclasts, allowing the cavity to increase in size, and at the same time osteoblasts from the periosteum produce new compact bone to cover the outer surface of the bone. The growth in length is known as endochondral growth, which takes place in the epiphyseal plates until their ossification. The cartilage in the epiphysis is replaced by bone from the shaft side and this is matched by the production of new cartilage from the epiphyseal plate. This process continues until early adulthood when hormones cause the cartilage in the epiphyseal plate to ossify.

Bone growth is influenced by:

- nutrition
- sunlight
- hormones
- exercise.

Bone is constantly remodelling and re-appropriating its matrix and minerals along lines of mechanical stress, allowing worn or damaged bone to be removed and replaced with new tissue. Bone also stores calcium and phosphorous. There is a delicate homeostasis maintained between the action of osteoclasts removing calcium and collagen from the bone and osteoblasts depositing calcium and collagen. If too much tissue or calcium is removed, the bones become weakened and break easily, leading to osteoporosis.

There are a number of other hormones involved in the metabolism of bone:

- vitamin D (calcitriol) regulates calcium and phosphorous levels, and the mineralisation of bone
- calcitonin inhibits the action of osteoclasts, thus inhibiting the removal of calcium from bone
- parathyroid hormone increases the number and activity of the osteoclasts which release calcium and phosphate from bones into blood
- oestrogens inhibit the activity of osteoclasts, protecting the bones from excessive bone turnover
- human growth hormone is responsible for the general growth of bones at the epiphyseal plates.

Skeletal Muscle

Skeletal muscle appears striated (striped) and has the fastest contraction rate under voluntary control of all muscles. It is controlled by the central and autonomic nervous system and provides force and power for movement. Muscles then contract and relax to bring about movement and perform three main functions:

1) movement (voluntary and reflex) through the actions of bones, joints and the skeletal muscles attached to the bones

2) maintenance of posture through the contraction of muscles to support the body in a stationary position

3) heat production: contraction produces most of the body's heat.

Skeletal muscles are composed of collections of striated muscle fibres and some connective tissues such as blood vessels and nerves. Deep fascia is a dense connective tissue that lines the body wall and extremities as well as holding muscles together and separating them into functioning groups. The entire muscle is wrapped with a fibrous connective tissue called the epimysium. Bundles of muscle fibres called fasciculi are covered by fibrous connective tissue known as perimysium and endomysium, fibrous connective tissue that penetrates into the interior of each fascicle and surrounds and separates the muscle fibres. Individual muscle fibres are long and cylindrical structures with multiple nuclei and their length and width vary depending on the function and purpose of each muscle. Each muscle fibre contains thousands of microscopic contractile units known as myofibrils that bring about contraction following electrical stimulation in a complex process of sliding filaments within the myofibrils.

Muscles are named according to their shape, location or a combination of both and according to function, e.g. flexion, extension or rotation.

Skeletal Muscle Attachment

Skeletal muscles produce movement by exerting force on tendons, which in turn pull on bones. When a muscle contracts it draws one articulating bone towards the other. The attachment of a muscle tendon to the stationary bone is called the *origin*. The attachment of the other muscle tendon to the moveable bone is known as *insertion*. Levers are created by the bones, and joints and tendons attach muscles to the bone and act on the skeleton by contracting and shortening or relaxing to allow two bones to move closer or move away.

Ligaments, Tendons and Cartilage

Ligaments, tendons and cartilage connect bones, joints and muscles, and guide and protect movement that has been initiated by muscles.

Ligaments and tendons are formed from regularly arranged dense connective tissue with strong parallel fibres that attach muscles to bone. Aponeoroses are the flattened sheet-like tendons which connect muscle to bone or muscle to muscle. Large fibrous sacs known as bursae protect some tendons such as those at the hip, knee and elbow.

Ligament elasticity allows stretch and stabilises the joint to ensure movement remains within its normal planes.

Dense irregular connective tissue forms cartilage. Fibres are arranged irregularly, allowing them to endure more stress than ligaments and tendons. There is no blood or nerve supply to cartilage and it has minimal ability to heal. There are two types of cartilage that relate to the skeletal system:

- hyaline cartilage is the most abundant type found at joints over the ends of the long bones as articular cartilage. It provides flexibility and support, absorbs shock and reduces friction.
- fibrocartilage allows greater resistance to compression and tension due to its fibrous structure. It can be found at the symphysis pubis, the intervertebral discs between vertebrae and the menisci of the knee.

Neurovascular Supply

Bone has a rich nerve and blood supply, supplying the nutrients for bone growth and muscle contraction and supporting biofeedback systems.

Bone has a rich blood supply from which it acquires nutrients required for growth, remodelling and repair. Large nutrient arteries enter bones through holes known as nutrient foramen into the diaphysis of the bone and then divide into the proximal and distal branches and supply the head of the bone. Blood vessels and capillaries divide from the nutrient artery and enter the central/Haversian canals to supply the compact bone. Perforating canals within the compact bone allow entry of the capillaries into the cancellous bone, supplying the nutrients required for bone cell and bone marrow activity. The central canal of long bones and central area of flat bones contain red marrow (haematopoietic tissue), which is responsible for the production of red blood cells.

Nerves are prolific throughout bone, allowing communication with the central nervous system and providing feedback as well as being responsible for some of the pain felt when there is bone disease or injury. Blood vessels and nerves run side by side and are most prolific in the ends of long bones, where they provide autonomic feedback/proprioception from the joints.

Joints

Bones are held together at joints by flexible connective tissue, where all movement takes place. The structure of the joint determines how it functions. Some joints permit no movement, whilst others permit slight or considerable movement. The structural classification of joints is based on whether there is a synovial cavity and the type of connective tissue that binds the bones together. Structurally joints are classified as:

- *Fibrous joints* lack a synovial cavity and the articulating bones fit very closely together. There is little or no movement. There are three types:
  - Sutures lie between the bones of the skull. The bones are united by a thin layer of dense fibrous connective tissue. The irregular structure of sutures gives added strength and decreases the chance of fracture. Some sutures present during growth are replaced by bone in the adult and these are called synostoses.
  - Syndesmosis is a fibrous joint where the fibrous connective tissue is present in a greater amount than in a suture but the fit between the bones is not quite as tight. The fibrous connective tissue forms an interosseous membrane or ligament. The syndesmosis is slightly moveable because the bones are separated more than in a suture and some flexibility is permitted by the interosseous membrane, e.g. the talofibular joint.
  - Gomphosis is a type of fibrous joint where a cone-shaped peg fits into a socket, e.g. the articulation of the roots of teeth with the sockets.
- *Cartilagenous joints* have no synovial cavity and articulating bones are tightly connected by cartilage, allowing little or no movement. There are two types:
  - Synchondrosis: the connecting tissue is hyaline cartilage. The most common type is the epiphyseal plate found between the epiphysis and diaphysis of a growing bone. The joint is eventually replaced by bone when growth ceases, synostosis, e.g. the joint between the first rib and the sternum.
  - Symphysis: a cartilaginous joint in which the connecting material is a broad flat disc of fibrocartilage, e.g. between the bodies of the vertebrae and the symphysis pubis. These joints are slightly moveable, amphiarthrotic.
- *Synovial joints* are the most common joints. They have a space known as the synovial cavity between the articulating bones and are freely moveable. Synovial joints have five main features:
  - Joint cavity: the space between articulating bones providing the space for movement.
  - Articular cartilage: covers the surfaces of the articulating bones and is formed of hyaline cartilage. Prevents friction and absorbs shock.
  - Articular capsule: synovial joints are surrounded by a sleeve-like structure enclosing the synovial cavity and uniting the articulating bones. It is composed of two layers, the fibrous capsule and the synovial membrane. The fibrous capsule consists of dense connective tissue and is attached to the periosteum at a

variable distance from the edge of the articular cartilage. The flexibility of the fibrous capsule allows for movement at the joint while its tensile strength resists dislocation.

- Synovial membrane is the inner layer of the articular capsule and covers all surfaces of the joint not already covered by articular cartilage. It is composed of loose connective tissue and secretes synovial fluid.
- Synovial fluid is secreted by the synovial membrane, fills the joint cavity, lubricates the joint, provides nourishment for the articular cartilage, reduces friction, supplies nutrients and removes metabolic wastes from the cells of the articular cartilage. Synovial fluid contains phagocytic cells, which remove microbes and debris from wear and tear in the joint.

Synovial joints are further classified by their movement and the structures of the articulating bones:

- Hinge joint: the convex surface of one bone fits into the concave surface of another bone. The movement is in a single plane and is similar to that of a hinged door, e.g. the knee, elbow and interphalangeal joints where the movement allowed is flexion and extension.
- Ball and socket joint: a ball-like surface of one bone fits into a cuplike depression of another bone, allowing movement in three planes: flexion/extension, abduction/adduction and rotation/circumduction, e.g. the shoulder joint and hip joint. The stability of the joint depends on how deep the socket is and the fit of the ball within the socket.
- Plane joint (gliding): the articulating surfaces glide against each other in one plane only and are usually flat, allowing only limited movement, e.g. the joints between the carpal bones, tarsal bones and the sternum and clavicle.
- Pivot joint: the conical surface of one bone articulates within a ring formed partly by another bone and a ligament, allowing rotation, e.g. the joint between the atlas and axis allowing rotation of the head.
- Condyloid joint: an oval-shaped condyle of one bone fits into an elliptical cavity of another bone, allowing side to side and back and forth movements and allowing flexion/extension, abduction/adduction and circumduction, e.g. the joint at the wrist between the radius and carpals.
- Saddle joint: the articular surface of one bone is saddle shaped and the other articular surface is shaped like a rider sitting in the saddle, a modified condyloid joint with freer movement. Movements are side to side and back and forth, e.g. the joint between the trapezium and the metacarpal of the thumb. Figure 4.4 illustrates the different types of synovial joints.

The Cranium (the Skull)

The bony skeleton of the head (cranium) supports the structure of the face and forms a cavity for the brain. It is thin, light and solid, and is usually described via the eight bones that make it up (Table 4.3), sometimes referred to as the neurocranium. The inner surfaces attach to membranes that position and stabilise the brain, blood vessels and nerves. The outer surfaces act as an attachment for muscles so the head can move in various ways.

The cranium is proportionally more developed at birth and grows more quickly during the first years of life than the rest of the skeleton. To allow flexion so that childbirth can take place, the bones of the cranium at birth are connected by non-ossified membranous regions (fontanelles). Ossification closes the fontanelles usually by a child's second birthday. Where the bones meet they become connected to each other by immobile solid fibrous articulations called cranial sutures.

The cranium has four main functions:

- protection of the brain
- contains and supports the eyes and the face
- fixes the distance between the eyes to allow stereoscopic vision
- fixes the ears into position to help the brain use auditory cues to judge direction and distance of sounds.

There are 14 facial bones, which hold the eyes in place and form the facial features. The face is sometimes referred to as the splanchnocranium and makes the cranium into the skull. These bones meet with the cranial bones to give each face a unique individual form.

The hyoid bone is one further bone. It stands alone and is located in the neck below the tongue. It is held in place by the ligaments and muscles of the styloid process of the temporal bone.

The Spine

The vertebral column (the backbone or spine) extends from the base of the skull to the pelvis and has five distinct regions:

- cervical spine (seven vertebrae) is the neck, and supports the head and allows for nodding and shaking the head
- thoracic spine (12 vertebrae) attaches the ribs
- lumbar spine (five vertebrae) forms the lower back, carrying most of the weight of the upper body and providing a stable centre of gravity
- sacrum (five fused vertebrae) makes up the posterior wall of the pelvis
- coccyx (four small fused bones) sits at the base of the spine.

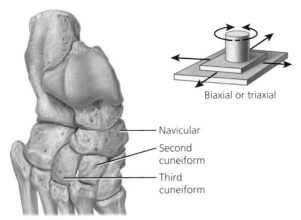

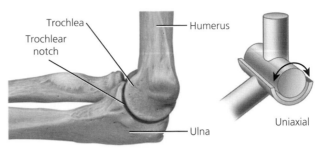

(a) Plane joint between navicular and second and third cuneiforms of tarsus in foot

(b) Hinge joint between trochlea of humerus and trochlear notch of ulna at the elbow

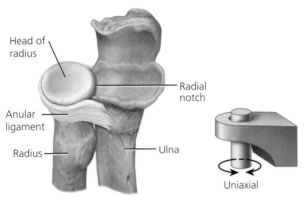

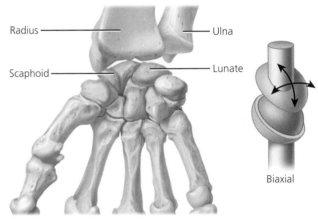

(c) Pivot joint between head of radius and radial notch of ulna

(d) Condyloid joint between radius and scaphoid and lunate bones of carpus (wrist)

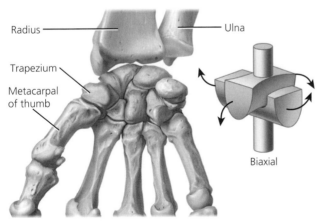

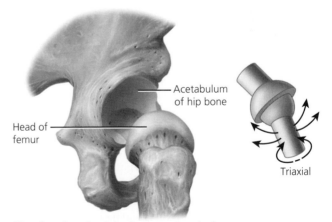

(e) Saddle joint between trapezium of carpus (wrist) and metacarpal of thumb

(f) Ball-and-socket joint between head of femur and acetabulum of hip bone

Figure 4.4 Types of synovial joint. *Source:* Tortora, G.J. and Derrickson, B.H., *Essentials of Anatomy and Physiology*, 2018, Wiley. Reproduced with permission of John Wiley & Sons.

Table 4.3 The function of the bones of the skull.

Bones	Function
Frontal	Situated at the front of the head forming the forehead, the roof of the eye sockets and nasal cavity as well as the base of the anterior of the skull.
Occipital	Situated at the rear of the skull just above the nape of the neck. It has a hole at the base which is the channel of the spinal cord between skull and the spinal column. The occipital bone is connected to the top two vertebrae (atlas and axis), allowing the head to move freely.
Sphenoid	A wing-shaped bone situated at the base of the skull in front of the temporal bones. It is the only bone that articulates with the other seven bones of the skull. It spans the skull laterally and helps form the base of the cranium, the sides of the skull, and the floors and sides of the eye sockets. The central body has two sinuses within it which lie side by side and are separated by a bony septum that projects downward into the nasal cavity and forms channels for the optic nerve and other nerves.
Ethmoid	Separates the nasal cavity from the brain. It is spongy and light, can be easily damaged and is situated between the eye sockets at the roof of the nose. The external walls contain small sinuses.
Temporal × 2	Found on each side of the skull and form part of the sides and the base. Each is divided anatomically into four parts: the mastoid, petrous, squamous and tympanic. It is closely involved in the anatomy of the ear. They also form a projection from the cheekbone to the eye (the zygoma).
Parietal × 2	Two of the largest bones of the skull that form the sides and roof. In the front each parietal bone adjoins the frontal bone, in the back, the occipital bone, and below, the temporal and sphenoid bones.

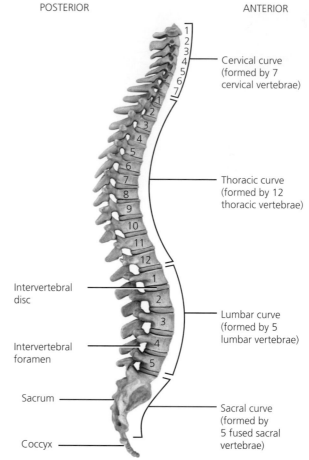

POSTERIOR   ANTERIOR

Cervical curve (formed by 7 cervical vertebrae)

Thoracic curve (formed by 12 thoracic vertebrae)

Intervertebral disc

Lumbar curve (formed by 5 lumbar vertebrae)

Intervertebral foramen

Sacrum

Sacral curve (formed by 5 fused sacral vertebrae)

Coccyx

Right lateral view showing four normal curves

Figure 4.5 The spine. *Source:* Tortora, G.J. and Derrickson, B.H., *Essentials of Anatomy and Physiology*, 2018, Wiley. Reproduced with permission of John Wiley & Sons.

The spine provides strong flexible support for the head and body, and keeps the trunk straight whilst allowing the torso to move. It protects the spinal cord and acts as an attachment point for the ribs, the pelvic girdle and the muscles of the back. The strength and mobility of the spine is enhanced by four curves of the spine, two concave at the cervical and lumbar levels (lordosis/lordoses) and two convex at the dorsal and sacral areas (kyphosis/kyphoses). Figure 4.5 shows the overall structure of the spine.

The main functions of the spine are:

- protection of the spinal cord and nerve roots
- supports and balances the body in an upright position with the help of surrounding muscles and ligaments
- attachment for the ribs, pelvic girdle, muscles, ligaments and tendons
- mobility of the vertebrae and the intervertebral discs allows mobility in the trunk of the body.

The Vertebrae

The vertebrae are named by using the initial of the area concerned, i.e. C = cervical, D (or T) = dorsal (or thoracic) etc. and the number according to the vertebra's position in the spine, i.e. C3 is the third cervical vertebra. Figure 4.6 illustrates the structure of a typical vertebra. The basic structure is the same at all levels and consists of the following:

- A vertebral body, which is the thickest and load-bearing part of the vertebrae. Rough surfaces provide excellent adhesion for the intervertebral discs. It also contains two foramina that allow blood vessels to pass through.

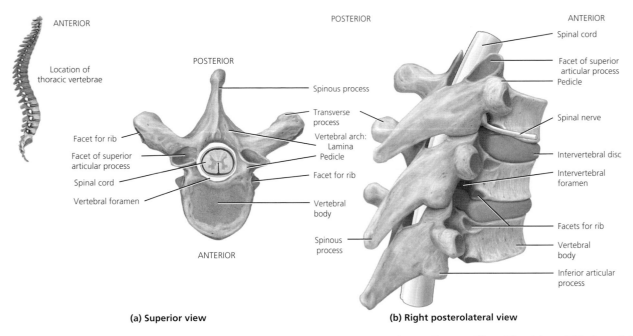

(a) Superior view   **(b) Right posterolateral view**

Figure 4.6 Structure of a typical vertebrae (illustrated by a thoracic vertebra). *Source:* Tortora, G.J. and Derrickson, B.H., *Essentials of Anatomy and Physiology*, 2018, Wiley. Reproduced with permission of John Wiley & Sons.

- A vertebral arch composed of two thick projections (vertebral pedicles) and two flat sections of bone (vertebral laminae) and completed by the vertebral body. This forms the vertebral foramen that encloses the spinal cord. Once the vertebrae are stacked on each other the vertebral foramen form the vertebral canal. The stacked pedicles create a gap on each side, each allowing for the passage of a spinal nerve.
- Seven processes commence from the vertebral arch: two transverse, four articular and one spinous process. The four articular processes are covered in hyaline cartilage and articulate with the vertebrae above and below.

The vertebrae are different depending on the level of the spine they correspond to (see Table 4.4), but two vertebrae are unique: C1 and C2.

- C1 (atlas) supports the head and is a ring of bone with two transverse processes. It has articular facets on its upper side that are concave and articulate with the occipital condyles, allowing the head to move up and down. On the lower surfaces it articulates with the second vertebra.
- C2 (the axis) has a characteristic protrusion on the upper surface known as the dens. This serves as a pivot for the rotation of the atlas and the head, allowing it to rotate from side to side.

Table 4.4 The characteristics of vertebrae.

Vertebral position	Size and structure	Characteristics
Cervical (C1–C7)	Smaller than other vertebrae but with wider arches	• Form the bony structure of the neck, includes C1 and C2 • Three foramina: one vertebral, which accommodates the spinal cord, and two transverse, which allow the vertebral artery to pass through with its corresponding vein and nerve
Thoracic (T1–T12)	Large and robust except for T11, T12, T1 and T2, which have longer transverse processes	• At the back of the thoracic cavity and articulate with the ribs
Lumbar (L1–L5)	Largest and most robust vertebrae with short thick processes	• Carry most of the body weight and support the lower back
Sacrum	Five fused vertebrae	• Forms a triangle and part of the posterior wall of the pelvic cavity • It is wider in women than in men
Coccyx	Four fused vertebrae	• Forms a smaller triangle and the posterior portion of the bones of the pelvis • Connected to the sacrum

Soft Tissues of the Spine

Intervertebral discs have two functions:

- to attach the vertebrae to one another
- to absorb and dampen shock to the spine.

All the vertebrae are separated by the intervertebral discs except for C1 and C2 and the coccyx. These are made of varying thickness of cartilage, the thickest occurring in the lumbar vertebrae, which take the most stress.

The annulus fibrosus of the disc is a strong outer structure made up of concentric sheets of collagen fibres connected to the vertebral end plates. This encloses the nucleus pulposus, which contains gel-like matter full of water that resists compression; the amount of water in the nucleus varies throughout the day depending on activity (see Figure 4.7).

The ligaments of the spine (listed in Table 4.5) connect bone to bone and are fibrous connective tissues made up of densely packed collagen fibres. These help to provide structural stability and a natural brace along with the tendons and muscles, which help to protect the spine from injury. There are two primary ligament systems in the spine. The intrasegmental system includes the ligamentum flavum, and interspinous and intertransverse ligaments, which hold many of the vertebrae together. The intersegmental system includes the anterior and posterior longitudinal ligaments, and the supraspinous ligaments.

The primary function of the complex muscle and tendon system of the spine is to support and stabilise the structure. Specific muscles are associated with movement of parts of the anatomy and have very important roles. For example, the sternocleidomastoid muscle (neck area) assists with movement of the head, while the spinalis thoracis is associated with extension of the vertebral column.

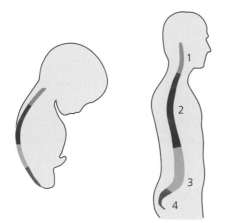

Single curve in fetus   Four curves in adult

Fetal and adult curves

Functions of the vertebral column

1. Permits movement.
2. Encloses and protects the spinal cord.
3. Serves as a point of attachment for the ribs and muscles of the back.

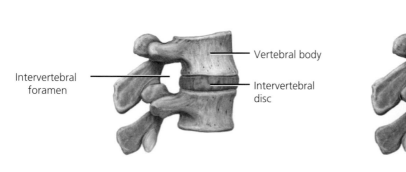

Intervertebral foramen — Vertebral body — Intervertebral disc

Normal intervertebral disc   Compressed intervertebral disc in a weight-bearing situation

Intervertebral disc

Figure 4.7   Intervertebral discs. *Source:* Tortora, G.J. and Derrickson, B.H., *Essentials of Anatomy and Physiology*, 2018, Wiley. Reproduced with permission of John Wiley & Sons.

Table 4.5 The ligaments of the spine.

Ligament name	System	Description
Anterior longitudinal ligament	Intersegmental system	• One of the primary spine stabilisers that runs the entire length of the spine from the base of the skull to the sacrum • Connects the front (anterior) of the vertebral body to the front of the annulus fibrosis
Posterior longitudinal ligament	Intersegmental system	• Another primary spine stabiliser that runs the entire length of the spine from the base of the skull to the sacrum • Connects the back (posterior) of the vertebral body to the back of the annulus fibrosus
Supraspinous ligament	Intrasegmental system	• Attaches the tip of each spinous process to the next one
Interspinous ligament	Intrasegmental system	• A thin ligament • Attaches to the ligamentum flavum, which runs deep into the spinal column
Ligamentum flavum	Intrasegmental system	• The strongest ligament • Runs from the base of the skull to the pelvis, in front of and between the lamina, and in front of the facet joint capsules • Protects the spinal cord and nerves

The Spinal Cord and Spinal/ Vertebral Nerves

The spinal cord consists of millions of nerve fibres, which transmit electrical information to and from the brain to the limbs, trunk and organs of the body. The spinal cord descends through the vertebral foramen of each vertebra down to the cauda equina. The brain and the spinal cord are surrounded by the meninges, which have three distinct layers:

• the dura mater: strong connective grey outer layer
• the arachnoid mater; a thinner layer resembling a loosely woven fabric of arteries and veins
• the pia mater: a delicate inner layer of highly vascular membrane providing blood to the neural structures.

The space between the arachnoid mater and pia mater (subarachnoid space) is filled with cerebrospinal fluid (CSF), a clear fluid found in the ventricles, spinal canal and spinal cord that is secreted from a vascular part of the ventricles in the brain, the choroid plexus. This acts as a shock absorber to protect against injury and contains different electrolytes, proteins and glucose.

The communication system from the spinal cord is via spinal nerves that link to the peripheral nervous system, then branch off and pass out from the cord through the foramen of the vertebra. Figure 4.8 shows the spinal cord and spinal nerves. There are four main groups of spinal nerves, which exit different levels of the spinal cord:

• cervical nerves: supply movement and feeling to the arms, neck and upper trunk and control breathing
• thoracic nerves: supply the trunk and abdomen
• lumbar and sacral nerves: supply the legs, bladder, bowel and sexual organs.

The spinal nerves carry information to and from different levels (segments) in the spinal cord. Both the nerves and the segments in the spinal cord are numbered in a similar way to the vertebrae, e.g. T3. There are 31 pairs of spinal nerves in the cervical region of the spinal cord. The spinal nerves exit above the vertebrae, but this changes below the C7 vertebra where there is an eighth cervical spinal nerve, although there is no eighth cervical vertebra. From the first thoracic vertebra all spinal nerves exit below their equivalent numbered vertebrae.

The Upper Limb

The pectoral or shoulder girdle attaches the bones of the upper limb to the axial skeleton. Each of the two pectoral girdles consists of a clavicle (collar bone) and a scapula (shoulder blade). The anterior component is the clavicle, which articulates with the sternum at the sternoclavicular joint. The posterior component is the scapula, which articulates with the clavicle at the acromion process and the humerus at the glenoid cavity. The scapula is a flat, triangular bone that lies over the ribs at the back of the rib cage and is held within a complex group of muscle attachments.

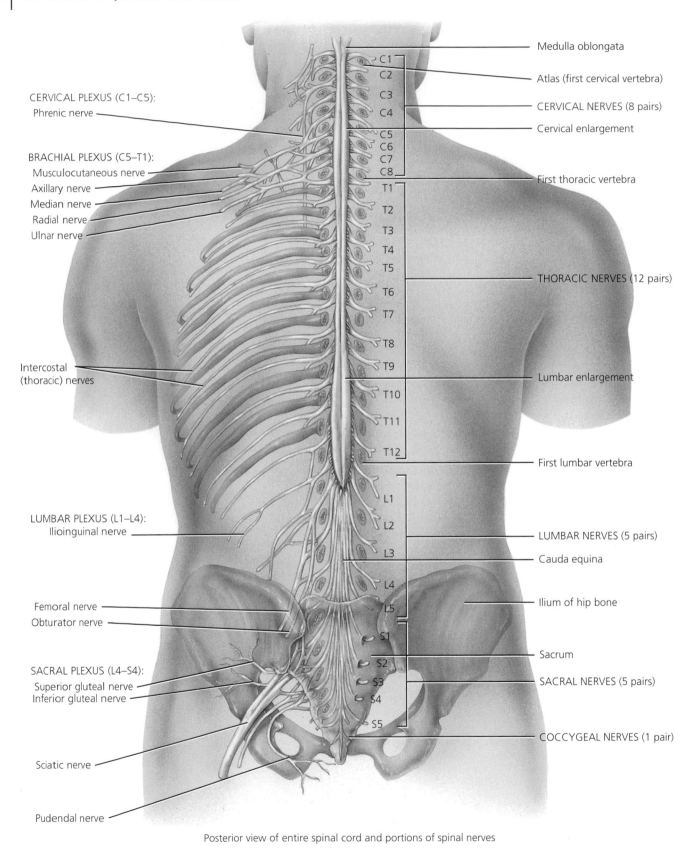

CERVICAL PLEXUS (C1–C5):
  Phrenic nerve

BRACHIAL PLEXUS (C5–T1):
  Musculocutaneous nerve
  Axillary nerve
  Median nerve
  Radial nerve
  Ulnar nerve

Intercostal
(thoracic) nerves

LUMBAR PLEXUS (L1–L4):
  Ilioinguinal nerve

Femoral nerve
Obturator nerve

SACRAL PLEXUS (L4–S4):
  Superior gluteal nerve
  Inferior gluteal nerve

Sciatic nerve

Pudendal nerve

Medulla oblongata
Atlas (first cervical vertebra)
CERVICAL NERVES (8 pairs)
Cervical enlargement

First thoracic vertebra

THORACIC NERVES (12 pairs)

Lumbar enlargement

First lumbar vertebra

LUMBAR NERVES (5 pairs)
Cauda equina

Ilium of hip bone

Sacrum

SACRAL NERVES (5 pairs)

COCCYGEAL NERVES (1 pair)

C1
C2
C3
C4
C5
C6
C7
C8
T1
T2
T3
T4
T5
T6
T7
T8
T9
T10
T11
T12
L1
L2
L3
L4
L5
S1
S2
S3
S4
S5

Posterior view of entire spinal cord and portions of spinal nerves

Figure 4.8 Spinal cord and spinal nerves. *Source:* Tortora, G.J. and Derrickson, B.H., *Essentials of Anatomy and Physiology*, 2018, Wiley. Reproduced with permission of John Wiley & Sons.

The pectoral girdles do not articulate with the vertebral column.

The clavicle (collarbone) is a long slender bone with a double curve that lies horizontally in the superior anterior part of the thorax. The medial end articulates with the sternum at the sternoclavicular joint and the lateral end articulates with the acromion of the scapula at the acromioclavicular joint. The clavicle transmits forces from the upper limb to the trunk of the body.

The scapula (shoulder blade) is a large triangular flat bone that sits posteriorly over the thoracic cage between the levels of the second and seventh rib. A sharp spine runs diagonally across the posterior surface and ends at a flattened projection known as the acromion, which articulates with the clavicle at the acromioclavicular joint and can easily be felt as the high point of the shoulder. Below the acromion, the glenoid cavity articulates with the humerus to form the shoulder joint. Figure 4.9 shows the right upper limb.

The ball and socket joint of the shoulder (glenohumeral joint) is freely moveable in many directions but is relatively unstable because the glenoid cavity is very shallow. The rim is slightly deepened by cartilage but has little effect on the stability of the joint. A number of ligaments and tendons help to secure the humeral head in the joint cavity along with the series of four tendons (subscapularis, supraspinatus, infraspinatus and teres minor) which make up the rotator cuff.

The humerus is the longest and largest bone of the upper limb. The proximal end consists of a head that articulates with the glenoid cavity and it has an anatomical neck just distal to the head. The neck of the humerus is a constricted area just distal to the greater and lesser tubercles, and is liable to fracture. The shaft of the humerus is cylindrical but gradually becomes flattened and triangular at its distal end.

The elbow is a synovial hinge joint that allows flexion and extension, and is important to the flexibility and function of the upper limb. Supination and pronation of the forearm take place at the proximal radioulnar joint contained within the elbow joint capsule. The distal end of the humerus articulates with the proximal end of the ulna and radius. At the distal end of the humerus:

- the capitulum is a rounded knob that articulates with the head of the radius
- the radial fossa is a depression which receives the head of the radius when the elbow is flexed
- the trochlea is the surface that articulates with the ulna
- an anterior depression known as the coronoid fossa receives the ulna head when the forearm is flexed
- the olecranon fossa is a posterior depression that receives the olecranon of the ulna when the elbow is extended.

Most of the muscles of the forearm are attached to the distal end of the humerus at the medial and lateral epicondyles, and the ulnar nerve lies on the posterior surface of the medial epicondyle.

The radius is the lateral bone of the forearm situated on the thumb side and the ulna is the medial bone of the forearm situated on the little finger side. The head of the radius articulates with the capitulum of the humerus and the radial notch of the ulna. The shaft of the radius widens at its distal end and articulates with two of the wrist bones, the lunate and scaphoid. At the proximal end of the ulna the olecranon process forms the point of the elbow. The elbow is stabilised by ligaments which prevent rotation and provide stability and strength.

The wrist and hand are capable of very fine, flexible movements. The wrist consists of eight small bones: the carpals, in two transverse rows with four bones in each row, united by ligaments. The proximal row of carpal bones (from lateral to medial) are the scaphoid, lunate, triquetrum and pisiform. The distal row (from lateral to medial) are the trapezium, trapezoid, capitate and hamate. A passageway on the palmar side of the carpal bones known as the carpal tunnel provides a conduit through which the median nerve and flexor tendons of the hand pass. The nerve supply to the arm and hand, with specific reference to the brachial plexus, is considered in some detail in Chapter 20.

The metacarpals which form the palm of the hand each consist of a proximal base which articulates with the distal row of carpal bones, and a shaft and a distal head which articulate with the proximal phalanges of the fingers. The metacarpal bones are numbered 1–5. The phalanges are the bones of the fingers and there are 14 in each hand: two in the pollex (thumb) and three in each of the remaining four fingers. A single bone of the finger is referred to as a phalanx. The articulations between the metacarpal bones and the phalanges are referred to as the metacarpophalangeal (MCP) joints, which flex and extend the fingers and thumb. The two joints in the fingers are known as the interphalangeal joints: the joint closest to the MCP joint is referred to as the proximal interphalangeal joint (PIP) and the joint near the end of the finger is called the distal interphalangeal joint (DIP). The thumb has only one interphalangeal joint.

The Pelvis

The pelvis is a bowl-shaped ring of bones that transmits weight from the spine through the legs. Its two (right and left) innominate bones are made up of three bones, the ilium, ischium and pubis, which fuse together at puberty. The pelvic girdle consists of the innominate bones connected at the

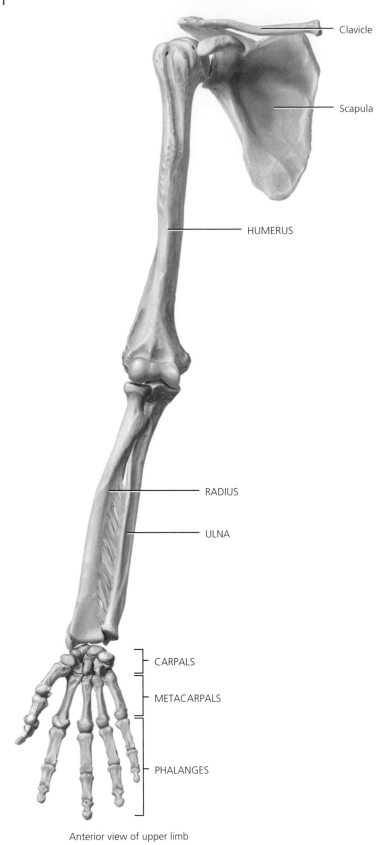

Clavicle

Scapula

HUMERUS

RADIUS

ULNA

CARPALS

METACARPALS

PHALANGES

Anterior view of upper limb

Figure 4.9 Right upper limb. *Source:* Kuntzman and Tortora 2010 / with permission of John Wiley & Sons.

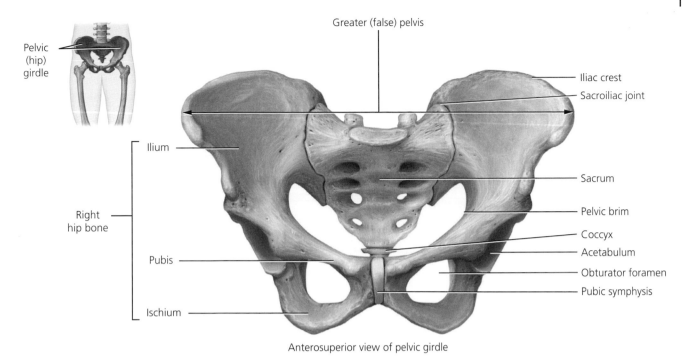

Pelvic (hip) girdle

Greater (false) pelvis

Iliac crest

Sacroiliac joint

Ilium

Right hip bone

Pubis

Ischium

Sacrum

Pelvic brim

Coccyx

Acetabulum

Obturator foramen

Pubic symphysis

Anterosuperior view of pelvic girdle

Figure 4.10   The female pelvis – anterior view. *Source:* Tortora, G.J. and Derrickson, B.H., *Essentials of Anatomy and Physiology*, 2018, Wiley. Reproduced with permission of John Wiley & Sons.

> **Box 4.4   Functions of The Pelvis**
>
> - Weight bearing: bears the weight of the upper body in sitting and standing
> - Transfer: transfers weight from the axial skeleton to the appendicular skeleton in standing and walking
> - Attachments: provides attachments for and withstands the forces of the muscles used for posture and movement
> - Protection: contains and protects the pelvic and abdominopelvic viscera.

pubic symphysis anteriorly and the sacrum posteriorly at the sacroiliac joint to form the highly stable but immobile pelvic ring (see Figure 4.10). The pelvic cavity contains the reproductive organs, bladder and rectum. The female pelvis is wider and shallower than the male to facilitate childbirth. The functions of the pelvis are summarised in Box 4.4

The Lower Limb

The lower limbs are composed of 60 bones (see Figures 4.11 and 4.12). Each limb includes the femur, patella, tibia, fibula, tarsals, metatarsals and phalanges.

The ball and socket arrangement of the hip joint allows flexion/extension, adduction/abduction and medial/lateral rotation, and is central to the transfer of weight from the trunk and upper body to the legs. The proximal end, or head, of the femur articulates with the acetabulum of the innominate bone. The neck of the femur is a constricted region distal to the head. The greater and lesser trochanters are projections that serve as points for the attachment of some of the thigh and buttock muscles. The joint is supported by a series of strong muscles and ligaments with a main nerve supply from the femoral and obturator nerves formed from the lumbar plexus. The main blood supply comes from the femoral artery.

The femur is the longest and heaviest bone of the body and distally articulates with the tibia at the knee joint. The diaphysis of the femur has a rough vertical ridge on its posterior surface, which serves as the attachment for several thigh muscles. The distal end of the femur expands and includes the medial and lateral condyles.

The knee is the largest joint. It is a hinge joint allowing flexion and extension supported by a complex system of ligaments and made up of three joints: the lateral and medial femorotibial and the patellofemoral. The two femorotibial joints are articulations between the lateral and medial condyles of the femur and the tibial condyles, separated by the intercondylar eminence. The patella is a small triangular sesamoid bone that sits in the quadriceps tendon anterior to the knee joint and provides protection to the knee joint during kneeling, and glides over the distal femur during flexion and extension of the knee forming the patellofemoral joint.

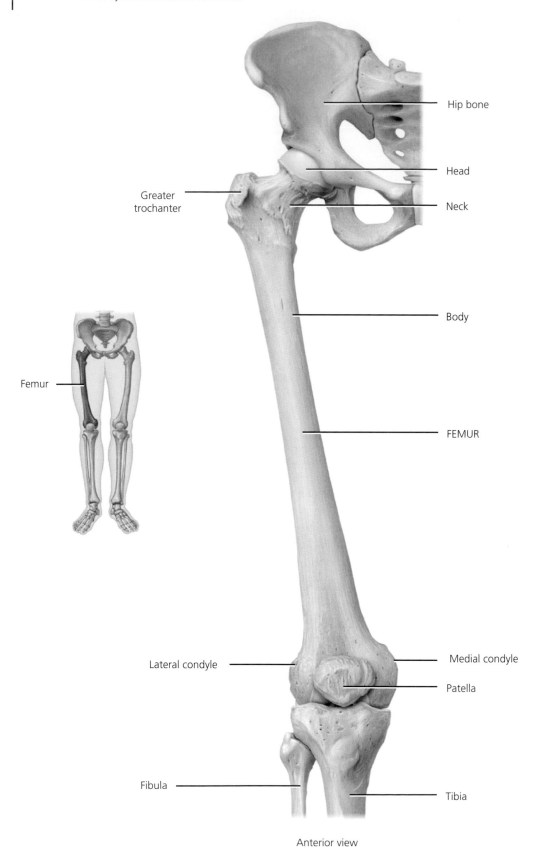

Anterior view

Figure 4.11 Lower limb – hip to knee. *Source:* Tortora, G.J. and Derrickson, B.H., *Essentials of Anatomy and Physiology*, 2018, Wiley. Reproduced with permission of John Wiley & Sons.

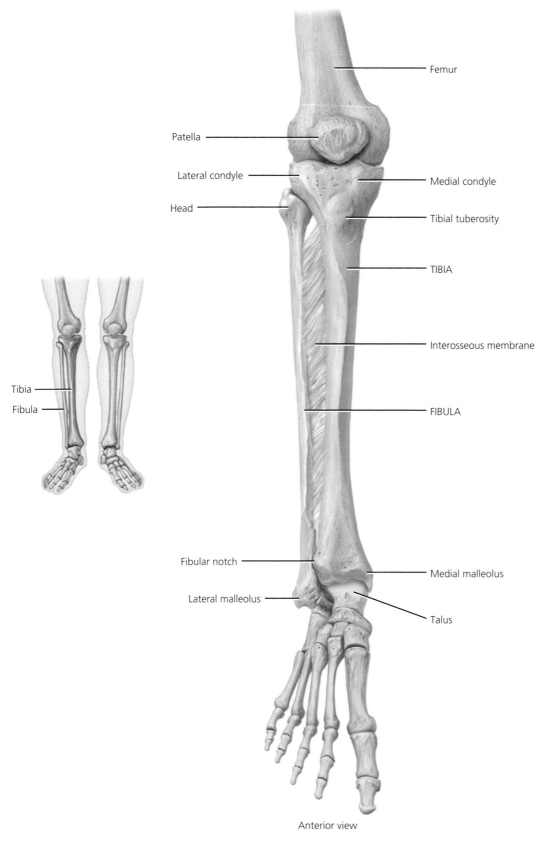

Anterior view

Figure 4.12 Lower limb – knee to foot. *Source:* Tortora, G.J. and Derrickson, B.H., *Essentials of Anatomy and Physiology*, 2018, Wiley. Reproduced with permission of John Wiley & Sons.

Stability is provided by the ligaments, cartilage and tendons of the joint, particularly the cruciate ligaments in the centre of the knee, but these are vulnerable to injury especially under excessive rotational forces. Two cartilage shock absorbers, the menisci, sit on the medial and lateral tibial condyles. The medial and lateral collateral ligaments lie external to the joint capsule and attach the medial and lateral femoral condyles to the medial tibial condyle and the head of the fibula laterally to prevent rotation.

There are 28 bones in the foot and ankle, allowing adaptation to various surfaces, providing balance, mobility and weight-bearing stability and shock absorbency. The ankle joint is the articulation between the distal ends of the tibia and fibula and the talus bone. During walking, the talus initially bears the entire weight of the body and half of that weight is then transferred to the calcaneus. The remaining weight is transmitted to the other tarsal bones: cuboid, navicular and three cuneiform bones. The talus and calcaneum are located at the posterior part of the foot and the rest of the tarsal bones are located anteriorly. The cuneiform bone and cuboid bone articulate with the metatarsals. There are five metatarsals each consisting of a proximal base, shaft and distal head. Distally the metatarsals articulate with the proximal row of phalanges, which consist of a proximal base, middle shaft and distal head. The hallux (big toe) has two large heavy phalanges while the other four toes each have three phalanges: proximal, middle and distal. The bones of the foot are arranged in two arches, which enable the foot to support and distribute weight. The arches of the foot are maintained by the bones, ligaments and tendons of the foot; these are not rigid, but yield when weight is applied and spring back when the weight is released.

Tendons and ligaments are vital to the foot for flexibility and movement, and the muscles of the foot work in partnership with those of the lower leg. There are many nerves within the foot which permit sensation, particularly feeling the surface when walking.

Conclusion

A fundamental guide to musculoskeletal anatomy and physiology has been provided in this chapter. It is recognised, however, that considerable further detailed knowledge is required to support expert and effective practice, and this can be gained from further reading. This should include a deeper review of muscle anatomy and physiology than has been possible to include here.

Anatomy and physiology acts as part of the diverse evidence base that underpins musculoskeletal care. Practitioners cannot understand what has gone wrong with a system and meet patients' needs if they do not know how it works when it is undamaged. To understand musculoskeletal diseases and disorders, and the care and treatment associated with these health problems, the practitioner must have, as a priority, an in-depth working knowledge of the anatomy and physiology of the musculoskeletal system along with a general knowledge of other systems. Orthopaedic and trauma care covers the full span of life and most people will access some form of orthopaedic and trauma service in their lifetime. A knowledge of anatomy and physiology is essential in facilitating prompt assessment and treatment as well as providing the tools for post-injury education of the patient.

Further Reading

Kuntzman, A.J. and Tortora, G.J. (2010). *Anatomy and Physiology for the Manual Therapies*. New Jersey: Wiley.

Palastanga, N. and Soames, R.W. (2012). *Anatomy and Human Movement: Structure and Function*, 6e. Edinburgh: Churchill Livingstone.

Tortora, G.J. and Derrickson, B.H. (2018). *Tortora's Principles of Anatomy and Physiology*, 15e. Wiley.

References

Kuntzman, A.J. and Tortora, G.J. (2010). *Anatomy and Physiology for the Manual Therapies*, Wiley.

Tortora, G.J. and Derrickson, B.H. (2018). *Essentials of Anatomy and Physiology*, Wiley.

5

The Team Approach and Nursing Roles in Orthopaedic and Musculoskeletal Trauma Care

Sandra Flynn

University of Chester, UK

Introduction

The aim of this chapter is to introduce the notion of multidisciplinary team working and the disciplines that make up the team within orthopaedic and trauma care. The term 'multidisciplinary' is used to describe the collaborative work of the various health professional groups (Finn et al. 2010) who are drawn together to use their knowledge and skills within a specialist field towards a common patient goal (Choi and Pak 2007; Solheim et al. 2007).

Lemieux-Charles and McGuire (2006, p. 265) state that, 'A team is a multi-dimensional construct and team structures and processes can vary widely depending on the membership, work, tasks and interactions'.

Models of care define the way in which healthcare is delivered to the patient. Healthcare professionals may interact and collaborate in ways that aim to optimise the skills and efficiency of the workforce (Choi and Pak 2006; Kaltner et al. 2017). The term multiprofessional is used to describe the structural component of a team and the setting in which they work. The team is interchangable according to the needs of the patient (Chamberlain-Salaun et al. 2013; Jovanovic et al. 2020). The terms multidisciplinary, interdisciplinary and transdisciplinary are used interchangeably in the literature and are considered distinct conceptual models of team-working (Ellis and Sevdalis 2019).

Choi and Pak (2006), propose that the terms multidisciplinary, interdisciplinary, and transdisciplinary should only be used when 'the exact nature of a multiple disciplinary effort is known' (p. 359), otherwise the term 'multiple disciplinary' should be used.

Multidisciplinary teams comprise various healthcare professionals who assess patients on an individual basis. Team members adhere to their disciplinary boundaries so that care is provided from a separate but interrelated role perspective. This approach to care is considered non-integrative (see Chapter 6).

Interdisciplinary teams involve the unification of a group of practitioners with different skills working together to develop and achieve a management plan for the patient. Individual practitioners maintain their professional identities, but closer integration is observed (Kaini 2017).

Transdisciplinary teams are composed of interdisciplinary team members who share and acquire new disciplinary role functions. This concept represents the notion of the multiskilled, flexible health practitioner. Disciplinary boundaries are blurred, allowing team members to share their skills, knowledge and responsibilities about their respective disciplines so that each may function in the other's role when required (Van Bewer 2017).

A collaborative and reliable multidisciplinary team approach to person-centred care plays a key role in supporting individuals to make informed decisions about their own unique health and healthcare needs (Fazio et al. 2018). Delivering healthcare is an intricate and interdependent process traversing political, organisational, disciplinary, technical, social and cultural boundaries (Rosen et al. 2018). Promoting person-centred practice also requires a demonstration of humanity and kindness to ensure people are treated with dignity, compassion and respect (Jemal et al. 2021). Improving the patient experience and the delivery of safe, high-quality person-centred care is key to minimising preventable morbidity and mortality (Rosen et al. 2018; Burton et al. 2020), and helping to ensure that the unique needs of the patient, family and carer are fully met. Healthcare professionals assume responsibility for promoting and restoring health, preventing illness and relieving suffering. Clinical expertise that is based on sound clinical knowledge, employing discretionary judgement,

Orthopaedic and Trauma Nursing: An Evidence-based Approach to Musculoskeletal Care, Second Edition. Edited by Sonya Clarke and Mary Drozd.
© 2023 John Wiley & Sons Ltd. Published 2023 by John Wiley & Sons Ltd.

understanding illness and its trajectory, and appreciating the varied human response to illness is central to professional healthcare practice.

The Team and Importance of a Multidisciplinary Approach

Establishing a culture of safety is necessary to improve the quality and delivery of healthcare and reduce patient harm (Klevens et al. 2007; Miake-Lye et al. 2013; Howell et al. 2014). The complexity of chronic conditions and the expanding development in medical care and treatment options available has led to the need for effective and efficient healthcare teams (Rosen et al. 2018) and a multidisciplinary approach to the provision of care and rehabilitation. A team culture is created when a group of individuals who possess shared beliefs, values and behavioural norms (Sacks et al. 2015) are committed to a shared purpose in the best care of the patient with musculoskeletal conditions or injuries. Teams vary in size and composition both in primary and secondary care settings, from dyadic interactions and shared decision making between primary care providers and patients, to extensive specialist multiprofessional team systems (Weaver et al. 2014). A common approach and focus on teamwork consists of several key dimensions relating to team coordination, including effective communication, shared knowledge, complex problem solving, diagnosis, planning, treatment and management (Gittell et al. 2000, 2008; Rosen et al. 2018).

Teamwork involves a highly complex and interdependent collaboration amongst team members who may work together for short or long periods of time (Hughes et al. 2016). The intricate and often transient nature of teamwork makes it difficult to apply to all situations (Cunninghan et al. 2018). It does, however, offer a flexible and fluid approach to the delivery of healthcare.

Research does highlight the often-intricate balance of working collaboratively while maintaining the professional identity of individual health and care workers. This is important for several reasons: it acknowledges their unique skills and attributes, it retains professional identity and it fosters team integration (Wald 2015; Gilburt 2016).

It is important for orthopaedic and trauma practitioners to understand and engage the varied roles of the multidisciplinary team so that they complement each other and work together to deliver a high-quality service and the provision of care designed around the diverse needs of the patient within the trauma and orthopaedic clinical settings.

In addition to promoting better outcomes for patients, research has demonstrated that multidisciplinary collaborative working affords opportunities to enhance skills and

knowledge, contribute to decision-making processes, service design and development, and provide informal education as well as promoting a culture of respect and understanding of each other's roles and abilities (Tzenalis and Sotiriadou 2010; Academy of Medical Royal Colleges 2020).

The role of the multidisciplinary team includes:

- assessment
- treatment/management of conditions
- education/advocacy
- referral/collaboration
- research and clinical audit.

Musculoskeletal pathways of care differ from patient to patient and the number of healthcare professionals involved in an individual pathway of care will vary according to the complexity of their needs (Jester et al. 2021). Care needs to be personcentred, and a team approach helps to ensure services are delivered in partnership with the patient and their family/carer.

Team Roles

Optimal management and care of patients with musculoskeletal conditions requires the expertise of specialists from different disciplines. Collectively the multidisciplinary team provides a holistic, seamless service over the full continuum of care. The individual practitioners who have roles within the musculoskeletal multidisciplinary team are discussed in the following section, but it is acknowledged that teams work within a complex healthcare system and may vary according to subspecialty, locality and context (Fulop and Robert 2015; Kringos et al. 2015) and that not all roles may be represented.

Nursing Roles in Orthopaedic and Trauma Care

Nursing roles within the specialty of trauma and orthopaedics are diverse and found in a variety of settings within primary and secondary care services. Nursing areas of practice include, but are not limited to, adult and paediatric orthopaedic units, trauma units, outpatient departments, day surgery centres, operating theatres, emergency departments and rehabilitation units. Nursing staff provide an important link within the team, working with the patient and other healthcare professionals to develop, plan, implement, coordinate and evaluate plans of care. Nursing roles include:

- healthcare assistant/healthcare support worker
- registered nurse
- nursing associate
- ward/unit/department manager
- matron
- pre-assessment nurse
- casting room nurse
- theatre nurse
- clinical nurse specialist
- nurse practitioner
- advanced nurse practitioner
- orthopaedic trauma coordinator
- surgical care practitioner
- consultant nurse.

A brief description of some roles is given below.

- Healthcare assistants are trained in basic nursing skills and work under the guidance of a healthcare professional such as a registered nurse. They work as part of the multidisciplinary team in hospitals, health centres, general practice surgeries and nursing homes.
- Healthcare support workers are also trained in basic nursing skills, supporting patients to manage daily activities and helping the multidisciplinary team deliver care and treatment.
- Nursing associate is a role in the UK regulated by the Nursing and Midwifery Council (NMC). Nursing associates work alongside registered nurses, healthcare assistants and support workers to provide care (NMC 2020).

Advanced and Specialist Nursing Roles

The notions of 'advanced' and 'specialist' practice/practitioner encompass several job titles and roles within the specialty of trauma and orthopaedic nursing. Each role is multifaceted and exhibits contrasting quantities of clinical activity, education, management, leadership, collaboration and research, depending on the individual job profile and client/service requirements. Advanced level nursing is concerned with a higher level of clinical practice, regardless of specialist area or role, which is beyond that of first-level registration (Department of Health 2010) and is continually evolving while remaining firmly rooted in the provision of direct care or clinical work with patients, families and populations. The capabilities of advanced clinical practice lie within four domains or pillars of practice (Health Education England 2017):

- clinical practice
- leadership and management
- education
- research.

Consultant Nurse

In 2000, the role of nurse consultant was established in the UK with the following aim (*Department of Health* 1999):

> . . . help to provide better outcomes for patients by improving services and quality, to strengthen leadership and to provide a new career opportunity to help retain expert nurses . . .

The nurse consultant provides highly specialised professional advice, consultancy, clinical expertise and leadership to patients, carers and colleagues in collaboration with medical, nursing and allied health professional colleagues. The nurse consultant develops and delivers highly specialised care using advanced skills and competencies. An essential component of the role in musculoskeletal care is to initiate research in the field of orthopaedic and trauma nursing to ensure evidence-based practice is embedded in all aspects of care and treatment. The role is structured around four core functions:

- clinical/professional leadership
- expert practice
- policy and service development, research and evaluation
- education and professional development.

Nurse consultants are seen as an influential force, generating and sustaining change (The King's Fund 2018), contributing to the ongoing development and delivery of health and wellbeing services in many countries around the world.

Orthopaedic Trauma Coordinator

The orthopaedic trauma coordinator is a registered nurse with clinical expertise and specialist knowledge. Working as an integral member of the orthopaedic trauma team, the coordinator collaborates with the multidisciplinary team and the patient to plan and implement care and treatment to maximise best clinical outcomes. Postholder responsibilities vary and can include the coordination of a specific service or services within the specialty, such as virtual fracture clinics and patient flow through orthopaedic trauma pathways. The orthopaedic trauma coordinator provides a primary point of contact within the specialty for health professionals and patients.

Surgical Care Practitioner

The Curriculum Framework for the Surgical Care Practitioner (Royal College of Surgeons 2014) defines the role of the surgical care practitioner (SCP) as:

A registered non-medical practitioner who has completed a Royal Colleage of Surgeons accredited programme, working in clinical practice as a member of the extended surgical team, who performs surgical intervention, pre-operative care and post-operative care under the direction and supervision of a Consultant Surgeon (p. 11).

The SCP is a trained clinical professional such as a theatre nurse or operating department practitioner who completes an accredited programme of training to extend their scope of practice (Royal College of Surgeons 2014). Working as part of the surgical team the SCP provides care in clinics, on the wards and in the operating theatre. The role is varied and responsibilities include:

- pre-operative assessment and physical examination
- the consent process following GMC guidelines
- assisting with the preparation of patients for surgery
- assisting with surgical procedures in the operating theatre under the supervision and direction of the operating surgeon
- acting as first or second assistant at operations
- ordering of pre- and post-operative investigations
- post-operative care and identification of the acute deterioration of patients
- documentation of operation notes and taking of ward round notes
- research, audit, education and development within the surgical specialty.

Nursing roles are continually evolving in response to the increasing healthcare needs of the patient requiring orthopaedic and trauma care, and in response to a transforming healthcare system.

Medical Roles in Orthopaedic and Trauma Care

Orthopaedic surgeons and supporting medical staff are concerned with all aspects of healthcare relating to the patient requiring elective orthopaedic and orthopaedic trauma care be it conservative or surgical. Medical, physical and rehabilitative methods as well as surgery are employed to provide the most appropriate treatment. Surgery may be indicated when it is the best option for restoring function following injury or disease of bones, joints and related soft tissues. Medical staff work closely with the multidisciplinary team, playing an important role in diagnosis and decision making, and in prescribing and delivering musculoskeletal treatment and care.

Medical staffing roles include:

- general practitioners with a specialist interest in musculoskeletal conditions (primary care)
- secondary care

- orthopaedic consultants (specialist interest) leading their own team of doctors and administration staff
- orthogeriatricians, who focus on the management of older patients with fragility fractures usually in the acute phase of management. The orthogeriatrician comanages the patient working alongside the orthopaedic multidisciplinary team. The role addresses the dual problem of bone fragility and patient frailty (Falaschi and Marsh 2020).
- physician associate, a rapidly expanding and professionally regulated role that forms part of the multidisciplinary frontline workforce. The physician associate profession was developed in the United States in the 1960s to improve and expand healthcare, and similar roles now exist in healthcare systems worldwide. Physician associates are medically trained to work alongside doctors and are an integral part of the multidisciplinary team in both primary and secondary healthcare settings.

Allied Health Professional Roles in Orthopaedic and Trauma Care

Allied health professionals are other clinical staff uniquely placed to provide a wide range of specific services that include diagnostic, therapeutic and direct patient care. They work closely with other healthcare professionals to ensure an integrated and coordinated service to patients and service users (Department of Health 2010).

In the UK these roles play a significant part in recent NHS England service development aimed at ensuring patients are seen by 'the right person, in the right place, first time' (NHS England 2017). These include musculoskeletal triage and review services, such as first-contact practitioner services, which help to accelerate musculoskeletal assessment, investigation, treatment and referral. Patients have the option to see a first-contact practitioner rather than their general practitioner (Langridge 2019). With an ageing population and people experiencing long-term musculoskeletal conditions, these services expand capacity to help meet patient demand (Health Education England 2018).

Within the specialty of orthopaedics and musculoskeletal trauma in many countries, allied healthcare professionals include:

- physiotherapists, including physiotherapy extended-scope practitioners
- occupational therapists
- advanced clinical practitioners
- orthopaedic plaster technicians
- diagnostic radiologists

- clinical specialist biomechanical podiatrists
- orthotists
- prosthetists
- dieticians.

Physiotherapists in musculoskeletal care are concerned with identifying, maximising and maintaining movement and the functional ability and potential of the patient by focusing on health promotion, disease or injury prevention as well as treatment and rehabilitation (Chartered Society of Physiotherapists 2018). The role of the physiotherapist has evolved considerably in recent years along with a range of skills in assessment, diagnosis and management. The emergence of the physiotherapy extended scope practitioner has enabled and improved the treatment of patients, where appropriate, with many extended scope practitioners qualified to request radiological and pathological investigations, interpret results, prescribe medications and refer to other services (Langridge et al. 2015).

Occupational therapists play a fundamental role in recovery and vocational rehabilitation (Blas et al. 2018), working with the orthopaedic multidisciplinary team to meet treatment goals. The role of the occupational therapist in musculoskeletal care is to perform a thorough assessment that facilitates and provides advice to assist the patient to live and work as independently as possible (World Federation of Occupational Therapy 2019). Physical strength and stamina, proper movement and ability can be affected following musculoskeletal disease or injury and subsequent treatment, and occupational therapists work with individuals to promote maximum functional ability so that activities of daily living can be maintained. The occupational therapist will obtain information about the patient's lifestyle abilities prior to injury, illness or surgery to develop a plan of care that will assist the patient in adjusting to their current physical condition. There may be a need for the individual to learn new skills or adapt the way in which they live and/or work to address disability, for example where joint and limb function has been impaired. This is achieved by assisting patients to overcome and manage limitations resulting from their conditions (Prior 2018).

Pharmacists are healthcare professionals who are experts in medicines and how they work, and are concerned with the safe and effective use of medication. Their role encompasses an understanding of the biochemical mechanisms of the action of drugs, the way medicines are selected and supplied, therapeutic roles, side effects, potential drug interactions and monitoring. Pharmacists are directly involved in patient care and use their expertise to work collaboratively within the team to ensure patient safety, experience and outcomes, and improve the quality of all medicine-related practices (Health Education England 2019). Pharmacists may function as

advanced clinical practitioners, undertaking further training to attain skills that include non-medical prescribing, advanced patient assessment, clinical reasoning, decision making and diagnostics (Health Education England 2020).

Musculoskeletal radiology is concerned with the diagnostic imaging and diagnosis of the skeleton and associated soft tissue. Imaging includes X-rays, computed tomography (CT), ultrasound and magnetic resonance imaging (MRI). Radiologists are healthcare professionals who are experts in obtaining and interpreting medical images. They work with other clinicians by reporting findings of examinations and tests, and confer with referring medical staff to recommend further examinations or treatments.

Clinical specialist biomechanical podiatrists perform the biomechanical assessment and examination of lower limb function and gait to look for abnormalities that may cause pain or discomfort resulting from sports injuries, trauma and congenital abnormalities. They can advise on treatment such as orthotics, exercise and footwear to improve lower limb strength and flexibility.

Orthotics and prosthetics are dynamic and diverse allied healthcare professions. They are applied physical disciplines that use assessment, diagnosis and management of the body to address neuromuscular and structural skeletal problems through orthotic appliances and prostheses, including artificial limbs. The orthotist and prosthetist liaise directly with members of the multidisciplinary orthopaedic team to achieve maximum function, prevent further disability and facilitate improved body image and play an important role in advising on the rehabilitation of patients with physical challenges and disabilities (World Health Organisation 2017). Orthoses, usually a brace, splint or special footwear, are designed to provide one or more of the following:

- relieve pressure on a diseased joint or stress in a bone weakened by disease or injury
- correct or prevent physical deformity
- stabilise a joint or several joints
- improve mobility
- protect the joint from further injury.

A member of the multidisciplinary team formulates an orthotic prescription and the orthotist will assess the patient's needs, take measurements, design the orthosis, and then fit and adjust it. This can be an ongoing process for many patients but more so for children and young people due to their growing and changing immature skeletal frame. An essential part of the role is to educate the individual and/or carer in the fitting and using of the device.

The prosthetist provides artificial replacements for individuals who have lost or were born without all or part of a limb and may face disability. The prosthetist will design and select the most suitable prosthesis from a range of components with the aim of enabling the individual to lead a normal life.

Dietitians are regulated health professionals who use "sound evidence, practice, and reasoning" (British Dietetic Association 2017, p.4) to apply expert knowledge of nutrition to support individuals in understanding and applying the principles of healthy eating and maximising nutrition throughout their lifespan. They assess patients' nutritional needs, developing and implementing nutrition programs, thus contributing to health promotion and illness-prevention strategies (British Dietetic Association 2017).

Additional Supporting Team Members

Additional members of the healthcare team that are central to patient care include the following:

- Casting/plaster technicians are members of the wider healthcare team trained in the application, adaptation and removal of casts and splints. At the request of a doctor or appropriate practitioner, a cast or splint may be applied following surgery for orthopaedic conditions or trauma. The post-holder, in consultation with other members of the team, will assess, plan, implement and evaluate epsiodes of care across orthopaedic and trauma services (British Orthopaedic Association 2015).
- Operating department practitioners are an integral part of the operating department multiprofessional team, helping to ensure effective and safe peri-operative care. This incorporates the anaesthetic, surgical and recovery stages of the patient pathway in orthopaedic and trauma care (see Chapter 14).
- Social workers collaborate with the multidisciplinary team on discharge planning to ensure that patients' needs are met in order that they may be discharged from hospital in a safe and timely fashion. They connect patients with support needs and their families to appropriate resources and support to protect them from harm (International Federation of Social Workers 2021).
- Clinical psychologists work mainly in health and social care settings and assist in the assessment of the mental health needs of the patient. They form part of the healthcare team providing expert psychological assessment and strategies where patients require assistance through

---

Box 5.1 Evidence digest: Interventions to improve team effectiveness within health care: a systematic review of the past decade (Buljac-Samardzic et al. 2020).

A systematic review was conducted by the authors to review the literature and assess the impact of all team interventions associated with improving the effectiveness of teams working within healthcare organisations. The authors placed no restrictions on the type or setting of the interventions or the research design employed.

Only peer-reviewed journal articles published in English were included, with a review timeline of between 2008 and July 2018.

The review authors searched seven databases and found 297 relevant articles across acute hospital settings. Primary and other care setting were poorly represented.

The authors conclude that many studies provided a low level of evidence and evaluated interventions focused on improving non-technical skills and provided evidence of improvements.

Four main categories of interventions were identified: training, tools, organisation (re) design and programme.

Training was the principal intervention evaluated and was subdivided to represent (i) predefined principles, such as team resource management, (ii) a specific method such as simulation and (iii) general team training.

Tools focused on the methods employed to structure (SBAR, situation, background, assessment and recommendation), facilitate (communication technology) or trigger (monitoring) teamwork.

Organisational intervention was concerned with the stimulation of team processes and function by redesign, and finally programmes comprise a combination of all three interventions.

The authors conclude that the number of research studies on interventions to improve team effectiveness within healthcare has increased over the past decade.

The authors recommend that future research in this field should:

- include wider healthcare settings
- include alternative interventions which better reflect practice
- explore the long-term effects of these interventions to generate a more informed understanding of factors that influence sustainability
- provide more detail on how interventions are implemented and in what context
- include less frequently used outcomes to help identify critical outcome combinations.

periods of emotional adjustment. This can follow a diagnosis of acute or chronic illness or traumatic injury, and where there is a need to promote, modify, or establish health-inducing behaviours (Beinart et al. 2009; British Psychological Society 2008).

- Multifaith workers ensure the provision of spiritual care, which is an important consideration and a multidisciplinary responsibility. Spiritual care encompasses emotional, psychological, social and pastoral support, together with a requirement to meet the religious needs of the patient.
- Orthopaedic research team delivers evidence-based research and innovation to improve patient care and treatment outcomes.

Conclusion

Healthcare professionals are transforming their practice in response to a rapidly evolving global healthcare system.

The last few decades have seen significant developments in the flexibility, expansion and extension of roles. The purpose of each remains unchanged, seeking to optimise the health and wellbeing of the patient.

With the intension of providing safe, higher quality, patient-centred care, individual practitioners work together as a team to promote the sharing of ideas, values and common goals to execute their duties and responsibilities effectively.

Promoting a culture of teamwork within an organisation increases learning opportunities, accountability, productivity, communication and collaboration. Box 5.1 provides an evaluation and summary of interventions to improve the effectiveness of team working within health care.

Each role contributes a unique and equally important set of complementary skills to ensure the seamless and timely delivery of care. This division of labour allows for the development of specialised skills and knowledge so that the right person undertakes the right task at the right time across the continuum of orthopaedic and trauma pathways of care.

Further Reading

Drinka, T.J.K. and Clark, P.G. (2016). *Healthcare Teamwork: Interprofessional Practice and Education*, 2e. Praeger.

Firstenberg, M.S. and Stawicki, S.P. (ed.) (2021). *Teamwork in Healthcare*. IntechOpen ISBN 9781838810283.

McGee, P. and Inman, C. (2019). *Advanced Practice in Healthcare. Dynamic Developments in Nursing and the Allied Health Professions*, 4e. Oxford: Wiley Blackwell.

Zajac, S., Woods, A., Tannenbaum, S. et al. (2021). Overcoming challenges to teamwork in healthcare: a team effectiveness framework and evidence-based guidance. *Frontiers in Communication* 6: 1–20. https://www.frontiersin.org/article/10.3389/fcomm.2021.606445.

References

Academy of Medical Royal Colleges (2020). *Developing professional identity in multi-professional teams*. www.aomrc.org.uk/wpcontent/uploads/2020/05/Developing_professional_identity_inmulti-professional_teams_0520.pdf (accessed 17 July 2021).

Beinart, H., Kennedy, P., and Llewelyn, S. (2009). *Clinical Psychology in Practice*. Oxford: Blackwell.

Blas, A.J.T., Beltran, K.M.B., and Martinez, P.G.V. et al. (2018). Enabling Work: Occupational Therapy Interventions for Persons with Occupational Injuries and Diseases: A Scoping Review. *Journal of Occupational Rehabilitation* 28: 201–214.

British Dietetic Association (2017). *Code of Professional Conduct*. www.bda.uk.com/uploads/assets/ef8656c5-320e-4d8d-b5c7ff7c82519d47/Code-of-Conduct.pdf.

British Orthopaedic Association (2015). *Casting Standards*. www.boa.ac.uk/uploads/assets/uploaded/

83dcfe25-307e-4e82-abf362976f08a3ae.pdf (accessed 19 September 2021).

British Psychological Society (2008). *Briefing paper No. 27. Clinical Health Psychologists in the NHS*. The British Psychological Society.

Buljac-Samardzic, M., Doekhie, K.D., and van Wijngaarden, J. (2020). Interventions to improve team effectiveness within health care: a systematic review of the past decade. *Human Resources for Health* 18 (1): 2. doi: 10.1186/s12960-019-0411-3.

Burton, A., Davis, C.M., Boateng, H. et al. (2020). A multidisciplinary approach to expedite surgical hip fracture care. *Geriatric Orthopaedic Surgery & Rehabilitation* 11: 1–9.

Chamberlain-Salaun, J., Mills, J., and Usher, K. (2013). Terminology used to describe health care teams: an integrative review of the literature. *Journal of Multidisciplinary Healthcare* 6: 65–74.

Chartered Society of Physiotherpay (2018) First Contact Posts in General Practice: An implementation guide. www.csp. org.uk/system/files?file=001404_fcp_guidance_england_ 2018.pdf.

Choi, B.C.K. and Pak, A.W.P. (2006). Multidisciplinarity, interdisciplinarity and transdisciplinarity in health research, services, education and policy: 1. Definitions, objectives, and evidence of effectiveness. *Clinical and Investigative Medicine* 29 (6): 351–364.

Choi, B.C.K. and Pak, A.W.P. (2007). Multidisciplinarity, interdisciplinarity and transdisciplinarity in health research, services, education and policy: 2. Promotors, barriers and strategies of enhancement. *Clinical and Investigative Medicine* 30 (6): 224–232.

Cunninghan, U., Ward, M.E., De Brún, A., and McAuliffe, E. (2018). Team interventions in acute hospital contexts: a systematic search of the literature using realist synthesis. *BMC Health Services Research* 18: 536.

(1999). Department of Health. In: *Nurse, Midwife and Health Visitor Consultants. Establishing Posts and Making Appointments. Health Service Circular*. London: Department of Health.

Department of Health (2010). *Advanced Level Nursing: A Position Statement*. London: Department of Health.

Ellis, G. and Sevdalis, N. (2019). Understanding and improving multidisciplinary team working in geriatric medicine. *Age and Ageing* 48: 498–505. https://doi. org/10.1093/ageing/afz021.

Falaschi, P. and Marsh, D. (ed.) (2020). *Orthogeriatrics: The Management of Older Patients with Fragility Fractures*, 2e. Cham: Springer.

Fazio, S., Pace, D., Flinner, J., and Kallmyer, B. (2018). The fundamentals of person-centred care for individuals with dementia. *The Gerontologist* 58 (suppl_1): 10–19.

Finn, R., Learmonth, M., and Reedy, P. (2010). Some unintended effects of teamwork in healthcare. *Social Science and Medicine* 70 (8): 1148–1154.

Fulop, N. and Robert, G. (2015). *Context for Successful Quality Improvement*. London: The Health Foundation.

Gilburt, H. (2016). Supporting integration through new roles and working across boundaries. King's Fund, London. https://www.Kingsfund.org.uk/publications/ supporting-integration-new-roles-boundaries.

Gittell, J.H., Fairfield, K.M., Bierbaum, B. et al. (2000). Impact of relational co-ordination on quality of care, post-operative pain and functioning and length of stay: a nine hospital study of surgical patients. *Medical Care* 38 (8): 807–819.

Gittell, J.H., Weinberg, D., Pfefferle, S., and Bishop, C. (2008). Impact of relational coordination on job satisfaction and quality outcomes: a study of nursing homes. *Human Resource Management Journal* 18: 154–170.

Health Education England (2017). *Multi-professional framework for advanced practice in England* (Online). https://www.hee.nhs.uk/sites/default/files/documents/ multi-professionalframeworkforadvancedclinicalpracticein england.pdf.

Health Education England (2018). *Musculoskeletal First Contact Services Implementation Guide*. https://www.hee. nhs.uk/sites/default/files/documents/FCP%20How%20 to%20Guide%20v21%20040919%20-%202.pdf.

Health Education England (2019). *Advancing pharmacy education and training: a review* (Online). https://www. hee.nhs.uk/sites/default/files/documents/Advancing%20 Pharmacy%20Education%20and%20Training%20 Review.pdf.

Health Education England (2020). *Navigating advanced pharmacist practice*. https://psnc.org.uk/sheffield-Ipc./ wp-content/uploads/sites/79/2021/03/Advanced- pharmacist-Practice-Handbook-Dec-2020-2.pdf.

Howell, A.M., Panesar, S.S., Burns, E.M. et al. (2014). Reducing the burden of surgical harm: a systematic review of the interventions used to reduce adverse events in surgery. *Annals of Surgery* 259: 630–641. PubMed: 24368639.

Hughes, A.M., Gregory, M.E., Joseph, D.L. et al. (2016). Saving lives: a meta-analysis of team training in healthcare. *Journal of Applied Psychology* 101: 1266.

Internationl Federwtion of Social Workers (2021). *Global definition of social work*. Retrieved from http://ifsw.org/ policies/definition-of-social-work.

Jemal, K., Hailu, D., Mekonnen, M. et al. (2021). The importance of compassion and respectful care for the health workforce: a mixed-methods study. *Journal of Public Health* 1–12. https://doi.org/10.1007/s10389-021-01495-0.

Jester, R., Santy, J., and Rogers, J. (2021). *Oxford Handbook of Trauma and Orthopaedic Nursing*, 2e. Oxford: Oxford University Press.

Jovanovic, S., Stankovic, M., Kilibarda, T. et al. (2020). The terminology use to describe teamwork in the health care system. *A Literature Review. Acta Medica Medianae* 59 (4): 13–19.

Kaltner, M., Murtagh, D., Bennetts, M. et al. (2017). Randomised control trial of a transprofessional healthcare role interventionin an acute medical setting. *Journal of Interprofessional Care* 31 (2): 190–198.

Kaini, B.K. (2017). Interprofessional Team Collaboration in Health Care. *Global Journal of Medical Research* 17 (2). Version 1.0. Online ISSN 2249-4618 & Print ISSN 0975-5888.

Klevens, R.M., Edwards, J.R., Richards, C.L. Jr. et al. (2007). Estimating health care-associated infections and deaths in US hospitals, 2002. *Public Health Reports* 122: 160–166. PubMed: 17357358.

Kringos, D.S., Sunol, R., Wagner, C. et al. (2015). The influence of context on the effectiveness of hospital quality improvement strategies: a review of systematic reviews. *BMC Health Services Research* 15: 277.

Langridge, N. (2019). The skills, knowledge and attributes needed as a first-contact physiotherapist in musculoskeletal healthcare. *Musculoskeletal Care* 17: 253–260.

Langridge, N., Roberts, L., and Pope, C. (2015). The clinical reasoning processes of extended scope physiotherapists assessing patients with low back pain. *Manual Therapy* 20 (6): 745–750.

Lemieux-Charles, L. and McGuire, W.L. (2006). What do we know about health care team effectiveness? A review of the literature. *Medical Care Research and Review* 63: 263–300.

Miake-Lye, I.M., Hempel, S., Ganz, D.A., and Shekelle, P.G. (2013). Inpatient fall prevention programs as a patient safety strategy: a systematic review. *Annals of Internal Medicine* 158: 390–396. PubMed: 23460095.

NHS England (2017). *Transforming musculoskeletal and orthopaedic elective care services. A handbook for local health and care systems.* https://www.england.nhs.uk/wp-content/uploads/2017/11/msk-orthopaedic-elective-care-handbook-v2.pdf (accessed 10 August 2021).

Nursing and Midwifery Council (2020). *Standards of Proficiency for Registered Nursing Associates.* London: Nursing and Midwifery Council www.nmc.org.uk (accessed 17 July 2021).

Prior, Y. (2018). The contribution of occupational therapy in the care of people with musculoskeletal diseases. *Rheumatology* 57 (3): https://doi.org/10.1093/rheumatology/key075.072.

Rosen, M.A., DiazGranados, D., Dietz, A.S. et al. (2018). Teamwork in healthcare: key discoveries enabling safer, high quality care. *American Psychology* 73 (4): 433–450.

Royal College of Surgeons (2014). *The Curriculum Framework for the Surgical Care Practitioner.* http://accreditation.rcseng.ac.uk/pdf/SCP%20Curriculum%20Framework%202014.pdf (accessed 15 September 2021).

Sacks, G.D., Shannon, E.M., Dawes, A.J. et al. (2015). Teamwork, communication and safety climate: a systematic review of interventions to improve surgical culture. *BMJ Quality and Safety* 0: 1–10.

Solheim, K., McElmurray, B., and Kim, M. (2007). Multidisciplinary teamwork in US primary health care. *Social Science and Medicine* 65 (3): 622–634.

The King's Fund (2018). *Transformational change in health and care reports from the field.* www.kingsfund.org.uk/sites/default/files/2018-05/Transformational_change_King's_Fund_May_2018_0.pdf.

Tzenalis, A. and Sotiriadou, C. (2010). Health promotion as multi-professional and multi-disciplinary work. *International Journal of Caring Sciences* 3 (2): 49–55.

Van Bewer, V. (2017). Transdisciplinarity in health care: a concept analysis. *Nursing Forum* 52 (4): 339–347.

Wald, H.S. (2015). Professional identity (trans)formation in medical education. *Academic Medicine* 90 (6): 701–706. https://doi.org/10.1097/ACM.000000000000073.

Weaver, S.J., Dy, S.M., and Rosen, M.A. (2014). Team-training in healthcare: a narrative synthesis of the literature. *British Medical Journal Quality & Safety* 23: 359–372.

World Federation of Occupational Therapy (2019). *Position Statement: Occupational Therapy and Rehabilitation.* World Federation of Occupational Therapy. https://www.wfot.org/ResourceCentre.aspx.

World Health Organization (2017). *Rehabilitation 2030: A call for action.* Meeting report. World Health Organization, Geneva. https://www.who.int/disabilities/care/Rehab2030MeetingReport2.pdf?ua=1 (accessed 8 November 2021).

6

Rehabilitation and the Orthopaedic and Musculoskeletal Trauma Patient

Rebecca Jester

Royal College of Surgeons Ireland Medical University, Manama, Bahrain

Introduction

The aim of this chapter is to provide an evidence-based discussion of rehabilitation of the orthopaedic and trauma patient. There are many patients who require and will benefit from prehabilitation and/or rehabilitation and some specific examples will be provided within this chapter and within other condition-specific chapters. Where robust evidence exists, there will be a critical application of research to approaches to rehabilitation. However, to date there is limited high-level evidence to support many aspects of patient rehabilitation within trauma and orthopaedics. There are five relevant Cochrane systematic reviews relating to rehabilitation for trauma/orthopaedic patients. Cameron et al.' (2009) review compared coordinated multidisciplinary approaches to rehabilitation of older patients with proximal femoral fractures to usual orthopaedic care, and Smith et al. (2020) compared enhanced rehabilitation and care models for adults with dementia following hip fracture surgery (these reviews are discussed in more detail in Box 6.1). Mason et al.'s (2012) review included two trials related to rehabilitation following hamstring injuries, Handoll and Elliot (2015) examined rehabilitation following distal radial fractures in adults and Peters et al. (2021) studied rehabilitation following surgery for flexor tendon injuries of the hand (these reviews are discussed in more detail in Boxes 6.2 and 6.3).

Rehabilitation for orthopaedic and trauma patients is a very broad topic and to facilitate a manageable search for evidence the key words (and synonyms and truncation terms) rehabilitation, orthopaedic, trauma, settings, enhanced recovery pathways and pre-habilitation were used in the Cochrane database and Web of Science. The information within this chapter is therefore based on evidence from the following sources: Cochrane reviews, systematic reviews and meta-analyses, individual research papers from Web of Science, formal education, symposia, conference presentations, non-research publications, expert opinion and reflections on clinical experience (of the author and other clinical experts).

History and Context of Rehabilitation

Rehabilitation is a process that aims to optimise a patient's full recovery potential following an episode of illness, trauma or surgery. Mauk (2012) offers the following definition:

> Rehabilitation is a process of adaptation or recovery through which an individual suffering from a disabling or functionally limiting condition, whether temporary or irreversible, participates to regain maximal function, independence and restoration. (p. 2)

There are two key misconceptions about rehabilitation to be cognisant of. First, rehabilitation is not a place, it is a process. Hence, to state 'the patient is waiting to go to rehabilitation' is a misnomer and furthermore is detrimental to the patient as the rehabilitation process should begin as soon as the patient is medically stable. Second, there is frequently a misconception that rehabilitation is about restoring the individual to their pre-injury/surgery status. This is not always possible, and a significant aspect of rehabilitation is to support the patient and their family to adapt to a change in their functional ability. Rehabilitation has several key goals, including:

- restoration of optimum function (physical, social and psychological)
- to promote and sustain maximum independence and provide assistance where care deficits exist
- facilitation of adaptation when return to former health status or function is not possible

- psychological support for the patient and their family who have experienced trauma, change or loss (in the context of the loss of the former self)
- prevention and early detection of complications
- supporting the patient to meet their short-, medium- and long-term goals
- creating enabling environments to facilitate independence and social integration
- education of the patient and informal carers to understand their condition and ongoing treatment and management strategies
- promote self-management and patient empowerment
- optimising health and quality of life (including pain management).

The concept of rehabilitation in healthcare is not a new phenomenon. The importance of restoring function following trauma has been evident over many centuries, particularly during war and conflict. Florence Nightingale pioneered rehabilitation as a nursing concept during the Crimean War. Many developments in prosthetics, assistive devices, mobility aids, new treatments and therapies have been as a direct result of the need to support those wounded in conflict as either service men and women or civilian causalities and to facilitate, when possible, military personnel's return to active duty. Sadly, in contemporary society, the world continues to be plagued by conflict, war and terrorism, and the need for evidence-based rehabilitation has never been greater.

Prehabilitation

Prehabilitation is defined as the process of care initiated pre-operatively to optimise patients' physical, nutritional, physical and mental health prior to surgery with the aim of maximising post-operative outcomes and minimising complications. Prehabilitation has become increasingly utilised globally for patients undergoing procedures such as total hip arthroplasty (THA) and total knee arthroplasty (TKA), typically focusing on improving muscle strength around the hip/knee being replaced, and requires patients to participate in home- or outpatient-based exercise programmes for 4 to 8 weeks (Jahic et al. 2018). Evidence for the effectiveness of prehabilitation exercise and education is provided in Box 6.1.

Models of Care

Many of those requiring rehabilitation will have either a permanent or temporary disability. In recent years, there has been a realisation and acknowledgement that disabled people are not the problem, the problem is the way that

---

> **Box 6.1   Evidence of Efficacy of Prehabilitation for Patients Undergoing THA and TKA**
>
> A systematic review and meta-analysis by Moyer et al. (2017) reviewed 35 studies related to the longitudinal effects and efficacy of prehabilitation on postoperative outcomes following THA or TKA and concluded overall effect sizes for prehabilitation were small to moderate. In TKA patients significant improvements in function, quadriceps strength and length of stay were reported. In THA patients pain, function and length of stay were significantly improved.

society is organised to discriminate against those individuals with a disability (Jester 2007). In the UK (and reflected in the law in other parts of the world), the Disability Discrimination Act of 1995 has supported the view that it is a societal responsibility to prohibit less favourable treatment of people with a disability. The Act gave new rights in relation to access to goods, services and facilities, employment and buying or renting land or property and has supported the social model of disability where the onus is on society to make adjustments and support those with a disability. Crosby and Jackson (2000) summarised what disabled people have identified as their fundamental needs to be able to live independently:

- information about choices
- peer support and counselling
- appropriate housing, which you can access, move about in and live in, and which is in the right place
- equipment to support you to do the things you want to do
- personal assistance to facilitate independence
- accessible transport
- access to the built environment.

Healthcare practitioners have a key responsibility to provide information about enabling environments and patient's rights under the Disability Discrimination Act, and to signpost patients and their families to further information and services to optimise their independence. Apart from the social model of disability, practitioners need to have an applied working knowledge of frameworks and models that embrace maximising patient independence, promote a focus on health and wellbeing, and support patients and families to cope with change and make adaptations. Neuman's systems model (Neuman 1982) focuses on the impact of illness and disability on both the patient and the informal caregiver, and is based on their identification of inherent stressors and personal strengths, which can be recruited to aid coping and adaptation. Roy's adaptation model (Roy 1984) focuses on modes of adaptation, which include physiological role function, self-concept and interdependence modes. Both of these models lend themselves well to orthopaedic and trauma care generally, but are particularly pertinent in the rehabilitation phase.

There has been a realisation that it is both undesirable and unfeasible to promote paternalistic models of healthcare support for individuals with chronic disease and/or disability. A self-management model is preferable where individuals with chronic disease and/or disability embrace an internal locus of control for their own health and wellbeing. Self-management requires education and preparation of the individual and Redman (2004) suggests self-management programmes must use problem-based learning approaches and include skill development in problem solving, development of clinical judgement, self-efficacy building, and belief modification and symptom reinterpretation.

The Rehabilitation Process

Rehabilitation should begin as soon as the patient is medically stable enough to engage with it. It is important to emphasise that the patient and their family (if appropriate) are viewed as equal partners with practitioners within the rehabilitation process and not as passive recipients. Rehabilitation is best viewed as a cyclical process beginning with comprehensive assessment, agreeing short-, medium- and long-term goals, development of a collaborative plan to work towards the goals and evaluation of progress. As the patient achieves goals either partially or fully then the cycle begins again with reassessment.

Assessment

Comprehensive assessment is the first stage of the rehabilitation process. It is essential to gather data to form a baseline to measure progress against and ascertain the patient's support systems and home situation. The patient may be entering the rehabilitative phase within the same unit as their acute episode of treatment. In that case, the team will already have assessed the patient and have relevant information about the health status and social situation. If the patient is transferred from acute services to rehabilitation in another setting, a more comprehensive rehabilitation-focused assessment will be needed. A comprehensive discussion of assessment in trauma and orthopaedics is provided in Chapter 7, but an assessment within the context of rehabilitation needs to have a stronger psycho/social focus than the typical medical model. Hoeman (2008) suggests that assessment within the rehabilitation phase should have a specific focus on functional skills, psychosocial

status, environment and financial status. There are a number of models that lend themselves to rehabilitation, including Roy's adaptation model (Roy 1984) and Orem's (Orem 2001) self-care deficit model.

Goal Setting

Goal setting is not generally used in the acute care setting where the nursing process tends to focus on the identification of actual or potential patient problems. Goals have the following characteristics:

- Goals are positive statements of intent with associated time frames.
- Goals should be realistic and achievable, but at the same time provide appropriate challenge to the patient to give them something to strive and work towards.
- Goals should be discussed and agreed with the patient and family/significant others if appropriate and progress towards goals regularly reviewed and documented.

It is good practice for the goals to be a combination of short-, medium- and long-term as achievement of short-term goals can help to motivate the patient to push towards the medium- and long-term goals. For example, the patient with a traumatic amputation of a lower limb may have a short-term goal of being able to stand for a short period with their new/temporary prosthesis, a medium-term goal of walking up and down stairs with their prosthetic limb and a long-term goal of returning to a sport such as horse riding using their prosthesis.

Developing an Implementation Plan and Evaluation

Once goals have been mutually agreed between the patient and multidisciplinary team (MDT), a plan to support the achievement of the goals needs to be developed and reviewed on a daily basis. The plan should make explicit the roles and required actions of the patient/family and each member of the MDT to achieve the goals. It must be agreed which member/s of the team has the best skills and expertise to support the patient with each particular goal (Jester 2007). Often nurses will have an important continuing function with all of the goals due to their 24-hour presence with the patient. Realistic time scales should also be agreed between the MDT and the patient and then documented. It is important that the plan minimises the use of jargon and is understandable to the lay person. Treatment and therapies planned should be evidence-based and advantages, potential disadvantages and associated risk should be discussed with the patient for their consent to participate to be considered informed.

Progress towards achievement of the agreed goals needs to be reviewed on a regular basis. The process of evaluation should be shared between the MDT, patient and family where appropriate. Evaluation involves the gathering of both objective and subjective measurements to make an informed decision regarding change in the patient's function and status. Subjective data include seeking the patient's own perceptions, typically through self-reported generic health-related quality of life and disease-specific measures (which are discussed later within this chapter and are defined in Chapter 7) along with pain assessment. Objective data include clinician-measured function, movement and physiological parameters; examples of these are provided later within this chapter. Once evaluation has been completed new goals can be set or adjustments made to existing goals.

Team Approaches to Rehabilitation

Effective team working is one of the most important factors in successful rehabilitation, but it is important to understand what is meant by team working and the different approaches such as multidisciplinary, interdisciplinary and transdisciplinary, and their cognate advantages and disadvantages (see Box 6.2). A description and comparison of these approaches is provided in Table 6.1. There is a move away from multidisciplinary working towards transdisciplinary and interdisciplinary because increasingly rehabilitation is provided in the community setting, which requires team members to have a wider repertoire of skills than the traditional professional-specific model. Multiskilling between nurses and therapists is becoming common, particularly in 'hospital at home' schemes, as it is not cost-effective or desirable for the patient for discreet professions to make multiple visits. The team involved in rehabilitation of the trauma/orthopaedic patient typically involves nurses, healthcare and therapy assistants, physiotherapists, occupational therapists, social workers, medical practitioners and orthotists. Other professionals such as dieticians and psychologists may be included if the patient's goals require their input. It is essential that practitioners fully embrace the patient and if appropriate family or informal carers as legitimate members of the team.

The Role of the Nurse

Nurses make a unique contribution to the rehabilitation process and yet continue to struggle to articulate what their contributions and roles are. Conversely, the contribution of

---

Box 6.2 Evidence Digest: Multidisciplinary approaches for inpatient rehabilitation

Co-ordinated multidisciplinary approaches for inpatient rehabilitation of older patients with proximal femoral fractures (Review) (Cameron et al. 2009).

A Cochrane systematic review conducted by Cameron et al. (2009), which included nine trials, examined the effects of co-ordinated multidisciplinary inpatient rehabilitation, compared with usual (orthopaedic) care, for older patients with hip fracture and concluded there tended to be better combined outcomes (mortality and reduced function necessitating institutional care) for patients receiving co-ordinated inpatient rehabilitation, but the results were not statistically significant and the results were heterogeneous.

A Cochrane review carried out by O Smith et al. (2020) aimed to assess the effectiveness of models of care, including enhanced rehabilitation strategies designed specifically for people with dementia following hip fracture surgery, and included seven trials with 555 participants. The review reported there was low certainty that enhanced care and rehabilitation in hospital may reduce rates of postoperative delirium and very low certainty associating it with lower rates of some other complications. There was also low certainty that compared to orthopaedic-led management, geriatrician-led management may lead to shorter hospital stays. Further research is required to establish if rehabilitation models designed specifically for people with dementia are more effective than usual hip fracture rehabilitation services. This is an important aspect of evidence as 40% of hip fracture patients have dementia or cognitive impairment.

---

therapists, social workers, physicians and psychologists is well defined within the literature (Jester 2007). Waters (1996) considered the role of nurses to be secondary to that of other members of the MDT and comprise three main components:

- general maintenance, including overall ward management and maintenance of patients' physical wellbeing in terms of nutrition, hygiene and skin care
- expertise in areas such as tissue viability, continence and pain management
- carry-on role, i.e. nurses maintain the progress made by therapists over the 24-hour period, e.g. mobility and dressing practice.

The description of the nurse's role offered by Waters (1996) underestimates the essential nature of these fundamental aspects of the rehabilitation process. Specifically, the patient who has unmanaged pain or develops sepsis

Table 6.1 Description and summary of key differences between multidisciplinary, interdisciplinary and transdisciplinary approaches to team working

Multidisciplinary team	Interdisciplinary team	Transdisciplinary team
Independent profession-specific assessments of the patient	Shared assessment documentation and sharing of assessment data to avoid repetition	The primary clinician will lead the assessment but draw on the expertise of other team members as appropriate
Clearly demarcated role boundaries	Blurring of professional boundaries and more multiskilling between professional groups	Members of the team cross-train and develop a portfolio of skills that transcend traditional professional role descriptors
Communication is more vertical than lateral and team conferences do not usually take place	Regular communication in the form of goal review and case conferences	The primary clinician acts as the communication coordinator, but communication is open and non-hierarchal
Each member of the team usually works independently to achieve discipline-specific goals	Goals are patient-centred and shared with all members to work towards	Goals are patient-centred and team members are often cross-trained to work towards the goals
Each member of the team retains their own records for individual patients	Use of integrated care pathways and shared documentation	Records tend to be patient-held and updated in partnership with the patient and family
Team leader tends to nearly always be a medical doctor	Team leader not profession-specific, but based on the leader having the most appropriate experience, skills and leadership, and coordination abilities	One team member designated as the primary clinician for the patient, but is guided by other professionals as required

from pressure ulcers is not going to be able to fully commit to working towards their rehabilitation goals. Nurses also have a fundamental role in assessing and managing the risk of complications such as infection, pressure ulcers and venous thromboembolism, which pose a serious threat to the patient's wellbeing and ability to progress with their rehabilitation.

Nurses are still predominantly the only professional group to have a 24-hour presence and work over the 7-day week. This allows them to develop a strong therapeutic relationship with the patient and be sensitive and observant to small, but potentially significant changes in the patient's condition. Nurses are likely to be the only profession available to speak to and update families during visiting times about progress in the rehabilitation process. This unique 24-hour presence also enables the nurse to see how the patient functions over the 24-hour period. This can provide a valuable insight into the patient's readiness for discharge. For example, the patient who is safe and independent during the day may become disorientated and have a propensity to fall during the night.

Traditionally nurses working with patients in the acute phase of their care provide assistance with the activities of daily living that the patient is too unwell to do for themselves. Within the restorative phase, however, the nurse needs to optimise independence and to encourage the patient to do as much for themselves as possible. The transition from direct caring to a more supportive 'hands-off' approach can be difficult for both patients and nurses to come to terms with. A study by Ellul et al. (1993) reported that when nurses incorporated the skills patients were learning in therapy sessions into everyday aspects of the patient's care, it resulted in a 55% increase in the time that patients spent engaged in meaningful therapeutic activity contributing towards achievement of their goals.

To date the nursing role in rehabilitation remains underdeveloped, partly through a relatively low emphasis on rehabilitation within the pre-qualifying nursing curriculum and few opportunities at postgraduate/post-registration level. This may also be due to nursing being unable to clearly articulate the value of its role in rehabilitation compared to other professionals such as therapists. However, rehabilitation as a specialism is gaining momentum. The potential role of nurses in rehabilitation, if they were afforded better support and education to develop the requisite skills, was summarised in the work of Nolan et al. (1997), who suggested the following role contributions:

- assessment of physical condition, delivery of evidence-based care and prevention of complications
- education/counselling
- psychosocial interventions
- support and education of family carers
- coordinating, liaison and facilitating transition.

Clare (2018) described the rôle of the nurse in stroke rehabilitation and emphasised that providing support to families and carers is a particularly important element of caring for people who have experienced a stroke. This can equally apply to nurses supporting patients' rehabilitation after orthopaedic interventions and trauma.

The Royal College of Nursing (2007) guidance on the role of the rehabilitation nurse outlines eight categories where the nurse can positively influence rehabilitation:

- essential nursing skills
- therapeutic practice
- coordination
- education
- empowerment and advocacy
- clinical governance
- political awareness
- advice and counselling.

Psychological Support in Rehabilitation

Both the work of Nolan et al. (1997) and the Royal College of Nursing guidelines (2007) have emphasised the importance of the nurse in providing psychological support to patients engaged in rehabilitation. Many trauma and orthopaedic patients who require rehabilitation will have some degree of altered body image. Body image is defined by Schilder (1935) as:

> the picture of our body which we form in our mind, that is to say the way in which our body appears to ourselves (p. 17)

Price (1990) identified dimensions of body image (perception, cognition, social and aesthetic) and proposed a five-dimensional model of body image comprising three body concepts (Table 6.2) and two mitigating personal responses to change or threat to the body concepts: personal coping strategies and our social support network.

Price (1990) recommends that for the individual to have an acceptable self-body image, an equilibrium needs to be maintained between the three concepts and two personal responses. The trauma and orthopaedic patient may have severe threats to their body concepts due to temporary or permanent changes to their body such as scoliosis, limb shortening due to hip pathology, amputation, scarring from surgery or trauma, need for an

Table 6.2 Body concepts (Price 1990)

Body concepts
1) Body reality: the body as it really is
2) Body ideal: beliefs about how the body should be
3) Body presentation: how the body is presented to the outside world (how we dress, use of cosmetics, wigs, etc.)

external fixator, casts and the use of walking/mobility aids. The impact of alterations of body image should be explored with the patient and appropriate support put in place. This may be to empower the patient to optimise self-help and informal support through support groups and family/social support or referral to counselling and psychotherapy.

Trauma and Orthopaedic Conditions Requiring Rehabilitation

The need for rehabilitation will exponentially rise as the demographic profile of the population continues to age. Those requiring trauma and orthopaedic care will range from the very young child to older people. For example, the infant born with congenital orthopaedic conditions such as osteogenesis imperfecta (brittle bone disease) will need lifelong support to optimise function and minimise disability. Broadly, the type of conditions that require rehabilitation to optimise function can be categorised as:

- acute onset, for example fractures, bone tumours, osteomyelitis and soft tissue injury such as ligament ruptures
- gradual onset with relapsing course, for example rheumatoid arthritis and low back pain
- acute onset with constant course, such as spinal cord injury, traumatic amputation and ankylosing spondylitis
- gradual onset and progressive course, such as osteoarthritis (OA), bone and joint tuberculosis and degenerative spondylolisthesis.

Nurses working within trauma and orthopaedics with very young infants through to older people require knowledge, skills and competence in rehabilitation no matter where the care setting might be. Boxes 6.3 and 6.4 provide examples of evidence-based rehabilitation following acute onset conditions.

Rehabilitation Settings

Traditionally, rehabilitation for trauma and orthopaedic patients was delivered within the in-patient setting either within the same unit as the acute phase of care or following transfer to a specialist rehabilitation facility. The second of these options frequently led to the rehabilitation phase not being instigated until the patient was transferred and had a deleterious impact on patient outcomes and length of stay. There has been an increasing emphasis on shortening hospital length of stay for many patients following procedures such as joint replacement surgery or surgical fixation for hip fractures by the implementation

---

Box 6.3   Evidence Digest

Handoll and Elliot's (2015) Cochrane review of 26 randomised controlled trials (RCTs) examined the effects of rehabilitation interventions for adults with distal radial fractures treated conservatively or surgically. They concluded the level of evidence across included trials was low or very low quality based on GRADE criteria indicating considerable uncertainty about the findings. Rehabilitation started during immobilisation of the fracture in seven of the RCTs and post-immobilisation in the remaining 19 trials. There was very low quality evidence of improved hand function for patients that received hand therapy during immobilisation compared to patients who received instruction only at 4 days following cast removal. There was low quality evidence that patients who received physiotherapy post-immobilisation had better short-term hand function compared to patients receiving just instruction on home exercise from a surgeon or a progressive home exercise programme.

Box 6.4   Evidence Digest

Peters et al. (2021) reviewed 16 RCTs and one quasi RCT which focused on any post-operative rehabilitation intervention compared to another rehabilitation intervention, placebo, control or no intervention for patients who had undergone surgery for flexor tendon injuries of the hand. Ten studies evaluated one each of eight different hand exercise programmes. The other seven studies evaluated a variety of other rehabilitation approaches, such as laser therapy, in which light is directed at the tendons to encourage healing, ultrasound, in which sound waves are directed at the tendons to encourage healing, and a wearable machine (exoskeleton) designed to assist people in their movements. The review concluded there was very little evidence about the benefits and risks of different rehabilitation approaches and further robust RCTs are required.

---

of enhanced recovery pathways sometimes referred to as fast-track pathways. Fast-track is a multidisciplinary process beginning before surgery that continues after discharge and has become a predictable and safe reality (Specht et al. 2018). Fast-track aims to supply best evidence practice and seeks to optimise pre-operative patient information, multimodal opioid-sparing analgesia, fluid management/nutrition and rehabilitation (Husted 2012). Although fast-track has been found to be highly effective, Specht et al. (2018) reported patients in the home stage of the process were not sufficiently involved in their discharge planning and this led to feelings of uncertainty and being left on their own after discharge, which affected their pain management and concordance with exercise regimens at home. Models of care such as fast-track have further increased the shift of rehabilitation into patients' homes and outpatient settings (Jester et al. 2021). This shift has, in part, been due to a systematic reduction in the number of hospital beds available and the realisation that prolonged hospitalisation is not therapeutically beneficial for many, specifically children and older adults. Another influencing factor is that community rehabilitation is less costly and is also more realistic in the patient's own home (Jester 2007).

There appears to be a growing body of evidence to support home-based rehabilitation compared to hospital-based alternatives. A summary of the evidence is provided in Box 6.5. However, it is important to remember that home-based interventions often require the patient to have sufficient family/informal carer support to be eligible for 'hospital at home' schemes. Smith (1999) recommended that decisions about location of rehabilitation services should consider:

- appropriateness or relevance of the service for the patient, for example home-based rehabilitation may be more realistic for some individuals, but for others their levels of social support may present risk for home-based interventions
- equity: there should be equal access to rehabilitation that is not dependent on locality
- accessibility: this relates to issues of physical accessibility as discussed earlier within this chapter and issues such as waiting times for specialist rehabilitation services
- acceptability: the degree to which the rehabilitation service meets the expectations of the patient.

Within contemporary healthcare, commissioners often make decisions about setting up or discontinuation of services based on cost-effectiveness and patient choice, and preference may not always be considered. Jester (2003) urged that decisions regarding rehabilitation setting following joint arthroplasty of the knee and hip should take into consideration patient preference, their locus of control and support systems, and that the orthopaedic nurse has a key role in advocating for patient choice regarding location of their rehabilitation.

Home-based rehabilitation means that patients are often required to exercise unsupervised and this can lead to feelings of uncertainty or a lack of motivation

Box 6.5 Evidence Digest: The Setting for Rehabilitation

A study by Jester and Hicks (2003a) of 'hospital at home' (HaH) services and inpatient units in the rehabilitation phase following hip and knee replacement surgery (THR and TKR) reported that HaH was found to be significantly more effective in terms of patient satisfaction and reduced joint stiffness and at least as effective as in patient care in relation to levels of joint pain, joint function and incidence of post-operative complications. The study also included the views of family carers and reported that of the 21 family carers interviewed all would choose HaH in preference to inpatient care. Jester and Hicks (2003b) also reported HaH was more cost-effective than inpatient models because of a reduction of hospital bed days offset against community service costs. An RCT by Siggeirsdottir et al. (2005) also reported home-based rehabilitation was safer and more effective in improving function and quality of life after THR than in-patient rehabilitation.

Mahomed et al. (2008) concluded from a comparison of home- and hospital-based rehabilitation following primary THR and TKR in Canada that there was no difference in pain, functional outcomes or patient satisfaction between patients receiving home-based rehabilitation and those that had inpatient rehabilitation, but found the home-based intervention to be more cost-effective.

Grant et al. (2005) compared home- and hospital-based rehabilitation programmes for patients undergoing anterior cruciate ligament reconstruction and reported improved outcomes at 3 months post-operatively for the home-based rehabilitation group.

(Specht et al. 2018). The nurse has an important role in both patient education about their rehabilitation activities and optimising patient concordance. Checking on patients' progress, concordance and motivation can be achieved by regular phonecalls between nurses and patients rehabilitating at home (Chen et al. 2016). Lack of adherence to exercise and rehabilitation processes will have a deleterious impact on patients' achievement of their rehabilitation goals and increase the risk of complications such as deep vein thrombosis, joint stiffness and reduced range of joint movement (Pozzi et al. 2013). Technology can also assist in supporting patients with rehabilitation in the home setting and this is discussed in further detail below.

The Use of Technology to Support Rehabilitation

There is an increasing use of technology such as applications (apps), Skype and exegames to support patients through their rehabilitation, particularly for patients who are home-based supported by HaH schemes or via outpatient visits. An exergame is played on a video game system and requires the player to move his body to interact with an avatar involved in a movement activity. Digital healthcare devices for rehabilitation have grown exponentially in recent years (Kungwengwe and Evans 2020). They allow patients to practice their own exercises and provide direct feedback during their performance, and motivate them to train more (Ficklscherer et al. 2016). Non-face or virtual support has proliferated due to the COVID-19 pandemic and many rehabilitation services previously delivered on a face-to-face basis have used telehealth interventions to support patients. However, the evidence base for the effectiveness of technology in supporting rehabilitation is still emerging and further long-term research is needed (see Box 6.6). Technology such as apps, Skype and exegames may be used as either standalone rehabilitation modalities or as an adjunct to therapist/nurse interventions. Patients and staff both require training to learn how to use technology modalities in the rehabilitation process and assessment of patients' readiness, ability and willingness is essential.

Summary

This chapter has aimed to demonstrate that most trauma and orthopaedic patients will require some form of rehabilitation and therefore the nurse needs to optimise their role and contribution to the rehabilitation process. Rehabilitation has been defined as a goal-orientated process that should be begin as soon as the patient is medically stable following trauma or elective interventions. A relatively strong evidence base has been presented regarding the choice of rehabilitation settings, with home-based models proving a more cost-effective alternative to inpatient approaches, although the importance of patient choice and consideration of suitability were emphasised. Nurses need to work across the interface of hospital and community settings to support patients through the rehabilitation journey and should ensure they have the requisite skills and knowledge to facilitate this. In addition, the benefits of transdisciplinary team working have been explored where nurses and therapists share and expand their collective repertoire of skills and underpinning knowledge.

Box 6.6   Use of Technology to Support Home-based Rehabilitation

Hinman et al. (2017) conducted a qualitative study of 12 patients with knee OA who received physical therapist-prescribed exercises over Skype. In-depth interviews with patient participants and the physiotherapists administering the intervention described mostly positive experiences using Skype as an intervention model for physical therapist-supervised exercise management of moderate knee OA and concluded Skype is feasible and acceptable, with the potential to increase access to supervised exercise management for people with knee OA, either individually or in combination with traditional in-clinic visits.

Jensen et al. (2019) used a qualitative participatory approach to work in partnership with older hip fracture patients to develop a smart phone application 'app' designed to support the needs of patients following a hip fracture by empowering them to self-care. Twenty hip-fracture patients were educated and supported with their health literacy with the app during their hospital admission and for 3–4 weeks after their discharge. The key findings were that the participants would not have downloaded the app themselves, but found the app being presented for them on a tablet to take home helpful in supporting their rehabilitation following discharge. The study demonstrated that older people who may not be technology minded can benefit from technology to support their health literacy, rehabilitation outcomes and be empowered.

Reis et al. (2019) conducted an umbrella review of previous systematic reviews, meta-analysis and literature reviews that investigated exergame interventions on outcomes such as balance, gait, limb movements and muscle strength in healthy and non-healthy older adults. The review concluded exergaming had a positive effect on balance, gait, muscle strength, upper limb function and dexterity when used as a standalone intervention and when compared to traditional physiotherapy.

Further Reading

Hoeman, S. (2008). *Rehabilitation Nursing: Prevention, Intervention and Outcomes*, 4e. St Louis: Mosby Elsevier.

Jester, R. (2007). *Advancing Practice in Rehabilitation Nursing*. Oxford: Wiley Blackwell.

Mauk, K. (2012). *Rehabilitation Nursing: A Contemporary Approach to Practice*. Sudbury, MA: Jones and Bartlett.

References

Cameron, I., Handoll, H., Finnegan, T. et al. (2009). *Co-ordinated multidisciplinary approaches for inpatient rehabilitation of older patients with proximal femoral fractures (review)*. John Wiley and Sons Ltd. *Cochrane Database of Systematic Reviews* (4).

Chen, M., Li, P., and Lin, F. (2016). Influence of structured telephone follow-up on patient compliance with rehabilitation after total knee arthroplasty. *Patient Preference and Adherence* 10: 257–264. https://doi.org/10.2147/PPA.S102156.

Clare, C.S. (2018). Role of the nurse in stroke rehabilitation. *Nursing Standard* https://doi.org/10.7748/ns.2018.e11194.

Crosby, N. and Jackson, R. (2000). *The Seven Needs and the Social Model of Disability*. Derbyshire: Coalition for Inclusive Living.

Ellul, J., Watkins, C., Ferguson, N., and Barer, D. (1993). Increasing patient engagement in rehabilitation activities. *Clinical Rehabilitation* 7: 297–302.

Ficklscherer, A., Stapf, J., Michael Meissner, K. et al. (2016). Testing the feasibility and safety of the Nintendo Wii gaming console in orthopedic rehabilitation: a pilot randomized controlled study. *Archives of Medical Science* 12 (6): 1273–1278.

Grant, J.A., Mohtadi, N.G., Maitland, M.E., and Zernicke, R.F. (2005). Comparison of home versus physical therapy-supervised rehabilitation programs after anterior cruciate ligament reconstruction: a randomized clinical trial. *The American Journal of Sports Medicine* 33 (9): 1288–1297.

Handoll, H. and Elliot, J. (2015). Rehabilitation for distal radial fractures in adults. *Cochrane Database of Systematic Reviews* (9).

Hinman, R., Nelligan, R., Bennell, K., and Delaney, C. (2017). Sounds a bit crazy, but it was almost more personal: a qualitative study of patient and clinician experiences of physical therapist-prescribed exercise for knee osteoarthritis via Skype. *Arthritis Care & Research* 69 (12): 1834–1844.

Hoeman, S. (2008). *Rehabilitation Nursing: Prevention, Intervention and Outcomes*, 4the. St Louis: Mosby Elsevier.

Husted, H. (2012). Fast-track hip and knee arthroplasty: clinical and organizational aspects. *Acta Orthopaedica Supplement* 83: 1–39. https://doi.org/10.3109/1745367 4.2012.700593.

Jahic, D., Omerovic, D., Tanovic, A. et al. (2018). The effect of prehabilitation on postoperative outcome in patients following primary total knee replacement arthroplasty. *Medical Archives* 72 (6): 439–443.

Jensen, C., Overgaard, S., Kock Wiil, U., and Clemensen, J. (2019). Can tele-health support self-care and empowerment? A qualitative study of hip fracture patients' experiences with testing an "App". *Sage Open Nursing* 5: 1–11.

Jester, R. (2003). Early discharge to hospital at home: should it be a matter of choice? *Journal of Orthopaedic Nursing* 7, 2: 64–69.

Jester, R. (2007). *Advancing Practice in Rehabilitation Nursing*. Oxford: Wiley Blackwell.

Jester, R. and Hicks, C. (2003a). Using cost-effectiveness analysis to compare hospital at home and in-patient interventions. Part 1. *Journal of Clinical Nursing* 12: 13–19.

Jester, R. and Hicks, C. (2003b). Using cost-effectiveness and analysis to compare hospital at home and in-patient interventions. Part 2. *Journal of Clinical Nursing* 12: 20–27.

Jester, R., Santy-Tomlinson, J., and Rogers, J. (2021). *Oxford Handbook of Trauma and Orthopaedic Nursing*. Oxford: Oxford University Press.

Kungwengwe, T. and Evans, R. (2020). Sana: A gamified rehabilitation management 348 system for anterior cruciate ligament reconstruction recovery. *Applied Sciences* 349 (10). 4868. https://doi.org/10.3390/app10144868.

Mahomed, N.N., Davis, A.M., Hawker, G. et al. (2008). Inpatient compared with home-based rehabilitation following primary unilateral total hip or knee replacement: a randomized controlled trial. *The Journal of Bone and Joint Surgery (American)* 90 (8): 1673–1680.

Mason, D., Dickens, V., and Vail, A. (2012). Rehabilitation for hamstring injuries. *Cochrane Database of Systematic Reviews* 12: CD004575. https://doi.org/10.1002/14651858. CD004575. pub3.

Mauk, K. (2012). *Rehabilitation Nursing: A Contemporary Approach to Practice*. Sudbury, MA: Jones and Bartlett.

Moyer, R., Ikert, K., Long, K., and Marsh, J. (2017). The value of preoperative exercise and education for patients undergoing total hip and knee arthroplasty: a systematic review and meta-analysis. *JBJS Reviews* 5 (12): e2. https://doi.org/10.2106/JBJS.RVW.17.00015 PMID: 29232265.

Neuman, B. (1982). *The Neuman Systems Model: Application to Nursing Education and Practice*. Norwalk, CT: Appleton Century Crofts.

Nolan, M., Booth, A., and Nolan, J. (1997). *New Directions in Rehabilitation: Exploring the Nursing Contribution*, Research Report Series No 6. London: English National Board for Nursing, Midwifery and Health Visiting.

Orem, D.E. (2001). *Nursing: Concepts of Practice*, 6the. London: Mosby.

Peters, S., Jha, B., and Ross, M. (2021). Rehabilitation following surgery for flexor tendon injuries of the hand. *Cochrane Database of Systematic Reviews* (1): CD012479. https://doi.org/10.1002/14651858.CD012479.pub2.

Pozzi, F., Snyder-Mackler, L., and Zeni, J. (2013). Physical exercise after knee arthroplasty: a systematic review of controlled trials. *European Journal of Physical and Rehabilitation Medicine* 49 (6): 877–892.

Price, B. (1990). *Body image: Nursing Concepts and Care*. London: Prentice Hall.

Redman, B.K. (2004). *Patient Self Management for People with Chronic Diseases*. Sudbury, MA: Jones and Bartlett.

Reis, E., Postolache, G., Teixeira, L. et al. (2019). Exergames for motor rehabilitation in older adults: an umbrella review. *Physical Therapy Reviews* 24 (3–4): 84–99. https://doi.org/10.1080/10833196.2019.1639012.

Roy, C. (1984). *Introduction to Nursing: An Adaptation Model*, 2e. Englewood Cliffs, NJ: Prentice Hall.

Royal College of Nursing (2007). *The Role of the Rehabilitation Nurse: RCN Guidance*. London: Royal College of Nursing Publishing.

Schilder, P. (1935). *Image and Appearance of the Human Body*. London: Kegan Paul.

Siggeirsdottir, K., Olafsson, O., Jonsson, H. et al. (2005). Short hospital stay augmented with education and home-based rehabilitation improves function and quality of life after hip replacement: randomized study of 50 patients with 6 months of follow-up. *Acta Orthopaedica* 76 (4): 555–562.

Smith, M. (1999). *Rehabilitation in Adult Nursing Practice*. Edinburgh: Churchill Livingstone.

Smith, T., Gilbert, A., Sreekanta, A. et al. (2020). Enhanced rehabilitation and care models for adults with dementia following hip fracture surgery. *Cochrane Data Base of Systematic Reviews* (2).

Specht, K., Agerskov, H., Kjaersgaard-Andersen, P. et al. (2018). Patients' experiences during the first 12 weeks after discharge in fast-track hip and knee arthroplasty – a qualitative study. *International Journal of Trauma and Orthopaedic Nursing* 31: https://doi.org/10.1016/j.ijotn.2018.08.002.

Waters, K. (1996). Rehabilitation: core themes in gerontological nursing. In: *A Textbook of Gerontological Nursing: Perspectives on Practice* (ed. L. Wade and K. Waters). London: Baillere-Tindall.

Part II

Specialist and Advanced Practice

7

Clinical Assessment of the Orthopaedic and Trauma Patient

Rebecca Jester

Royal College of Surgeons Ireland Medical University, Bahrain

Introduction

The aim of this chapter is to provide an evidence-based discussion of assessment of the orthopaedic and trauma patient. The chapter adopts a person-centred approach to the subject of assessment, as it is important to remember that, although a person's chief complaint will be a musculoskeletal problem, most are likely to have comorbidities and psycho/social issues that relate to their problem. Practitioners will be using their assessment skills throughout the patient's journey from initial presentation in primary care, emergency room or outpatient's department to ongoing evaluation following intervention or change in medical status. There has been a significant shift towards virtual consultations due to the COVID pandemic and this requires a change in how patient assessment is conducted. Throughout the chapter, where robust evidence exists, there will be critical application of research to approaches to assessment and examination. However, to date there is very little high-level evidence to support many aspects of patient assessment/clinical diagnostics within trauma and orthopaedics affirmed by a dearth of systematic reviews. Therefore, the information within this chapter is in the main based on evidence from the following sources: formal education, symposia, conference presentations, non-research publications, expert opinion and reflections on clinical experience (the author and other clinical experts).

Principles of Clinical Assessment

Clinical assessment can be defined as gathering both objective and subjective data for the purposes of generating differential diagnoses, evaluating progress following a specific procedure or course of treatment and evaluating the impact of a specific disease process. Examples of objective and subjective data can be found in Table 7.1.

There are some important key principles related to assessment, including:

- introducing yourself
- confirming the patient's identity
- explaining what the assessment is going to involve
- gaining the patient's consent for the assessment
- establishing if the patient wants a family member or carer to be present during the assessment
- good hand hygiene prior to and on completion of assessment/examination.

It is important to establish, either prior to or early in the assessment, if the patient has any degree of cognitive dysfunction. Communicating with patients with impaired cognition requires management of the immediate environment to reduce accessory noise and constant reorientation to what you are doing and why. It is also important to establish that the patient has the mental capacity to consent to the assessment before proceeding. People with learning disabilities often are not supported well in acute hospitals (Drozd et al. 2020). Thoughtful communication involves minimising healthcare jargon, use of pictorial aids if appropriate and including a family carer. These can all help to alleviate anxiety during the assessment process. Non-verbal and para-verbal communication play a key role in putting patients with cognitive impairment or learning difficulties at ease during the assessment and enhancing the accuracy and quality of information elicited during the assessment.

It is important to do the following:

- Ensure the patient is comfortable and their privacy and dignity are maintained at all times during the assessment. Patients of either sex should be asked if they would like a chaperone present during any physical examination and

Table 7.1 Types of subjective and objective data

Subjective data	Objective data
History – dependent on accuracy of patient and/or family as historians	Radiographic and other clinical investigations such as blood tests, MRI and CT
Patient reported outcome measures, patients' subjective perceptions of their symptoms and the impact on their quality of life and functional ability, mental health status	Measurement of range of movement using goniometry
	Baseline observations such as blood pressure, weight, height, body mass index, temperature and heart rate
Pain assessment	Measurements of limb length and muscle strength
	Physical assessment including muscle, strength, palpation, auscultation and inspection
	Clinician measures, such as timed get up and go test

unless the patient refuses (this should be documented) a chaperone should always be present during intimate examinations of patients of the opposite sex. The name and signature of any chaperone should be clearly documented.

- Check the patient is not in pain, thirsty, hungry or needing the toilet prior to embarking on the assessment process. Also, be mindful not to overtire older or frail patients with prolonged questioning, examination and clinical investigations. Patients may require a break and the assessment process may need to be phased to accommodate their needs.
- When documenting the assessment ensure you record negative as well as positive findings. For example, 'Patient reports no locking or giving way of the knee joint'.

Models and Frameworks of Patient Assessment

It is important to adopt a systematic approach to patient assessment to avoid missing valuable information and to minimise repetition. Patient assessment should be inter-professional and a shared assessment document adopted. This approach enables the multidisciplinary team (MDT) to share information and avoid wasting the patient's time by several healthcare professionals attempting to collect the same information. Approaches to patient assessment will vary depending upon patient needs, for example

whether the patient is presenting as an emergency with multiple trauma or a non-emergency with a painful joint/s or musculoskeletal dysfunction.

Emergency Presentation

The patient presenting in the emergency department (ED) with severe or multiple injuries must have an urgent and systematic assessment to identify life-threatening issues using the (C)ABCDE approach (Parker and Magnusson 2016):

- (C)atastrophic haemorrhage
- Airway with spinal protection
- Breathing
- Circulation
- Disability (neurological)
- Exposure and environment

In most healthcare organisations, these observations will be recorded on an early warning score (EWS) chart, such as the National Early Warning Score (NEWS2) (RCP 2017). See Chapter 16 for further detail regarding assessment of the patient following trauma.

Non-emergency, Elective or Planned Presentation

Within orthopaedic care, the medical model of assessment has predominated, with the main aim of the assessment being to understand the patient's chief complaint/problem and arrive at a differential diagnosis. Traditionally, this has been solely within the remit of the medical profession, but in recent years a growing number of specialist and advanced nurse and physiotherapy practitioners have taken on this role. The medical model comprises:

- taking a history to elicit the chief complaint or presenting problem
- observation and inspection
- physical examination using palpation, percussion and auscultation
- assessing movement and strength
- clinical investigations.

The medical model lends itself to the patient who is presenting with a clearly defined orthopaedic problem with minimal comorbidities or without complex social or psychological issues. However, many patients within the orthopaedic setting have more problems than just a single chief complaint and require a more person-centred rather than disease-centred approach to their assessment. The medical model of assessment tends to focus on the disease process rather than the impact of the disease on an individual and the ideology of holistic health assessment is to review the individual as a whole, with a focus on their overall health needs rather than the disease.

There are several assessment frameworks or models that lend themselves to the person with multiple physical, social and psychological issues and which nurses may find useful to structure their assessment. Assessment is the first part of the nursing process (comprising assessment, planning, implementation and evaluation of care). Nursing models and theories seem to have lost favour in contemporary clinical practice, which has become mainly target-orientated, but it remains important that nurses promote a holistic approach to assessment and care. An overview of the assessment component of these nursing or psychological models is presented below.

Roy's Adaptation Model

This model, developed by Roy (1984), is based on four modes: physiologic, self-concept (including body image and self-concept), role function and interdependence. This model lends itself particularly well to patients who are in the restorative phase following musculoskeletal trauma or spinal cord injury or those suffering with chronic conditions such as back pain and arthritis (see Chapter 6 for further reading on rehabilitation). The model focuses on assessing the patient's behaviour and stimuli towards adaptation in each of the four modes. The physiologic mode includes:

- oxygenation
- nutrition
- elimination
- activity and rest
- skin integrity
- the senses
- fluid and electrolytes
- neurological function
- endocrine function.

The role function model includes:

- primary role (age, sex, development level)
- secondary role (relatively permanent positions requiring performance such as spouse, parent, sibling)
- tertiary role (freely chosen and relatively temporary such as employee, student).

The self-concept mode includes:

- the physical self
- body image
- body sensations
- the personal self, comprising self-ideal and self-expectancy
- the moral–ethical–spiritual self.

The interdependence mode is about support systems, both intrinsic and extrinsic to the individual, and their receptive/contributive behaviours.

Wellness Framework

The wellness framework (Pinnell and de Meneses 1986) can be used to provide a systematic approach to data collection during the assessment process. It focuses on health and wellness rather than disease or ill-health and uses the following categories:

- Degree of fitness: exercise patterns, muscle strength, muscle and joint flexibility, body proportions (fat and muscle).
- Level of nutrition: analysis of nutritional intake, patient's knowledge of healthy nutrition, sociocultural beliefs about diet.
- Risk appraisal/level of life stress: identification of patient's risk factors to health, identification of sources of stress to the patient, the patient's perception of stress and their coping patterns.
- Lifestyle and personal health habits: habits regarding health behaviours, regular health screening, dental checks, alcohol/drug/smoking consumption, sleep and weight management.

The role of the nurse in orthopaedic care must incorporate promotion of healthy lifestyles and supporting patients to minimise risk such as the link between obesity and joint problems, and the wellness framework lends itself well to this aspect of orthopaedic assessment.

Maslow's Hierarchy of Needs

Maslow (1954) first developed the theory of motivation and personality. From this seminal work, a hierarchy of needs can be used to structure the assessment process. The needs are arranged in a pyramid based on the premise that until the lowest or most fundamental needs of the individual are addressed, they are unable to move to higher levels of functioning. These levels of need are presented below in order (lowest to highest):

- Physiological (survival needs): assessment of oxygenation, nutrition status, fluid balance, body temperature, elimination, shelter (home conditions and support) and sex (assessing individual's concerns about resuming sexual activity following procedures such as spinal fusion or hip arthroplasty).
- Safety and security (need to be safe and comfortable): physical safety, i.e. assess risk of falls, pressure sores, infection, venous thromboembolism and pain assessment. Psychological security should be assessed in terms

of the patient's need for information and inclusion in decisions about their care and treatment.

- Love and belonging: elicit information about the patient's social and family support.
- Esteem and self-esteem: assess issues around body image, adaptation and coping, and elicit what the patient's goals are.
- Self-actualisation: assess the extent to which the patient's full potential is being reached, their levels of autonomy and motivation.

The Medical Model

History-taking

Taking a history has three principal functions:

- provision of data to inform decision making around differential diagnosis and treatment planning
- initiate a medium by which a therapeutic bond is formed between patient and practitioner
- create a forum for education.

The importance of thorough and accurate history-taking has been recognised for many years. It is very tempting for busy practitioners to try and steer the patient's presenting signs and symptoms to fit a particular disease pattern by asking leading questions, but this can lead to an inaccurate diagnosis (Flynn et al. 2015).

History-taking comprises 10 stages, which should be followed in order:

1) *Chief complaint*: Elicit the chief complaint, using an open-ended question such as 'What brings you here today'?
2) *History* of the chief complaint:
   P Provocative or palliative: what makes it worse or better?
   Q Quantity or quality: how often do you experience the problem?
   R Region or radiation: is the problem localised or more diffuse?
   S Severity or scale: how would you rate your problem?
   T Timing: is there a particular time of the day or night associated with your problem? When was the onset of your problem and has it been constant or intermittent?
3) *Recapitulation*: Reaffirm with the patient at this stage that you have understood what their main problem is and the history of that problem as this allows any misconceptions to be resolved before proceeding further with the history.
4) *Family history*: Some musculoskeletal conditions have a genetic disposition, such as rheumatoid arthritis.

A genogram is the most systematic and succinct way to record a family history.

5) *Past medical history*: This should include all major illnesses, surgery and treatments. Patients may often forget significant aspects of their past medical history and you may need to triangulate information with accessory information from the patient's notes, further questioning based on their medication and findings from inspection such as scarring indicating previous trauma or surgery.
6) *Psychosocial and occupational history*: Frequently musculoskeletal problems can be associated with patients' previous or current occupation, for example often severe osteoarthritis of the knee is related to occupations such as HGV driving, climbing up and down ladders or carpet fitting. Repetitive strain injury of the wrists and hands is often found in people who use computers for long periods of time on a daily basis. A social history will elicit what the patient's home situation is in terms of living accommodation and support from family and friends. This is very important for discharge planning and ascertaining if any adaptations to the home or work environment are needed to alleviate the patient's symptoms and increase independence.
7) *Review of symptoms*: Although the patient will be presenting with a chief complaint of a musculoskeletal problem/s, in certain situations, such as preoperative assessment, it is necessary to review all the body systems to rule out any comorbidities that may present as a risk during surgery/anaesthesia (see Chapter 5 for further detail on pre-operative assessment). The review of systems should also include a review of the individual in terms of rest and sleep patterns, smoking and alcohol habits. Table 7.2 provides guidance on reviewing the body systems. To review the systems in a systematic way it is best to take a head-to-toe approach.
8) *Allergies*: Ascertain if the patient has any known allergies to medications, dressings/adhesive or latex. Historically patients were tested for sensitivity to nickel, cobalt or chromium, but the clinical significance of metal sensitivities following prosthetic replacements is questionable and therefore routine metal allergy testing is no longer recommended. However, it is still important to question patients about metal skin sensitivity, specifically nickel, as the patient may have a skin reaction from clips or staples following surgery. The evidence base for the value of routine metal allergy testing is equivocal, as a study by Frigerio et al. (2011) concluded that objective determination of metal sensitivity at pre-operative assessment should be considered when planning joint arthroplasty as it would help the surgeon determine the most appropriate prosthesis.

Table 7.2 Review of systems

Body system	Example questions
Integmentary	Do you have any skin lesions, sores, unhealed wounds, pressure sores, rashes or fungal infections of nails?
Mental health/ psychological wellbeing	Do you currently suffer with anxiety or depression?
Neurological	Do you suffer with fits, faints, blackouts, headaches, muscle weakness/wasting or altered or loss of sensation?
Respiratory	Do you suffer with shortness of breath either at rest or on exertion or suffer with wheezing, bronchitis, asthma, chest infections or dry or productive cough?
Cardiovascular	Do you have any problems with chest pain, circulatory problems, leg ulcers, blood clots or varicose veins?
Musculoskeletal (The chief complaint will have been explored earlier in the history, but additional musculoskeletal problems may be present)	Do you have any joint pain, swelling, locking or giving way, limitations to movement, fractures or muscle/tendon/ ligament injury?
Gastrointestinal	Do you have any gastric bleeding, ulcers, abdominal pain, oesophageal reflux, loss of appetite or unintentional weight loss or gain? (Ascertain bowel habits and if there has been any recent change)
Genitourinary	Do you have any problems passing urine such as urgency, frequency, incontinence, hesitancy, nocturia or urine infection?

9) *Medications*: Include prescribed, over-the-counter and homoeopathic medicines. Patients can often be unsure of the names, doses and function of their medications so it is important to cross-verify with accessory information such as prescription printouts.

10) *Education*: This stage of the history-taking process facilitates the opportunity for the patient and/or their family if present to ask questions and also to provide health promotion advice. For example, if the patient reports smoking then smoking cessation advice can be provided. In addition, if the patient is obese or morbidly obese, information and support for weight reduction can be offered. It is also important to offer the patient and/or family member the opportunity to ask any questions or raise any issues they feel have not been covered during the history-taking/assessment.

Principles of Physical Examination

Based on information gained during the history, the practitioner can then be focused in the physical examination. Which body systems to include in the assessment will depend on both information from the history and the nature of the assessment. For example, if the patient is presenting post-operatively with deteriorating vital signs, a thorough examination of several systems, including cardiovascular, respiratory, neurological and abdominal, may be needed. If the patient is presenting in the orthopaedic or primary care clinic with a specific localised musculoskeletal problem then the examination can focus on the joint of concern, bearing in mind that musculoskeletal pain can often be referred and therefore it is important to include examination of joints above the specific site of the problem and to always compare both limbs. The important principle is to have a sound rationale for which systems and specific elements of systems you decide to include and exclude, and this should be documented within your assessment.

It is important to use all senses during assessment, including sight, smell, hearing and touch. There are several techniques used within physical examination: observation, inspection, palpation, percussion, auscultation and measurement.

Observation

The first step of assessing a patient is through observation of them. Observation involves the senses of sight, smell and hearing. A good tip is to start observing the patient as you approach them (or them you) to observe:

- how they rise from a chair, transfer from bed to chair, etc.
- facial expressions indicating pain/discomfort, anxiety or low mood
- use of a walking aid and if they are using it correctly
- gait analysis, e.g. Trendelenburg gait indicating a potential hip problem, stiff knee gait or a drop foot
- crepitus from movement of the joints or wheezing/rattles from the chest
- does the patient look flushed, hot, pale, sweaty or jaundiced?
- does the patient look well cared for or unkempt?
- smell of acetone from the breath indicating ketosis
- smell of urine or faeces.

Your initial observations should be recorded within the assessment and explored with the patient during the history.

Inspection

Inspection is much more detailed than general observation and focuses on detecting specific issues in musculoskeletal examination such as the presence or absence of swelling, bruising, scarring, skin discoloration, oedema, muscle wasting, alteration of shape, posture or deformity.

Inspection for swelling/s should note if it is localised or diffuse and confined to the joint or extending beyond the joint. Swelling confined to the joint itself can indicate either effusion due to excessive synovial fluid or non-pyogenic conditions such as rheumatoid or osteoarthritis. Swelling beyond the joint may indicate infection of the limb such as cellulitis, tumours, vascular or lymphatic problems. It is important to be precise in recording the location and extent of any swelling observed and to affirm by further questioning the onset, duration and pattern of swelling, e.g. intermittent, fluctuating in severity, relieving or exacerbating factors. There are specific tests to confirm swelling which are discussed under palpation and special tests.

Inspection should also include the identification of any bruising or abrasions suggesting recent trauma and scarring from previous surgery or trauma. Changes to skin colour should also be noted, specifically erythema (redness), which may indicate a localised response to trauma or infection, or pallor possibly indicating compromised vascular function. Any muscle wasting should be noted, usually indicating limited use due to pain or injury or impaired nerve supply (denervation). For example, muscle wasting of the quadriceps can be very common in patients with knee trauma or pathology, and wasting of the thenar eminence (of the thumb) in conditions of the hand/wrist such as carpal tunnel syndrome (median nerve compression). Inspection should also be used to detect deformity, altered posture or shortening, which can result from a congenital abnormality, trauma or destructive joint disease.

Palpation

Palpation should be used to detect changes in the temperature of the limbs/joints/spine and detect any tenderness. The back of the hand rather than the practitioner's palms should be used to detect localised or diffuse changes in temperature. Increased heat over a joint is indicative of inflammatory processes, whereas diffuse heat away from the joint may indicate a tumour or infection such as cellulitis. Coolness of a limb is generally indicative of arterial pathology such as atherosclerosis.

Identifying the exact location of tenderness is important in identifying precisely which underlying structures may be involved. Observing the patient for signs of distress or discomfort during palpation is important as is documenting precisely the exact location and extent of tenderness and/or alteration in skin temperature.

Assessing Movement

Many orthopaedic conditions result in loss or restriction of movement. Assessing the range of joint movement requires knowledge of the normal range possible (Chapter 4). Restriction in movement can be due to contraction of joint capsules, tendons and muscles or lodging of loose bodies between the articulations of the joint. A resultant fixed flexion deformity of the joint can occur, most commonly an inability to fully flex the joint. Movement of the joint controlled by the patient is known as active range of movement and passive movement is when the practitioner controls the movement of the joint; the latter being appropriate when the muscles responsible for movement of the joint are paralysed. It is important to observe and listen to the patient when conducting measurement of range of movement, observing for signs of pain and distress. There is an unequivocal evidence base regarding the best method of measuring range of joint movement.

Assessing Muscle Strength

Assessing strength of muscle contraction is indicative of the strength of each joint movement and therefore should be included within the examination process. A scale developed by the Medical Research Council 1975 is used to record muscle strength and is shown in Box 7.1.

Assessing for Shortening of the Lower Limbs

As part of examination of the hip and lower limb, it is important to determine the presence or absence of shortening (McRae 2010). True shortening, where the limb is physically shorter, may be caused by a number of pathologies, including loss of articular cartilages caused by arthritis, displaced hip fracture, dislocation of the hip, epiphyseal trauma and old fractures of the tibia or femur. In apparent shortening, the limb length is not altered but appears shorter because of contracture of the adductor muscles

---

Box 7.1 Medical Research Council Scale for Recording Muscle Power (Medical Research Council 1975)

0 = no muscle power
1 = flicker of activity
2 = movement with effect of gravity eliminated, i.e. in a place at right angles to gravity but not against resistance
3 = movement against gravity but not against applied resistance
4 = movement against applied resistance but less than full power
5 = normal power

resulting in tilting of the pelvis. To measure for true shortening the first stage is to ask the patient to lie flat on a couch with the pelvis positioned squarely and both legs stretched out as straight as possible with heels flat to the couch. In the normal patient, the heels and the anterior iliac spines are level. If a discrepancy is noted by this visual check, it is necessary to measure the limbs with a tape measure, which should be of material that does not stretch. Measure from the inferior edge of the anterior superior iliac spine to the middle of the medial malleolus and then extend the measurement down to the bottom of the heel with the ankle in the neutral position. Compare both sides and repeat the measurements until accuracy is assured. To measure for apparent shortening, measure between the umbilicus or xiphisternum down to the middle of both medial malleoli.

Gait Assessment

There are many causes of abnormal gait patterns, including neurological and musculoskeletal disorders. There are a number of orthopaedic conditions that may produce gait abnormalities, including Trendelenburg gait (waddling gait) due to hip pathology, stiff knee gait due to knee pathology and drop foot gait due to damage to the nerves responsible for dorsi-flexion of the foot. Gait analysis is most commonly undertaken by the physiotherapist or orthopaedic surgeon, but nurses working within specialist or advanced roles may carry out gait analysis as part of their assessments.

Special Tests

There are a number of specific tests that may be included as part of the examination of the patient. Clinical reasoning based on the patient history and prior aspects of the examination, including observation, inspection, palpation and measurement of motion, will determine if special tests are required to assist in making a differential diagnosis. The most common of these include testing for valgus instability of the knee joint using the anterior draw test, testing for varus instability using the Lachman test and the Trendelenburg test for weakness of the abductor muscles of the hip. The Trendelenburg test involves the patient standing on one leg and then the tilt of the pelvis on the opposite side is observed: if the pelvis drops below the horizontal plane then the test is said to be positive.

Assessing Deep Tendon Reflexes

Deep tendon reflexes are tested by gently tapping over a tendon using a patellar hammer and observing for movement of the associated muscles. When examining the spine for suspected prolapsed intervertebral disc, both the knee and ankle reflexes should be tested. When testing the knee reflex, the knee should be supported by the clinician's arm and the infra patellar tendon gently tapped, observing for contraction of the quadriceps. A diminished or absent contraction indicates a possible prolapse at the level of L3/L4. The ankle reflex is assessed by positioning the ankle in the mid position, knee bent and hip slightly externally rotated then lightly tapping the Achilles tendon and observing for plantar flexion of the foot. An absent or diminished ankle reflex is indicative of pathology at vertebrae S1/S2. It is important when assessing deep tendon reflexes that there is no muscle contraction in the area being assessed so the patient must be relaxed. Reflexes are recorded as follows:

0 = absent
+ = reduced
++ = normal
+++ = increased
++++ = increased with clonus

Clinical Investigations

Once the history and examination have been completed, the practitioner needs to decide what clinical investigations are needed to arrive at a differential diagnosis and/or treatment plan. Clinical investigations including X-rays, magnetic resonance imaging (MRI) and computed tomography (CT) scans or blood investigations have associated costs and risks to the patient, e.g. cumulative doses of radiation, and so should be requested only with a clear justification of their need. Nurses working in trauma and orthopaedics should have an understanding of the common investigations to offer support and explanation to the patient. Nurses working in specialist and advanced roles often undertake the requesting and interpretation of clinical tests within their scope of practice. The most common investigations include the following:

- Radiographic imaging (X-rays): This is the most commonly used diagnostic imaging in trauma and orthopaedics. AP and lateral views are the most frequently requested view, but other views include comparison images, oblique views, localised views and stress films. All clinicians requesting X-rays must undertake specific radiology safety training and be judicious in requesting X-rays in relation to the cumulative dose of radiation the patient is receiving.
- CT scan: This technique also uses beams of radiation, but provides a more detailed view of tissue slices from different angles and more detailed differentiation of different tissue types.
- MRI: Avoids any exposure to radiation, using high strength magnetic fields and electrical impulses to create detailed images of bone and soft tissue. MRI is increasingly used in the investigation of spinal problems such as suspected prolapsed intervertebral discs and damaged structures such as meniscal and ligament tears in the knee and shoulder.

- Ultrasound imaging: Regarded as being risk-free and comparatively inexpensive. Its main value is to detect fluid in and around joints and therefore it is useful in identifying heamarthrosis or the presence of infected or inflamed tissue.
- Dual-energy X-ray absorptiometry: A non-invasive scan to test the density of bones for diagnosis of osteoporosis.
- Common haematological investigations: These include full blood count (FBC) (which includes red and white cells and platelets) and tests for inflammatory processes including C-reactive protein (CRP), erythrocyte sedimentation rate (ESR) and plasma viscosity (PV). It should be noted that these markers of inflammation can also be present due to infection. Serum uric acid and serum calcium, phosphate and alkaline phosphate may also be requested.

Boxes 7.2 and 7.3 provide examples of the underpinning evidence for two modes of physical assessment.

Box 7.2   Evidence Digest: Goniometry

Goniometry has for many years been considered the gold standard in measuring the range of joint movement, indeed if performed correctly it provides a very accurate measure of joint motion. Watkins et al. (1991) reported that use of a long-armed goniometer (LAG) in measuring flexion and extension of the knee joint had greater accuracy and interrater reliability than visual estimations. The measurements are obtained by placing the parts of the measuring instrument along the proximal and distal bones adjacent to the joint concerned and the movement should be free of any muscle contraction. It is important to align the goniometer carefully with appropriate anatomical landmarks such as the greater trochanter of the femur and lateral malleous to measure the motion of the knee joint and to ensure the goniometer stays in position as the patient moves their joint. The measurement should be taken three times and the average range of movement recorded to 5° increments. However, new technologies are being introduced to further improve accuracy in measuring joint movement. A study by Hambly et al. (2012) compared the accuracy of the traditional LAG and a new novel smart phone application (iGoniometer) in measuring active knee flexion in a healthy adult population, and reported that the iGoniometer demonstrated high relative and absolute reliability, although they recommended that further evaluation was required on a population with knee pathology.

Box 7.3   Evidence Digest Assessment Findings

A 3-year prospective longitudinal study of 68 patients with osteoarthritis of the knee joint reported a significant correlation between diminished joint space width and patient-reported symptoms of pain, but found no correlation between increased osteophyte formation visible on X-ray and patient-reported symptoms (Fukui et al. 2010). An earlier study by Neogi et al. (2009) also reported a strong correlation between radiographic evidence of diminished joint space in patients with osteoarthritis knee and pain symptoms, but did not find a significant relationship between osteophyte changes on X-ray and patient-reported symptoms. This research emphasises the need to use self-reported outcome measures to gain the subjective perspective of the patient regarding the impact of the pathology on their quality of life and functional ability, and also their view on their health status following a particular treatment or procedure.

Assessing the Impact of Disease on the Individual

It is important, as part of the assessment process, to evaluate the impact of a particular disease on the individual to inform the treatment or management plan. There may be little correlation between what clinical investigations and examination reveal and the perception of the individual. Patients with severe osteoarthritic changes on X-ray may report minimal disruption to their activities of daily living. Conversely, patients with minimal radiographic changes may report their symptoms to be intolerable, with a dramatic impact on their quality of life and functional ability (Swagerty and Hellinger 2001). This is explored in more detail in Box 7.4.

Box 7.4   The Abbreviated Mental Test Score

- How old are you?
- What is the time to the nearest hour?
- Name the place.
- Recognition of two persons, e.g. a nurse and a doctor.
- Date and month of birth.
- Date of First World War (start or end).
- Queen's name.
- Count 20–1 backwards.
- Five-minute recall of a full street address.

Source: Qureshi and Hodkinson (1974). Reproduced with permission from Oxford University Press.

Self-reported outcome measures can be broadly categorised into general health-related quality of life (HRQoL) tools and disease-specific tools. HRQoL measures aim to measure the multifaceted nature of health, including physical, social and psychological health, and can be used across many different types of diseases and health issues (Jester et al. 2018). Their main limitation is that they lack the sensitivity to detect relatively small changes in health status for a particular disease process (Bowling 2001) and therefore should be used in conjunction with disease-specific measures. Examples of HRQoL measures include the Sickness Impact Profile, the Nottingham Health Profile and the Short-Form 36 Health Survey Questionnaire (SF36). There are many disease-specific self-report measures developed for patients with musculoskeletal conditions, including the Arthritis Impact Measurement Scale, the Oxford Hip and Knee Scores, the WOMAC index and the Harris Hip Score. The practitioner should ensure that any HRQoL or disease-specific measure used as part of the assessment process has undergone rigorous testing to ensure it is valid, reliable, sensitive, specific and patient-friendly.

Assessing Cognitive Function

A significant number of patients presenting with musculoskeletal problems may have a degree of cognitive dysfunction, which may already be noted in the patient's records. As part of a comprehensive assessment process, the nurse should ensure that cognitive dysfunction is detected and its cause investigated and managed. It should never be assumed that because a patient is elderly their confusion is due to dementia. It is vital to ascertain the onset of the patient's confusion, specifically if it is an established diagnosed problem due to dementia, head injury or stroke or whether there has been a recent onset. Acute confusional states must be thoroughly investigated by taking a history of the onset from the patient, if possible, family members or informal carers and then carrying out appropriate clinical investigations and observations to elicit the cause. Acute confusion (delirium) can be caused by many factors including urea and electrolyte (U&E) imbalance, sepsis, hyper- or hypoglycaemia, adverse reaction to prescribed medications, raised intracranial pressure and drug/alcohol related. The practitioner should inform the medical team of the onset of acute confusion and commence observations using the National Early Warning Score 2 (NEWS2) chart and Glasgow Coma Scale (Chapter 16) to determine if any vital signs fall outside of normal parameters. Then the practitioner, in collaboration with the medical team, should begin to collect information to contribute towards determining the cause of confusion including:

- blood tests for U&E, capillary blood sugar, liver function tests, blood cultures, CRP and ESR

- urinalysis for protein, ketones and glucose and send a midstream urine sample if a urine infection is suspected
- oxygen saturation rates
- accurate monitoring of fluid input and output
- review medication with medical and pharmacy team for possible interactions or adverse reactions.

Once delirium has been ruled out based on these investigations then the patient's cognitive status should be assessed using a valid and reliable tool such as the Abbreviated Mental Test Score (AMTS; Qureshi and Hodkinson 1974) or the Mini Mental State Examination (MMSE; Folstein et al. 1975). The AMTS comprises 10 items, as detailed in Box 7.4; the best possible score is 10/10 with each correct item scoring 1. The diagnostic cut-off point varies between authors, but generally <6 indicates cognitive dysfunction (Jester et al. 2011). Although widely used in clinical practice and well tested for their psychometric properties, both the MMSE and AMTS have their limitations as they are developed for a specific age and ethnic group. Explain to the patient why you are asking the questions comprising the MMSE and AMTS, and ensure privacy and an environment that has minimal background noise and disruption to get the best results.

Assessing Risk

An integral part of the assessment process is to assess the patient's risk of harm or injury, including risk of falls, pressure sores, malnutrition and venous thromboembolism. Specific risk assessment tools are presented and discussed within the related chapters of this text. However, the predictive accuracy of all risk assessment tools must be evaluated to ensure that the practice associated with them is evidence-based. Predictive accuracy is the ability of a tool to be both sensitive and specific to minimise the number of false positives (over prediction) and false negative (under prediction). A pilot study by Jester et al. (2005) found the predictive accuracy of two falls assessment tools (FRASE and STRATIFY) with older hip fracture patients to be poor, reporting Receiver Operator Characteristic scores to be 0.560 and 0.629, respectively, indicating significant over-prediction when using the tools.

Patient Assessment Using Telemedicine

The Covid-19 pandemic has necessitated that many patient assessments and examinations have moved from face-to-face patient/clinician interaction to virtual approaches such as telemedicine. This requires a new set of competencies and skills, and also preparation of patients as well as clinicians to ensure assessment via telemedicine is effective. Tanaka et al. (2020) suggest that although a non-face orthopaedic examination may lack the important elements of palpation and dynamic testing, available resources can be utilised to optimise the quality and outcome of a patient's virtual assessment. Patients will normally undergo clinical investigations such as X-rays, MRI scans and blood tests, and complete any relevant patient-reported outcome measure questionnaires prior to the virtual assessment, so results are available during the consultation. It is important that patients are fully informed about what the virtual assessment will entail and give consent to this format of assessment. The most effective mode of virtual assessment is to use video cameras and microphones as observation is then possible during the assessment, rather than reliance on telephone or verbal consultation only. Patients as part of the preparation for the virtual assessment will need guidance on proper positioning of their camera, location, lighting and clothing to allow for appropriate visibility and examination of the affected body part (Tanaka et al. 2020).

As with face-to-face assessment, it is vital to confirm the patient's identity and to introduce yourself and explain the assessment process. History-taking can follow the same process as used for face to face. Assessing patient's gait is possible using the camera and assessing ROM is possible using a virtual goniometer on the computer screen.

Not all patients will have access to a computer with video and microphone or feel competent in using them so it is important to assess a patient's readiness for assessment using telemedicine. Palpation and auscultation/percussion are clearly not possible using telemedicine, but patients can be instructed on how to feel for radiating heat over a joint or cool extremities and inform the clinician.

Summary

This chapter has discussed best practice in assessment of orthopaedic and trauma patients. The content has included the traditional medical approach to assessment, including physical examination, but has also offered a number of alternative models rooted in nursing and psychology theory. The use of telemedicine to conduct patient assessment has also been discussed. Where available there has been critical application of research and the deficit of high-level evidence to underpin clinical assessment has been highlighted. Good assessment skills are fundamental to nursing practice as they generate data from which our care and treatment is planned and implemented.

Further Reading

Jester, R., Santy, J. and Rogers, J. (2021) Oxford Handbook of Orthopaedic and Trauma Nursing, 2. Oxford University Press, Oxford.

Cleland, S., Koppenhaver, S. and Su, J. (2020) Netter's Orthopaedic Clinical Examination: An Evidence-based Approach, 4. Elsevier, London.

References

Bowling, A. (2001). *Measuring Disease*, 2e. Maidenhead: Open University Press.

Drozd, M., Chadwick, D., and Jester, R. (2020). A cross-case comparison of the trauma and orthopaedic hospital experiences of adults with intellectual disabilities using interpretative phenomenological analysis. *Nursing Open* https://doi.org/10.1002/nop2.693.

Flynn, S., Pugh, H., and Jester, R. (2015). Clinical assessment in trauma and orthopaedic nursing. *International Journal of Trauma and Orthopaedic Nursing* 19: 162–169.

Folstein, M., Folstein, S., and McHugh, P. (1975). 'Minimental state' a practical method for grading the cognitive state of patients for the clinician. *Journal of Psychiatric Research* 12: 189–198.

Frigerio, E., Pigatto, P., Guzzi, G., and Altonare, G. (2011). Metal sensitivity in patients with orthopaedic implants: a prospective study. *Contact Dermatitis* 64 (5): 273–279.

Fukui, N., Yamane, S., Ishida, S. et al. (2010). Relationship between radiographic changes and symptoms or physical examination findings in subjects with symptomatic medial knee osteoarthritis: a three-year prospective study. *BMC Musculoskeletal Disorders* 11: 269–279.

Hambly, K., Sibley, R., and Ockendon, M. (2012). Agreement between a novel smartphone application and a long arm goniometer for assessment of knee flexion. *International Journal of Physiotherapy and Rehabilitation* 54 (October): 4–6.

Jester, R., Wade, S., and Henderson, K. (2005). A pilot investigation of the efficacy of falls risk assessment tools and prevention strategies in an elderly hip fracture population. *Journal of Orthopaedic Nursing* 9 (1): 27–34.

Jester, R., Santy, J., and Rogers, J. (2011). *Oxford Handbook of Orthopaedic and Trauma Nursing*. UK: Oxford University Press.

Jester, R., Santy-Tomlinson, J., and Drozd, M. (2018). The use of patient reported outcome measures (PROMs) in clinical assessment. *International Journal of Orthopaedic and Trauma Nursing* 29: https://doi.org/10.1016/j.ijotn.2018.02.003.

Maslow, A. (1954). *Motivation and Personality*. New York: Harper.

McRae, R. (2010). *Clinical Orthopaedic Examination*, 6e. Edinburgh: Churchill Livingstone Elsevier.

Medical Research Council (1975). *Aids to the Investigation of Peripheral Nerve Injuries*. London: HMSO.

Neogi, T., Felson, D., Niu, J. et al. (2009). Association between radiographic features of knee osteoarthritis and pain, results from two cohort studies. *British Medical Journal* 339: b2844.

Parker, M. and Magnusson, C. (2016). Assessment of trauma. *International Journal of Trauma and Orthopaedic Nursing* 21: 21–30.

Pinnell, N. and de Meneses, M. (1986). *The Nursing Process: Theory*. Appleton-Lange, Norwalk, CT: Application and Related Processes.

Qureshi, K. and Hodkinson, H. (1974). Evaluation of a 10 question mental test in the institutionalized elderly. *Age and Ageing* 3: 152–157.

Roy, C. (1984). *Introduction to Nursing: An Adaptation Model*, 2e. New Jersey: Prentice-Hall.

Royal College of Physicians (2017). *National Early Warning Score (NEWS) 2 Standardising the Assessment of Acute-Illness Severity in the NHS*. London: Royal College of Physicians.

Swagerty, D. and Hellinger, D. (2001). Radiographic assessment of osteoarthritis. *American Family Physician* 64 (2): 279–287.

Tanaka, M., Oh, L., Martin, S., and Berkson, E. (2020). Telemedicine in the era of COVID-19: the virtual orthopaedic examination. *The American Journal of Bone and Joint Surgery* 102 (12): e57.

Watkins, M., Riddle, D., Lamb, R., and Personius, W. (1991). Reliability of goniometric measurements and visual estimates of knee range of motion obtained in a clinical setting. *Physical Therapy* 71: 90–96.

8

Key Musculoskeletal Interventions

Lynne Newton-Triggs[1], Jean Rogers[2], and Anna Timms[3]

[1] *Bedford Hospital, Bedford, UK*
[2] *Open University, Milton Keynes, UK*
[3] *Royal National Orthopaedic Hospital, Stanmore, Middlesex, UK*

Introduction

There are a number of key interventions used in the orthopaedic and trauma setting, mainly to support and immobilise limbs while bone and soft tissue healing take place. The three interventions most frequently met by the orthopaedic practitioner are casts, traction and external fixation. Caring for patients with any one of these interventions requires highly specialised, in-depth knowledge of the theory, application, care and complications so that safe, effective care can be provided. The following three sections consider casts, external fixation and traction with a focus on providing an overview of how each works and outlining the care and support required for safe, effective patient care whilst taking into account limitations in the evidence base.

The Principles of Casting

The aim of this section is to provide an overview of the principles of casting and care of the patient in a cast. The application of a cast is a specialised technical skill that requires education, training, practice and constant review of competence to ensure patients receive safe, high-quality care. Most casts should be applied by practitioners with specialist casting qualification and experience. It is important, however, that all practitioners working with patients with casts have an in-depth understanding of care needs once the cast has been applied so that any complications can be recognised and dealt with quickly.

A cast is a rigid device used to provide support and protection following injury and/or surgery and for other musculoskeletal conditions that require immobilisation (Table 8.1). Casts are constructed from flexible bandages impregnated with material which hardens when 'cured' following contact with water. The bandage is usually dipped in water, wrapped around the limb or body part and then held in position until the material hardens. This provides a firm support that follows the contours of the area it encases.

A number of materials are used for casting (Table 8.2). Plaster of Paris casts are most often used immediately following injury or surgery as they are relatively cheap and easy to apply. A lighter, more robust, synthetic cast can then be applied for a longer period of time once swelling has subsided. The choice of cast depends on applier preference and the instructions of the consulting surgeon.

Health and safety is an important consideration for both patients and staff whether a cast is applied in a casting room or other area. Employers and staff have a duty to ensure safety through systems that provide:

- training and education in safe cast application
- staff with the correct skills and experience
- appropriate, well-maintained equipment.

Ideally, casting should take place in a casting room where specialist facilities are available. Casting materials and equipment should always be used in accordance with the manufacturer's instructions and there should be a regular and recorded equipment maintenance programme. The application of casts involves the use of substances which might be hazardous to health. Appropriate risk assessment must therefore take place. Manufacturers of casting materials have a legal responsibility to provide information and guidance which must be adhered to. Important precautions include the following:

Orthopaedic and Trauma Nursing: An Evidence-based Approach to Musculoskeletal Care, Second Edition. Edited by Sonya Clarke and Mary Drozd.
© 2023 John Wiley & Sons Ltd. Published 2023 by John Wiley & Sons Ltd.

Table 8.1 The functions of casts.

Support	Supporting and restricting movement following fracture until healed
Rest	Resting soft tissues following fracture, strain or sprain to reduce swelling and muscle spasm
Immobilisation	To rest a joint in disease or hold a joint in place following dislocation, particularly if ligaments are damaged
	Also used following muscle or tendon surgery to aid healing
Positioning	To correct, stabilise and maintain alignment of a limb with a bone disorder or deformity
Prevention	To prevent bone deformity
Healing	To assist healing of wounds, i.e. leg ulcers
Comfort	For the comfort of patients to aid pain relief

Table 8.2 Types of casting materials.

Type of material	Properties	Advantages	Disadvantages
Plaster of Paris	Gauze bandages impregnated with powdered calcium carbonate	Relatively inexpensive Easily moulded Very strong Permeable, allowing the skin to breathe Supple at the edges	Poor strength-to-weight ratio Disintegrates when wet Requires 24 hours to fully set Affects the visibility of radiographs
Synthetic	Flexible fibreglass and polyester substrate impregnated with polyurethane resin	Lighter weight More durable Breathable and porous Radiolucent Water resistant Reaches full rigidity quickly	More expensive Abrasive and rough May cause skin reactions for patients and staff

- Plaster of Paris application and removal results in dust, which can be inhaled by patients and staff. Oscillating saws must be fitted with a vacuum, and staff and patients should wear a face mask.
- Gloves need to be worn, particularly when applying synthetic materials as the resin can cause irritation.
- The noise produced by the oscillating cast saw is below the required daily exposure limit for personnel. However, it becomes louder on contact with casting materials and ear defenders should be worn if the saw is to be used for prolonged periods of time.

There must be enough staff available to apply casts safely. Ideally, there should be one person to hold and position the patient's limb and reassure the patient whilst the other applies the cast.

Casting Technique

The basic principles of cast application are the same whether applying plaster of Paris or synthetic casts. Casting is a highly skilled and technical activity that requires great manual dexterity. It should only be undertaken by staff with the knowledge and skills required and who practice the skills regularly. Even so, all staff working in orthopaedic and trauma settings should have a working understanding of the principles of cast application.

A good cast should always:

- be applied in the recommended position, providing the best possible support of the limb
- be functional, not restricting joint movement unnecessarily and not restricting movement of joints that are not within the cast
- fit well to provide adequate splintage but not be too tight. Casts that are too tight restrict blood and nerve supply and must be smooth inside without ridges that could cause pressure.
- be 'just enough': sufficient casting material should be applied to achieve the support necessary whilst keeping the cast as light as possible
- be complete: the cast should not be a succession of layers but should be moulded so that the materials involved are fully bonded together.

Before applying a cast, it is essential to:

- check the patient's details and the written instructions for the cast
- prepare the area to be used and ensure all equipment is ready for use
- provide verbal and written information and gain consent
- provide reassurance and pain relief prior to any casting
- position and support the patient and limb correctly and comfortably
- maintain privacy and dignity
- assess the condition of the patient's skin
- ensure that jewellery has been removed from the limb to be casted.

Cast application follows general principles:

- Stockinette and appropriate padding is applied that is not excessive, but adequately protects bony prominences and vulnerable skin.
- Casting materials should be applied in accordance with the manufacturer's instructions for timings and water temperature.
- The casting material should be applied by starting at one end of the area to be covered and each turn of the casting bandage should be approximately one-third of the previous turn.
- All the bandages should be applied carefully, but rapidly, smoothing continuously so that the cast layers laminate together.
- The cast should be applied without tension so that it is not too tight or too loose.
- The cast is then moulded to the shape of the area. This should be done with the palm of the hand and not the fingers, which can cause indentations, leading to pressure under the cast.
- Once the cast has set, the edges should be trimmed and the stockinette should be folded back and secured with casting material.

Application of a synthetic cast is very similar but with the following exceptions:

- Padding is used but stockinette is not required.
- Extra strips of adhesive padding are applied at the ends where the cast will start and terminate so that it can be turned back over the edges of the cast.
- The bandages are rolled out covering half of the previous turn with controlled tension.
- During the final moulding the cast needs to be held in place until set, otherwise the shape will not be held.

Following completion of the cast:

- The patient's skin should be cleansed and dried.

- Cast edges should be checked and trimmed as necessary to ensure that joints maintain their full range of movement and that edges do not rub the skin. The edges should then be padded and the stockinette secured in place.
- Cast setting depends on the type of cast applied and the patient should be advised how long this will take and instructed to rest the area and not bear weight on the cast during this time. All limbs in casts should be elevated and rested on pillows.
- The cast should be left uncovered for 48 hours to allow it to dry and should be handled as little as possible to prevent denting and cracking.
- Neurovascular assessment should be undertaken for all limb casts (see Chapter 9) and clearly documented.
- Documentation of any assessment, intervention and follow-up must be clear and precise.
- All advice given verbally should also be given in written format to the patient and carer. It should include care of the cast to prevent complications and exercise sheets.
- If equipment such as crutches is required, advice and demonstration/practice should be given in writing and verbally on how to use them both. A physiotherapy referral may be advised.

Cast Complications

If a cast is poorly or inappropriately applied, the patient is at risk of injury and professional and legal action could be taken. A good-quality cast is the best way to make sure that complications do not occur. The complications of casts along with mode of recognition and management are listed in Table 8.3. These complications can also be prevented by making sure the patient knows how to seek help immediately if they have any problems at all.

Table 8.3 Complications of casts.

Complication	Recognition	Management
Cracking, softening, breakdown	The cast has not been applied or treated correctly Patients and carers must be given clear verbal and written instructions	- Observe the cast hourly until dry - Reapply or reinforce only following medical review
Bleeding through the cast	If the cast is over an open or surgical wound or if the cast is causing a sore	- Seepage through a cast to be marked and observed - Excessive or odorous seepage requires medical review - Removal or bi-valving may be necessary

Table 8.3 (Continued)

Complication	Recognition	Management
Pressure or cast sores	Caused by a poorly fitted cast or because the patient has tried to relieve itching under the plaster using foreign objects There may be burning under the cast and/or localised heat, with possible swelling and discharge from the cast Sleep is often disturbed	• Easing back of the edge of the cast for observation may be possible • Splitting or bi-valving may be necessary • Remove the cast on medical advice if there is a severe sore or a foreign body is retained inside the cast
Circulatory and/or nerve impairment	Causes: • the cast is too tight • swelling within the cast These can lead to increased pressure within the limb	• Patient and carers must know what to look for and when and who to report any change to • Hourly colour, movement and sensation and capillary refill monitoring • Immediate medical advice must be sought • Removal or bi-valving of the cast may be necessary • Elevation of the limb unless compartment syndrome is suspected • Gentle exercise of the joints above and below the cast to improve circulation
Cast syndrome (fluid volume deficit)	A patient with a body cast may exhibit nausea, vomiting and abdominal pain Caused by hyperextension of the spine, causing the duodenum to be compressed between the superior mesenteric artery and the aorta, which can lead to intestinal obstruction Can occur weeks or months after the cast has been applied	• Information to patients and carers about how to recognise the condition • Immediate medical attention • Cut a hole in the plaster (window) or bi-valve the cast to allow for abdominal distention • The patient should be positioned onto their abdomen • If the patient is vomiting a nasogastric tube may be required
Joint stiffness	Patient complains of pain and stiffness on movement at a joint	• Clear verbal/written instructions for exercising affected and unaffected joints
Skin reactions	Patient complains of itching or has non-localising burning pains or rashes The skin can also blister This is unusual and is generally a reaction to the padding	• Medical advice must be sought and the cast may need to be removed and different padding and material applied

Living with a Cast

It is important that practitioners have an understanding of how a patient will cope with life in a cast (Box 8.1). A comprehensive assessment by the multidisciplinary (MDT) team may be required to ensure the patient will be able to manage safely after discharge. This will depend on previous levels of independence, the ability to accept a different level of self-care than before, availability of assistance from others and the practical advice they are given.

Assistance may be required with some activities of daily living, including the following:

Toileting: a stool to place the leg on if in a long leg cast and a commode and/or hoist if mobility is poor.

Eating and drinking: food and fluids within easy reach; making sure the patient has their food cut up if their arms are in casts; equipment such as non-slip mats and adapted cutlery.

Dressing: advice on the best clothing to wear or adaptations to be made, such as Velcro fastenings.

Mobility: assessment of mobility and aids required with instructions for use.

Sleeping can be difficult. Extra pillows and bed cradles may help along with short-term medication to help re-establish a sleep pattern.

Socialising: living with a cast can result in significant isolation and additional support is needed in leaving the home, such as temporary use of a wheelchair and contact with voluntary organisations to provide transportation.

Box 8.1   Evidence Digest

Living in a plaster cast

The number of casts applied in any orthopaedic department each year is enormous, but there is only a very limited evidence base regarding supporting and caring for patients living with a cast. A qualitative research study by Williams (2010) describes the patient's experiences of living in a below-knee cast. Data were collected from patients who had been in a lower limb cast for at least 4 weeks using unstructured interviews and transcriptions were analysed using interpretive phenomenological analysis. Seven main themes were identified: 'hard work' illustrated how difficult everyday tasks became; 'it gets you down' described how the participants began to feel frustrated and sorry for themselves; 'different circumstances' showed how participants put their situation in context to cope. Other themes were 'making it better', 'back to normal', 'pain' and 'getting through it'. It is important that practitioners have an understanding of this experience from the patient's perspective and such qualitative research is an ideal medium for this.

Cast Removal, Splitting and Bi-valving

Casts may be removed or bi-valved at the end of treatment, when a new cast is needed or if there is a problem with the cast or limb causing neurovascular compromise. Every orthopaedic practitioner should be able to safely remove or bi-valve a cast. Bi-valving involves cutting the cast in half along both sides so that one half of the cast can be removed whilst the limb is still supported with the other half. The same process should be used when removing a cast, allowing the bottom half of the cast to be used as a splint while the limb is inspected. The limb can then be carefully lifted out of the cast for removal.

Casts are bi-valved or removed using either plaster shears or an oscillating plaster saw. Practitioners must receive training and be competent in the use of either piece of equipment. Prior to cutting, the cast should be marked on the medial and lateral sides so that the cutting lines do not pass over any bony prominences or fragile skin.

Before removing a cast it is important to:

- check the patient's details and the written instructions for removal
- prepare the area and equipment to be used
- give verbal information to gain the patient's cooperation and consent

- demonstrate the equipment to be used on the patient prior to allay anxiety
- provide adequate pain relief
- position the patient comfortably and support the part of the body to have the cast removed in the correct position
- maintain privacy and dignity at all times
- assess the patient's cast carefully to ensure the correct equipment is used for cast removal
- mark the cutting area medially and laterally, avoiding bony prominences
- give written information to the patient following cast removal.

All types of casts can be removed with plaster shears or an oscillating saw. Synthetic casts require special saw blades made of tungsten.

Plaster shears are blunt and crush plaster of Paris between two hinged 'jaws'. The blade of the shears should be passed between the cast and the padding with the hand nearest the cast being kept parallel to the limb and kept still. If the shears are tilted they can dig in or catch the patient's skin. The other hand is then used to push the shears together to cut through the cast. Once the cast is cut through on both sides, it can be opened with the plaster spreaders and the padding cut all the way through with bandage scissors. Shears are often used to remove children's casts as the oscillating plaster saw may frighten them. Shears are often not effective with synthetic casts.

Plaster saws have an oscillating circular blade which vibrates back and forth at high speed, rubbing through the casting material. It must have a vacuum attached to ensure the dust is collected in keeping with health and safety regulations. The blade is held at right angles to the cast and light pressure is applied to make it cut without dragging the saw along the cast. The blade is then removed and reapplied above or below the original cut in an in-and-out motion. The saw must not be used by someone with wet hands and care must be taken as the blade can become hot and burn the skin if:

- a dragging motion is used instead of the in-and-out motion
- the saw is used continually for a long period of time
- if there is a large cast and it is taking a long time to remove it

Even in normal use the patient may feel the heat through the padding.

The patient's skin can also be damaged if:

- the cast is bloodstained and the padding and gauze has hardened

- the patient's skin is taught through swelling
- the blade of the saw is blunt or damaged
- the cast is unpadded as extra care then needs to be taken to avoid damaging the patient's skin.

The patient's limb should be placed back in the remaining half of the cast until it has been assessed and permission is given to remove it.

It is important that the patient is warned that their skin will have flaky yellow scales where the upper layers have been unable to shed. The limb will also appear thin and withered as muscles lose their tone from lack of use. The skin should be carefully inspected and assessed, and any signs of pressure or soreness should be reported and documented. The patient should be encouraged to wash and dry the area gently and if the skin is very dry, oils or emollient cream can be applied. The skin will be more sensitive to sunlight.

Orthotics, Braces, Prosthetics and Appliances

Orthotics is a specialty that deals with the design, manufacture and supply of orthoses, a general term for splints, appliances and braces. These are externally applied devices that are used to modify the structural or functional characteristics of the neuromuscular and skeletal systems (British Association of Prosthetists and Orthotists 2020). They can be used for acute injuries, chronic conditions and prevention of injury. Prosthetics are devices used to replace either a whole or part of an absent or deficient limb. An orthosis may be used to:

- control, guide or immobilise a limb, joint or body segment
- restrict movement in a given direction
- assist movement and/or posture
- reduce weight-bearing forces for a particular purpose
- assist with rehabilitation following fractures after the removal of a cast
- provide easier movement capability or reduce pain by correcting the shape and/or function of the body
- act as part of fixed or balanced traction
- prevent or correct deformity
- act prophylactically for athletes in contact sports.

The orthotist is a healthcare professional with a key role in an orthopaedic and trauma MDT (Chapter 5). They design and fit a variety of orthoses under prescription from a licenced healthcare provider. Orthotists also provide ongoing support and information to the patient and the carers.

Caring for a patient with an orthosis is very much like caring for a patient in a cast. Patients and carers can be taught to undertake their own skin care and advised how to seek help if there are problems. Advice also needs to be given regarding preventing and recognising neurovascular problems, exercising and mobilising safely using the orthosis or prosthesis to prevent joint stiffness and swelling. Verbal and written information and advice on how to care for the orthosis and how to recognise complications must be given to both patients and carers. Adjustments to any orthosis should only be undertaken by staff that have the knowledge and skills required. The complications that can occur for patients with an orthosis are related to poorly fitted devices and are similar to those experienced with casts.

External Fixation and Pin Site Care

External fixation is a powerful surgical technique, which involves the use of pins and tensioned wires attached to an external scaffolding framework to hold bones in place. The types of frames used in limb reconstruction correct deformity in children and adults, stabilise high-energy fractures in near-fatal trauma and grow bone lost due to trauma or bone tumours where the only other alternative is amputation.

Stabilisation of fractures using external fixation has been in use for thousands of years and mummified remains of humans with long bone fractures with external splintage have been found. It evolved in the 1950s to include deformity correction following the work of Gavril Abramovich Ilizarov (1921–1992), who first used circular frames with threaded rods and wires to help post-war amputees to overcome flexion contractures. One such patient had an undiagnosed fracture. Rather than distracting the contracture itself, distraction occurred at the fracture site. Subsequent X-rays showed bone formation in the gap. This was termed *distraction osteogenesis*, a previously unknown phenomenon. Bone actively forms in the endosteum, periosteum and bone marrow when compression and distraction are applied in the presence of a stable external fixation. Connective tissue only forms bone by distraction osteogenesis; this is the process by which fibroblasts lay down type 1 collagen, orientated along the line of tension. The tension is supplied through the external fixator gradually distracting the bone ends, normally at a rate of 1 mm per day. Osteoblasts then invade the periphery and start laying down bone in columns.

Types of Fixator

Many types of external fixator now exist, but they generally fall into two categories: *monolateral* and *circular*. Figures 8.1 and 8.2 illustrate just two of many different types of frames. Hybrid fixators are a combination of both

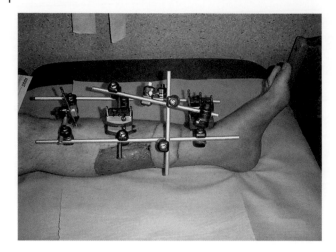

Figure 8.1 Hoffman (monolateral) external fixator frame.

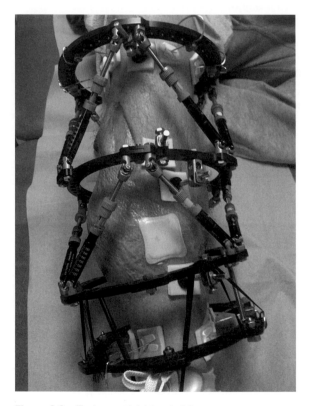

Figure 8.2 Taylor spatial (circular) frame.

circular and monolateral fixators. Monolateral fixators are biomechanically less stable than circular fixators.

Monolateral fixators (Figure 8.1) are usually modular devices used to stabilise a fracture. They enable the surgeon to build their own frame and position half pins away from any soft tissue injury. Some monolateral fixators can also be used for deformity correction; these usually involve a rail system. Often used for femoral lengthening, they are

arguably more comfortable for the patient than a circular fixator, but may not allow early weight bearing.

Circular external fixators (see Figure 8.2) are used for both fracture stabilisation and deformity correction. They can be used to correct:

- angulation
- rotation
- translation
- limb length discrepancy.

The circular frame is easily adjustable. Adding load, through early weight bearing to the already tensioned wires, stiffens the frame. Weight bearing increases blood flow to the limb and promotes healing. There are two main types of circular fixator: the *Ilizarov* and the *hexapod*. The Ilizarov has straight rods and hinges. The patient or their carer adjusts the fixator (usually with a set of spanners) in four increments per day of 0.25 mm. Hexapods are based on the Gough Stuart platform, which is also used in industry, for example in parallel robotics and aircraft simulators. Six telescopic struts are adjusted once daily according to a computer calculated prescription. Depending on the manufacturer of the fixator, it may be single or multi-use. The practitioner should establish if the equipment can be re-used and should the patient be transferred to another hospital, or in the case of death, it is important to ensure its return, as lost or mislaid equipment can lead to considerable financial loss (Timms et al. 2011).

Biomechanics

The biomechanical properties of the frame in addition to its fixation to the bone are important to the success of the treatment (Iobst 2017). A frame which is either unstable or too stiff can lead to non-union. The skill of the surgeon is of prime importance as poor application of the fixator will lead to failure of the treatment. The fixator can also become unstable due to failure of the hardware. Components of the fixator, wires and half pins may occasionally loosen or break. Pin loosening and pin site infections are known to be related (Kazmers et al. 2016). An unstable fixator needs urgent review. If the wire or pin breaks at the interface between the wire and the fixator, it may be possible to re-fix the wire. If the wire breaks at the interface with the bone, it will need to be removed and, depending on the stage of treatment, the patient may need further surgery to replace the broken wire or pin. The patient may describe:

- hearing the metal break
- the pin site becoming increasingly painful
- the wire moving freely depending on where it has broken
- the fixator feeling unstable.

It is important to inform the surgeon of this as one broken wire affects the overall fixator stability, which may lead to further wire or pin breakage and a failure of the fixator.

Complications

Pain

Pain is an anticipated result of limb reconstruction and patients should be prepared to deal with some degree of discomfort, particularly in the early stages. Modern analgesic drugs allow much more control of pain and offer several alternatives if a particular drug is found to be unsuitable.

Pin Site Infection

This is arguably the second most likely complication after pain (Kazmers et al. 2016) and should take up a large part of pre-operative counselling. Teaching patients to recognise the signs and symptoms of infection is essential as following discharge from hospital it is unlikely that the patient will see a health professional daily. It is important to explain that should infection occur it is not a failing on the patient's or clinician's part, but rather a common outcome of having metal work penetrating the protective barrier of the skin for prolonged periods of time (see pin site care below).

Joint Stiffness

Prolonged periods of immobility will lead to joint stiffness. Patients should be encouraged, with physiotherapist support, to mobilise and exercise joints not constrained by the frame. In some cases the frame will span a joint – most commonly the knee or ankle – because of the fracture site and it is important to inform the patient that following frame removal a great deal of work will be necessary to regain joint function. Managing expectations is very important, as the joint in question may never be as flexible as it was pre-injury.

Swelling

The majority of patients will experience some swelling during the treatment. This is partly a natural biophysical reaction to the presence of metalwork within the body. With lower limb frames, most commonly the swelling is due to the loss of the pumping action supplied by the calf muscles when mobilising. Weight bearing through the affected limb can help reduce this. In some circumstances,

the limb may swell to a degree that the rings are in contact with the skin and steps must be taken to protect the area from pressure damage.

Nerve and Blood Vessel Injury

A complication of any orthopaedic surgery where a wire or pin has been inserted is that it may need to be removed or possibly re-sited.

Compartment Syndrome

Because frame surgery is often minimally invasive, compartment syndrome is rare. However, the same neurovascular assessments should be undertaken throughout treatment and the immediate post-operative period with frame surgery as any other orthopaedic procedure (Chapter 9). Some of the temporary, monolateral fixators are applied following high-impact trauma, where risk is greatly increased.

Venousthromoboembolism

Any procedure that limits mobility and function puts the patient at risk of VTE (Chapter 9). Pre-operative preparation gives the clinician the opportunity to advise the patient on the signs and symptoms to look out for.

Re-fracture

Although X-rays may look adequate and the patient is reporting positively, a frame is sometimes removed too early. This can result in re-fracture. This will present in a gradual 'bend' at the fracture/regenerate site and increased pain. This is why many surgeons are now opting to remove the interlocking struts for a couple of weeks prior to complete removal; if bending occurs the struts can be reinserted and the limb can be left to heal for longer. Others will choose to protect the limb in a cast or orthotic for a few weeks preceding removal. It is considered preferable to remove the frame late rather than too early.

Nursing Care

Nursing care for patients with frames can be time-intensive and both physically and emotionally draining for both the patient and carers. Pre-operative counselling improves patient understanding and acceptance, but in cases of new trauma this is not an option. Those with chronic injuries may be facing the decision of having a frame fitted or amputation, raising a discussion about when to abandon limb salvage treatment and offer amputation. This involves intense psychological support, especially given that the patient may have many months or years of treatment in a frame for it to then fail, with the end result being amputation. Therefore, it is worth bearing in mind the work of the Lower Extremity Assessment Project (LEAP) (MacKenzie and Bosse 2006), demonstrating the importance of managing patients' expectations (See Box 8.2). Patients should be made aware that following severe trauma, the function of the affected limb may never return to its pre-injury state.

Patients, with support from family and friends, will cope with limb reconstruction better than those without a support network, especially concerning factors such as reduced mobility, fixator adjustments and getting to multiple hospital appointments. Patient support groups are not widespread, so many will turn to websites and social networking for information. Whilst this should be encouraged, patients should be made aware that much of this information is opinion and not evidence based.

Another consideration is the frequent X-rays required to monitor bone regeneration. Poor regeneration may result in the need to reduce the rate of adjustment or distraction, or it may be appropriate to speed up the adjustment process. Where regeneration is slow or in patients having treatment for non-union, it is especially important to advise on the effects of smoking and non-steroidal anti-inflammatory use. Cigarette smoke contains toxic chemicals which affect both respiratory parenchyma and the fracture healing process as nicotine in the blood supply causes the vessels to constrict by approximately 25% of

---

Box 8.2   Evidence Digest

Factors influencing outcome following limb salvage surgery and amputation

MacKenzie and Bosse (2006)
Factors Influencing Outcome Following Limb-Threatening Lower Limb Trauma: Lessons Learned From the Lower Extremity Assessment Project (LEAP).

At 2- and 7-year follow-ups, the LEAP study found no difference in functional outcome between patients who underwent either limb salvage surgery or amputation. However, outcomes on average were poor for both groups. This study and others provide evidence of wide-ranging variations in outcome following major limb trauma, with a substantial proportion of patients experiencing long-term disability. Outcomes are often more affected by the patient's economic, social and personal resources than by the initial treatment of the injury, specifically amputation or reconstruction and level of amputation.

Box 8.3   Evidence Digest

Smoking and bony union after ulna-shortening osteotomy

A study examined the relationship between cigarette use and occurrence of delayed union and non-union after ulna-shortening osteotomy for ulnar impaction syndrome. Chen et al. (2001) examined healing data from 39 patients who had undergone wrist surgery in 40 wrists. The mean union rates were 7.1 months in smokers and 4.1 months in non-smokers. Six smokers (30%) and no non-smokers experienced delayed union or non-union. Given the adverse effects of smoking on bony union, they recommend that smoking history be considered when selecting patients for such procedures.

---

normal diameter and decreased levels of nutrients are supplied to the bones. This is potentially catastrophic for a patient undergoing further surgery for a non-union. See Box 8.3 for further discussion.

Non-steroidal anti-inflammatory drugs (NSAIDs) are commonly used in orthopaedic trauma and surgery. A lesser known side effect is that of decreased fracture healing. Although much of the available literature is based on animal studies, it demonstrates that NSAID administration in the early stages of fracture healing delays the process (Dodwell et al. 2010), causing decreased osteoblastic activity, although there is also some dispute of this (Utvag et al. 2010; Yates et al. 2011). NSAIDs also reduce the synthesis of type I collagen (Ou et al. 2012) and osteocalcin mRNA and diminish angiogenesis (Jones et al. 1999), so many surgeons are now recommending that patients avoid these drugs for a period of time after injury. This may be difficult for patients and it is important that patients are informed of the rationale. A sound knowledge of other analgesics which could be offered as an alternative is important and specialist pain practitioners should be sought.

Mobilising

With the majority of circular frames, the patient will be able to fully weight bear and this should be encouraged as controlled stress at the fracture site stimulates fracture healing. Mobilisation also contributes to the patient's psychological wellbeing at a time when patients may be suffering with feelings of loss of control. It will take time for a patient to be able to fully weight bear through an affected limb, ranging from days to months. Often a good place to build up confidence is in a swimming pool, although this needs to be timed with pin site care.

Work

Returning to work will have a positive psychological impact but may not be practical and a thorough social history will assist in being able to provide advice. Someone who is desk-based is more likely to be able to return to work than a builder, but care will still have to be taken that the environment is suitable, for example the patient must be able to elevate the limb throughout the day and perhaps alter their method of transport to work.

Sleeping

Sleep can be severely affected following application of a frame. Support of the limb, comfort measures and good pain management may help. Care should also be taken to protect the rest of the body from the frame using padding.

Sexual Activity

Patients sometimes have a frame for a substantial period of time and may have undergone years of failed treatments, placing considerable strain on relationships. The patient should be given the opportunity to discuss this openly. They may enquire about sexual activity during treatment. It is important the nurse is prepared for this and can offer appropriate guidance when required.

Pin Site Wounds

The pin site is the point at which the pin or wire penetrates the soft tissues. The nature of the pin site is affected by many biopsychosocial factors and can be influenced by all members of the MDT and the patient. These factors include the following:

- The patient or their carers need to commit to caring for their limb and the fixator through self-care, allowing others into their home and/or attending their GP surgery and hospital appointments on a regular basis.
- Pins and wires should be inserted using a slow pulsed technique to prevent the wire becoming overheated and causing thermal necrosis to the soft tissues and bone, providing an ideal environment for bacteria to flourish. Untensioned wires, frames and loose pins are also known to be related to pin site infection (Saithna 2011).
- The nurse is the majority stakeholder in the patient's care so needs to ensure the patient and their carers feel confident with basic frame care through assessment and education.
- The physiotherapist ensures mobility is maintained wherever possible and educates the patient on the prevention of contractures. Exercise may irritate the pin sites and strategies such as applying more padding with compression to the sites may help alleviate this.
- The occupational therapist assesses the patient and provides aids such as a shower seat to help maintain the patient's hygiene needs. This is important because there is evidence that a patient's skin is a major source of bacterial infection contributing to postoperative wound infection (Florman and Nichols 2007).

Pin Site Infection

The prevention, identification and treatment of any infection is of prime importance. With pins and wires passing through the skin, muscle and bone, pin site infection is a constant risk. The presence of a foreign body in the wound interrupts the normal healing process, Parallels between the general infection guidelines and the 2010 Royal College of Nursing pin site guidance can be seen (Box 8.3). Pin site care is an area lacking in sufficient high-quality research (Walker 2018). Cochrane systematic reviews (Lethaby et al. 2013) have concluded that there is little or no evidence on which to base practice. In the absence of such research, practitioners should implement strategies to minimise infection. Despite there being limited literature regarding pin site infection, there is currently no validated assessment tool. This is important because it affects the validity and comparison of research trials. There is some consensus amongst practitioners (Clint et al. 2010; Santy-Tomlinson et al. 2011) that pin sites appear to fall into three categories:

- A healthy, 'calm' or 'good' pin site is not inflamed, is dry and resembles a piercing.
- An infected or 'ugly' pin site is painful, inflamed and heavily discharging, possibly with frank pus.
- The third category is the hardest to quantify but lies at an unknown point between the other two. Santy-Tomlinson et al. (2011) describe these sites as being 'irritated'.

Wound swabs do not help in the distinction between 'irritated' and 'infected' sites, as they do not distinguish between colonisation and infection. See Box 8.4 for a summary of recommendations for the care of pin sites.

Box 8.4   Evidence Digest

Pin site care

Guidance on pin site care. Report and recommendations from the 2010 consensus project on pin site care (Timms et al. 2011). This consensus study is based on expert opinion. Although the lowest form of evidence, the lack of high-quality studies makes this an appropriate way to guide practice. The recommendations from the consensus reflect current infection control guidance for percutaneous insertion sites as well as findings from studies cited in the Cochrane review.

The recommendations of the consensus are as follows:

- In the absence of allergy or skin sensitivity, pin sites should be cleaned once weekly using an alcoholic chlorhexidine solution and non-shedding gauze.
- The frequency of dressing changes should be increased if infection is confirmed or suspected or if strikethrough occurs on the pin site dressing.
- Pin sites should be kept covered with a dressing that is non-shedding and which also keeps excess exudate away from the wound.
- Dressings should be held in situ with a clip attached to the wire or half pin to apply light compression.
- Patients with pin sites should not soak in a bath of water, but may shower immediately prior to dressing changes.
- Infection should be diagnosed using patient-reported signs and symptoms, and patient perceptions of the presence of infection should be taken seriously.
- Increasing pain at the pin site, decreased mobility, spreading erythema, increased swelling and discharge are indicators of the presence of infection.

Contemporary Traction

Traction is now used much less commonly due to improved implants and surgical techniques for the treatment of fractures. The result of this is that the skills needed to care for patients with traction are often not maintained. However, management by traction remains essential for those patients whose age or condition means that surgical treatment is not appropriate. It is vital that orthopaedic nurses have a basic understanding of the principles of traction, the ability to apply the most common types of traction and the knowledge to care for patients with traction. The evidence base for both the benefits of traction and the care required is very limited because it is now such a small, but important, part of

orthopaedic care. This presents the practitioner with little evidence-based guidance and much advice is based on experience and trial and error.

Principles of Traction

Traction is the application of a pulling force to a part or parts of the body for the treatment of bone and muscle disorders or injuries. Traction in the opposite direction, *counter-traction*, is also necessary in accordance with Newton's third law of motion: that for every action there is an equal and opposite reaction. Control of the injured part by traction facilitates bone and soft tissue healing based on simple mechanical principles but this can lead to complications (Royal College of Nursing 2021). Traction can be used to:

- relieve pain due to muscle spasm
- restore and maintain alignment of bone following fracture or dislocation
- rest injured or inflamed joints whilst maintaining a functional position
- allow movement of joints during fracture healing
- prevent or gradually correct deformities due to contraction of soft tissue caused by disease or injury.

Methods of Application

To apply traction a satisfactory grip must be obtained on a part of the patient's body via the skin or bone for a specified period of time. This can be achieved manually or via skin or skeletal traction:

- *Manual*: The pulling force is applied manually usually by the hands, for example when the fracture is being reduced or held in alignment while a cast or a more permanent form of traction is applied. Manual traction is also required during any adjustments to the traction arrangement which necessitate the temporary release of the traction weight.
- *Skin*: The application of a traction force over a large area of skin, which is then transmitted via the soft tissues to the bone. The maximum pull should not exceed that recommended by the manufacturer of the traction appliance. The grip on the body is less secure than with skeletal traction. Skin traction can be adhesive or non-adhesive. Non-adhesive traction is preferable if the traction is only to be on for a short period of time. Adhesive traction should not be used with fragile or damaged skin as removal may cause further skin injury.
- *Skeletal*: The application of a traction force directly to the bone through metal pins or wires allowing large forces to

be transmitted directly to the bone. It is used if traction is to be maintained for a significant amount of time and when greater weight is required. Sites for the insertion of metal pins for skeletal traction include the proximal end of the tibia, the calcaneum, the distal femur, the skull and the olecranon.

There are two mechanisms that can be used for skin and skeletal traction:

- *Fixed*: The pull is between two fixed points, such as Thomas splint traction (Figure 8.3).
- *Balanced or sliding*: The pull is between the weights and the body weight of the patient (Figure 8.4).

These two forms of traction can be applied in several ways: fixed or sliding skin traction, fixed or sliding skeletal traction, combined fixed and balanced traction, and modified skeletal traction. The method that is chosen depends on the condition or injury being treated.

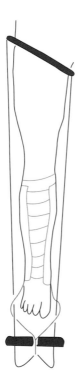

Figure 8.3   Fixed skin traction with a Thomas splint.

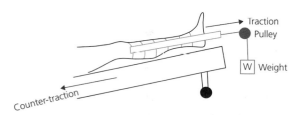

Figure 8.4   Skin traction.

Principles of Applying Traction

Some essential principles must be observed if traction is to be effective:

- the grip or hold on the body must be secure
- there must be counter-traction
- the weights used should be prescribed and documented
- there must be minimal friction from cords and pulleys frequent checks of the patient and traction equipment should be made and documented to ensure that:
  - the traction setup is functioning as planned and is safe
  - the patient is not suffering any injury or deterioration due to the traction treatment
  - the traction system once set up is maintained at all times.

Traction that is poorly or incorrectly applied and maintained can cause discomfort and further injury.

Mechanics of Traction

Traction systems have a number of mechanical components that it is important to understand when providing care:

- *Counter-traction*: It is essential in any traction system that there is a pull in the opposite direction to overcome muscle spasm and to prevent the patient from being dragged towards the traction pull. Counter-traction can be achieved in two ways: balanced sliding traction or fixed traction.
  - *Balanced (sliding) traction*: A system of weights and pulleys is used to apply and direct the traction pull. Counter-traction is exerted by the weight of the patient aided by gravity when the bed is tilted away from the traction pull by elevating the foot or head end of the bed (Figure 8.4).
  - *Fixed traction*: Traction and counter-traction are exerted between two fixed points. An appliance such as the Thomas splint is used to gain purchase on the body proximally to the muscles in spasm/injury. Skin extensions on the leg are then tied firmly to the end of the Thomas splint and counter-traction forces are transmitted up the sides of the Thomas splint to the ring encircling the limb. This is a self-contained system that does not require weights or bed elevation to achieve traction and counter-traction (see Figure 8.3). It can be used when transferring patients. A balanced system is sometimes added to elevate the limb and for ease of movement of the patient.

- *Position of pulleys*: The position of pulleys within the traction system determines the direction of the traction pull and the angle. The number of pulleys used and their position affect the amount of pull that is exerted. For example, in a single pulley system the amount of traction pull is virtually equal to the amount of traction weight used, whereas two pulleys in the line of the same traction weight almost doubles the pull exerted because of the block-and-tackle effect. This can be seen in Hamilton Russell traction, where the amount of horizontal pull exerted on the leg is double that of the weight applied (Figure 8.5).
- *Vector forces*: Traction forces in two different, but not opposite, directions to the same body part create a resultant force. The direction of the resultant force is determined by the position of the pulleys which direct the traction cords to the weight. In Hamilton Russell traction, for example, one force – the weight – is broken up into multiple forces to achieve a specific resultant force on the fracture site. The vector forces created can only act in the direction of the traction cords and include an upward force applied directly to the knee by means of the sling and two forces distal to the foot, which reaches the femur through the leg (Figure 8.5). Changes and adjustments can be made by altering the weights or the position of the pulleys.
- *Friction*: The force that acts between any two surfaces and is present within the traction system. It gives resistance to the traction pull and reduces the efficiency of the traction force. Friction cannot be eliminated but can be minimised by ensuring that:
  - the pulley wheel runs freely
  - the traction cord runs centrally over the groove of the pulley
  - the weights are not resting against the bed or on the floor
  - the bedclothes are not resting against the traction cords.

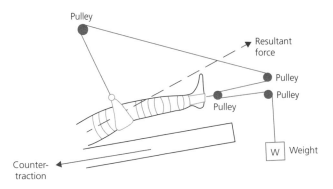

Figure 8.5 Hamilton Russell traction.

Care of Traction

In addition to the fundamental holistic care of the patient with traction there are a number of checks that should be made on the traction system. These checks should be carried out by a practitioner who has appropriate competence, skill and knowledge:

- Traction equipment should be checked daily to ensure that beams and clamps have not become loose.
- Traction should be checked at least once every shift and following interventions such as movement of the patient, physiotherapy and X-ray as the traction system may have been inadvertently altered.
- Traction cords must be attached securely using standard non-slip knots such as the clove-hitch or two-half-hitches. Only traction cord should be used as it is designed not to stretch and the ends of the cords should be short and bound back on themselves to prevent fraying. The knot should not be covered. Short cords should not be joined together by knots as this prevents the smooth running over pulleys.
- The alignment of the cords should be checked to ensure the maintenance of the appropriate pulling forces and the cord should run freely over the groove.
- The pulleys must be checked at least once each shift to ensure they are running freely to minimise friction and that the cords are sitting in the groove. There should only be one traction cord per pulley wheel.
- Weights should be hanging freely and not resting on the floor or any other surface as this compromises the efficiency of the traction system. They should also be securely attached.
- Weights should not be hung directly over the patient.
- Bed cradles should be in use to prevent bed clothes from interfering with the free running of traction cords.
- Counter-traction should be maintained at all times.
- If skin traction is in use the skin should be checked at least 4-hourly for rubbing or sore areas and the bandages should be monitored to ensure they are not too tight and do not become loose or slip.
- If skeletal traction is being used the sharp ends of the pins should be covered to prevent injury and the pins should be checked to ensure they have not become loose or moved. In addition, the pin sites should be checked for signs of infection as discussed above.
- If a Thomas splint is in use it should fit correctly. Skin under the ring should be kept clean and dry, and should be checked and gently moved to prevent skin injury. The traction system may need to be adjusted to avoid increasing pressure under the ring.

Common Types of Traction

Hamilton Russell Traction

A balanced traction system using vectors to effect a pull along the long axis of the femur (Figure 8.5). It is used to:

- maintain the joint space at the hip
- manage fractures of the acetabulum
- support fractures of the shaft of femur.

Traction can be applied using below-knee skin traction or a skeletal pin.

Gallows/Bryant Traction

This is used in the management of fractures of the shaft of femur in very young children and in the preliminary management of congenital dislocation of the hip. It is only safe to use for children who are under 2 years of age and weigh less than 14 kg due to the risk of vascular complications. Traction is exerted by full-length skin extensions to both legs and the child is positioned with the hips flexed to 90° and both legs are suspended vertically. Enough weight is applied so that the child's pelvis is lifted just clear of the mattress ensuring that counter-traction is provided by the weight of the child's body (Figure 8.6). Due to the risk of vascular complications a set of baseline neurovascular observations should be documented prior to the application of the traction and these should be repeated hourly for the first 24 hours, then 2-hourly for a further 24 hours and then 2–4-hourly thereafter. The feet should be checked for colour, temperature, capillary return, pulses and active/passive movement.

Thomas Splint Traction

The Thomas splint is used in conjunction with skin or skeletal traction to immobilise and position fractures of the femur. It can be used in all age groups. It is a long leg splint with a ring at the hip and extends to beyond the foot

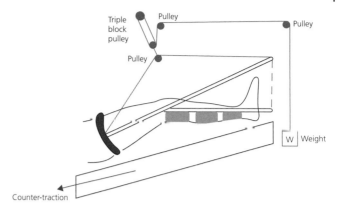

Figure 8.7 Balanced Thomas splint traction with Pearson attachment.

(Figure 8.3). The Thomas splint can be suspended in a balanced system using skin or skeletal traction either as a sliding system of traction or as fixed traction. This type of traction allows the injured limb to be maintained and moved in a gravity-free environment (Figure 8.7). The Thomas splint can also be used with fixed traction to transport patients between wards/departments and hospitals.

Dunlop Traction

Dunlop traction is now rarely used for the gradual reduction of supracondylar and transcondylar fractures of the humerus in children and adolescents. The shoulder is abducted 45° and the elbow is flexed to 45°. Lateral pull is exerted on the forearm via the skin extensions and a second force is directed downwards on the distal humerus by the use of a weighted sling. These two forces act in different but not opposite directions and counter-traction is achieved by the weight of the patient's body when the side of the bed or mattress is elevated (Figure 8.8).

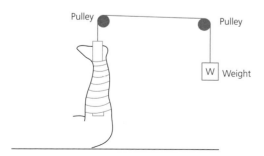

Figure 8.6 Bryants/Gallows traction.

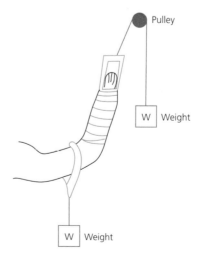

Figure 8.8 Dunlop traction.

Further Reading

Jester, R., Santy, J., and Rogers, J. (2021). *Oxford Handbook of Orthopaedic and Trauma Nursing*, 2e. Oxford: Oxford University Press.

References

British Association of Prosthetists and Orthotists (2020). *Guidelines for Best Practice*. Paisley: British Association of Prosthetists and Orthotists.

Chen, F., Osterman, A.L., and Mahony, K. (2001). Smoking and bony union after ulna-shortening osteotomy. *American Journal of Orthopaedics* 30 (6): 486–489.

Clint, S.A., Eastwood, D.M., Chasseaud, M. et al. (2010). The "good, bad and ugly" pin site grading system: a reliable and memorable method for documenting and monitoring ring fixator pin sites. *Injury* 14 (2): 147–150.

Dodwell, E.R., Latorre, J.G., Parsini, E. et al. (2010). NSAD exposure and risk of non-union: a meta-analysis of case control cohort studies. *Calcific Tissue International* 87: 193–202.

Florman, S. and Nichols, R.L. (2007). Current approaches for the prevention of surgical site infections. *American Journal of Infectious Diseases* 3 (1): 51–61.

Healy, A., Farmer, S., Pandyan, A., Chockalingam, N. (2018). A systematic review of randomised controlled trials assessing effectiveness of prosthetic and orthotic interventions. *PLoS One* 13 (3): e0192094. doi: 10.1371/journal.pone.0192094. PMID: 29538382; PMCID: PMC5851539.

Iobst, C.A. (2017). Pin-track infections: past, present, and future. *Journal of Limb Lengthening Reconstruction* [serial online] 3: 78–84. https://www.jlimblengthrecon.org/text. asp?2017/3/2/78/213563.

Kazmers, N.H., Fragomen, A.T., and Rozbruch, S.R. (2016). Prevention of pin site infection in external fixation: a review of the literature. *Strategies in Trauma and Limb Reconstruction* 11: 75–85.

Leggett, H., Scantlebury, A., Byrne, A. et al. (2021) Exploring what is important to patients with regards to quality of life after experiencing a lower limb reconstructive procedure: a qualitative evidence synthesis. *Health Qual Life Outcomes* 19 (1): 158. doi: 10.1186/s12955-021-01795-9.

Lethaby, A., Temple, J., and Santy-Tomlinson, J. (2013). Pin site care for preventing infections associated with external bone fixators and pins. *Cochrane Database of Systematic Reviews* (12): CD004551. https://doi.org/10.1002/14651858. CD004551.pub3.

Ou, Y.S., Tan, C., An, H. et al. (2012). The effects of NSAIDs on types I, II, and III collagen metabolism in a rat osteoarthritis model. *Rheumatology International* 32 (8): 2401–2405.

Royal College of Nursing (2021). *Traction Principles and Application*. London: Royal College of Nursing.

Santy-Tomlinson, J., Vincent, M., Glossop, N. et al. (2011). Calm, irritated or infected? The experience of the inflammatory states and symptoms of pin site infection and irritation during external fixation. A grounded theory study. *Journal of Clinical Nursing* 20 (21/22): 3163–3173.

Timms, A., Vincent, M., Santy-Tomlinson, J. and Hertz, K. (2011) *RCN guidance on pin site care*. Report and recommendations from the 2010 Consensus Project on Pin Site Care. Royal College of Nursing. www.rcn.org. uk/__data/assets/pdf_file/0009/413982 004137.pdf (accessed 30 March 2014).

Utvag, S.E., Fuskevag, O.M., Shegarfi, H., and Reikeras, O. (2010). Short-term treatment with COX-2 inhibitors does not impair fracture healing. *Journal of Investigative Surgery* 23: 257–261.

Walker, J. (2018). Assessing and managing pin sites in patients with external fixation. *Nursing Times* 114 (1): 18–21.

Williams, M. (2010). The patient's experience in a plaster cast. *International Journal of Orthopaedic and Trauma Nursing* 14 (3): 132–141.

Yates, J.E., Shah, S.H., and Blackwell, J.C. (2011). Do NSAIDs impede fracture healing? *The Journal of Family Practice* 60 (1): 41–42.

9

The Complications of Musculoskeletal Conditions and Trauma: Preventing Harm

Julie Santy-Tomlinson[1], Sonya Clarke[2], and Peter Davis[3]

[1] *International Journal of Orthopaedic and Trauma Nursing*
[2] *Queen's University Belfast, Belfast, UK*
[3] *Newark, Nottinghamshire, UK*

Introduction

Patient harm during healthcare is a leading cause of morbidity and mortality, and early detection and prevention of patient harm is a priority (Panagioti et al. 2019). This includes preventable complications following orthopaedic and trauma care. The aim of this chapter is to provide evidence-based guidance for the identification of risk, detection, prevention and management of those complications which are significant risks for the orthopaedic and trauma patient. Preventable complications are major causes of both morbidity (complications) and mortality (death), and are of considerable significance in providing evidence-based care. Harm to a patient following musculoskeletal care and procedures is almost always the result of one or more complications which can also lead to poorer outcomes, patient distress and discomfort, significant delays in recovery and increased costs. Much care provided in both the acute, rehabilitation and community setting is aimed at minimising the potentially harmful effects of four factors that lead to complications:

- *tissue injury* to bone and/or soft tissue due to trauma or surgery
- *surgery*, i.e. the effects of anaesthesia and surgical procedures
- *reduced mobility* because of musculoskeletal conditions, injury or surgery and associated care
- *stasis* of major body systems because of reduced mobility.

It is worth noting poor life choices may predispose patients to an increased risk of complications, delayed recovery and death when musculoskeletal conditions and trauma occur. For example, lack of activity/exercise, stress, reduced sleep, poor nutrition and hydration, excessive alcohol and smoking. This chapter describes appropriate nursing interventions based on Roper et al.'s (2000) activities of daily living. This model is still used to identify and direct nursing care today even though it was first described in the 1970s. Those activities relevant to this chapter are:

1) breathing
2) eating food and drinking fluids
3) eliminating body waste
4) mobilising
5) sleeping.

Finally, while there are many potential complications for the orthopaedic and trauma patient, this chapter will focus on those which are either the most common or likely to result in the most significant harm: infection, shock, venous thromboembolism (VTE), fat embolism syndrome (FES), acute compartment syndrome (ACS), urinary retention, urinary tract infection (UTI), respiratory tract infection and constipation.

Infection

The human body is constantly exposed to microorganisms from the environment. The immune system provides a range of defence mechanisms against infection, which include physical, chemical, innate and adaptive responses to attack by organisms. A large and diverse community of commensal organisms (which inhabit human mucosa and skin without causing harm) play an important role in defence against pathogenic (causing diseases) organisms.

Infections can occur when damaged or vulnerable tissue is exposed to harmful pathogens (such as bacteria, viruses and fungi), leading to a complex tissue response brought about by the multiplication of and attack by such microorganisms. This depends on the susceptibility of the patient and the virulence of the organism. Potentially harmful organisms such as bacteria, viruses and fungi may *contaminate* tissue. Multiplication of the organisms may then lead to *colonisation*. Infection is not, however, considered to be present until attack from a pathogenic organism results in an acute or chronic tissue reaction. Bacteria may contaminate or colonise tissue without causing infection. When the patient's immune system is compromised due to factors such as age, ill-health or depleted nutrition, colonisation is more likely to progress to *infection* and host defences are less effective in fighting infection.

Both tissue injury and infection result in an inflammatory reaction, which is part of the immune response; a distinct reaction brought about by both chemical and physical phenomena which results in the 'cardinal' signs of inflammation/infection: redness, pain, swelling and heat. There may also be increased exudate. If the organism causing infection is 'pyogenic' (pus producing) collections of pus may also form as abscesses.

Infection is best diagnosed by observing the tissue response to microbial invasion and the subsequent symptoms of infection as a manifestation of the inflammatory response. This response will vary depending on the infecting organisms and the tissue or system affected. They can include:

- pain, swelling, redness and heat at the site of infection, in the surrounding area or deep within the tissues
- loss of function of the area affected, particularly if pain and/or swelling affect joints and other musculoskeletal structures
- tissue exudate, which may or may not contain pus
- pyrexia and/or
- generally feeling unwell, with malaise or lethargy.

A diagnosis of infection should be made based on the symptoms reported by the patient. This can be augmented, but not replaced by, microbiological culture and analysis of wound samples in the laboratory.

The orthopaedic and trauma patient is particularly vulnerable to the following types of infection:

- wound infection (Chapter 12): categorised as either surgical site infection (SSI) or traumatic wound infection
- bone infection (osteomyelitis) and joint infection (infective arthritis) (Chapter 13)
- UTI
- respiratory tract infection.

Healthcare-associated infection is the main cause of infection in orthopaedic and trauma patients, acquired by transfer from one person or surface to another. The way by which an infection can spread involves five links in the chain of infection (Public Health England 2017). Understanding how the links are made is important in understanding the ways in which the chain can be broken and infection prevented:

1) *A causative organism*: a pathogenic organism is present which can cause infection
2) *A reservoir of infection*: a place (human or environmental) which provides conditions for the organism to multiply
3) *A portal of exit*: allows the organism to leave the reservoir, e.g. in body fluids, on the skin (particularly the hands) and in various body fluids such as respiratory droplets
4) *A mode of transmission*: a method through which the organism is spread to another person, e.g. through body fluids, the hands of patients and healthcare workers, ingestion and airborne transmission
5) *A susceptible patient*: vulnerable to infection because their immune response is compromised, e.g. hospitalised patients, the injured, surgery, the very young, the very old (and frail) and those with concurrent medical conditions and malnutrition.

A significant concern is also the ability of remote infections such as UTIs and SSIs to transfer to sites of orthopaedic implants because of 'seeding' of bacteria to implant sites. The prevention of infections in orthopaedic patients is particularly important because of the potentially devastating consequences of transfer of infection to bone and subsequent osteomyelitis, which is difficult to eradicate and results in long-term pain and distress; the avoidance of this is a central aim of infection control in orthopaedic settings. Infection may also lead to life-threatening sepsis (see Sepsis and septic shock section).

Infection Prevention

Prevention of infection measures has been standardised because of a large body of amassed evidence that demonstrates the most effective approaches (see Box 9.1 for an example of evidence-based guidelines), which include the following interventions (Loveday et al. 2014):

- *Hospital environmental hygiene* through rigorous cleaning processes and assessment of cleanliness, equipment decontamination.
- *Hand hygiene/hand decontamination*: many healthcare-associated infections are transferred from one person to the other on the hands of healthcare staff.

Box 9.1 Evidence Digest

Evidence-based guidelines for preventing healthcare-associated infections

Many counties have developed national guidelines for the prevention of healthcare-associated infection. The epic 3 guidelines (Loveday et al. 2014) provide an example from England. These were commissioned by the Department of Health (England) and revised, reviewed and updated for a second time in 2014. They were created by a nurse-led multiprofessional team who undertook extensive consultation using multiple systematic reviews of the evidence and other guidelines as well as expert opinion, demonstrating use of all levels of evidence available at that time. The guidelines are freely available as open access at https://doi.org/10.1016/S0195-6701(13)60012-2.

The guidelines describe in detail the interventions and precautions practitioners should take to prevent healthcare-associated infection, which include the recommendations outlined in Loveday et al. (2014). These precautions are designed to break the chain of infection. The authors point out that effective infection prevention and control are essential in ensuring patient safety and preventing harm. The orthopaedic and trauma team must incorporate such national, regional and local guidelines into everyday practice to reduce infection risk during care and intervention.

Box 9.2 Evidence Digest

Hand hygiene compliance: what the evidence says

Hand decontamination is a universally accepted elementary method for infection prevention. It is easy, cheap and quick to perform. Remarkably, compliance with the five moments of hand hygiene (HH) (WHO 2009) is consistently poor among all health professionals in every setting. A systematic review conducted by Erasmus et al. (2010) found that 60% of HH opportunities are missed. Some studies have already been conducted which show that even during the COVID-19 pandemic healthcare workers returned to poor compliance levels surprisingly quickly (Stangerup et al. 2021). The reasons for poor HH compliance among practitioners are complex and every practitioner will be subtly aware of their own reasons for such failures in safe practice.

Many studies have also been conducted which consider the interventions most likely to improve HH compliance. Researchers in the USA (Sands and Aunger 2020) conducted a survey that considered the factors, barriers and levers that influence HH among nurses. They found the following situations were associated with higher compliance:

- leadership
- conducting tasks perceived as dirty
- access to HH facilities and materials
- availability of alcohol rub/gel
- good practice examples of other team members
- feedback on performance.

However, a systematic review by Doronina et al. (2017) found that education regarding HH is forgotten as little as a month later. While all staff should undergo regular education to support compliance and to ensure that skills are up to date and embedded in their practice, there is a need to consider how this can be maintained during daily practice.

- The use of *personal protective equipment* to provide a barrier between the healthcare provider and a source of infection.
- The *safe use and disposal of sharps*: there is a high risk of blood-borne infection from accidental inoculation with contaminated sharps.
- Preventing infections associated with the use of *short-term indwelling urethral catheters*, which provide a major portal for infection.
- Preventing infections associated with *central venous catheters*, which are linked with blood-borne infection.

Evidence has shown that effective hand hygiene is the most effective method of preventing the transfer of infection. National and international guidelines emphasise the importance of adherence to hand hygiene guidance and provide an overview of the barriers and factors that influence hand hygiene compliance (Loveday et al. 2014). Compliance is much lower than the target of 100%

(Box 9.2) and measures are needed to ensure that compliance is as high as possible (Tromp et al. 2012).

There are three common healthcare-associated infections of particular concern to the orthopaedic and trauma patient: SSI, respiratory tract infection and UTI. Several evidence-based guidelines exist globally which provide the practitioner with best practice advice for the prevention and management of each of these types of infections. Some of these are listed in Box 9.3.

Box 9.3 Evidence-based Guidance for the Prevention and Management of Surgical Site Infection and Respiratory Tract Infection

Surgical site infection

Centers for Disease Control and Prevention (CDC) (2017) Guideline for the Prevention of Surgical Site Infection. https://jamanetwork.com/journals/jamasurgery/fullarticle/2623725.

Ling, M.L., Apisarnthanarak, A., Abbas, A. et al. APSIC guidelines for the prevention of surgical site infections. Antimicrob Resist Infect Control 8, 174 (2019). https://doi.org/10.1186/s13756-019-0638-8.

National Institute for Health and Care Excellence (NICE) (2019) Surgical site infections: prevention and treatment. NICE Guideline NG12G. www.nice.org.uk/guidance/ng125.

World Health Organisation (2018). Global guidelines for the prevention of surgical site infection, 2nd edn. World Health Organisation. https://apps.who.int/iris/handle/10665/277399.

Respiratory tract infection

NICE (2019) Pneumonia (hospital-acquired): antimicrobial prescribing. NICE guideline [NG139]. www.nice.org.uk/guidance/NG139. (Note: NICE withdrew their guideline Pneumonia in adults: diagnosis and management. Clinical guideline [CG191] in 2019 during the COVID pandemic and stated that they are reviewing the recommendations.)

Pássaro, L., Harbarth, S. & Landelle, C. Prevention of hospital-acquired pneumonia in non-ventilated adult patients: a narrative review. Antimicrob Resist Infect Control 5, 43 (2016). https://doi.org/10.1186/s13756-016-0150-3.

Urinary tract infection

Centers for Disease Control and Prevention (CDC) (2009) Guideline for Prevention of Catheter-Associated Urinary Tract Infections. https://www.cdc.gov/infectioncontrol/guidelines/cauti/index.html.

Surgical Site Infection

SSI is a major risk of orthopaedic surgery, particularly following implantation of, for example, internal fixation devices or arthroplasty. After internal fixation of fractures SSI rates have been reported to be as high as 3.6% (Bai et al. 2019) and 10% after hip fracture surgery (de Jong et al. 2017). Patients with SSI have longer hospitals stays, more readmissions and higher mortality. SSI following orthopaedic surgery can lead to poorer outcomes from surgery, functional loss, implant failure and amputation (Copanitsanou 2020).

Prevention of SSI is an interdisciplinary team priority. Prevention should be focused on adherence to infection prevention guidelines (see previous section) and up-to-date evidence-based guidance as outlined in Box 9.3. Prophylactic prevention of infection using antibiotics in the orthopaedic and trauma setting is standard practice and has been shown to reduce rates of infection where risk is high, such as in traumatic wounds and surgery which involves implantation (Gillespie and Walenkamp 2010). However, resistance is an increasing problem across all healthcare settings and the careful and prudent use of antibiotic therapy is increasingly important. This reinforces the need for measures that minimise all infections (Bryson et al. 2016).

Urinary Tract Infection

The urinary tract is the most common source of healthcare-associated infection. Because of stasis in the urinary system during anaesthesia, surgery and post-operative recovery, the risk is high in all surgical patients and in those with restricted mobility. The risk of infection is significantly increased by bladder catheterisation, so this should be avoided in orthopaedic patients because of the link between bacteriuria and implant site infection (Meddings et al. 2019).

Guidance for the prevention of healthcare-associated UTI is provided in Box 9.4. Engaging all clinical staff in measures to prevent UTI, particularly urinary catheter-associated UTI, is essential (Thakker et al. 2018).

Respiratory Tract Infection (Pneumonia)

Pneumonia (lower respiratory tract infection) is a potentially fatal hospital-acquired infection. It is a significant cause of death for orthopaedic patients, particularly following fragility hip fracture. Mucosal surfaces in the respiratory tract contain large numbers of resident flora, which combat pathogenic attack. Hypostatic pneumonia is a risk when mechanisms such as the cough reflex are suppressed due to anaesthesia and sedation, and patient mobility problems mean that respiratory ventilation is decreased, particularly in older and frail patients and those with concurrent medical conditions.

Box 9.4   Guidance for the Prevention of Healthcare-associated UTI

Avoid unnecessary placement of indwelling urinary catheters

Removal of urinary catheters as early as possible, preferably within 24 hours

Use of closed drainage systems and aseptic management of catheters and systems

Avoidance of dehydration

Early mobilisation to prevent urinary stasis and return to normal toileting habits as soon as possible

Evidence-based continence management without the use of indwelling urinary catheters where required

High standards of perineal/penile hygiene

Early identification and treatment of UTI and good hydration

Measures for prevention of respiratory tract infection in the orthopaedic patient include:

- avoidance of elective surgery in patients with pre-existing respiratory infections (usually viral) through preoperative screening
- post-operative pain relief to facilitate coughing and deep breathing
- early post-operative mobilisation
- since chest infection is often hospital-acquired, universal infection control precautions are an essential aspect of prevention.

Observation of the at-risk patient for symptoms of pneumonia is essential in enabling early management. Symptoms may be insidious or develop quite suddenly and include:

- shortness of breath/rapid and/or shallow breathing
- a cough which may or may not be productive initially
- sputum which may be yellow, green, brown or blood stained; a specimen should be obtained for culture
- chest pain
- pyrexia
- tachycardia
- acute confusion
- general malaise and fatigue
- loss of appetite.

A diagnosis of pneumonia is made based on the above symptoms along with chest auscultation (abnormal lung sounds can be heard) and chest X-ray (demonstrating lung consolidation). There will also be a raised white cell count. A positive sputum culture will help to identify the causative organism and direct treatment.

Management of pneumonia should be commenced immediately due to the potentially life-threatening nature of the infection. This should include the following considerations:

- Antibiotic therapy according to the nature and sensitivity of the pathogen causing the pneumonia. The timeliness and appropriateness of this is central to the recovery of the patient along with other supporting measures but may be complex if a resistant strain of bacteria is the causative organism.
- Constant monitoring of the vital signs of the patient with a view to detecting and acting on any further deterioration.
- Maintenance of hydration using intravenous infusion of fluids if necessary.
- Optimum nutrition using nutritional supplementation, nasogastric or enteral feeding as necessary.
- The patient should be cared for sitting up or in the semi-recumbent position, providing it is aligned with their orthopaedic condition.
- Deep-breathing exercises and chest physiotherapy.

Sepsis and Septic Shock

Sepsis is a leading cause of avoidable death. It is a clinical syndrome in which immune and coagulation responses are triggered by an infection. Sepsis can lead to septic shock, a life-threatening condition that occurs when sepsis leads to low blood pressure and low blood flow that can result in organ failure (NICE 2016) (as described in the section considering shock). Sepsis can be caused by any source of infection, including cellulitis and wound infections, UTIs, respiratory infections, septicaemia, septic arthritis and osteomyelitis, meaning that the orthopaedic patients is at significant risk. The mortality rate is estimated to be as much as 56% (Bauer et al. 2020).

Early recognition may be difficult and the practitioner's role is central in recognising changes in patient condition and seeking medical attention. The person may present with similar signs to hypovolemic shock (see below) but without a potential source of bleeding. There may also be hypotension, altered coagulation, inflammation, impaired circulation, anaerobic metabolism and changes in mental status. NICE (2016) provide a series of tools/algorithms for the identification of those who could be presenting with sepsis (see Box 9.5).

Shock

Shock is a complex life-threatening physiological syndrome resulting from a significant reduction in systemic tissue perfusion, and subsequent hypotension and reduced

---

Box 9.5   Could this Be Sepsis? Sepsis: Risk Stratification Tools (NICE 2016)

Could this be sepsis?

For a person of any age with a possible infection:

- Think – could this be sepsis? Does the person have signs or symptoms that indicate infection, even if they do not have a high temperature?
- Be aware that people with sepsis may have non-specific, non-localised presentations (e.g. feeling very unwell).
- Pay particular attention to concerns expressed by the person and their family or carer.
- Take particular care in the assessment of people who might have sepsis if they, or their parents or carers, are unable to give a good history (e.g. people with English as a second language, people with communication problems).

Assessment

- Assess people with suspected infection to identify:
  - Possible source of infection
  - Risk factors for sepsis (see below)
  - Indicators of clinical concern such as new onset abnormalities of behaviour, circulation or respiration.

Risk factors for sepsis

- The very young (under 1 year) and older people (over 75 years) or very frail people.
- Recent trauma or surgery or invasive procedure (within the last 6 weeks).

- Impaired immunity due to illness (e.g. diabetes) or drugs (e.g. people receiving long-term steroids, chemotherapy or immunosuppressants).
- Indwelling lines, catheters, intravenous drug misusers, any breach of skin integrity (e.g. any cuts, burns, blisters or skin infections).

Management of sepsis and associated septic shock includes (NICE 2016):

- urgent medical review
- structured face-to-face assessment and observation (essential in both recognising sepsis and in monitoring the patient with sepsis) at least every 30 minutes, and using an early warning score and recording system
- early administration of broad-spectrum antibiotics until the source and microbiology of infection is identified
- identification and medical treatment of the source of infection
- intravenous fluid resuscitation according to recent guidance
- referral to critical care services for ongoing treatment and monitoring.

The UK Sepsis Trust (www.sepsistrust.org) provides resources to help clinicians learn about recognising and managing sepsis, including education resources and guidelines.

---

oxygen (O_2) delivery to the tissues. Early recognition and management are vital in increasing the odds of survival. Poor perfusion of cells leads to an imbalance between O_2 delivery and O_2 consumption. Oxygen deprivation (hypoxia) causes cellular hypoxia and disruption of critical cellular processes, including failure to meet the demands of cell metabolism and removal of waste. Without intervention, the result is sequential cell death, multisystem organ failure and death (Archbold and Naish 2015). There are several types of shock with different causes and presentations. The focus here will be on hypovolaemic shock (having considered septic shock above) since this is most relevant to the orthopaedic/trauma practitioner.

There are four stages of shock, which are initially reversible but then rapidly become irreversible:

Stage 1 Initial stage of shock: This is reversible, but easily missed as there are very few signs. Cardiac output is reduced and metabolism switches from aerobic to anaerobic, potentially leading to lactic acidosis (due to the inadequate clearance of lactic acid from the blood).

Stage 2 Compensatory stage of shock: The sympathetic nervous system produces catecholamine in an attempt to regain homeostasis and improve the perfusion of tissues by dilating the bronchi and constricting peripheral blood vessels. Water conservation is initiated by the release of aldosterone by the adrenal/renal system. Changes to vital signs will occur.

Stage 3 Progressive stage of shock: The compensatory mechanisms that sustain the perfusion of tissues are lost, resulting in metabolic and repository acidosis along with electrolyte imbalance. A visible deterioration in the patient's condition is seen.

Stage 4 Refractory stage of shock: There is irreversible cellular and organ damage. The condition becomes unresponsive to treatment and death is imminent (Tait et al. 2015).

Hypovolaemic Shock

Hypovolaemic shock (HS) is a life-threatening condition in which a reduction in blood volume leads to insufficient oxygen and nutrient supply to the cells. Uncontrolled bleeding is the leading cause of HS (Mutschler et al. 2014) and the most common cause in the orthopaedic patient is blood loss following trauma or surgery.

Trauma to both soft tissue and bone can lead to significant bleeding. If injuries are superficial, bleeding may be obvious, alerting the practitioner to potential hypovolaemia early. However, trauma to major skeletal structures and associated soft-tissue damage can lead to bleeding that is not immediately obvious. Fractures of the femoral shaft, for example, are usually the result of high-energy trauma and bleeding at the fracture site can be a significant cause of hypovolaemia without obvious external signs. Pelvic fractures have a particularly high risk of haemorrhage because the mechanism of injury is usually crushing of the pelvis with subsequent potential damage to the structures contained in the pelvic cavity, including major blood vessels.

In the patient undergoing elective orthopaedic or emergency trauma surgery, there is always a risk of postoperative haemorrhage, not only from the surgical site itself, but also 'hidden' losses from the surrounding tissues. Early warning score systems and modified versions are likely to be helpful in enabling collection of observation data and recognising the deteriorating patient so that management of shock can be initiated (Qin et al. 2017).

Early detection of uncontrolled bleeding and shock involves close observation of the person who has recently sustained trauma or undergone orthopaedic surgery. Understanding the nature and progression of the signs and symptoms of HS assists the practitioner in recognising the need for intervention. The ATLS® (American College of Surgeons 2008; Mutschler et al. 2014) (see Table 9.1)

classification of HS provides an overview of the observation/vital sign parameters that are seen as shock progresses and represent the physiological mechanisms which try to maintain homeostasis. These parameters reflect decreasing circulatory volume and blood flow, hypoxia, altered cognition due to decreased cerebral perfusion, sympathetic nervous system outflow and acidosis. Changes in skin appearance such as mottling, coolness or clamminess may also be evident due to reduced peripheral perfusion. Progression of symptoms indicates increasing blood and fluid loss, worsening the potential outcome, so identifying early subtle signs is essential.

Management of hypovolaemia in both the trauma and orthopaedic surgery patient follows similar principles:

- senior medical assessment for sources of bleeding and prompt action to control bleeding, including surgery/further surgery
- close monitoring and recording of patient vital signs and condition using an evidence-based early warning score tool
- supplementary oxygen therapy as prescribed
- assessment of blood levels of arterial blood gases, electrolytes, haemoglobin, lactate and haematocrit to identify deficits
- optimal fluid resuscitation according to most recent evidence-based guidelines, including use of blood and plasma replacement products, usually a combination of plasma, platelets and red blood cells (Holcomb et al. 2015).

Venous Thromboembolism

VTE is a condition in which a blood clot (thrombus) forms in a vein. Blood flow through the affected vein can be restricted by the clot, leading to swelling and pain.

Table 9.1 ATLS® classification of hypovolaemic shock (American College of Surgeons 2008; Mutschler et al. 2014).

	Class I	Class II	Class III	Class IV
Blood loss in % of total volume	<15	15–30	30–40	>40
Pulse rate	Normal	Normal	Decreased	Greatly decreased
Blood pressure	Normal	Normal	Decreased	Greatly decreased
Pulse pressure	Normal or increased	Decreased	Decreased	Decreased
Respiratory rate	14–20	20–30	30–40	>35
Mental status	Slightly anxious	Mildly anxious	Anxious, confused	Confused, lethargic
Urine output (ml/h)	>30	20–30	5–15	Minimal

Venous thrombosis usually occurs in the deep veins of the leg or pelvis, known as a deep vein thrombosis (DVT). An embolism can occur if all or part of the clot breaks off from the site where it has formed and then travels through the venous system. If the clot lodges in the lung, a serious and sometimes fatal condition, pulmonary embolism (PE), occurs.

Venous thrombosis can occur in any part of the venous system, but DVT and PE are the most common manifestations of this. The term VTE embraces both the acute conditions of DVT and PE as well as the chronic conditions that can occur after acute VTE, such as post-thrombotic syndrome and pulmonary hypertension, problems associated with significant ill-health and disability.

Risk Factors for VTE

The three main underlying factors that lead to VTE were first described by Rudolph Virchow in 1853 and are commonly referred to as Virchow's triad:

> venous stasis
> vein injury
> changes in blood chemistry.

It is accepted that it is usually a combination of these factors that causes a thrombus to form, rather than one factor in isolation. The inherent impaired physical mobility and activity intolerance that affects orthopaedic patients gives rise to circulatory stasis. If they also have existing conditions of, or have experienced trauma to, the circulatory system as well as alterations in blood coagulation, then they are in danger of developing VTE (Davis 2004a).

Orthopaedic patients are at significant risk of developing VTE due to the nature of their condition and its management. The most significant general risk factors for VTE are listed in Box 9.6. Many of these apply specifically to orthopaedic patients.

Risk Assessment

Most hospitalised orthopaedic patients should be considered at risk of developing a VTE so that they can receive appropriate prophylactic interventions. Those in the community or following discharge are also at risk. Assessment is based on some, but not all, of the predisposing factors referred to previously and listed in Box 9.3. NICE guidelines (2018) recommend that all hospitalised patients should receive a risk assessment for VTE at pre-admission, on admission and at every point that their condition changes, especially for trauma and surgical patients. Various risk assessment tools are available to support practitioners in undertaking and recording risk

---

Box 9.6   General Risk Factors for VTE

- Immobility
- Major surgery, including orthopaedic surgery
- Major fractures of the pelvis, lower limb and long bones
- Multiple trauma
- Cancer
- Cancer treatment, including chemotherapy and surgery
- Age over 60 years
- Known thrombophilias
- Dehydration
- Obesity
- Close family history of VTE
- Varicose veins with associated phlebitis
- Oestrogen contraceptive therapy
- Hormone replacement therapy
- One or more signify ant comorbidities (e.g. heart disease, metabolic, endocrine or respiratory conditions, acute infections, inflammatory conditions)

---

assessment, and local guidance should be followed in this respect. NICE (2010) have provided an example of a risk assessment proforma that begins with an assessment of mobility (www.nice.org.uk/guidance/ng89/resources/department-of-health-vte-risk-assessment-tool-pdf-4787149213).

Methods of Prevention

VTE is a leading cause of adverse events, disability and death directly due to hospital admission (International Society on Thrombosis Haemostasis 2018) although the true incidence of DVT, PE and related deaths is difficult to calculate. Importantly, however, VTE is a preventable condition. There have been numerous research studies that provide evidence of the effectiveness of methods to prevent VTE; this evidence-base is constantly progressing. Regularly updated guidance exists that identifies those preventative methods most likely to be successful. Some of the latest guidelines are listed in Box 9.7.

Prevention interventions for VTE fall into three main categories: (i) pharmacological, (ii) mechanical and (iii) care.

Pharmacological Interventions

Pharmacological measures for VTE prevention focus on the inhibition of thrombus formation by acting on clotting mechanisms. These measures are recommended for all orthopaedic patients assessed as at risk of VTE. NICE (2018) currently recommends prophylaxis with low molecular weight heparin (LMWH) or fondaparinux sodium for

Box 9.7   Evidence Digest

Examples of recent evidence-based guidelines for the prevention of VTE in hospitalised patients

Australian Commission on safety and quality and health-care (2020) Venous Thromboembolism Prevention Clinical Care Standard. www.safetyandquality.gov.au/publications-and-resources/resource-library/venous-thromboembolism-prevention-clinical-care-standard.

Afshari, A., Ageno, W., Ahmed, A., Duranteau, J., Faraoni, D., Kozek-Langenecker, S., Llau, J., Nizard, J., Solca, M., Stensballe, J., Thienpont, E., Tsiridis, E., Venclauskas, L., Samama, C.M, for the ESA VTE Guidelines Task Force European Guidelines on perioperative venous thromboembolism prophylaxis, European Journal of Anaesthesiology. February 2018, Volume 35, Issue 2, p. 77–83. Doi: 10.1097/EJA.0000000000000729.

NICE (2018).www.nice.org.uk/guidance/ng89/resources/venous-thromboembolism-in-over-16s-reducing-the-risk-of-hospitalacquired-deep-vein-thrombosis-or-pulmonary-embolism-pdf-1837703092165.

people with lower limb immobilisation or having lower limb or spinal surgery and those with pelvic, lower limb or spinal fractures or spinal injury. A medical decision needs to be made about whether the risk of VTE outweighs the additional risk of bleeding resulting from the administration of anticoagulation therapy.

Mechanical Interventions

There are three main evidence-based mechanical methods for VTE prophylaxis. The main advantage of such interventions is that they do not increase the risk of bleeding as pharmacological methods do.

1) Graduated compression stockings/hosiery (also known as anti-embolic stockings, AES) are designed and manufactured to exert pressure on the limb with the aim of improving the efficiency of the circulation. The stockings exert the greatest degree of compression at the ankle and the level of compression gradually decreases up the garment. Sachdeva et al. (2018) found high-quality evidence that graduated compression stockings are effective in reducing the risk of DVT in hospitalised patients who have undergone general and orthopaedic surgery. Wellington et al. (2015) provide guidance for the assessment, fitting, application and ongoing safe care of the patient with compression/AES stockings.
2) Intermittent pneumatic compression (IPC) devices involve inflatable garments (boots or stockings, thigh or knee-length) which are wrapped around both legs. A pneumatic air pump inflates and deflates the garments in cycles, which intermittently apply and release pressure on the limb, helping to improve the venous circulation in the legs with the aim of preventing thrombosis formation. This inflation–deflation cycle 'simulates the thigh, calf and foot's normal ambulatory pump action, thus increasing both the volume and rate of blood flow, eliminating venous stasis and replicating the effects of the natural muscle pump. Intermittent pneumatic compression devices can be thigh- or knee-length sleeves that are wrapped around the leg, or a garment that can be wrapped around or worn on the foot that is designed to mimic the actions of walking' (NICE 2018, p. 33). This has been shown to decrease the incidence of VTE both as a single measure and combined with other measures (Pavon et al. 2016). NICE (2018) recommend the use of IPC in patients undergoing major orthopaedic surgery that places them at risk of VTE when other methods of VTE prophylaxis are not feasible or contraindicated, particularly in patients with fragility fractures and those undergoing total knee arthroplasty. The device should continue to be used until the patient is fully mobile, so they may need to continue at home. However, compliance with this method of VTE prophylaxis has been found to be low due to issues such as: patient discomfort, patient knowledge, healthcare professional knowledge and behaviours, use of guidelines, mobilisation issues, equipment availability and, prescribing issues (Greenall and Davis 2020). Practitioners can therefore help to improve compliance by ensuring that patients are well educated about the need for and use of the devices.

Care Interventions

Two important factors in prevention include the fact that modern orthopaedic care means that patients now have less invasive surgery and great emphasis is placed on early mobilisation and early discharge from hospital. Some clinicians believe that DVT and PE are less prevalent than they used to be in surgical patients, but this may be hidden due to enhanced recovery pathways, and many DVTs occur after discharge.

The two most important nursing interventions for VTE prevention are:

1) Early mobilisation and leg exercises
2) Hydration (but through the oral route, not intravenous).

Current guidelines recommend the use of these interventions in combination. They also increasingly highlight the patient's view such as the difficulty and discomfort associated with graduated compression stockings (NICE 2010). All prophylactic interventions carry risk as well as benefit and this must be balanced in any care decisions for individual patients. The risk of bleeding is an example with pharmacological interventions for VTE.

The linking of evidence through an evidence-based practice approach to orthopaedic nursing practice is well illustrated by the issue of VTE. Research, such as in areas of early mobilisation and hydration, is often lacking or so poor quality that it cannot be relied on to direct practice decisions. Even when evidence is strong, it has to be applied consistently and with knowledge and understanding. Davis (2004b) discusses ways in which the problems of translation and utilisation can be overcome with respect to VTE.

NICE (2020) have developed a three-page visual summary of the recommendations on diagnosis and anticoagulation treatments for venous thromboembolism (www.nice.org.uk/guidance/ng158/resources/visual-summary-pdf-870909145).

Fat Embolism Syndrome

FES is a life-threatening condition that can lead to respiratory failure in orthopaedic patients. It is a medical emergency that requires immediate recognition and action.

The term 'fat embolism' (FE) refers to the presence of fat globules in the peripheral circulation and lung parenchyma most commonly following fracture of long bones, the pelvis or other major trauma, although it can also occur following major implant surgery that involves reaming of bone. The condition is usually asymptomatic and may not become evident unless it develops further. Fat embolism syndrome is a severe and life-threatening manifestation of FE that usually occurs within 24–72 hours of injury or surgery to a long bone. The patient presents with a collection of clinical symptoms, including dyspnoea, hypoxaemia, mental confusion (due to hypoxia) and petechial rash. Some patients will develop signs and symptoms of multiorgan dysfunction, particularly involving the lungs, brain and skin.

The clinical signs/symptoms and course of FES are a result of a series of pathological processes (Jain et al. 2008; Kosova et al. 2015; Rothberg and Makarewich 2019). Fat emboli are released from the marrow of long bones following fracture or reaming of bone.

The trauma responses at the injury (or surgery) site release chemical mediators, which bring about various coagulation events, including coagulation of circulating lipids, which result in the development of fat emboli large enough to occlude pulmonary vessels. Emboli obstruct the capillaries of major organs (most commonly the lungs, but also the brain and kidneys). The ensuing inflammatory response results in acute respiratory distress syndrome (ARDS) and signs of dysfunction in other organs.

Box 9.8   Signs of Fat Embolism Syndrome (Gurd and Wilson 1974.

Major signs:
- petechial rash
- respiratory insufficiency
- cerebral involvement.

Minor signs:
- tachycardia >120 bpm
- fever >39.4 °C
- retinal signs – fat or petechiae
- jaundice
- renal signs – anuria/oliguria.

There is evidence that the incidence of FES has reduced over the last few decades due to improvements in fracture management (Lempert et al. 2021), suggesting that prevention should be focused on fracture care.

The clinical team caring for patients in the first few days following injury or surgery to long bones needs a high level of suspicion in recognising the early signs of FES so that respiratory support can be instigated early. As part of the general observation of the patient following trauma/surgery, nurses should observe for any signs listed in Gurd and Wilson's (1974) diagnostic criteria (shown in Box 9.8), which are still considered relevant today (Kosova et al. 2015).

Any of these clinical signs should be reported to a senior clinician as an emergency. Because of the risk of respiratory and multiple organ failure, patients with clinical signs of FES require emergency management, respiratory support and fluid resuscitation in a critical/intensive care facility or high-dependency unit. Supplemental oxygenation should be prescribed and administered early on, and mechanical ventilation may be necessary along with constant monitoring of vital signs. If early and effective emergency and intensive care is provided, outcomes are good (Kosova et al. 2015).

Acute Compartment Syndrome

ACS is a clinical condition that occurs when there is an increase in pressure and/or a decrease in the size of a muscle compartment resulting in reduced capillary blood flow and leading to cell death. It is an orthopaedic emergency because if the pressure is not relieved within hours, irreversible damage to the tissues and nerves may result in contractures, paralysis, loss of sensation and amputation (Ali et al. 2014). This can lead to muscle ischaemia, infarction, and necrosis and rhabdomyolysis, a life-threatening condition in which toxins released from ischaemic/necrotic muscle into the circulation can lead to organ failure.

The most common site of ACS is the anterior compartment of the lower leg. Any compartment, however, can be affected, although most cases present following a tibial fracture. The condition can be difficult to diagnose in all patients, including children, with delays in diagnosis leading to disastrous outcomes (Bae et al. 2001). Although ACS is an uncommon condition, it is dangerous and life threatening, so the clinician needs to be able to recognise it immediately so that it can be treated.

The orthopaedic patient (including children) can present with ACS following:

- *trauma*: fracture, haematoma, vascular damage, electrical injuries, particularly to the lower leg and forearm
- *surgery* to the lower or upper limb
- *external compression* due to casts or restricting bandages.

In acute limb compartment syndrome (ALCS), limb compression leads to local pressure with local tamponade (blockage). This results in capillary necrosis and oedema with increased compartment pressure and muscle ischaemia. This then leads to compartment tamponade, nerve injury and muscle infarction.

The British Orthopaedic Association (BOA)/British Association of Plastic Reconstructive and Aesthetic Surgeons provide standards for the diagnosis and management of compartment syndrome of the limbs (BOA/BAPRAS 2014). They state that the key clinical indicators of ACS in the conscious patient are:

- pain out of proportion to the associated injury
- pain on passive movement of the muscles of the involved compartments.

It is pain that is the earliest sign of ACS and it is this on which the practitioner should focus. While neurological symptoms such as tingling (paraesthesia) and numbness, and circulatory symptoms such as changes in colour and warmth should be recorded, these are late signs and do not contribute to early diagnosis of the condition (BOA/BAPRAS 2014). These late signs demonstrate that neurovascular and muscle damage have already occurred and the priority for the practitioner is to recognise the condition from the early signs so that permanent damage can be prevented. Monitoring of compartment pressure is considered helpful in the unconscious patient but is not available in many units (Ali et al. 2014).

Bandages and dressings should be removed if ACS is suspected, and the limb should not be elevated even though this is a common principle of care for the orthopaedic/trauma patient with swelling and pain.

Neurovascular Assessment

All patients who have a musculoskeletal injury, undergone orthopaedic surgery or have cast immobilisation of a limb are at risk of developing neurovascular compromise, which can lead to compartment syndrome. Such neurovascular compromise can include ALCS as well as other damage to neurovascular structures in the limbs due to injury, surgery and other procedures, and swelling (Box 9.9).

Peripheral neurovascular assessment involves the systematic assessment of the neurological and vascular integrity of a limb, with the aim of recognising any neurovascular deficit promptly (Judge 2007). Tissue damage deteriorates with time, so prompt identification and intervention are necessary. The optimum frequency of assessment is unclear but should reflect the acute nature of the patients' recent injury/procedure and the potential for compromise to occur with the rationale recorded. The main parameters of neurovascular assessment are listed, with their rationale, in Box 9.10. These parameters should be recorded in a neurovascular assessment chart – sometimes included in early warning score charts – so that comparisons can be made and deterioration identified quickly. Shields and Clarke (2011) recommended the use of a dedicated chart to record pain intensity and type, alongside warmth, sensation, colour, capillary refill time and the movement of the affected

---

Box 9.9   Evidence Digest

Royal College of Nursing guidelines for peripheral neurovascular observations for acute limb compartment syndrome

Peripheral neurovascular observations for acute limb compartment syndrome. RCN consensus guidance

Royal College of Nursing (2014) Peripheral neurovascular observations for acute limb compartment syndrome RCN consensus guidance. Royal College of Nursing. London. Available at: www.rcn.org.uk/professional-development/publications/pub-004685.

The Royal College of Nursing's Society of Orthopaedic and Trauma Nursing published these guidelines following a 3-year project to develop consensus regarding best practice in the early identification of ALCS, reducing its risk, the role of clinical observation and compartment pressure measurement in early detection.

Following a literature review (Ali et al. 2014) which found that the evidence was insufficient to guide best practice, the guideline development group held a consensus conference to develop guidance for practice by seeking the consensus of expert clinicians.

Box 9.10	Neurovascular Assessment Parameters for Patients with Limb Injuries, Surgery or Casts
Parameter	Rationale
Pain (priority sign)	Both vascular (depleted blood supply leading to ischaemia) and neurological (damaged nerve conduction) damage result in a pain response. This is always (except in the unconscious patient) the earliest sign of damage. Practitioners should take any reports of pain in the area around and/or peripheral to the injury seriously and report this to a medical practitioner immediately. Pain is unresolved by analgesia.
Pulses	Pulses peripheral to the site of injury/surgery provide an assessment of the circulation (vascular) at the site. Absence of pulses, however, is a late sign of vascular injury/occlusion.
Capillary refill	Capillary refill time provides an assessment of the perfusion to an area peripheral to an injury/surgical site. It is conducted by applying pressure to the finger-tip/nail or toe-tip/nail for 5 seconds with enough pressure to cause blanching as the blood is pushed out of the tissues. The pressure is then released and the time taken for the tissue to return to the same colour as that around it. Normal refill time is considered to be 2 seconds or less.
Pallor/discoloration/temperature	Paleness, discolouration (blue/mottled) and/or coolness of the skin are signs of vascular compromise indicating that peripheral tissues have no, or insufficient, blood supply. This is also a very late sign of vascular injury/occlusion.
Paraesthesia	Paraesthesia is a patient-reported perception of abnormal sensation, which can include 'pins and needles', tingling, pricking or crawling. This is a potential sign of peripheral nerve damage (neuropathy).
Loss of sensation and/or paralysis	Both loss of sensation and paralysis of a limb or section of a limb indicate lack of nerve supply to bring about movement or sensation.

and unaffected limb as an important method of collecting and comparing data from baseline onwards.

Shields and Clarke (2011) also recommend the use of a dedicated chart to record pain intensity and type alongside warmth, sensation, colour, capillary refill time and the movement of the affected and unaffected limbs as an important method of collecting and comparing data from baseline onwards.

A central aspect of care of the patient with suspected ALCS, or other form of neurovascular compromise, is to treat any suspicion as a medical emergency requiring immediate medical attention. It is essential that the practitioner inform a senior member of medical staff immediately so that intervention can be instigated.

Fasciotomy is the management option of choice for ALCS; the fascia is divided along the length of the compartment to release pressure. The pressure at which fasciotomy is performed is based on the clinical picture/rising pressure. Following the procedure, the wound is usually left open for approximately 5 days until the soft tissues have recovered and swelling has begun to subside. Muscle and skin grafting may be required.

Urinary Retention

A significant reason for urinary catheterisation in the orthopaedic patient is post-operative urinary retention, which is frequently reported following orthopaedic surgery. It has been reported to occur in up to 84% of patients following total hip arthroplasty (Lawrie et al. 2017). It is defined as an inability to pass urine even though the patient has a full bladder. This can result in pain and distress for the patient and can lead to bladder distention. Retention can also lead to UTI, adverse autonomic responses such as vomiting, hypotension and cardiac dysrhythmia, and permanent damage to the bladder with resultant future urinary problems (Baldini et al. 2009). Early recognition of the problem is therefore essential and should be included as an aim for all postoperative care. There is no evidence that routine catheterisation intraoperatively as a method of prevention is beneficial and the risk of haematogenous spread of infection to the surgical site is too great for this to be advised (Crain et al. 2021).

The main symptom of urinary retention is pain and discomfort in the lower part of the abdomen in a patient who is unable to pass urine despite good fluid balance. This can, however, be masked post-operatively by the effects of general and regional anaesthesia, nerve blockade and analgesia. Bladder catheterisation can also be used as a method of assessing bladder volume and diagnosing retention through measurement of the residual volume of urine. This, however, carries with it the risk of infection associated with per urethral catheterisation. The literature suggests that the use of nurse-led ultrasound to assess bladder volume is a relatively simple and appropriate way for the practitioner to monitor bladder volume and identify retention whilst avoiding unnecessary catheterisation (Crain et al. 2021).

Once retention has been identified, the treatment usually involves bladder catheterisation. It is recommended that this is done as an in-out (intermittent) catheterisation rather than with an indwelling catheter and that antibiotic prophylaxis is essential (Baldini et al. 2009). It may be necessary for the bladder volume to be monitored for up to 48 hours post-operatively, but most problems tend to resolve once the patient begins to mobilise and is able to visit the toilet to void.

Constipation

Constipation is a very common and significant complication that can be either acute or chronic. In the orthopaedic and trauma patient, it is often caused by a decrease in bowel action due to a combination of factors that lead to hard, dry stools that are difficult and/or painful to pass. The problem is defined by the patient and may include what they feel to be 'unsatisfactory' or incomplete defecation. Although it is thought there is a link between the incidence of constipation and increasing age, this is most likely because of the greater incidence of other precipitating factors in older people. Some other common causes of constipation in the orthopaedic and trauma patient include:

- *dehydration*, leading to desiccated stools
- *reduced mobility*, resulting in weakness in the accessory muscles, which help bowel evacuation
- *reduced or changed dietary intake*, resulting in a diet that is depleted or lacking in fibre
- *pharmacological agents*: one of the main side effects of many drugs is constipation and in the orthopaedic and trauma patient both opioid and non-opioid analgesic agents are implicated (known as opioid-induced constipation; Sonneborn and Bui 2019), but other drugs such as antidepressants can also contribute because of the slowing effect on peristaltic action.

Hospitalised patients and those reliant on others for toileting needs often resist the urge to pass bowel movements because of embarrassment or pain associated with the required activity, particularly if they require a bedpan (Cohen 2009). Because of embarrassment, patients may not be willing to inform a health professional of the problem. These are issues that it is essential the practitioner is sensitive to.

Impaction, where faeces become trapped in the lower part of the large bowel, is very distressing for the patient. The most serious consequence of untreated constipation and impaction is bowel obstruction by a volvulus, which becomes a surgical emergency and can be fatal. It is essential that this be avoided through careful assessment and prevention.

The most important aspect of the prevention and management of constipation is the early and continuous assessment of bowel activity. Because nearly all orthopaedic and trauma patients have at least one risk factor for constipation and because of the reluctance of patients to discuss difficulties with the nurse, it is essential that a proactive daily assessment of bowel activity is made. 'Normal' bowel habits vary from one person to another and the practitioner must take this into account when assessing bowel function, considering the patients' normal frequency of opening their bowels. If constipation lasts more than a few weeks and/or is associated with other symptoms such as abdominal mass/pain or blood in the stools, then a medical referral is made to rule out other more serious causes.

Proactive prevention of constipation is an important aspect of the care of the orthopaedic and trauma patient. It is important that this is incorporated into the standard care of all patients at risk of constipation and is not left until constipation has begun to occur. Prevention involves management of the causes and risk factors for constipation. This generally includes helping to provide conditions for toileting routines that are as near normal for the patient as possible with due consideration of privacy and position:

- *monitor*: daily assessment and recording of bowel activity
- *diet*: ensuring the diet contains or is supplemented with foodstuffs high in dietary fibre
- *hydration*: ensuring that the patient takes plenty of oral fluids
- *exercise*: within the limits and abilities of the patient; when unable to walk there may be benefit from abdominal exercise such as pelvic tilt (Joanna Briggs Institute 2008).

It is important that any tendency to constipation be managed as soon as possible after symptoms occur. The management of constipation generally involves the use of pharmacological laxatives. There are several different types of laxative, which work in different ways:

Box 9.11   Evidence Digest: Nurse-led Management and Prevention of Opioid-induced Constipation

Sonneborn, O. and Bui, T. (2019) Opioid induced constipation management in orthopaedic and trauma patients: treatment and the potential of nurse-initiated management, *International Journal of Orthopaedic and Trauma Nursing*, 34, pp. 16–20. https://doi.org/10.1016/j.ijotn.2019.03.002.

Sonneborn and Bui (2019) point out that opioid analgesics, used to treat moderate to severe pain, are associated with common side effects, such as constipation. Orthopaedic and trauma patients are at high risk of developing opioid-induced constipation (OIC) because their mobility is reduced and there is a need for opioids such as codeine to manage pain.

The authors' aim was to 'examine the evidence base to guide clinicians on the most effective or tolerated laxative regimen for the management of OIC and nurse-initiated management of OIC'.

They conducted a review of the literature, searching several databases to identify studies regarding OIC, laxatives and nurse-initiated management.

The review findings concluded the following:

1) Laxatives do not address the underlying cause of OIC and there is currently insufficient evidence to guide clinicians on the most effective or tolerated laxative regimen for the management of OIC.
2) The use of peripheral acting mu-opioid receptor antagonists (PAMORAs) could be considered in those for whom regular use of a combination of laxatives has not been successful, and nurses should take a broader role in the assessment of symptoms and response to treatment.

The authors conclude that there is an important balance between adequate analgesia and minimising OIC symptoms, making this an ongoing challenge for clinicians and an area of patient care where nurses could be leading management.

- *bulking agents* contain fibrous material that absorbs water in the bowel and makes stools softer
- *peristaltic stimulants* are useful where peristaltic action is reduced
- *osmotic laxatives* encourage the absorption of fluid into the stools
- *stool softeners* lubricate and moisten stools.

When constipation is opioid-induced it is advisable to begin treatment with a combination of an osmotic laxative and a peristaltic stimulant (see Box 9.11). If this treatment fails to resolve constipation or faecal impact is suspected, treatment with suppositories or enemas along with peristaltic stimulants may be required.

Further Reading

Donalson, L., Ricciardi, W., Sheridan, S. and Tartaglia, R. (eds) (2021) Textbook of Patient Safety and Clinical Risk Management (open access eBook). Springer. https://doi.org/10.1007/978-3-030-59403-9.

References

Ali, P., Santy-Tomlinson, J., and Watson, R. (2014). Assessment and diagnosis of acute limb compartment syndrome: a literature review. *International Journal of Orthopaedic and Trauma Nursing* 18 (4): 180–190. https://doi.org/10.1016/j.ijotn.2014.01.002.

American College of Surgeons Committee on Trauma (2008). *Advanced Trauma Life Support for Doctors–Student Course Mannual*, 8e. Chicago.: American College of Surgeons.

Archbold, A. and Naish, J. (2015). *The Cardiovascular System* (ed. J. Naish and D. Syndercombe-Court), 493–562. Medical Sciences.

Bae, D., Kadiyala, K., and Waters, P. (2001). Acute compartment syndrome in children: contemporary diagnosis, treatment, and outcome. *Journal of Pediatric Orthopaedics* 21 (5): 680–688.

Bai, Y., Zhang, X., Tian, Y. et al. (2019). Incidence of surgical-site infection following open reduction and internal fixation of a distal femur fracture. *Medicine* 98 (7): e14547. https://doi.org/10.1097/MD.0000000000014547.

Baldini, G., Hema, B., Aprikian, A., and Carli, F. (2009). Postoperative urinary retention: anaesthetic and perioperative considerations. *Anesthesiology* 110 (5): 1139–1157.

Bauer, M., Gerlach, H., Vogelmann, T. et al. (2020). Mortality in sepsis and septic shock in Europe, North America and Australia between 2009 and 2019.: Results from a systematic review and meta-analysis. *Critical Care* 24: 239. https://doi.org/10.1186/s13054-020-02950-2.

BOA/BAPRAS (2014). *Diagnosis and management of compartment syndrome of the limbs*. BOAST. www.boa.ac.uk/uploads/assets/0d37694f-1cad-40d5-b4c1032eef7486ff/de4cfbe1-6ef3-443d-a7f2a0ee491d2229/diagnosis%20and%20management%20of%20compartment%20syndrome%20of%20the%20limbs.pdf.

Bryson, D.J., Morris, D.L.J., Shivji, F.S. et al. (2016). Antibiotic prophylaxis in orthopaedic surgery. *The Bone & Joint Journal* 98-B (8): 1014–1019. https://doi.org/10.1302/0301-620X.98B8.37359.

Cohen, S. (2009). Orthopaedic patient's perceptions of using a bed pan. *Journal of Orthopaedic Nursing* 13 (2): 78–84.

Copanitsanou, P. (2020). Recognising and preventing surgical site infection after orthopaedic surgery. *International Journal of Orthopaedic and Trauma Nursing* 37: https://doi.org/10.1016/j.ijotn.2019.100751.

Crain, N.A., Goharderakhshan, R.Z., Reddy, N.C. et al. (2021). The role of intraoperative urinary catheters on postoperative urinary retention after total joint arthroplasty: a multi-hospital retrospective study on 9,580 patients. *The Archives of Bone and Joint Surgery* 9 (5): 480–486. https://doi.org/10.22038/abjs.2020.49205.2441.

Davis, P. (2004a). Venous thromboembolism prevention – an update. *Journal of Orthopaedic Nursing* 8: 50–56.

Davis, P. (2004b). A critical exploration of practice improvement with reference to VTE prevention. *Journal of Orthopaedic Nursing* 8: 208–214.

Doronina, O., Jones, D., Martello, M. et al. (2017). A systematic review on the effectiveness of interventions to improve hand hygiene compliance of nurses in the hospital setting. *Journal of Nursing Scholarship* 49 (2): 143–152. https://doi.org/10.1111/jnu.12274. Epub 2017 Jan 23. PMID: 28114724.

Erasmus, V., Daha, T., Brug, H. et al. (2010). Systematic review of studies on compliance with hand hygiene guidelines in hospital care. *Infection Control and Hospital Epidemiology* 31 (3): 283–294. https://doi.org/10.1086/650451.

Gillespie, W.J. and Walenkamp, G.H.I.M. (2010). Antibiotic prophylaxis for surgery for proximal femoral and other closed long bone fractures. *Cochrane Database of Systematic Reviews* 3: CD000244. https://doi.org/10.1002/14651858.CD000244.pub2.

Greenall, R. and Davis, R.E. (2020). Intermittent pneumatic compression for venous thromboembolism prevention: a systematic review on factors affecting adherence. *BMJ Open* 10: e037036. https://doi.org/10.1136/bmjopen-2020-037036.

Gurd, A.R. and Wilson, R.E. (1974). The FES. *Journal of Bone and Joint Surgery (British)* 56: 408–416.

Holcomb, J.B., Tilley, B.C., Baraniuk, S. et al. (2015). Transfusion of plasma, platelets, and red blood cells in a 1:1:1 vs a 1:1:1 ratio and mortality in patients with severe trauma: The PROPPR randomized clinical trial. *Journal of the American Medical Association* 313 (5): 471–482. https://doi.org/10.1001/jama.2015.12.

International Society on Thrombosis Haemostasis (2018). *Time to Deliver: Third UN high level meeting on on-communicable diseases*. https://www.who.int/ncds/governance/high-level-commission/International-Society-for-Thrombosis-and-Haemostasis.pdf.

Jain, S., Nagpure, P.S., Singh, R., and Garg, D. (2008). Minor trauma triggering cervicofacial necrotizing fasciitis from odontogenic abscess. *Journal of Emergency Trauma Shock* 1: 114–118.

Joanna Briggs Institute (2008). *Management of Constipation in Older Adults*. Best Practice 12(7). http://connect.jbiconnectplus.org/ViewSourceFile.aspx?0=45 (accessed 30 March 2014).

de Jong, L., Klem, T.M.A.L., Kuijper, T.M., and Roukema, G.R. (2017). Factors affecting the rate of surgical site infection in patients after hemi arthroplasty of the hip following a fracture of the neck of the femur. *Bone and Joint Journal* 99-B (8): 1088–1094. https://doi.org/10.1302/0301-620X.99B8.BJJ-2016-1119.R1. PMID: 28768787.

Judge, N.L. (2007). Neurovascular assessment. *Nursing Standard* 21 (45): 39–44.

Kosova, E., Bergmark, B., and Piazza, G. (2015). Fat embolism syndrome. *Circulation* 131 (3): 317–320. https://doi.org/10.1161/CIRCULATIONAHA.114.010835.

Lawrie, C.M., Ong, A.C., Hernandez, V.H. et al. (2017). Incidence and risk factors for postoperative urinary retention in total hip arthroplasty performed under spinal anesthesia. *The Journal of Arthroplasty* 32 (12): 3748–3751. https://doi.org/10.1016/j.arth.2017.07.009.

Lempert, M., Halvachizadeh, S., Ellanti, P. et al. (2021). Incidence of fat embolism syndrome in femur fractures and its associated risk factors over time – a systematic review. *Journal of Clinical Medicine* 10: 2733. https://doi.org/10.3390/jcm10122733.

Loveday, H.P., Wilson, J.A., Pratt, R.J. et al. (2014). epic3: National evidence-based guidelines for preventing healthcare-associated infections in NHS hospitals in England. *Journal of Hospital Infection* 86 (1): S1–S70. https://doi.org/10.1016/S0195-6701(13)60012-2.

Meddings, J., Skolarus, T.A., Fowler, K.E. et al. (2019). Michigan appropriate perioperative (MAP) criteria for urinary catheter use in common general and orthopaedic surgeries: results obtained using the RAND/UCLA appropriateness method. *BMJ Quality and Safety* 28: 56–66.

Mutschler, M., Paffrath, T., Wölfl, C. et al. (2014). The ATLS® classification of hypovolaemic shock: a well-established teaching tool on the edge? *Injury* 45 (Suppl 3): S35–S38. https://doi.org/10.1016/j.injury.2014.08.015.

NICE (2010). *Risk assessment for venous thromboembolism*. NICE guideline NG89. www.nice.org.uk/guidance/ng89/resources/department-of-health-vte-risk-assessment-tool-pdf-4787149213.

NICE (2016). *Sepsis: recognition, diagnosis and early management*. NICE guideline NG51. www.nice.org.uk/guidance/ng51.

NICE (2018). *Venous thromboembolism in over 16s: reducing the risk of hospital-acquired deep vein thrombosis or pulmonary embolism*. NICE guideline NG89. www.nice.org.uk/guidance/ng89.

NICE (2020). *Venous thromboembolic diseases: diagnosis, management and thrombophilia testing*. NICE guideline NG158. www.nice.org.uk/guidance/ng158.

Panagioti, M., Khan, K., Keers, R.N. et al. (2019). Prevalence, severity, and nature of preventable patient harm across medical care settings: systematic review and meta-analysis. *BMJ* 366: l4185. https://doi.org/10.1136/bmj.l4185.

Pavon, J.M., Adam, S.S., Razouki, Z.A. et al. (2016). Effectiveness of intermittent pneumatic compression devices for venous thromboembolism prophylaxis in high-risk surgical patients: a systematic review. *Journal of Arthroplasty* 31: 524–532.

Public Health England (2017). *Guidance: Health Matters: Preventing infections and reducing antimicrobial resistance*. https://www.gov.uk/government/publications/health-matters-preventing-infections-and-reducing-amr/health-matters-preventing-infections-and-reducing-antimicrobial-resistance.

Qin, Q., Xia, Y., and Cao, Y. (2017). Clinical study of a new modified early warning system scoring system for rapidly evaluating shock in adults. *Journal of Critical Care* 37: 50–55. https://doi.org/10.1016/j.jcrc.2016.08.025.

Roper, N., Logan, W., and Tierney, A.J. (2000). *The Roper-Logan-Tierney Model of Nursing: Based on Activities of Living*. Churchill Livingstone.

Rothberg, D.L. and Makarewich, C.A. (2019). Fat embolism and fat embolism syndrome. *The Journal of the American Academy of Orthopaedic Surgeons* 27 (8): e346–e355. https://doi.org/10.5435/JAAOS-D-17-00571.

Sachdeva, A., Dalton, M., and Lees, T. (2018). Graduated compression stockings for prevention of deep vein thrombosis. *Cochrane Database of Systematic Reviews* (11): CD001484. https://doi.org/10.1002/14651858.CD001484.pub4.

Sands, M. and Aunger, R. (2020). Determinants of hand hygiene compliance among nurses in US hospitals: a formative research study. *PLoS One* 15 (4): e0230573. https://doi.org/10.1371/journal.pone.0230573.

Shields, C. and Clarke, S. (2011). Neurovascular observation and documentation for children within accident and emergency: a critical review. *International Journal of Orthopaedic and Trauma Nursing* 15 (1): 3–10.

Sonneborn, O. and Bui, T. (2019). Opioid induced constipation management in orthopaedic and trauma patients: treatment and the potential of nurse-initiated management. *International Journal of Orthopaedic and Trauma Nursing* 34: 16–20. https://doi.org/10.1016/j.ijotn.2019.03.002.

Stangerup, M., Hansen, M.,.B., Hansen, R. et al. (2021). Hand hygiene compliance of healthcare workers before and during the COVID-19 pandemic: a long-term follow-up study. *American Journal of Infection Control* 49 (9): 1118–1122. https://doi.org/10.1016/j.ajic.2021.06.014.

Tait, D., James, J., Williams, C., and Barton, D. (2015). *Acute and Critical Care in Adult Nursing*. Learning Matters.

Thakker, A., Briggs, N., Maeda, A. et al. (2018). Reducing the rate of post-surgical urinary tract infections in orthopedic patients. *BMJ Open Quality* 7: e000177. https://doi.org/10.1136/bmjoq-2017-000177.

Tromp, M., Huis, A., de Guchteneire, I. et al. (2012). The short-term and long-term effectiveness of a multidisciplinary hand hygiene improvement program. *Am J Infect Control.* 40 (8): 732–736. https://doi.org/10.1016/j.ajic.2011.09.009.

Wellington, B., Flynn, S., and Duperouzel, W. (2015). Anti-embolic stockings for the prevention of VTE in orthopaedic patients: a practice update. *International Journal of Orthopaedic and Trauma Nursing* 19 (1): 45–49. https://doi.org/10.1016/j.ijotn.2014.11.005.

World Health Organization (2009). *WHO guidelines on hand hygiene in healthcare*. http://whqlibdoc.who.int/publications/2009/9789241597906_eng.pdf.

10

Nutrition and Hydration

Rosemary Masterson

National Orthopaedic Hospital, Cappagh, Dublin, Ireland

Introduction

Nutrition and hydration vary across the globe and are influenced by many factors, including personal and psychological factors (e.g. beliefs, attitudes, emotions), biological and physiological factors (e.g. age, gender, pregnancy, activity), socioeconomic factors (e.g. availability and cost), cultural and religious factors, educational factors (e.g. nutritional knowledge), extrinsic factors (e.g. media, time, foods in season) and food factors (taste and appearance) (Kearney and Pot 2017). A detailed discussion of all of these factors is outside the scope of this chapter but where relevant to the discussion they will be included.

Good nutrition plays an important role in recovery from planned orthopaedic surgery or traumatic injury. Musculoskeletal health can be impacted by poor nutrition, e.g. failure to get enough nutrients can lead to poor development or rickets while the impact of a poor quality diet can contribute to obesity or osteoporosis. In the orthopaedic patient, poor nutrition can delay wound healing and fracture repair, increase the risk of infection, decrease muscle strength, lead to the development of constipation and ultimately delay recovery. Endo et al. (2018) identified eight essential factors that predicted inpatient mortality after fracture neck of femur and noted weight loss as one of these, thus highlighting the need for attention in this area. This in turn can prolong the treatment for the patient and may prevent the patient returning to work or to independent living. Delayed discharge from hospital increases the cost to the patient and the health service.

Maintaining good hydration is also critical to maintaining good health. It becomes even more important as we age. Poor hydration can lead to multiple problems such as tendons and ligaments becoming less resilient, constipation, repeated urinary tract infections and fatigue. In the orthopaedic patient recovering from surgery or injury, dehydration can delay recovery and discharge.

This chapter will examine the role of diet in musculoskeletal health, discuss the metabolic response of the body to trauma and surgery, and analyse the importance of a nutritional assessment and the subsequent interventions plus the role of hydration and dehydration. A summary will follow.

Diet and Musculoskeletal Health

A balanced diet is essential for health. It provides the appropriate amount of all nutrients to meet the requirements of the body. This can be achieved by eating a variety of foods. No single food has the correct proportions of all essential nutrients. If a deficiency or an excess of a nutrient is consumed, it can have an impact on one's health, e.g. obesity, anaemia, rickets or osteoporosis. The role of hydration will be dealt with in Section 10.5.

Healthy eating requires planning and knowledge. Consideration should be given to the amount of energy required to meet the individual's requirements. Several factors can influence the daily energy requirement, such as age, gender, activity levels and basal metabolic rate. In relation to musculoskeletal health, a well-balanced diet containing the major components is important in preventing disease, promoting recovery and healing.

Our basal metabolic rate refers to activity in our bodies that maintains life (e.g. respiratory function, cardiac function, body temperature) and is affected by metabolism, catabolism and anabolism. Metabolism is the processing of nutrients within our bodies while catabolism is the reactions that release energy and anabolism is the building of new tissue. Energy requirements will increase depending on the demands placed on the body, e.g. in the event of a fracture which is healing or an infection that might be present, therefore a balance of nutrients is vital for maintaining health. The recommended daily amounts are based on the average healthy adult and will need to be adjusted for the individual who is facing challenges (e.g. recovering from a traumatic injury such as a hip fracture).

Six major components are considered essential in our diet: carbohydrates, proteins, fats, vitamins, minerals and water. Carbohydrates, proteins and fat are called macronutrients and are required in larger amounts than the micronutrients (vitamins and minerals). Although the micronutrients are required in smaller amounts, they are essential for metabolism, normal growth and wellbeing.

As part of national approaches to promote healthier eating, national agencies have produced diagrammatic evidence to assist in this endeavour. The food pyramid was first introduced in Sweden in the early 1970s and was adopted by national agencies in a number of countries, including the USA, the UK and Ireland, over recent decades. The aim of the food pyramid is to provide a practical visual graph of what a healthy diet should consist of. Approximately 10 years ago, the food circle or plate model was designed. This showed a plate illustrating how much you need to eat of each food group, replacing the previous campaign. Following a review, Public Health England devised the 'Eatwell Guide' which it considered would resonated with the public better. While there are similarities with the food plate, there are some distinct differences, such as the removal of the knife and fork, drawn images instead of photographs, updated food segment names, resizing of food groups and the inclusion of a hydration message (Public Health England 2018). The British Nutrition Foundation (2019) published a guide entitled 'Find your balance' which aims to give guidance on portion size for adults. This is reflected in a publication by the Department of Health in Ireland (2021), who updated their guidance with the launch of 'Healthy Food for Life', a toolkit which includes a new food pyramid and guidance material to help make choices to maintain a healthy balanced diet reflecting best national and international advice.

Carbohydrates, Proteins and Fats

Carbohydrates are made up of mainly sugars and starches. They are essential in providing energy and heat, in sparing the use of protein to provide energy and in the provision of an energy store (as glycogen and fat) when eaten in excess of the body's needs.

Proteins are essential for growth and repair of the tissues and body cells. Proteins also have a role to play in the production of enzymes, plasma proteins, immunoglobulins and some hormones. They also are involved in the provision of energy (when there is not enough carbohydrate in the diet).

Fats are made up of different types of fatty acids, some of which are essential for health in small amounts. Fatty acids are usually classified as saturated, monounsaturated or polyunsaturated depending on their structure. Fat provides energy (Gordon and Jin 2017). It is a carrier of fat-soluble vitamins and is necessary for their absorption. A high intake of saturated or trans fatty acids can have adverse effects on health as it can contribute to comorbidities (British Nutrition Foundation 2021).

Vitamins

Vitamins are chemical compounds required in small quantities that are essential for normal functioning and health. They are divided into two groups, the fat-soluble vitamins (D, A, E and K) and the water-soluble vitamins (B and C). For the purpose of this discussion, the vitamins relevant to musculoskeletal health are discussed.

Vitamin D regulates calcium and phosphate metabolism by increasing their absorption from the gut and stimulating their retention by the kidneys, therefore promoting the calcification of bones. A deficiency of this vitamin in children can cause rickets and in adults can cause osteomalacia (refer to Chapter 23). This may occur as a result of impaired absorption or defective metabolism. It can be manufactured in the skin as a result of exposure to sunlight and/or obtained in the diet from sources such as fat spreads, cereal products and oily fish. Some groups of people, e.g. those of Asian descent, black people, older, institutionalised and housebound people, and those who habitually cover the skin (for religious reasons) are vulnerable to vitamin D deficiency as a result of limited exposure to sunlight. In a systematic review of vitamin D status in populations worldwide, Hilger et al. (2014) noted that mean population 23-hydroxyvitamin D (25(OH)D) levels varied considerably, with the highest levels in North America. From analyses, they suggested that newborns and the institutionalised elderly from several regions worldwide appeared to be at generally higher risk of exhibiting lower values. To reduce the risk of the potential health consequences of an inadequate vitamin D status, substantial details on worldwide patterns of vitamin D status are needed to inform public health policy.

Vitamin A (retinol/carotenoids) is found in whole milk, egg yolks, liver, fish oil, cheese, butter, carrots, dark-green leafy vegetables and orange-coloured fruits such as mangoes and apricots. It is responsible for cell growth and differentiation (e.g. epithelial cells), promotion of immunity, as a defence against infection and for the promotion of growth in bones. Some food products are now fortified with vitamin A, such as margarine and reduced-fat spreads.

Vitamin B complex is broken down into B_1, B_2, B_3, B_6, B_{12}, folate, pantothenic acid and biotin. Thiamin (vitamin B_1) is found in bread and breakfast cereals, vegetables (especially potatoes), meat and meat products. A deficiency can result in severe muscle wasting, delayed growth in children and increase susceptibility to infections. Riboflavin (vitamin B_2) deficiency can cause angular stomatitis (cracking of the skin around the mouth) and glossitis (inflammation of the tongue). Ribiflavin is found in milk and milk products, meat and meat products, breakfast cereals and beverages (especially beer). A deficiency in vitamin B_3 (niacin) can cause anorexia, nausea, dysphagia, inflammation of the oral mucosa and cognitive issues such as delirium, mental disturbance and dementia. It is found in bread and breakfast cereals, meat and meat products, vegetables and milk and milk products. While these vitamins do not impact directly on musculoskeletal health, the impact of stomatitis, glossitis, anorexia, nausea, dysphagia, inflammation of the oral mucosa and cognitive issues could influence nutritional intake. Vitamin B_{12} (cobalamin) is necessary for DNA synthesis and a deficiency can lead to megaloblastic anaemia. Again, it is found in meat and meat products, milk and milk products, fish eggs and egg dishes. Vitamin B_6 (pyridoxine), folic acid (folate), pantothenic acid and biotin are not dealt with in this discussion.

Vitamin C is found in fresh fruit, nuts and green vegetables. It is associated with protein metabolism, e.g. laying down of collagen fibres in connective tissue. A deficiency can delay wound healing and inhibit bone repair (Kearney and Pot 2017).

Minerals

Minerals are inorganic substances required by the body in small amounts for a variety of different functions. They are involved in the formation of bones and teeth, are essential constituents of body fluids and tissues, and are components of enzyme systems. They are also involved in normal nerve function. Minerals relevant to the discussion on musculoskeletal health are discussed here.

Calcium is the most abundant mineral in the human body and is found in dairy products (e.g. milk, cheese, yoghurts), eggs, green vegetables and some fish (e.g. sardines) (Kearney and Pot 2017). An adequate supply should be obtained from a well-balanced diet but certain groups can require more, such as teenagers and pregnant or nursing mothers. Calcium is absorbed from our intestines and is an essential structural component of our bones and teeth. That is where we find approximately 99% of our calcium with the other 1% found in blood. Calcium is required for vascular contraction and

vasodilation, muscle function, nerve transmission, intracellular activity and hormonal secretion. It provides rigidity in bones in the form of calcium phosphate (also known as hydroxyapatite). Calcium regulation is controlled by the action of the parathyroid hormone, vitamin D and calcitonin (Sharp 2017), with less than 1% needed to support metabolic function. As it is tightly regulated, the levels in the body do not fluctuate with dietary changes, instead the body uses bone tissue as a source of calcium to maintain concentrations. A negative calcium balance occurs when net calcium absorption fails to compensate for urinary calcium losses. Signs of calcium deficiency include stunted growth, poor quality bones and teeth, and bone malformation. Bone undergoes continuous remodelling, with constant resorption and deposition into new bone. The balance between these two actions can change with age. In periods of growth (in children and adolescents), formation exceeds absorption. In adulthood both actions are relatively equal but in the ageing population, particularly post-menopausal women, bone resorption exceeds formation, resulting in bone loss and an increased risk of osteoporosis. During these periods, this results in a change in the recommended daily intake. Recommended daily calcium intakes vary from country to country and the recommended daily intakes for the USA and the UK are shown in Tables 10.1 and 10.2.

Luliano et al. (2021) carried out a study to assess the anti-fracture efficacy and safety of a nutritional intervention in institutional older adults replete in vitamin D but with mean intakes of 600 mg/day of calcium and <1 g/kg body weight of protein/day and concluded that improving calcium and protein intakes by using dairy foods is a readily accessible intervention that reduces the risk of falls and fractures commonly occurring in aged-care residents.

Table 10.1 Daily recommended intake of calcium in healthy subjects (National Institute of Health 2021).

Age	Calcium intake (mg) per day	
	Male	**Female**
0–6 mo	200	200
7–12 mo	260	260
1–3 years	700	700
4–8 yr	1000	1000
9–13 yr	1300	1300
14–18 yr	1300	1300
19–50 yr	1000	1000
51–70 yr	1000	1200
71 plus	1200	1200

Table 10.2 Daily recommended intake of calcium (British Dietetic Association 2021a).

Age	Calcium intake (mg) per day
Under 1	525
1–3 yr	350
4–6 yr	450
7–10 yr	550
11–18 yr (girls)	800
11–18 yr (boys)	1000
19+	700
Breastfeeding women	1250
Women past the menopause	1200
Men over 55	1200
Coeliac disease (19+)	1000–1500
Osteoporosis (19+)	1000
Inflammatory bowel disease (19+)	1000

Cheese, oatmeal, liver and kidney provide a supply of phosphorus. It is also added to foods and drinks such as cola as polyphosphates or phosphoric acid. Where there is a normal level of calcium, it is unlikely that a deficiency of phosphorus will be found. Bone mineral consists of calcium phosphate and therefore a supply of phosphorus is essential for skeletal development. Along with calcium and vitamin D, phosphorus is involved in the hardening of bones (Waugh and Grant 2010). Excessive phosphorus lowers the excretion of calcium in the urine and lowers the absorption of calcium from the diet.

Iron is an essential trace element and is found in beef, kidneys, liver, green vegetables and wholemeal bread. Our diet contains between 9 and 15 g of iron but only a small proportion of this is absorbed (less than 15%). The levels of iron do not directly influence the skeletal system but are essential for the formation of haemoglobin (the oxygen-carrying component of our blood) in our red blood cells. Certain groups require increased intake, such as teenagers and pregnant women. In excess, iron is extremely toxic to our cells and therefore it is essential that the amount is regulated. Iron deficiency is a condition that causes anaemia if iron stores are depleted and is the most common nutritional deficiency (Sharp 2017). Whilst mild anaemia in many individuals is of little health consequence due to compensatory mechanisms in the body (such as increased cardiac output, diversion of blood flow and increased release of oxygen from haemoglobin), the body cannot compensate in severe anaemia. This results in poorer oxygen delivery to the tissues and

impacts on body function. Work performance is limited and this will influence the participation of patients in rehabilitation post-injury and after surgery. It is essential that when planning a rehabilitation programme or in planned surgery, that the patient's haemoglobin is within an acceptable range. Where emergency surgery is necessary, again a work-up for surgery should include haemoglobin measurement and necessary corrections can take place if required.

According to Barker and Blumsohn (2017), there is very limited evidence that dietary zinc is important for the skeleton, although its undernutrition is proposed as a risk factor for osteoporosis. Zinc can be obtained from shellfish, meat and whole grains, with a recommended intake of between 5.5 and 7.3 mg daily (Geissler and Powers 2017) in the UK. It is noted by Barker and Blumsohn that elderly people consume zinc-deficient diets and they report on other studies that highlight post-menopausal osteoporotic women having elevated urinary zinc levels in comparison to healthy controls but conclude that the link between zinc status and osteoporosis risk is tenuous.

Sodium is found in most foods, e.g. eggs, fish, meat, milk and processed foods. It is also added to food during preparation and prior to eating (table salt). Sodium helps to regulate water content in the body. A diet high in sodium increases urinary calcium excretion. Sodium occurs as an extracellular cation and is involved in muscle contraction, transmission of nerve impulses along the axons, and water and electrolyte balance. The Food Safety Authority of Ireland (2016) and the British Heart Foundation (2018) recommend a salt intake (sodium chloride) of no more than 6 g daily (1 teaspoon). Currently intakes of sodium are too high and although some is essential, most people need to reduce their intake substantially. Potassium is found in fruit, vegetables and other foods. As with sodium, it is involved in muscle contraction, transmission of nerve impulses, and water and electrolyte balance, and it occurs as an intracellular cation.

Today, fluoride is present in drinking water and the majority of foods. Fluoride increases the activity of the osteoblasts. Adding fluoride to drinking water is controversial, with highly inconsistent findings in studies. Barker and Blumsohn (2017) reported a link to fractures with high-dose fluoride therapy in osteoporotic patients.

Magnesium is important in calcium homeostasis. It is also important in the metabolism and/or action of vitamin D and is essential for the synthesis and secretion of the parathyroid hormone. A deficiency therefore results in impaired parathyroid hormone secretion and disturbed calcium homeostasis, and hypocalcaemia is a common symptom of a moderate to severe deficiency (Expert Group on Vitamins and Minerals 2003).

Aluminium toxicity occurs in chronic renal failure or in patients receiving parenteral nutrition. Osteoblast function is impaired in this toxic environment and there is reduced bone remodelling and osteomalacia. Boron supplements are sold by advertising their skeletal benefits but according to Barker and Blumsohn (2017) human studies are rare, limited in scope and contradictory.

A number of other trace elements are identified as part of a nutritious diet. These include copper, chromium, boron and strontium. A deficiency in copper is rarely reported due to its availability from our diet, but skeletal problems can result from a deficiency. A severe deficiency is associated with skeletal disease. Chromium supplements are also advertised as having beneficial skeletal effects. There are conflicting reports on whether the musculoskeletal system can benefit from a normal intake (Barker and Blumsohn 2017). According to the Expert Group on Vitamins and Minerals (2003), boron deficiency has not been observed in human populations but they suggest that it could contribute to Kashin–Beck disease, which is a deficiency that can result in severe joint deformity. The relevance of dietary strontium in relation to skeletal health is unknown, with a higher incidence of rickets noted in geographical areas where strontium soil levels are high (Barker and Blumsohn 2017). Fibre is found in cereal, beans, pulses, fruit and vegetables, and although not a nutrient, it improves movement in the gut and helps prevent constipation (refer to Chapter 9).

Other Components

Other dietary components can influence bone health. Abusing alcohol can compromise bone quality and increase the risk of fracture. The latest advice is that it is safest for men and women not to drink more than 14 units a week on a regular basis (Drinkaware 2021). The Scottish Intercollegiate Guideline Network (SIGN 2021) note that an alcohol intake of more than 3.5 units per day may alter a person's underlying risk for fragility fractures, therefore they advise maintaining intake within recommended guidelines. There is a suggested link between an increased intake of caffeine and fracture risk in osteoporosis. SIGN (2021) suggest that it may be prudent to restrict intake of coffee to no more than four cups a day, particularly if dietary calcium intakes are low.

A high intake of carbonated cola-type drinks is associated with a low bone mineral density in observational studies carried out on teenagers, but according to Barker and Blumsohn (2017) there have been few reports of studies in adults and they are inconsistent, and this is supported by SIGN (2021).

Metabolic Response to Trauma, Surgery and Other Issues

The metabolic effect of trauma and/or surgery is one of catabolism of stored body fuels. The size and time span of the response is proportional to the injury and any complications, e.g sepsis, that might develop (Desborough 2000), therefore energy requirements will increase depending on body demands. It is important that the nutritional needs of the patient are considered in the pre-operative, peri-operative and post-operative periods. Nutritional assessment can play an important role (refer to Section 10.4), alongside patient fasting (refer to Section 10.5). The increased demands placed on the body during recovery from surgery, injury and occurring complications warrants careful consideration by the multidisciplinary team.

The dietary needs of the child and adolescent must be considered in light of their age, growth and development, and this can make them susceptible to nutritional imbalance and deficiencies. Consideration must be given to nutritional needs when demands are placed on the body by exercise, sport and training programmes. As a person ages, the risk of chronic disease increases and nutrition can play a role in the development of or susceptibility to and outcome of disease. Other groups who experience a risk include those with learning disabilities and dementia. Undernutrition can be a particular problem and the need for nutritional assessment becomes extremely important. The need for guidance for families and staff in the area of dementia is highlighted by Lee and Kolassa (2011). They identify some of the common symptoms of feeding problems in advanced Alzheimer's, assisted feeding methods and behaviours that affect individuals with Alzheimer's receiving adequate nutrition.

Nutrition Assessment and Intervention

Kneale (2005) stated that nutrition deprivation does not imply a lack of food but the provision of a diet that does not meet the physiological needs of the patient, which may vary during a period of hospitalisation.

Malnutrition broadly refers to deficiencies, excesses or imbalances in a person's intake of energy and/or nutrients. Undernutrition includes energy or macronutrient deficiencies (protein-energy malnutrition) and micronutrient deficiencies or insufficiencies, while overnutrition is routinely associated with overweight, obesity and diet-related non-communicable diseases (Geirsdóttir et al. 2021). The incidence of malnutrition and associated issues varies in publications, with Malafarina et al. (2018) noting in a review of hip fracture studies that 19% of patients were malnourished, 35% were at risk of malnutrition while the British Association for Parenteral and Enteral Nutrition (BAPEN 2021a) notes 25–34% of hospital admissions are at risk of malnutrition and 70% of patients weighed less on hospital discharge. The orthopaedic patient is at risk of malnutrition if their intake of nutrients is impacted by comorbidities, surgery or underlying problems that affect appetite or absorption of food. It is identified that malnutrition (undernutrition) can have a wide range of consequences, such as impaired immune response, reduced muscle fatigue and impaired wound healing and growth (BAPEN 2021a). In the acute setting, patients at risk of malnutrition remain inpatients for longer than those who are well nourished and are more likely to be discharged to alternative settings rather than their home. The risk of malnutrition is increased in the older person, with its presence leading to impaired coordination and an increased risk of falls that is heightened when osteoporosis is present. According to NICE (2017), nutritional support should be considered in those who are malnourished, i.e. a body mass index (BMI) of less than $18.5\,kg/m^2$, unintentional weight loss of greater than 10% in the last 3–6 months or a BMI of less than $20\,kg/m^2$ and an unintentional weight loss greater than 5% within 3–6 months.

Obesity is a common nutritional problem in many developed countries. It exists where there is an excess accumulation of body fat (Waugh and Grant 2010). Obesity is present when the BMI exceeds $29.9\,kg/m^2$ (see Table 10.3) and is associated with high morbidity and mortality rates. Obese patients may prove challenging during all phases of care due to an associated risk of complications. The role of the nurse during preparation for surgery is critical in providing support and advice with respect to achieving weight loss.

A study undertaken by the World Health Organisation (2003) between 1997 and 2003 generated new growth curves for assessing the growth and development of infants and young children around the world. The growth curves

Table 10.3 Body mass index, WHO classification.

Calculation of BMI

$$BMI = \frac{Weight\,(kg)}{Height\,(m^2)}$$

Interpretation of BMI

<16	Severely underweight
16–18.4	Underweight
18.5–24.9	Normal range
25–29.9	Overweight
30–39.9	Obese
>40	Severely obese

provide a single intervention standard that represents the best description of physiological growth for all children between birth and 5 years. Centile charts show the position of a measured parameter within a statistical distribution. They are useful for plotting parameters such as height or weight over time. If a problem is identified, e.g. childhood obesity or inadequate growth, a period of observation is required. Serial recordings of height and weight continue, an evaluation can be made of the evidence and an appropriate referral made.

Nutritional Assessment

Measuring nutritional status can be predictive of health outcomes with the assessment of nutritional intake required if it is thought there may be a need to provide advice to the person or more aggressive interventions such as enteral or parenteral support. Nutritional assessment approaches include dietary assessment, the use of anthropometry (the physical measurement of some or several aspects of human body size) and the use of biochemical, functional and clinical measures or indices.

Dietary assessment can be achieved by attaining a dietary history from the individual or their carer for the previous 24 hours or by giving the individual a questionnaire to determine the frequency of different food groups eaten over the previous week. Anthropometry can include the measurement of body weight and height from which BMI is calculated (Table 10.3). The percentage of body fat can be estimated by measuring the sum of the thickness of skinfolds over the biceps, triceps, subscapular and supra-iliac sites. The fat content varies with age and gender. It is now recognised that intra-abdominal fat measurement has a greater influence on the development of heart disease and diabetes than fat measurement in subcutaneous sites and is useful in orthopaedic assessment in preparation for surgery (Després 2012).

Biochemical status measures are defined for each nutrient and assess the concentration or its derivative in the body fluid while functional indices are an assessment of the metabolic processes that are nutritionally dependent. Finally, clinical indices are the signs and symptoms of a nutritional deficiency, e.g. rickets is a sign of vitamin D deficiency.

A range of screening and assessment tools exist and Roigk (2018) identifies the Malnutrition Universal Screening Tool (MUST) tool as one that is valid and reliable. It was developed in 2003 by a subgroup of the British Association for Parenteral and Enteral Nutrition. Using MUST involves five steps; the first three steps include gathering nutritional measurements, noting the percentage of unplanned weight loss and considering the effect of acute disease, which are all scored. An overall risk score or category of malnutrition is determined by adding the score obtained from steps 1 to 3 (step 4). The patient is then considered at either low risk, medium risk or high risk. Step 5 involves using guidelines and/or local policy to form an appropriate action plan for the patient (BAPEN 2021b). Actions can involve repeat screening (for those at low risk), observation and nutritional support (for those at medium risk), and referral to a dietician, regular monitoring and nutritional support (for those at high risk). It is essential that those in all categories have any underlying condition treated and are provided with help and advice on food choices and with eating and drinking. Training for staff on the use of such a tool is an important part of its implementation.

Methods to improve or maintain nutritional intake are classified as nutrition support and may be as simple as assistance at mealtimes or the provision of a diet deemed appropriate to the patient's needs after a nutritional assessment. As part of this dietary plan, the nutritional support can include oral nutrition supplements, enteral tube feeding, e.g. via the nasogastric route/percutaneous endoscopic gastrostomy, or parenteral nutrition. NICE (2017) provide a protocol for nutritional, anthropometric and clinical monitoring of nutritional support. This includes provision of nutrients, monitoring weight and BMI, observing gastrointestinal function, monitoring feeding tubes or catheter entry sites, observing the patient's clinical condition, setting goals and laboratory monitoring.

Multidisciplinary Assessment

Once an assessment has identified that the nutrition of a patient is compromised, a plan of care needs to be put in place. This can involve all or some of the multidisciplinary team depending on the needs of the patient, including the nursing team, dietician, speech therapist, occupational therapist, pharmacist and catering team.

Roigk (2018) notes that nurses are coordinators of the care process and can bring the other healthcare professionals together to collaboratively provide the care the patient requires. The nursing team also has the most contact with the patient. Observing and monitoring patients at mealtimes and providing assistance where appropriate can contribute to the provision of a balanced diet. Making sure patients are eating, recognising poor appetite, documenting any issues and reporting are essential. Within the ward environment, nurses can influence better nutrition for their patients, e.g. restricting visiting at mealtimes, ensuring that other nursing procedures are not carried out at mealtimes unless required for better patient outcomes, and avoiding the organisation of investigations or tests at

mealtimes. Each member of the nursing team (registered nurse, healthcare assistant) must be aware of his or her responsibilities so training is essential. Patients also need advice on a diet that is balanced to promote their individual recovery, which can be facilitated by nurses in conjunction with the dietician. Jester and Santy (2011) advocate such approaches and further suggest examples of good practice. They include the involvement of the multidisciplinary team, identifying and supporting at-risk patients, monitoring the intake of at-risk patients, giving help to those patients who need assistance, protecting mealtimes so that patients can focus on eating without unnecessary interruption, provision of appetising and attractive food and the availability of food, snacks and high calorific drinks around the clock.

Referral to the dietician is usually through locally agreed protocols. A dietician applies their knowledge of nutrition to promote health, prevent disease and aid in the treatment of illnesses. They can assess the nutritional status of the patient, advise on appropriate therapeutic diets or feeding regimens, and monitor and instigate appropriate changes in the nutritional care plan.

A speech therapist may be involved if the patient has problems swallowing or exhibits chewing difficulties or is considered at risk of aspiration. The occupational therapist's role involves assessing the patient's range of movement and mobility in relation to managing independence at home, e.g. preparing food, managing in the community and the provision of advice and appropriate aids, e.g. plate guards and customised cutlery, which can be used in hospital and the community. The pharmacist can provide support to the ward team when involved in the provision of dietary supplements, and enteral and parenteral feeds.

The catering team's role is to provide a variety of foods taking into account the nutritional value, the needs of the patient recovering from injury or surgery, or those with dietary restrictions in relation to medical conditions, and the cultural and religious issues that influence diet. The use of menu cards allows patients to experience a variety of foods. The presentation, texture and consistency of food produced by the team also contribute to a better service and patient outcome. The availability of food outside of designated mealtimes is also an important aspect of providing a good service. A balanced diet can be achieved by working with the other members of the multidisciplinary team. A member of the catering team meeting with patients on a regular basis can provide good feedback on which aspects of the service should continue or provide information that can lead to improvements.

The move towards creating a healthier environment in hospitals with respect to nutrition is advocated. The Council of Europe (2003) identified 10 key characteristics of good nutritional care in hospitals and these have been endorsed by many organisations, such as the Department of Health in the UK and Ireland.

In the drive to improve standards, national governments have got involved. One such example is the essence of care, which identified 12 benchmarks to address the fundamentals of care and these continue to be relevant (Box 10.1).

The Health Service Executive (2019) and the Royal College of Nursing (2021) have published advice on maintaining standards in relation to malnutrition, which are accessible online. While having best practice recommendations is important, measuring standards of care delivery within our hospitals is recognised as contributing to improving practice. Quality care metrics is one such example providing a framework to identify gaps in care delivery, thus enabling planning for quality improvement and a mechanism for accountability in care delivery (Health Service Executive 2018).

Oral health problems, such as dental caries, oral disease, gum disease and infection, can all affect food choices and ultimately nutritional status. Ill-fitting dentures may be a sign of recent weight loss. Healthcare professionals can help their patients by asking about oral health problems and recommended referral for a dental consultation where appropriate. Other interventions can include inspection of the oral cavity, noting any ulceration or abnormality. The plan should include frequent oral hygiene, cleaning of dentures and use of a mouthwash.

Hydration and Dehydration: Assessment and Intervention

Hydration is the process of drinking enough liquids to keep fluid levels in the body topped up, ensuring bodily functions can take place normally (British Dietetic Association 2021b). Dehydration occurs when you lose or use more fluid that you take in and as a result the body cannot carry out its normal functions (Mayo Clinic 2021).

Maintaining good hydration is critical to maintaining good health, which becomes even more important as we age. Poor hydration can lead to multiple problems, such as tendons and ligaments becoming less resilient, constipation, dry and itchy skin, acne, nose bleeds, repeated urinary tract infections, dry coughs, sneezing, sinus pressure, headaches, confusion and falls, which can be the result of toxins building up in our bodies. It can also weaken the body's immune system and leads to chemical, nutritional and pH imbalances. Being insufficiently hydrated is also a cause of daytime fatigue.

Hydration is essential for peak athletic performance. When you do not consume enough liquid or fresh fruits

---

Box 10.1   Essence of Care (Department of Health 2010)

Essence of care was first published in the UK in 2001 and revised in 2010 (Department of Health 2010). This document provides benchmarks for the management of food and drink in the healthcare setting and the community. Ten factors are set out with best practice statements. Indicators for achieving the best practice statements are listed and it allows for the addition of local practice indicators. A set of general indicators is given at the beginning of the document, and these need to be considered with each of the factors. These are the people's experience, diversity and individual needs, effectiveness, and consent and confidentiality.

Factor	Benchmark of best practice
1) Promoting health	People are encouraged to eat and drink in a way that promotes health
2) Information	People and carers have sufficient information to enable them to obtain their food and drink
3) Availability	People can access food and drink at any time according to their needs and preferences
4) Provision	People are provided with food and drink that meets their individual needs and preferences
5) Presentation	People's food and drink is presented in a way that is appealing to them
6) Environment	People feel the environment is conducive to eating and drinking
7) Screening and assessment	People who are screened on initial contact and identified as at-risk receive full nutritional assessment
8) Planning implantation evaluation and revision of care	People's care is planned, implemented, continuously evaluated and revised to meet individual needs and preference to food and drink
9) Assistance	People receive care and assistance when required with eating and drinking
10) Monitoring	People's food and drink intake is monitored and recorded

and vegetables to stay properly hydrated, you end up thirsty and light-headed. Insufficient hydration fatigues your muscles, reduces your coordination and causes muscle cramps. While working out or playing sports, dehydration compromises the body's ability to cool itself through sweating. This leads to heat exhaustion and in extreme cases a potentially life-threatening condition called heat stroke.

Water is essential for life. It makes up about 60% of the body weight of men and about 55% of the body weight in women (Waugh and Grant 2010). Adequate fluid intake is essential for healthy organ function, including our muscles. We lose water when we breathe (about 300–400ml per day) and urinate (1–2l per day with a general rule of thumb of 1ml/kg body weight/h with boundaries of 0.5–2ml/kg/h). Water is also lost through the skin by evaporation (600ml per day) and faeces (100–200ml per day). How much water we lose depends on our age, body size, physical activity, health and environmental conditions. It is normally balanced by our intake of food and water. Water has many functions, incorporating the moistening of food for swallowing, regulation of body temperature, transport of substances around our bodies, as a medium for excretion of waste products, dilution of water products in the body, provision of a moist environment required by our living cells and the provision of conditions where metabolic reactions can take place.

The recommended fluid intake is 1.2l–1.6l a day for adults. The British Nutrition Foundation (2021) has published guides to fluid intake for different age ranges. For children, the recommended fluid intake changes with age (NICE 2010) (Table 10.4).

Fluid and electrolyte balance can be affected by the physiological response of the body to the stress of surgery or injury. Glucocortoid secretion increases reabsorption of sodium and water in the kidney with a corresponding loss of potassium and hydrogen ions. Increased levels of the antidiuretic hormone also increase water reabsorption while high aldosterone levels further increase sodium reabsorption to maintain circulating volumes and renal perfusion. As a result of trauma to the tissue from injury or surgery, intracellular potassium is released, resulting in an exchange for retained sodium. Levels of potassium need careful monitoring and should be replaced as appropriate (Alexander et al. 2019).

Nausea and Vomiting

Post-operative nausea and vomiting (PONV) is a common unpleasant experience, with patients at risk of aspiration, electrolyte imbalance, pain, increased length of stay and reduction in patient satisfaction. Risk factors identified for PONV include obesity, older age, female gender, children, prior history, anxiety, inadequate pain relief, prolonged fasting and post-operative hypotension. This issue needs to be identified and managed appropriately. Hatfield and Tronson (2009) promote simple measures such as hydration, supplemental oxygen, sitting the patient upright and wheeling feet first when being transferred back to the ward from theatre as very effective, with the appropriate use of antiemetics recommended. With an increase in patients undergoing day case joint replacement surgery, this issue is of critical importance. Stephenson et al. (2021) advocate adherence to pre-operative risk stratification and a standard anti-emetic prophylactic protocol to significantly reduce the prevalence of nausea and vomiting. The enhanced recovery after surgery programme (Department of Health 2011) details principles that can contribute to less nausea and vomiting, earlier participation in rehabilitation and the achievement of recovery goals and earlier discharge (Box 10.2). Wainwright et al. (2020) suggest in their consensus statement that evidence supports the use of screening for PONV and multimodal PONV prophylaxis and treatment for patients undergoing total hip and knee replacement.

Table 10.4 Recommended daily fluid intake for children.

Age	Sex	Total daily intake (ml)
4–8 yr	Female	1000–1400
	Male	1000–1400
9–13 yr	Female	1200–2100
	Male	1400–2300
14–18 yr	Female	1400–2500
	Male	2100–3200

Box 10.2 Enhanced Recovery after Surgery (Department of Health 2011)

Enhanced recovery is a growing movement within surgery which aims, through a variety of methods, to help patients to get better sooner after major surgery.

The programme was established to support the NHS to implement and realise the benefits in major surgeries, including musculoskeletal procedures. It is based on the following premises:

1) The patient is in the best possible condition for surgery.
2) The patient has the best possible management during and after his/her operation.
3) The patient experiences the best post-operative rehabilitation.

Key principles
Patient education/communication

- Starts at outpatient appointment
- Continues at pre-operative assessment
- A weekly education session is held (alternate education sessions: one week for prospective hip replacement patients, alternate week for prospective knee replacement patients; this could vary depending on service need)
- Over 2 hours, cover what to expect, pain relief, physiotherapy, occupational therapy
- Alleviating patient worries: know what to expect, meet ward staff, sleep better before surgery

Anaesthetic factors

- Avoidance of premedication
- Individualised goal, directed fluid therapy (carbohydrate loading)
- Regional anaesthesia
- Short-acting anaesthetic agents
- Prevention of hypothermia
- Effective opiate-sparing analgesia
- Minimise post-operative nausea and vomiting

Surgical factors

- Minimally invasive approaches
- Reduced tourniquet time
- Careful haemostasis
- Careful tissue handling
- Local anaesthetic infiltration
- Leave dressing in situ for at least 48 hours
- Training

Nutrition

- Maximising patient's pre-operative hydration
- Individualised and targeted prevention of nausea and vomiting
- Early post-operative hydration

Rehabilitation

- Front loading
- Same-day mobilisation
- 365-day service
- Encouragement of patient self-care
- Own clothes (and make-up!)

Process

- Admit patients on the day of surgery
- Planned discharge criteria
- Telephone and follow-up support immediately post discharge, 48-hour call from the nurse
- Auditing and monitoring of outcomes

Fasting

Historically, surgical patients were fasted routinely from food and drink for long periods (up to 12 hours) before anaesthesia to reduce the risk of aspiration and pneumonitis at anaesthesia. Despite evidence that a shorter pre-operative fast does not increase the risk of this complication, practice across Europe varies. Long fasting times for surgery can impact on hydration and nutrition, therefore surgery should be planned to ensure fasting/starvation times can be kept to a minimum and intravenous hydration considered.

Pre-operative fasting is often in excess of the recommended 2 hours for fluids and 6 hours for milk or food (Royal College of Nursing 2005). This is also supported by NICE (2020), who also note the contribution of this to reducing headaches and nausea and vomiting. The 2–6 rule applies to adults where water can be drunk up to 2 hours before induction of anaesthesia and there is a minimal pre-operative fasting time of 6 hours for food (solids, milk and milk-containing drinks). The volume of administered fluid does not appear to have an impact on patients' residual gastric volume and gastric pH when compared to a standard fasting regime (Royal College of Nursing 2005). It is suggested that the anaesthetic team should consider further interventions for patients at the highest risk of regurgitation and aspiration. For children, the 2–4–6 rule applies. The intake of water should cease 2 hours before induction of anaesthesia, with breast-feeding ceasing 4 hours before anaesthesia. Formula milk, cow's milk or other solids should cease 6 hours before anaesthesia. Translation of these recommendations into clinical practice is still noted as poor (Hewson and Moppett 2020) with 'risk aversion on the part of staff and patients that pulmonary aspiration may occur despite following guidance'. There is now consideration being given to shortening fasting times for fluids from 2 hours to 1 hour as gastric emptying in unmedicated healthy adults is quick and exponential. Wainwright et al. (2020) note that the use of carbohydrate loading may improve patient wellbeing and metabolism, but as it has not been shown to accelerate the achievement of discharge criteria or reduce complications, it is not currently recommended by this group as an essential routine intervention. NICE (2020) would concur with this.

Fluid Replacement

Minimising the length of fasting times combined with appropriate fluid management during surgery is considered a key factor during major surgery and can improve surgical outcomes. Post-operative patients should be encouraged to drink when ready providing there are no contraindications (Royal College of Nursing 2005).

Intravenous replacement should be provided as prescribed and discontinued when the patient is drinking adequate fluids. Other evidence-based strategies are documented by Roigk (2018) and include availability of drinks (being constantly and readily available with 'drinks rounds' taking place), drinking pleasure (providing drinks based on individual preference, i.e. type, temperature, flavour), support and help to drink (offering individualised support and use of aids), and the monitoring and understanding of the necessity to drink (educating the patient on the importance of hydration and signs of dehydration).

Recording Fluid Intake/Output

Many serious fluid balance issues can be averted by keeping a careful eye on the intake and output of the patient and maintaining careful records (Roigk 2018). Fluid balance charting allows the healthcare professional to carefully monitor intake and output, and calculate a balance, usually completed over a 24-hour period. Accuracy in both measurement and documentation is fundamental to patient care and outcome, but this skill is often highlighted as substandard when undertaken by nurses. Output is often recorded as patient out to toilet or has passed urine ++ which is inaccurate and does not give a clear account of the patient's output.

Summary

Nutrition and hydration are important contributing factors to best practice in the management of the orthopaedic patient undergoing planned surgery or management of a trauma injury. This chapter provides an overview of the importance of nutrition and hydration, diet and musculoskeletal health, metabolic responses to trauma and surgery, nutritional assessment and intervention plus hydration and dehydration. Good nutrition plays a key role in patient recovery, with poor nutrition leading to a delay in the patient returning to their previous level of independence as a result of complications such as delayed healing or infection. The practitioner therefore needs to understand what good nutrition is and recognise how it and they can contribute to improved patient outcomes.

References

Alexander, M., Fawcett, J.N., and Runciman, P.J. (ed.) (2019). *Nursing Practice, Hospital and Home, the Adult*, 5e. Edinburgh: Churchill Livingstone Elsevier.

BAPEN (2021a) *Malnutrition.* http://www.bapen.org.uk/malnutrition-undernutrition/introduction-to-malnutrition. Accessed 17 October 2021.

BAPEN (2021b) *The MUST explanatory booklet.* http://www.bapen.org.uk. Accessed 17 October 2021.

Barker, M.E. and Blumsohn, A. (2017). *Nutrition and the skeleton.* In: *Human Nutrition*, 13e (ed. C. Geissler and H. Powers), 494–509. Oxford: Oxford University Press.

British Dietetic Association (2021a) *Calcium: Food fact sheet.* https://www.bda.uk.com/resource/calcium.html (accessed 17 October 2021).

British Dietetic Association (2021b) *The importance of hydration.* https://www.bda.uk.com/resource/the-importance-hydration.html (accessed 17 October 2021).

British Heart Foundation (2018) *Taking control of salt.* https://www.bhf.org.uk/-/media/files/publications/healthy-eating-and-drinking/taking-control-of-salt_download.pdf?

British Nutrition Foundation (2019) *Find your balance.* https://www.nutrition.org.uk/media/tfzieioa/bnf-1pp-a4-v5.pdf (accessed 17 October 2021).

British Nutrition Foundation (2021) *Hydration.* https://www.nutrition.org.uk/healthy-sustainable-diets/hydration/ (accessed 17 October 2021).

Council of Europe (2003) *Food and nutritional care in hospitals.* https://wcd.coe.int/ViewDoc.jsp?id=85747 (accessed 17 October 2021).

Department of Health (2010). *Essence of Care, Benchmarks for Food and Drink.* Norwich: The Stationery Office.

Department of Health (2011) *Enhanced recovery partnership programme.* http://www.dh.giv.uk/publications (accessed 26 October 2021).

Department of Health (2021) *Healthy food for life.* https://assets.gov.ie/7649/3049964a47cb405fa20ea8d96bf50c91.pdf.

Desborough, J.P. (2000). The stress response to surgery and trauma. *Br. J. Anesth.* 85 (1): 109–117.

Després, J.P. (2012). Body fat distribution and risk of cardiovascular disease an update. *Circulation* 126: 1301–1313.

Drinkaware (2021) http://www.drinkaware.co.uk/facts/alcoholic-drinks-and-units/how-much-alcohol-is-too-much (accessed 17 October 2021).

Endo, A., Baer, H., Nagao, M., and Weaver, M. (2018). Prediction model of inpatient mortality after hip fracture surgery. *J. Orthop. Trauma* 32 (1): 34–38. https://doi.org/10.1097/BOT.0000000000001026.

Expert Group on Vitamins and Minerals (2003). *Safe Upper Limits for Vitamins and Minerals.* London: Food Standards Agency.

Food Safety Authority of Ireland (2016) https://www.fsai.ie/science_and_health/salt_and_health/the_science_of_salt_and_health.html.

Geirsdóttir, Ó.G., Hertz, K., Santy-Tomlinson, J. et al. (2021). *Overview of nutrition care in geriatrics and orthogeriatrics*. In: *Interdisciplinary Nutritional Management and Care for Older Adults an Evidence Based Practical Guide for Nurses* (ed. Ó.G. Geirsdóttir and J.J. Bell), 3–18. Springer Open Access.

Geissler, C. and Powers, H. (2017). *Human Nutrition*, 13e, 494–509. Oxford: Oxford University Press.

Gordon, M.H. and Jin, Y. (2017). *Food and nutrient structure*. In: *Human Nutrition*, 13e (ed. C. Geissler and H. Powers), 24–47. Oxford: Oxford University Press.

Hatfield, A. and Tronson, M. (2009). *The Complete Recovery Room Book*, 4e. Oxford: Oxford University Press.

Health Service Executive (2018). *Nursing and Midwifery Quality Care Metrics: Acute Care Research Report*. Dublin: HSE Office of Nursing and Midwifery Services Director.

Health Service Executive (2019). Nutrition Standards for Food and Beverage Provision. https://www.hse.ie/eng/about/who/healthwellbeing/our-priority-programmes/heal/healthy-eating-guidelines/nutrition-standards-for-food-and-beverage-provision-for-staff-and-visitors-in-healthcare-settings.pdf.

Hewson, D. and Moppett, I. (2020). Preoperative fasting and prevention of pulmonary aspiration in adults: research feast, quality improvement famine. *Br. J. Anaesth.* https://10.1016/j.bja.2019.12.018.

Hilger, J., Friedal, A., Herr, R. et al. (2014). A systematic review of vitamin D status in populations worldwide. *Br. J. Nutr.* 111: 23–45.

Jester, R. and Santy, J. (2011). *Oxford Handbook of Orthopaedic and Trauma Nursing*. Oxford: Oxford University Press.

Kearney, J. and Pot, G. (2017). *Food and nutrition patterns*. In: *Human Nutrition*, 13e (ed. C. Geissler and H. Powers), 3–23. Oxford: Oxford University Press.

Kneale, J. (2005). The importance of nutrition. In: *Orthopaedic and Trauma Nursing*, 2e (ed. J. Kneale and P. Davis), 164–179. Edinburgh: Churchill Livingstone.

Lee, T. and Kolassa, K. (2011). Feeding the person with late stage Alzheimer's disease. *Nutr. Today* 46 (2): 75–79.

Luliano, S., Poon, S., Robbins, J. et al. (2021). Effect of dietary sources of calcium and protein on hip fractures and falls in older adults in residential care: cluster randomized controlled trial. *Br. Med. J.* 375: n2364. https://doi.org/10.1136/bmj.n2364.

Malafarina, V., Reginster, J.Y., Cabrerizo, S. et al. (2018). Nutritional status and nutritional treatment are related to outcomes and mortality in older adults with hip fracture. *Nutrients* 10 (5): 555. https://doi.org/10.3390/nu10050555.

Mayo Clinic (2021). Dehydration. https://www.mayoclinic.org/diseases-conditions/dehydration/symptoms-causes/syc-20354086 (accessed 26 October 2021).

National Institute of Health (2021) http://ods.od.nih.gov/factsheets/Calcium-HealthProfessional (accessed 8 October 2021).

NICE (2010). *Nocturnal Enuresis and Bedwetting in Children and Young People (CG111)*. London: National Institute for Health and Care Excellence.

NICE (2017). *Nutrition Support in Adults: Oral Nutrition Support, Enteral Tube Feeding and Parenteral Nutrition (CG32)*. London: National Institute for Health and Care Excellence.

NICE (2020). *Perioperative Care in Adults (CG180)*. London: National Institute for Health and Care Excellence.

Public Health England (2018) *The Eatwell Guide*. https://assets.publishing.service.gov.uk/government/uploads/system/uploads/attachment_data/file/742750/Eatwell_Guide_booklet_2018v4.pdf.

Roigk, P. (2018). Nutrition and hydration. In: *Fragility Fracture Nursing Holistic Care and Management of the Orthogeriatric Patient* (ed. K. Hertz and J. Santy-Tomlinson), 95–107. Springer Open Access.

Royal College of Nursing (2005). *Peri-Operative Fasting in Adults and Children*. London: Royal College of Nursing.

Royal College of Nursing (2021) *Nutrition and hydration*. www.rcn.org.uk/clinical-topics/nutrition-and-hydration. (accessed 17 October 2021).

Sharp, P. (2017). Minerals and trace elements. In: *Human Nutrition*, 13e (ed. C. Geissler and H. Powers), 288–308. Oxford: Oxford University Press.

SIGN (2021) *Management of osteoporosis and the prevention of fragility fractures, Guideline 142*. www.sign.ac.uk (accessed 17 October 2021).

Stephenson, S., Jiwanmall, M., Cherian, N.E. et al. (2021). Reduction in post-operative nausea and vomiting (PONV) by preoperative risk stratification and adherence to a standardized anti emetic prophylaxis protocol in the day care surgical population. *J. Fam. Med Prim. Care* 10 (2): 865–870.

Wainwright, T., Gill, M., McDonald, D.A. et al. (2020). Consensus statement for perioperative care in total hip replacement and total knee replacement surgery; enhanced recovery after surgery (ERAS) society recommendations. *Acta Orthop.* 91 (1): 3–19.

Waugh, A. and Grant, A. (2010). *Ross and Wilson, Anatomy and Physiology in Health and Illness*, 11e. Edinburgh: Elsevier Churchhill Livingstone.

World Health Organization (2003) *The WHO multicentre growth reference study (MGRS)*. http://www.who.int/nutrition/publications/serveremalnutrition/9789241598163/en/index.html (accessed 17 October 2021).

11

Pain Assessment and Management in Orthopaedic and Trauma Care

Carolyn Mackintosh-Franklin

Division of Nursing, Midwifery and Social Work, University of Manchester, Manchester, UK

Introduction

Pain is the most frequently reported initial symptom in 70–91% of all trauma patients and is the most common reason for self-referral to accident and emergency or community health services (Berben et al. 2008, 2011), with around 500 million people injured each year of which around 25% are orthopaedic trauma (Edgely et al. 2019). However, the high variability in pain experiences between individuals means that the extent of and reaction to pain is unpredictable. The individual and unique nature of this experience makes it essential for all patients to be rigorously assessed prior to initiating appropriate pain management treatments/techniques. To ensure optimal standards of patient care, this requires practitioners working with patients in pain to be fully informed of the evidence base for best practice in this area.

The Nature of Pain

Pain is frequently reported as having an elusive quality that is difficult to quantify and is highly variable between individuals. This has led to great difficulty in establishing explanations for pain as an emotion or a physical sensation.

The Gate Control Theory of Pain

In 1946, based on experiences in the Second World War, Dr H Beecher published a seminal paper which ignited debate on the nature of pain as a purely physical phenomenon and argued that the meaning of pain to the individual experiencing it was a key component (Beecher 1959). The first scientific evidence to support this was published by Melzack and Wall (1965) in their outline of what continues to be known as the gate control theory of pain (Figure 11.1). This has undergone a number of subsequent modifications, but the overall premise of the theory is generally accepted and provides a workable explanation for this complex phenomenon that marries mechanistic physiological explanations with myriad individual variables. It can be broken down into four key segments: peripheral sensitisation, spinal modulation, central modulation and conscious recognition. Together these are called nociception (Parsons and Preece 2010).

Peripheral Sensitisation

- At the point of trauma/injury the body's initial response is to initiate a chemical reaction known as an 'inflammatory response.'
- Once this reaches a critical threshold it activates a chain of nerve impulse reactions that propel the message towards the central body systems.
- Two key types of nerve fibres are specifically responsible for the transmission of pain messages: A-delta fibres and C fibres.
- A-delta fibres transmit 'fast' messages commonly associated with acute, sharp stabbing pain and reflex responses, and are present in large quantities in the somatic areas of the body.
- C fibres transmit 'slow' messages and are present in both the somatic areas of the body and the viscera, and are commonly associated with slower throbbing pain sensation and chronic pain conditions.
- A third peripheral nerve fibre, A-beta, is not involved in the transmission of pain but does play a role in moderating the pain experience.
- A-delta and C fibres are commonly referred to as nociceptors and they transmit noxious messages.

Orthopaedic and Trauma Nursing: An Evidence-based Approach to Musculoskeletal Care, Second Edition. Edited by Sonya Clarke and Mary Drozd.
© 2023 John Wiley & Sons Ltd. Published 2023 by John Wiley & Sons Ltd.

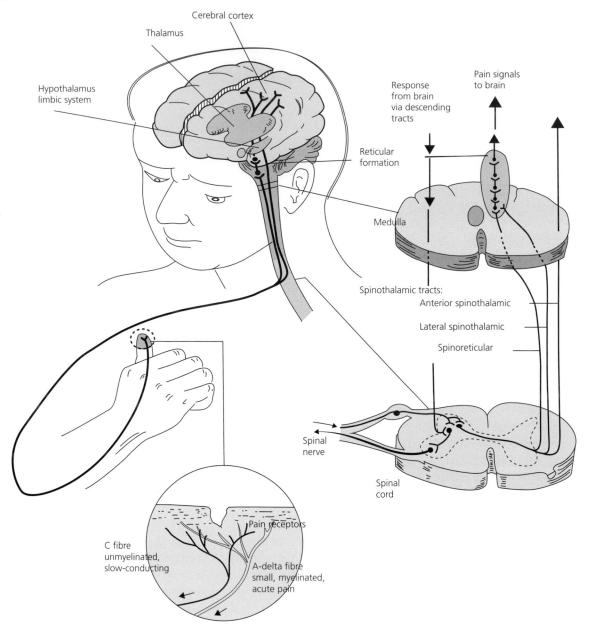

Figure 11.1 Gate control theory of pain.

Spinal Modulation

- Once messages from the peripheral nerves reach the spinal column they enter an area of the dorsal horn known as the substantia gelatinosa.
- Impulses cross over in the spinal tract and are sent upwards to the hypothalamus in the brain.
- Impulses may be modified on entry into the substantia gelatinosa and this can impact on the amount of pain experienced.
- Modification at this stage was initially hypothesised as a 'gate' similar to a garden gate which, when open, allows

unimpeded entry for nerve impulses to transmit messages upwards through the spinal tract. If closed, however, the gate prevents onward transmission and results in a lack of conscious awareness of pain.

- Melzack and Wall (1965) hypothesised that the gate could be closed by activating A-beta fibres to transmit non-noxious messages, which would result in a bottleneck through the gate that would prevent messages from the A-delta and C fibres getting through, e.g. rubbing your knee after banging it.
- They further hypothesised that the gate could also be closed by descending messages from the central nervous

system, e.g. reassurance, attribution and production of chemical modulators such as endogenous opioids.

Central Modulation

- Once nerve impulses reach the brain, they enter the hypothalamus, where C fibre impulses terminate.
- Impulses from A-delta fibres continue to be relayed to the higher centres of the brain and enter all areas of the brain matrix.
- Consciousness of pain is only gained once impulses have reached the brain and any intervention that prevents the onward and upward transmission of pain will ensure lack of awareness, e.g., spinal and epidural analgesia.

Conscious Recognition

- Only once an individual has become conscious of a painful sensation can recognition occur.
- Recognition is crucial in modulating the pain experience, as at this stage the individual will not only identify that they have pain, but place some form of value on it which will significantly affect their interpretation and behaviour.
- Acute pain (associated with trauma and orthopaedic surgery) may mean the pain is associated with a high anxiety or a highly emotional situation such as fear of death, making an individual highly vigilant about their pain, interpreting any pain sensations as severe and highly significant.
- Alternatively, pain could equally be interpreted as non-threatening and this may allow an individual to minimise the experience and treat symptoms lightly.
- It is hypothesised that this interpretation can lead to direct physiological modulation of pain impulses through changes to the inflammatory chemicals present in both the brain and the spinal tract (Parsons and Preece 2010).

The key learning points from the gate control theory which all healthcare workers should be aware of are the following:

1) Pain is highly individual.
2) There is no direct link between amount of tissue damage and amount of pain experienced.
3) Pain is the result of a combination of physiological, emotional and psychological factors.
4) The conscious experience of pain can be modulated at a number of points in the process.
5) Many physiological processes are still unproven, with many exact mechanisms unknown.

Although the gate control theory works relatively well to explain acute pain, the physiological processes underlying chronic pain are still subject to much debate.

Physiological Effects of Acute Pain

Aside from the actual process of nociception, acute pain also provokes a series of well-evidenced physiological responses known as the 'stress response.' This is generally considered a means by which the body can minimise or prevent further damage and is activated by sympathetic nervous activity. Prolonged stress such as that caused by unrelieved acute pain can result in a number of harmful effects across all major body systems (Table 11.1). It is especially important to recognise the effects of undertreated acute pain in the trauma patient, as many of the symptoms can also be caused by a range of other factors which may also be affecting the patient, e.g. hypovolaemia. Although action may be taken to correct one element, undertreated pain can reduce the effectiveness of any interventions.

Types of Pain

Acute pain is commonly associated with traumatic injury and orthopaedic surgery. It can be defined as pain of sudden specific onset of limited duration and is identified as having a number of key features:

- incident-specific
- serves a function
- objective clinical signs
- commonly associated with trauma

Table 11.1 Harmful effects of unrelieved pain

Body system	Harmful effect
Cardiovascular	Raised blood pressure and heart rate
Respiratory	Splinting: small tidal volumes, high inspiration and expiration pressures and decreased vital capacity, hypoxemia, pneumonia, and confusion
Endocrine	Release of hormones, carbohydrate, protein and fat catabolism, hyperglycaemia and increased inflammatory response
Gastrointestinal	Decrease in gastric emptying and motility, paralytic ileus
Reduced physical activity	Delayed mobilisation and increased inpatient stays

- of known duration
- responsive to a range of analgesics
- affects only the individual
- limited financial implications.

Acute pain is also commonly regarded as serving as an alarm warning about impending or actual bodily damage, motivation to escape from the cause of pain and to protect an injured area (Parsons and Preece 2010).

In contrast, chronic pain is associated with chronic musculoskeletal conditions and can be defined as pain of long or indeterminate duration which may persist beyond the time of normal healing or without specific causation (Mackintosh and Elson 2008). It can be identified as being:

- not incident-specific
- of uncertain causal factors
- of unknown duration
- of limited functionality
- unresponsive to a range of treatments
- affects a wider social group
- can have severe financial implications
- closely associated with depressive illness.

The clear difference between the two experiences can have a major impact on the individual pain sufferer and their family as well as affecting the central modulation of the pain experience (Mackintosh and Elson 2008). It is also important to note that acute and chronic pain do not necessarily occur in isolation from each other. Patients with chronic pain conditions can also suffer from acute pain episodes (e.g. hip fracture in a patient with osteoarthritis) and poorly treated acute pain is now a well-recognised precursor of chronic pain, with 25–60% of trauma patients reporting persistent injury-related pain 6–12 months after their trauma (Clay et al. 2010; Friedman et al. 2020).

Pain is also commonly classified into two major types (Parsons and Preece 2010):

1) Nociceptive pain: pain as a direct result of injury to somatic substances, e.g. skin, bone, muscle and connective tissues, and as a direct result of injury to the viscera, e.g. gastrointestinal obstruction, pancreatitis.
2) Neuropathic pain: pain as a direct result of damage to the sensory or peripheral nervous system; this can be centrally generated, i.e. sympathetically maintained pains (SMPs), or peripherally generated, e.g. nerve root compression.

These two types of pain do not occur in isolation and it is common for patients to experience both types of pain from the same trauma, e.g. both somatic and nerve damage from a compound fracture.

This means the orthopaedic/trauma practitioner will encounter patients experiencing a wide range of pain symptoms and reacting to these in highly variable and unpredictable ways. This places great importance on the individual assessment of pain to ensure treatment is both appropriate and effective.

Pain Assessment

The individual and highly variable nature of pain makes pain assessment an essential element of good-quality care. Without it the treatment and management of pain are likely to be ineffective. A large body of evidence continues to suggest that pain assessment is poorly and infrequently carried out. Reasons for the failure to adequately assess patients' pain are many and varied, including lack of knowledge of why or how to assess pain, pain assessment as a low priority, failure to believe patients' self-reports of pain and failure of patients to report pain (Gillaspie 2010).

Knowledge of how to assess pain is fundamental. Accurate assessment can provide many indicators that aid diagnosis of both the condition and the pain, and facilitate appropriate and effective treatment. Guidelines for the management of hip fractures and both primary and secondary chronic pain and trauma (NICE 2016, 2017, 2021) state that its vital to offer person-centred pain assessment followed immediately by offering analgesia to all patients with acute pain regardless of cognitive state, whilst working in a collaborative manner.

Nine key areas should be considered when taking a pain history (Australian and New Zealand College of Anaesthetists 2005):

1) site of pain: where it hurts
2) how the pain started
3) what the pain feels like: its character
4) how much it hurts: its intensity
5) symptoms associated with it: e.g. nausea
6) effect of pain on activities and sleep
7) any current treatment for the pain
8) any past medical history
9) other factors influencing symptoms: beliefs, expectations, coping mechanisms.

These can be used simply as direct questions when in conversation with a patient, but answers provide important clues to treatment and management. This is especially important if trying to differentiate between nociceptive pain and neuropathic pain. The patient's own descriptive words are essential. Nociceptive pain from somatic damage is commonly described as sharp, hot and vice-like, and is easily localised. Nociceptive pain (from viscera) is more likely to be described as dull, cramping or colicky and it is more difficult for the patient to identify the exact spot that hurts. Instead, it is characterised by a more generalised overall tenderness. Neuropathic pain may be described as burning, shooting and stabbing. It can happen spontaneously and can be associated with hypersensitivity of surrounding tissue (hyperalgesia).

Formal Pain Assessment

Although speaking directly to a patient to identify the nature of their pain is both common sense and best practice, because of the long history of failings in this area formalised pain assessment tools are now commonly used and there is clear evidence that they lead to improvements in patients' pain experiences (Parsons and Preece 2010), thus they are recommended in multiple National Institute for Health and Care Excellence (NICE) guidelines (2016, 2017, 2021). These take a variety of forms, measure a range of pain dimensions and have been developed for use across a wide range of different patients from pre-verbal infants to those with advanced dementia. Some of these tools focus on the patient's own self-report, whilst others use behavioural indicators to arrive at algorithmically derived measures of an individual's pain. It is generally accepted that using the patient's self-report of pain is best practice.

The most commonly used pain assessment tools in the acute setting are self-reported uni-dimensional tools, which measure one element of the pain experience, its intensity. These take three forms: descriptive scales, numerical scales and visual analogue scales (VASs) (Box 11.1).

Descriptive scales consist of a range of words which can be used to describe the intensity of pain along a continuum, e.g. from no pain to unbearable pain.

- Numerical scales require a patient to give their pain a rating based on a number, with 1 normally being the least and 10 the highest pain intensity.
- VASs consist of a 10-cm long line with no pain at one end and the worst pain imaginable at the other. The patient is asked to mark or indicate on the line where their pain currently sits.

Another commonly used uni-dimensional tool is the Wong Baker faces rating scale which consists of pictures of stylised faces ranging from smiling to crying, which can be used in children who are able to point to the appropriate picture.

The key advantage for these tools is:

- The speed with which they can be used (particularly for the patient following acute traumatic injury).
- They provide a baseline against which the effect of treatments can be measured.
- Their repeatability over a period of time/treatment.

Box 11.1 Example of Descriptive Scales, Visual Analogue Scale and Numerical Scales

Verbal rating scale

No pain	Mild pain	Moderate pain	Severe pain	Very severe pain

Pain intensity scale

0	No pain
1	Mild pain
2	Discomforting
3	Distressing
4	Horrible
5	Excruciating

Visual analogue scale

No pain _____ Worst pain imaginable
(Note: this line should be exactly 10 cm long when used in practice)

Verbal analogue scale

No pain	Mild pain	Moderate pain	Severe pain	Very severe pain

Numerical rating scale

1	2	3	4	5	6	7	8	9	10

They also suffer from a number of disadvantages (Parsons and Preece 2010):

- Their uni-dimensional nature severely limits their scope.
- Some patients have difficulty in conceptualising their pain as a number or a line on a rating scale.
- Some patients prefer to use their own choice of descriptive words and find others restricting.
- They commonly assume the patient has only one source of pain.
- They are entirely reliant on the patient's self-report.
- They cannot be used with a patient who is unable to communicate.
- They are not liked by some practitioners.

A useful adjunct to the uni-dimensional pain tool is the addition of body pictures, normally showing the front and back of the body. These allow either the patient or the nurse to draw exactly where the pain is, if it moves to indicate where this occurs and, where a patient has multiple sources of pain, to document each individually (Mackintosh and Elson 2008).

To overcome some of these disadvantages more complex multidimensional self-report pain assessment tools have been developed. A commonly used example of a more structured self-report scale is the McGill Pain Questionnaire (Mackintosh 2007), which assesses a range of aspects about the pain experience besides simple intensity. Its effectiveness in the acute situation is limited as it is lengthy to administer and is more commonly associated with chronic pain assessment.

In the UK chronic pain is now frequently assessed using the SF36 scale (available in the public domain from www.rand.org), which seeks to link quality of life with pain intensity and physical functionality, and has tended to replace the Brief Pain Inventory as the assessment tool of choice. Although these tools may be useful for assessing pain in the longer-term orthopaedic patient who has a complex trajectory of interventions and treatments, they are of little value in acute pain situations. They are also limited to use with patients who are able or willing to self-report. Where patients cannot self-report, a range of other tools have been developed focusing on two key groups: preverbal infants, and young children and patients who are cognitively impaired or suffer from dementia. These tools focus on observational data gained from analysis of the patient's behaviour and can include characteristics such as facial grimacing or frowning, agitation, aggression, verbal expressions such as moaning and physiological indicators of increased heart rate and raised blood pressure. The Abbey Dementia Scale is a commonly used example and is freely available from www.dementiacareaustralia.com. The effectiveness of these tools is hard to establish as they are used on a group of patients who are unlikely to provide feedback. Where these have been used to initiate improved pain management regimes for patients with dementia in care homes, there is evidence of decreased agitation and aggression, which is assumed to be evidence of reduced pain (Cunningham 2006).

When considering pain assessment tools, important points can be summarised as follows:

- Regular pain assessment using a tool improves acute pain management.
- Self-reporting of pain is best practice and should be used whenever possible.
- The pain assessment tool used should be appropriate to the individual patient.

Successful Pain Assessment

For pain assessment to be effective in minimising pain, it must focus beyond the use of a pain assessment tool and must be carried out frequently. It must be documented and

unacceptable levels of pain must result in action to alleviate the pain. Pain should be assessed immediately on presentation to the hospital and within 30 minutes of administering initial analgesia, followed by hourly pain assessment until settled and then assessed routinely (NICE 2017). The International Association for the Study of Pain (IASP) (Schugg 2011) has led a campaign since 2000 to have pain assessment included as the fifth vital sign in conjunction with routine temperature, blood pressure, heart rate and respiration rate (TPR), highlighting the importance of regular, routine pain assessment for all patients.

Parsons and Preece (2010) identify four key times when pain assessment should be carried out:

1) initially to gain a base line observation
2) at intervals following an intervention, e.g. 15–30 minutes
3) at regular intervals after a treatment begins
4) following any reported change in the description, location and intensity of the pain.

Parsons and Preece (2010, p. 75) also highlight six golden rules for pain assessment:

1) Always assess pain.
2) Always ask the patient.
3) Always use the same pain assessment tool on the same patient.
4) Always assess pain on movement or deep breathing or coughing and not just at rest.
5) Always document the patient's pain assessment.
6) Always evaluate the intervention using the same pain assessment tool.

All pain assessment that is reliant on the patient's self-report assumes that the patient's self-reports will be believed. As McCaffery (1979) is frequently quoted as saying 'pain is what the person says it is and exists when they say it does.' Unfortunately, a growing body of evidence suggests that, in many situations, practitioners are reluctant to believe patients and frequently use their own subjective judgements of a person's pain in preference to the patient's. Progress in pain assessment and management can only be made if practitioners are prepared to accept the patient's self-report and this is fundamental to all forms of pain assessment. Evidence focused on pain assessment is explored in Boxes 11.2 and 11.3.

Pain Management

Once pain has been assessed it can be managed in a number of ways, and it is now commonly accepted that in most instances a multi-modal or balanced approach towards pain management is likely to be the most effective (Malchow and

Box 11.2   Evidence Digest

Severe acute pain and persistent post-surgical pain in orthopaedic trauma patients: a cohort study (Edgley et al. 2019)

Orthopaedic trauma surgery is strongly associated with severe pain. Edgely et al.'s study aimed to investigate the risk factors associated with acute pain immediately following orthopaedic trauma and longer-term persistent pain. They collected data using a range of different self-report tools: an 11-point numerical rating scale (NRS), the modified Brief Pain Inventory (BPI), the Kessler Psychological distress scale, the WHO Disability Assessment Schedule (WHODAS) and the Pain Catastrophising Scale. Data were collected at three data collection points: within 2 hours prior to surgery, and 72 hours and 3 months after surgery from patients admitted to an Australian trauma unit.

Findings indicated 56% of participants experienced acute pain scored at 6 or more on the NRS preoperatively, whilst 65% reported persistent pain at the 3 months period. Three key risk factors were identified as the same for both severe acute pain and persistent pain 3 months after surgery: being female, having prior post-injury surgery and high pre-operative NRS scores. The authors suggest these findings could be used to target a range of pain management interventions at these specific groups who are at high risk of experiencing longer-term persistent pain.

Box 11.3   Evidence Digest

Communication and assessment of pain in hip fracture patients with dementia: experiences of healthcare professionals at an accident and emergency department in Sweden (Seffo et al. 2020).

It has been reported that around 20–30% of elderly people may suffer from dementia, with around 33% of patients admitted to hospital with a fractured neck of femur likely to suffer from some form of cognitive impairment. The assessment of pain in people with dementia is known to be exceedingly difficult and is compounded by the need for emergency department staff to work swiftly, consequently this qualitative Swedish study aimed to investigate the experience of emergency department staff and how they assessed pain in this group of patients.

Findings identified three categories: arrival at the emergency department, hip track, and handover to ward. Overall results indicated staff found assessment very difficult, exacerbated by communication difficulties, working in a stressful environment and shortage of staff and resources. Although emergency department staff stressed the importance of pain assessment, good communication and teamwork with other staff and relatives, the researchers were forced to conclude that the emergency department was not the best place to offer care for these patients, and additional resources are required to more fully meet current and future needs.

Black 2008; Gessner et al. 2020). A multi-modal approach involves treating the pain using a variety of approaches and methods designed to work on different components of the pain experience. A variety of models of treatment are used in practice, normally focusing on systemic analgesics, local and regional anaesthetics, adjuvant drugs and non-pharmacological management of pain. All of these approaches have some benefit to the management and treatment of acute traumatic and orthopaedic pain (Clark et al. 2009). An example of such benefits is explored in Box 11.4.

Pain Management Interventions at the Site of Trauma

Treatments to minimise pain can be focused at the site of trauma itself and can combine systemic, local and non-pharmacological techniques. Knowledge of pain physiology highlights the importance of the inflammatory response at the point of trauma and any intervention which reduces this response can produce pain relief.

The most common interventions which focus on the site of trauma are non-steroidal anti-inflammatory medications (NSAIDs) as these are particularly useful where there is extensive tissue damage or musculoskeletal pain. They can be taken orally, per rectum, in slow relief preparations or topically. However, NSAIDs are not inherently analgesics and provide pain relief simply through reducing the inflammatory response. This means that except in cases of mild pain, they should normally be used in combination with other forms of pain treatment for their opioid-sparing properties. NSAIDs work by reducing prostaglandin production through the inhibition of the cyclo-oxygenase (COX) system, and newer NSAIDs have been developed which work more selectively, targeting COX-2, which is associated with trauma-related inflammation, although due to gastrointestinal side effects NSAIDs should be used with caution and they should not be used in patients with a history of gastric ulceration. There is also some concern about the effect of NSAIDs on bone healing and this should be taken into account (Gessner et al. 2020).

Box 11.4 Evidence Digest

A comparison study: oral patient controlled analgesia versus traditional delivery of pain medication following orthopaedic procedures (Collins et al. 2020)

This study investigated the use of an oral wifi-operated patient-controlled analgesia (PCA) device that would enable patients to self-administer oral PRN pain medication based on previous evidence that suggests that the use of such a device can result in a significant decrease in pain levels reported by patients using it, as well as a saving in nursing time. This study focused primarily on a comparison of the nursing time taken to administer conventional oral PRN pain medication versus the PCA-administered oral self-medication, including initial pain assessment and reassessment for patients on an inpatient orthopaedic ward.

The findings indicated a significant nursing time saving for patients using the oral PRN PCA device, with each individual episode of analgesic medication administration taking on average 2.06 minutes when compared with 12.7 minutes for conventional oral PRN analgesic medication, an 84% overall time saving. As this also included time for pain assessment and reassessment, the authors argue that time saved through using this device could be better used to improve direct bedside nursing, which could include more thorough pain assessment.

Local anaesthetics can also be extremely useful for reducing pain at the site of trauma as their basic mode of action is to inhibit sodium influx preventing the nerve membrane from depolarising, hence preventing nerve impulses from achieving action potential and halting the onward transmission of pain messages to the dorsal horn of the spine. Infiltration is also a commonly used local anaesthetic method normally used during surgical procedures. A local anaesthetic agent is injected into a wound (surgical or traumatic) during suturing or wound closure and also has a longer-term effect of reducing the total amount of opioid analgesia required (Girdhari and Smith 2006; Gessner et al. 2020). Local anaesthetics can also be used to target specific nerve pathways through direct injection to create specific nerve blocks. A variety of these is available depending on the point of trauma, e.g. femoral nerve block for a hip fracture. They are normally limited to pain from trauma to a limb as blocks in the abdomen, pelvis and trunk are much more difficult to achieve.

Non-pharmacological methods for relieving pain at the site of trauma should also be attempted. These include a range of simple measures which could be utilised by all practitioners (Smith and Colvin 2005):

- positioning
- splinting/supporting
- application of heat or cold
- general comfort measures.

Pain Management Interventions to Block Onwards Transmission

As well as targeting the site of trauma, pain management interventions can also be used to prevent the onward and upward transmission of pain from the dorsal horn of the spine to the hypothalamus.

Although the use of transcutaneous electrical nerve stimulator (TENS) machines are not considered suitable for the relief of acute pain, they can have some efficacy once the initial acute phase has subsided and may be useful for patients with longer-term orthopaedic conditions. TENS machines are hypothesised to work by producing mild non-noxious (non-painful) stimuli in the form of electrical impulses. Electrodes are placed above the level of injury. A mild electrical impulse then stimulates A-beta fibres to activity and these messages enter the dorsal horn of the spinal column either at the same level or above that of the A-delta and C fibres in an attempt to 'crowd' the 'gate' and prevent onwards transmission of pain messages through the spinal tract. The efficacy of TENS machines is debatable, with limited evidence. As they have no known side effects and are considered effective by some patients, they are always worth consideration (Mackintosh and Elson 2008; Mummolo et al. 2020).

More commonly epidural or spinal analgesics are used to block onwards transmission of pain messages. Epidural analgesia produces pain relief by continuous administration of pharmacological agents into the epidural space via an indwelling catheter. For orthopaedic trauma and surgery, the catheter is commonly inserted into the lumbar epidural space, although it can also be inserted into the thoracic space following bowel and abdominal surgery and in patients with multiple rib fractures. Spinal or intrathecal analgesia differs from epidural as it is only used for short-term pain relief and normally as part of a surgical procedure (Gessner et al. 2020).

Commonly used pharmacological agents include local anaesthetics, normally in combination with an opioid analgesic. A range of combinations have been advocated and although it is now recognised that a combination of the two types of drugs achieves the highest efficacy for pain relief, the exact combination is subject to ongoing debate (Smith and Colvin 2005; Gessner et al. 2020).

Epidural and spinal analgesia can produce effective pain relief, but are subject to a number of constraints:

- They are both highly invasive techniques that require a skilled physician.
- They require carefully monitoring as serious side effects can occur.
- The nerve block achieved is non-discriminatory and although it will halt onward transmission of pain it also prevents all messages from reaching the higher senses, which means patients will be unable to mobilise or have reduced mobility, bladder and bowel emptying and need enhanced pressure area care.
- They cannot be used for prolonged periods of time.

Pain Management Interventions to Affect Conscious Recognition

Once pain messages have reached the higher centres of the brain, conscious recognition of the experience takes place. However, this awareness can be modulated through use of systemic analgesics, adjunctive analgesia and non-pharmacological methods.

Systemic Analgesia

Systemic analgesia is commonly used for the treatment of all pain types. This involves the use of paracetamol and opioids and inhalational analgesia such as nitrous oxide.

Paracetamol has limited anti-inflammatory action and should not be confused with aspirin, which is part of the NSAID family. It is useful in mild to moderate pain, can be safely used in combination with NSAIDs and opioids, and is considered to have opioid-sparing properties, i.e. when used in combination a lower opioid dose is required to achieve the same effect.

Opioids are the collective name for a group of drugs with opium-like properties which are similar to the endogenous substances the body is known to produce in response to pain. They have no peripheral action but bind to receptor sites in the central nervous system such as mu, kappa and delta receptors in the mid-brain and spinal cord, where they suppress or inhibit pain transmission. Morphine is the most common and most frequently used opioid analgesia and is the first-line systemic analgesic drug of choice for severe acute pain. It can be administered intravenously (IV), intramuscularly (IM), translingually, transdermally, orally and rectally (PR) as well as administered continuously in the form of an infusion or slow-release preparation or intermittently.

In acute pain, IV administration is the most effective way to produce fast-acting effective pain relief and should be the method of choice. IM administration should be avoided where possible as rate of take-up and action is slower and less certain than IV administration in acute situations. Once acute pain has been stabilised, transdermal or oral administration of morphine is preferred as its efficacy may be more closely monitored.

Individual opioid requirements vary up to a factor of 30, and for safe and effective use the dose should be titrated to the desired effect while minimising side effects. Side effects of systemic analgesia are frequently reported. Doses of paracetamol should be carefully monitored to ensure overdosing does not occur, as this can lead to irreversible liver damage. The use of opioids also engenders a range of side effects from the most commonly reported: constipation and gastric irritation, to sedation, confusion and respiratory depression. The more severe side effects are frequently over-represented and fears and misconceptions about these can lead to under-treatment of pain with opioids. Fear of addiction is also a factor which limits the appropriate and effective use of opioids in acute pain. This has arisen due to misconceptions and misinformation. Addiction is extremely unlikely to occur following use of opioids for acute pain management in opioid-naïve patients. It should only be considered as problematic in acute pain when a patient has had previous opioid use either prescribed or through illegal drug use. In either instance, where a patient has acute pain, it should not be withheld (Smith and Colvin 2005).

However, in chronic pain a number of concerns have now been raised about the use of long-term prescription opioid medication and links with addiction, and where possible long-term prescription opioids should be avoided, and instead a multimodal non-opioid medication regime may be more appropriate (Gessner et al. 2020).

Nitrous oxide is more commonly known as entonox in the UK and consists of a 50:50 mixture of oxygen and nitrous oxide which produces quick-acting, short-lasting pain relief. It is commonly used as a self-administered inhalation and is extremely useful for systemic pain relief when no other options are available, i.e. at an accident site or for relief of short-lasting incident-specific pain following a procedure, e.g. dressing change. It has minimal short-term side effects, but cannot be used as a long-term inhalation as nitrous oxide can lead to the breakdown of red blood cells.

Adjuvant analgesics may also have a place in the management of traumatic and orthopaedic pain, although their use is more commonly limited to patients with longer-term or chronic pain conditions thought to derive from underlying neuropathic damage. The exact mode of action of these drugs is not fully known and continues to be subject to extensive research, but they are well recognised as having an important effect in reducing the levels of pain reported by patients with neuropathic damage (Parsons and Preece 2010; Gessner et al. 2020). The two most common drug groups used are antiepileptic drugs and tricyclic antidepressants.

Carbamazapine is the most common of the antiepileptic drugs and has been used for the treatment of phantom limb pain. Amitriptyline has a long history of use in chronic pain, although it has now been superseded by a new generation of trycyclics, most notably gabapentin and pregabalin. Clinical guidelines for the use of these drugs are available from NICE (2021).

Both these groups of adjuvant drugs can take up to 2 weeks to have any noticeable effect on reducing pain, which means they are not suitable for the treatment of acute pain, but where neuropathic pain is suspected treatment should be initiated as soon as possible to allow for this delayed onset.

When considering the use of pharmacological preparations for pain management the relative efficacy of different drugs should also be considered (Table 11.2). This is especially important when amending prescriptions for patients who may have an existing analgesia regime (e.g. undergoing arthroplasty for osteoarthritis) or who require adjustment to gain optimum pain relief.

When considering pain management, the main points can be summarised as follows:

1) A multimodal or balanced approach will always produce the most effective pain relief.
2) This can be achieved by using management approaches that focus on managing pain, peripherally at the site of trauma, interfering with the transmission of pain and altering conscious perception of pain.

Table 11.2 Relative efficacy of commonly used analgesics

Drug	Number needed to treat
Paracetamol 1 g	4.6
Paracetamol 1 g + codeine 60 mg	2.2
Dihydrocedine 30 mg	10.0
Tramadol 100 mg	4.8
Diclofenac 50 mg	2.3
Ibuprofen 400 mg	2.4
Morphine 10 mg (IM)	2.9

Source: Adapted from Smith and Colvin 2005, p. 4.

3) Where pain management is suboptimal this is nearly always due to poor pain management practices and produces unnecessary suffering.

Summary

Pain assessment and management in orthopaedic and trauma patients adheres to the same principles regardless of the underlying condition. The varied nature of pain experienced by these patients ensures that all nurses involved in their care must be familiar with best practice across the full range of pain that an individual can experience. The management of pain is a humanistic imperative and poorly managed pain exposes patients to unnecessary suffering and is a symptom of poor practice, rather than a necessary consequence of physical trauma. Nurses should ensure that their practice reflects the current principles of best practice and that pain assessment and management for all patients is at optimum levels.

Further Reading

NICE (2020). *Perioperative care in adults.* NG180. National Institute for Health and Care Excellence, London. pp. 25–29. www.nice.org.uk/guidance/ng180/resources/perioperative-care-in-adults-pdf-66142014963397.

Parsons, G. and Preece, W. (2010). *Principles and Practice of Managing Pain.* McGraw Hill, Maidenhead: A Guide for Nurses and Allied Health Professionals.

References

Australian and New Zealand College of Anaesthetists and Faculty of Pain Medicine (2005). *Acute Pain Management: Scientific Evidence.* Canberra: National Health and Research Council.

Beecher, H.K. (1959). *Management of Subjective Responses.* New York: Oxford University Press.

Berben, S.A.A., Tineke, H.J.M., Meijs, R.T.M. et al. (2008). Pain prevalence and pain relief in trauma patients in the accident and emergency department. *Injury* 39: 578–585.

Berben, S.A.A., Schoonhoven, L., Tineke, H.J.M. et al. (2011). Prevalence and relief of pain in trauma patients in emergency medical services. *Clin. J. Pain.* 27 (7): 587–592.

Clark, M.E., Scholten, J.D., Walker, R.L., and Gironda, R.J. (2009). Assessment and treatment of pain associated with combat related polytrauma. *Pain Med.* 10 (3): 456–469.

Clay, F.J., Newstead, S.V., Watson, W.L. et al. (2010). Biopsychosocial determinants of persistent pain 6 months after non-life threatening acute orthopaedic trauma. *J. Pain* 11 (5): 420–430.

Collins, L., Cata, D.M., and Conely, N.S. (2020). A comparison study—oral patient controlled analgesia versus traditional delivery of pain medication following orthopaedic procedures. *Orthopaed. Nurs.* 39: 5.

Cunningham, C. (2006). Managing pain in patients with dementia in hospital. *Nursing Standard* 20 (46): 54–58.

Edgley, C., Hogg, M., De Silva, A. et al. (2019). Severe acute pain and persistent post-surgical pain in orthopaedic trauma patients: a cohort study. *British Journal of Anaesthesia* 123 (3): 350–359.

Friedman, B.W., Abril, L., Naeem, F. et al. (2020). Predicting the transition to chronic pain 6 months after an emergancy department visit for acute pain: a prospective cohort study. *J. Emerg. Med.* 59 (6): 805–811.

Gessner, D.M., Horna, J.L., and Lowenberg, D.W. (2020). Pain management in the orthopaedic trauma patient: non-opioid solutions. *Injury Int. J. Care. Injur.* S28–S36.

Gillaspie, M. (2010). Better pain management after total joint replacement surgery. A quality improvement approach. *Orthopaed. Nurs.* 29 (1): 20–24.

Girdhari, S. and Smith, S.K. (2006). Assisting older adults with orthopaedic outpatient acute pain management. *Orthopaed. Nurs.* 25 (3): 188–195.

Mackintosh, C. (2007). Assessment and management of patients with post-operative pain. *Nursing Standard* 22 (5): 49–55.

Mackintosh, C. and Elson, S. (2008). Chronic pain: clinical features, assessment and treatment. *Nursing Standard* 23 (5): 48–56.

Malchow, R.J. and Black, I.H. (2008). The evolution of pain management in the critically ill trauma patient: emerging concepts from the global war on terrorism. *Critic. Care Med.* 36 (7 suppl): S346–S357.

McCaffery, M. (1979). *Nursing Management of the Patient with Pain*, 2e. Philadelphia: Lippincott.

Melzack, R. and Wall, P.D. (1965). Pain mechanisms, a new theory. *Science* 150: 971–979.

Mummolo, S., Nota, A., Tecco, S. et al. (2020). Ultra-low-frequency transcutaneous electric nerve stimulation (ULF-TENS) in subjects with craniofacial pain: a retrospective study. *J. Craniomand. Sleep Pract.* 38 (6): 396–401.

NICE (2011). (Updated 2017) *Hip Fracture: The Management of Hip Fracture in Adults*. NCG 124. National Institute for Health and Care Excellence, London.

NICE (2016). *Major Trauma: Assessment and Initial Management. NG39*. London: National Institute for Health and Care Excellence.

NICE (2017) *Hip Fracture: Management.* National Institute for Health and Care Excellence, London.

NICE (2021). *Chronic pain (primary and secondary) in over 16s: assessment of all chronic pain and management of chronic primary pain*. NG 193. National Institute for Health and Care Excellence, London. www.nice.org.uk/guidance/ng193/resources/chronic-pain-primary-and-secondary-in-over-16s-assessment-of-all-chronic-pain-and-management-of-chronic-primary-pain-pdf-66142080468421.

Parsons, G. and Preece, W. (2010). *Principles and Practice of Managing Pain*. McGraw Hill, Maidenhead: A Guide for Nurses and Allied Health Professionals.

Schugg, S.A. (2011). 2011 – the global year against acute pain (editorial). *Anaesth. Intens. Care.* 39 (1): 11–14.

Seffo, N., Senorski, E.H., Westin, O. et al. (2020). Communication and assessment of pain in hip fracture patients with dementia - experiences of healthcare professionals at an accident and emergency department in Sweden. *Medicinski. Glasnik.* 17 (1): 224–233.

Smith, C.M. and Colvin, J.R. (2005). Control of acute pain in postoperative and post traumatic situations. *Anaesth. Intens. Care.* 6 (1): 2–6.

Online Resources

British Pain Society, http://www.britishpainsociety.org.

International Association for the Study of Pain, http://www. http://iasp-pain.org.

12

Wound Management, Tissue Viability and Infection

Jeannie Donnelly and Alison Collins

Tissue Viability Team, Belfast Health and Social Care Trust, Belfast, UK

Introduction

This chapter provides an outline of the knowledge and skills required by practitioners caring for patients with the main types of acute and chronic wounds in the field of trauma and orthopaedics. Recommendations for practice will often be pragmatic as empirical research is, in many instances, lacking. The chapter is divided into two sections. The first section focuses on the nursing management of wounds. This includes consideration of both surgical and traumatic wounds, an overview of the wound-healing process and discussion of the current thinking with regards to dressing techniques. The second section considers issues relating to the prevention and management of pressure ulceration.

Whilst all wound types move through the three main stages of wound healing (inflammation, proliferation and contraction), speed and efficiency of healing is affected by a range of local and systemic factors. Key factors (according to wound type) will be highlighted. These must not, however, be viewed as mutually exclusive as all factors, e.g. smoking and infection, affect all wound types.

Wound Management

Surgical Wounds

A simple surgical wound is a healthy and uncomplicated break in the continuity of the skin resulting from surgery. It is expected to follow a rapid and predictable pathway towards healing with minimal tissue loss, scarring and loss of function. Surgeons take great care to protect as much tissue as possible from injury, carefully considering the placement of the incision, managing blood loss (to prevent haemorrhage and haematoma) and considering the best way to bring each layer of tissue (muscle, fascia, subcutaneous tissue and skin) into approximation through wound closure (Coulthard et al., 2010). Approximation speeds time to healing, reduces scaring and helps prevent infection. The wound is said to heal by primary intention.

Traumatic Wounds

Traumatic wound care is an integral part of the care of the patient following musculoskeletal trauma as soft tissue wounds are often consistent with the rest of the pattern of injury. Such wounds present a number of additional challenges. A compound fracture wound with full thickness tissue loss, for example, requires careful assessment (as there may be damage to nerves, tendons or muscles) and debridement of devitalised tissue. Often the wound cannot be closed immediately due to the risk of or presence of infection or excessive oedema. Closing very oedematous tissue will result in a taut wound leading to stress, which can cause tissue ischaemia (reduced blood flow), particularly at the wound edge, potentially leading to tissue death or wound dehiscence (gaping or bursting open). To prevent this from happening body cavities and deeper structures are sutured closed and the layers of the skin left open to allow for free drainage of foreign material or pus or whilst waiting for swelling to decrease. The patient will normally return to surgery after 3–4 days for a further wound assessment, followed by irrigation and debridement and wound closure if it is safe to do so. This is known as delayed primary closure. The wound is said to heal by tertiary intention (Lorenz and Longaker 2008).

Some wounds cannot be closed using surgical techniques due to one or more of the following reasons: (i) the patient is not well enough to undergo surgery, (ii) the wound is small or superficial, (iii) the wound is heavily contaminated, infected

Orthopaedic and Trauma Nursing: An Evidence-based Approach to Musculoskeletal Care, Second Edition. Edited by Sonya Clarke and Mary Drozd.
© 2023 John Wiley & Sons Ltd. Published 2023 by John Wiley & Sons Ltd.

or chronic or (iv) the wound is deep, with a 'dead space' and lack of subcutaneous tissue. If the skin is left open, it is important to prevent the dead space filling with blood, as haematoma is the perfect medium for bacteria to multiply as it does not have a blood supply to initiate the immune system. Healing is by secondary intention.

The Wound-healing Process

Wound healing is the process by which damaged tissue is replaced and function restored. The wound-healing process is dynamic and can be divided into three overlapping phases: haemostasis/inflammation, proliferation and maturation (remodelling).

During haemostasis, damaged blood vessels constrict and blood leaking from them begins to coagulate. Platelets in the vicinity are 'activated' by collagen fibres in the damaged vessels and clump together, forming a relatively unstable plug. The activated platelets release vasoconstrictors and other chemicals, which stimulate the clotting cascade and attract other platelets to the area. The end result is a clot (platelets intertwined with fibrin).

The goal of the inflammatory phase of wound healing is to limit the amount of tissue damage and prepare the wound for healing by removing unhealthy tissue and foreign matter such as bacteria. White blood cells (basophils, neutrophils and monocytes) play a major role. Basophils release heparin and histamine. Neutrophils and monocytes (converted to macrophages) migrate from the blood vessels and congregate at the site of injury, engulfing and destroying microorganisms. The inflammatory process is a necessary part of healing. Visible signs of the process are redness, heat, swelling, pain, loss of function and increased exudate.

The goal of the proliferation phase is to close the defect as quickly as possible. The wound fills with granulation tissue (unless it is very superficial, in which case it will simply re-epithelialise), contracts down in size and epithelialises. Viable epidermal cells divide and migrate from the wound edges. Migration ceases when the epidermal cells come into contact with each other.

Granulation tissue is a network of collagen fibres, new blood vessels and white blood cells, and peaks between 5 and 9 days post-operatively, presenting as a 'healing ridge' along the margins of the wound (Doughty and Defriese 2007). New blood vessels form by the process of 'angiogenesis'. New capillaries (containing oxygen-rich blood and micronutrients) give the tissue a bright-red granular appearance. Oxygen is important for cellular activity and any condition that impedes oxygenation of the tissues (e.g. smoking, peripheral vascular disease) slows healing and can lead to wound breakdown (Knuutinen et al. 2002). Dark coloured granulation tissue, which bleeds easily, can be indicative of infection, poor perfusion or ischaemia.

Good nutrition (see Chapter 10) is central to successful wound healing. Malnutrition may involve a deficiency or excess (or imbalance) of energy, protein and other nutrients which can be a significant factor in wounds failing to heal or succumbing to infection.

Maturation occurs once the wound has re-epithelialised and strengthens the scar tissue. Weak type III collagen fibres (produced by fibroblasts during granulation) are changed into or replaced by strong type I collagen. As the wound has essentially healed there is a downturn in cellular activity and the need for extra oxygen and nutrients decreases.

In a simple surgical wound, the inflammatory phase is usually complete within 36–48 hours and the proliferative phase is complete in 28 days. Maturation can take around 100 days. A surgical wound is usually 'sealed' within 48 hours and will be dry (no bleeding or exudate) and can be exposed. The timeframe is variable and may be extended depending on the complexity of the surgery, local wound conditions and the health of the patient. A patient whose wound continues to produce a high amount of exudate 5 days post-operatively or who is complaining of increasing pain may have a surgical site infection (SSI). Wounds which are open or continue to 'weep' (exude) will need to be carefully monitored and dressed.

The phases of wound healing are dynamic; wounds may move forwards or backwards through each phase depending on the health of the patient. For example, a wound which was healing well (showing signs of granulation) but becomes infected will move back into the inflammatory stage. A chronic wound is often described as a wound which is 'stuck' in the inflammatory or proliferative phase of wound healing.

Factors Affecting Wound Healing

Factors affecting wound healing are often referred to as intrinsic (internal, specific to the individual) or extrinsic (external, applied to the individual). Any systemic condition that results in poor perfusion, a lack of essential micronutrients, an impaired ability to fight infection or tissue wasting/destruction can delay wound healing (Table 12.1).

To aid wound healing, the general health and wellbeing of the patient must be optimised. This is achieved by creating a care plan that takes into account relevant health and psychosocial issues. Nurses, as 'gatekeepers' of care, have a responsibility to use their knowledge of the patient's needs and refer to other practitioners when help is needed.

Table 12.1 Factors and conditions affecting wound healing.

Factor	Relevant conditions
Poor perfusion	• Respiratory and cardiovascular disorders • Arthrosclerosis, cardiovascular disorders such as cerebral vascular disease, angina and peripheral vascular disease • Diabetes: elevated blood glucose stiffens arteries and causes narrowing of the blood vessels, leading to decreased blood flow • Smoking (nicotine): causes blood vessels to constrict • Sepsis: leads to microvascular and macrovascular thrombosis • Medications: have a variety of effects on circulation • Poor social circumstances, especially homelessness, heat poverty • Stress: excess levels of noradrenaline are released, leading to vasoconstriction
Micronutrient deficiency	• Malabsorption disorders, e.g. ulcerative colitis • Inability to eat or drink effectively, e.g. swallowing difficulties • Poor diet due to poverty or poor dietary choices • Alcoholism • Malignancy/cancer, the body is in a state of catabolism, the patient may be malnourished (nausea and vomiting)
Immunodeficiency/ suppression	• Neonate • Advanced age • Rheumatoid arthritis • HIV, AIDS • Stress • Cushing's syndrome • Malignancy (myeloma, leukaemia, sarcoma etc.) • Diabetes: a high glucose level causes the immune cells to function ineffectively • Medications, e.g. cytotoxic drugs, corticosteroids
Tissue wasting/ destruction	• Malignancy • Diabetes: neuropathy leads to inflammation and degeneration of peripheral nerves, which may interfere with circulation • Multiple sclerosis, spinal injury • Some conditions, such as a stroke or spinal injury, may result in the patient being unable to reposition themselves, leading to pressure damage • Genetic disorders • Physical abuse, neglect or self-harm • Certain medicaments, e.g. nicorandil

Extrinsic factors that affect healing can be mechanical (pressure, shear, friction), chemical (wound exudate, cleansing solutions etc.) or thermal (heat, cold, radiation). Some of these factors (such as a moist wound environment) can aid healing, whilst others can delay healing.

Moist Wound Healing

Surgical wound dressings are applied to stem bleeding, absorb exudate and provide protection but there is constant debate about which dressing product best achieves such functions. Dry dressings may adhere to the wound (as fibres integrate into the clot matrix), causing pain and trauma on removal. Woven dressings are commonly used with the objective of absorbing wound moisture. It is claimed, however, that moist wounds heal more quickly than those left to dry out under textile-based dressings because epithelialisation is retarded by the formation of a dry scab (Winter 1962). A dressing that facilitates an optimal level of wound moisture, on the other hand, promotes wound healing (Harle et al. 2005). Orthopaedic wound dressings should therefore have the attributes of the ideal dressing (Box 12.1) in addition to being absorbent and protective. The ability of a wound dressing to stretch with movement to avoid restricting limb movement and accommodate post-operative oedema is also

---

Box 12.1   The Properties of an Ideal Dressing (Cosker et al. 2005)

Reproduced with permission from MA Healthcare Limited

- Permeability: to control the rate of air exposure and the gaseous exchange between the wound and the outside environment
- The ability to remain in situ during bathing
- Transparency: to allow the monitoring of any fluid accumulation and other complications
- Low adherence: to facilitate removal from susceptible thin skin
- The ability to act as a complete barrier to bacteria and water, but not to moisture vapour

---

Box 12.2   Evidence Digest: Wound Moisture Balance

Several studies examine the concept of moisture balance, facilitating an arthroplasty wound free of complications (Bhattacharyya et al. 2005; Cosker et al. 2005; Harle et al. 2005; Abuzakuk et al. 2006; Ravenscroft et al. 2006). According to Cosker et al. (2005) 'fabric plus film' island dressings perform better (in terms of less blistering) compared to adhesive central pad dressings, film dressings and traditional wound pads and tape alone. Bhattacharyya et al. (2005) noted a lower incidence of both postoperative blistering ($P = 0.24$) and superficial inflammation of surrounding skin ($P < 0.001$) when a 'fabric plus film' island dressing was used versus an adhesive central pad dressing post arthroscopy of the knee. This reduction in blister formation (whilst not statistically significant) is arguably clinically significant, given the association of peri-wound skin trauma with superficial wound infection (Harle et al. 2005; Polatsch et al. 2004) and the fact that minor wound sepsis potentially increases the risk of deep wound sepsis (Gaine et al. 2000). The use of a vapour-permeable film to retain a hydrofibre dressing also appears to offer clinical advantages (fewer skin injuries such as blistering and epidermal stripping) when compared with a conventional wound pad and tape (Harle et al. 2005) or adhesive central pad dressing (Abuzakuk et al. 2006; Ravenscroft et al. 2006).

---

important, especially after hip and knee arthroplasty, which requires a degree of force on behalf of the surgeon to position the prosthesis firmly, thereby resulting in post-operative bruising and swelling around the joint (Jester et al. 2000).

Permeability and Transparency

The permeability of a dressing refers to its ability to permit gaseous exchange (including water vapour) between the wound and the external environment. Transparent films allow wound exudate and peri-wound skin to be inspected without dressing removal, minimising the risk of accidental wound contamination and trauma. Exudate, however, can pool under film dressings and cause maceration of the wound and surrounding skin (Cutting and White 2002) and peri-wound blister formation (Harle et al., 2005). Absorbent central pad dressings with an adhesive border are quicker and easier to apply than traditional dressing pads, but offer no additional advantages in terms of permeability. Vapour-permeable film dressings transmit moisture away from the wound bed to varying degrees, but should not be applied as the primary dressing at sites of profuse drainage since absorbency is limited. 'Film plus fabric' dressings combine transpiration and absorbency, helping to prevent accumulation of fluid (Aindow and Butcher 2005). The moist and relatively hypoxic environment produced by semi-occlusive and occlusive dressings accelerates angiogenesis and promotes tissue repair (Holm et al. 1998). See Box 12.2 for further discussion of wound moisture balance.

Ability to Act as a Bacterial Barrier

Traditional absorbent dressings provide limited protection against microbial ingress and may shed fibres into the wound, causing a focal point for infection (Jones 2006). Microbes pass through the dressing rapidly when it is damp and are dispersed into the environment on dressing removal, increasing the risk of cross-infection (Cooper and Lawrence 1996). Vapour-permeable films, incorporated into a fabric-island dressing or used as a retention dressing, have the advantage of being impermeable to bacteria (Pudner 2001). Hydrocolloids protect the wound from exogenous bacteria and have the advantage of lowering the pH of wounds to slightly acidic, inhibiting the growth of microbes (Bryan 2004). Hydrofibre dressings protect the wound from bacterial invasion by absorbing and retaining large amounts of exudate (including microbes) (Clarke et al. 2009), reducing the need to change the dressing (Ravenscroft et al. 2006) and lessening dispersal of microbes on dressing removal (White 2001).

Bathing and Showering

There is a strong correlation between patient satisfaction with the post-operative dressing and ability to perform their usual personal hygiene routine (Bhattacharyya et al. 2005). There is arguably no need to apply any dressing to a surgical wound after the early post-operative period since a natural bacteria-proof barrier (fibrin seal) is quickly re-established. Patient hygiene is facilitated and worry about the wound reduced by use of a vapour-permeable film until the wound is sealed with fibrin and drainage has ceased. Environmental moisture has a minimal effect on waterproof dressings providing it does not migrate under the surface. For this reason, showering is preferable to bathing.

Ease of Removal

Patients may experience pain where traditional gauze dressings adhere to the wound bed. Paraffin tulle gras also has a tendency to dry out and may result in post-operative wound trauma (Voegeli 2008). According to Gupta et al. (2002), spirit-soaked gauze lifts off the wound as it dries. However, spirit-soaked gauze is likely to cause pain on contact with broken skin due to the astringent properties of alcohol-based preparations. Alcohol solutions delay wound healing and usage should be restricted to prophylactic skin disinfection (Morgan 2004). Ravenscroft et al. (2006) found removal of hydrofibre and film combined to be less painful than an adhesive fabric dressing.

Wounds can exhibit a wide combination of different characteristics, e.g. deep tissues may be exposed or the wound may be malodourous with a high or low exudate. There is no one product that is 'smart' enough to manage all of these. Characteristics change as wounds move through the healing continuum and practitioners must use their assessment to set realistic treatment objectives and make evidence-based dressing choices.

Wound Assessment

The first part of a wound assessment is to take a history of all factors leading to the cause of the wound. This information will provide clues to the underlying aetiology, the amount and type of tissue damage as well as potential complications such as infection. The five questions listed in Table 12.2 will help in this process. The second part of the assessment is to carefully observe the wound and the surrounding tissues to guide care and the choice of dressing. The results of the assessment should be recorded on a wound observation chart.

Table 12.2 Wound history questions for wound assessment.

Question	Rationale
Why is it there?	• Trauma due to a fall, surgery etc. – Following trauma, determine the type and amount of tissue damage by asking questions about the characteristics of the mechanism involved • When the aetiology is unclear further investigations should determine the cause, e.g. a tissue biopsy
Where is the wound?	• The position may suggest aetiology, e.g. a wound over a bony prominence may be linked to pressure damage • Wounds next to the anus may be at risk of faecal contamination • Wounds on the feet will raise issues around mobility • Wounds in awkward areas may be more difficult to dress, e.g. perineal area, joints, head • Accurate record keeping is essential, particularly if the patient has a number of wounds
When did it appear?	• The greater the time between wounding and good wound care, the greater the risk of infection, especially for traumatic wounds • To determine if the wound has become chronic or not progressing to healing
Who is looking after the patient/ client and their wound?	• It is important to communicate with practitioners, e.g. surgeons, district nurses, carers, who have been involved in the patient's care, particularly if the patient is a poor historian • They will provide important additional information about the patient's health and social status • Assess whether the patient's treatment regime is effective and identify allergies
What would the patient/client like to achieve?	• This is very important in establishing a realistic treatment objective, e.g. the patient may state that they want the wound healed in time for a special event. This may not be achievable and requires clarification so that the patient has time to accept the reality of their situation • This can help clarify the wound characteristic that is causing the patient the most distress, e.g. malodour, pain or exudate

Wound Measurement

The length, width and depth of the wound should be recorded as accurately as possible using a disposable tape measure (which must not touch the wound). The length and width of the wound should be measured using the body axes as a reference point (as opposed to the longest and shortest part of the wound). Dimensions can change rapidly and over time measurements can become confused. In a wound where depth is easily visualised, a sterile probe can be used to measure the distance from the bottom of the wound to the surface of the skin. Some wounds consist of extensive cavities or extremely narrow sinuses and the skin can be undermined, leading to exposure of fragile structures (blood vessels, nerves, organs). Wounds should not be probed unnecessarily as these fragile structures can be easily damaged. A surgeon or a tissue viability nurse may be able to map out the wound to assess the direction/depth of cavities. The dimensions of a wound which contains necrosis or slough will increase as 'dead' tissue is autolysed.

Wound Bed

The wound bed tends to be described by the colour of tissue observed (black/brown, yellow, red, and pink) (Table 12.3), indicating underlying problems such as ischaemia or tendon exposure. For example, if hard black necrosis is noted on the heel (Figure 12.1) it would be wise to assess the blood supply to the lower limb before wound debridement. If there is an impaired blood supply, tissue cannot regenerate or mount an effective host response to infection. Tendons, on the other hand, need to be kept moist to prevent desiccation and loss of function. If there is an impaired blood supply the practitioner should keep the wound dry and seek specialist help. As wounds can contain a mixture of tissues it can be difficult to accurately quantify what can be seen. Clinical judgement can be used to make a subjective calculation of each tissue type. This is then expressed as a percentage, e.g. 20% black, 50% yellow, 30% red. During dressing changes the percentages are recalculated and compared to the previous assessment. Changes help to determine improvement or deterioration. Photographs can also be useful in charting the progress of extensive wounds.

The practitioner must have an understanding of the evidence-based rationale behind dressing selection to enable setting realistic wound management objectives. Dressing products range from those that actively donate moisture to a wound (hydrogels) to those that absorb or contain moisture. Some are impregnated with

Table 12.3 Wound bed assessment: tissue colour.

Colour	Definition	Differential rationale
Black	Tissue is necrotic (dead). There is no blood supply. Hard black necrosis is called eschar.	Dressings and ointments which contain silver can stain the tissues a black colour but staining is superficial and temporary.
Yellow	This tissue is sloughy. Slough is made up of dead cells and wound debris.	Tendons, fascia, bone and fat can also appear yellow.
Red	This tissue is healthy. Granulating tissue is comprised of collagen fibres (type III) and new blood vessels. The new capillaries give the tissue its bright-red colour and slightly uneven 'bumpy' texture. Dark-red granulation tissue is a sign of poor perfusion or infection (Figure 12.2).	Muscles, organs (such as bowel) and dermis will also be red. Sometimes tissue can overgranulate, often referred to as 'proud flesh', as it sits above the level of the skin. It is often seen around trache and peg tube sites.
Pink	This tissue is healthy and is re-epithelialising.	The skin surrounding a wound can become very wet and macerated due to excess exudate. This skin can appear pinkish/white in colour.

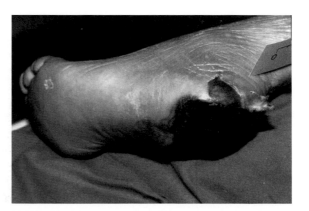

Figure 12.1 Heel pressure ulcer with necrosis and hard, black eschar.

antimicrobial agents which should not be used unless there are clinical signs of infection or the patient is immunocompromised and there is a very high risk of infection. It is also important that general advice and support is given to the patient with respect to promoting healing and preventing infection (Figure 12.2).

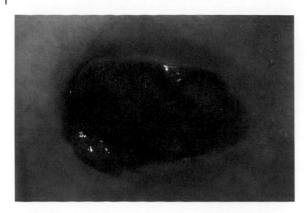

Figure 12.2 Wound containing overgranulation tissue.

Surgical Site Infection

Healthcare-associated infections (HAIs) collectively affect approximately one in 10 hospital patients every year (Department of Health 2006). Such infections are costly complications of heathcare that cause pain and discomfort, complicate and delay recovery, and sometimes lead to death (Srinivasaiah et al. 2007). SSI alone has been reported by National Institute for Clinical Excellence (NICE) (2008) to be responsible for over one-third of perioperative deaths, increased healthcare costs and a significant impact on patient quality of life. Surveillance and prevention of infection are a major focus of healthcare and are seen as a care quality indicator.

Any infection is the outcome of complex interactions between a host, a pathogen and the environment (European Wound Management Association 2005), and is defined as:

> The deposition of organisms in tissues and their subsequent growth and multiplication along with an associated tissue reaction.
>
> *(Ayliffe et al. 2001)*

Bacteria cannot penetrate intact skin, but can enter easily if the skin is damaged or an incision is made such as in the case of a surgical or traumatic wound. Infection is a painful and distressing complication that impairs the process of wound healing and is instrumental in delayed recovery. If it is allowed to progress it can lead to death through the spread of infection, septicaemia and organ failure.

The colonisation of any wound with microorganisms is unavoidable. The human body is host to a large number of bacteria and fungi that are part of the normal homeostatic mechanisms and are essential to many physiological processes. Harmful pathogenic organisms, however,

are ever-present on the human body, in the atmosphere and in the environment. Ordinarily, the human immune system prevents these potential pathogens from entering the human body and causing harm. Organisms that are normally relatively harmless can become problematic when conventional preventive mechanisms fail.

In the orthopaedic patient the major risk from the spread of infection is osteomyelitis (infection of bone tissue), which is extremely difficult to eradicate. Osteomyelitis is also associated with biofilms attached to implanted devices or haematogenous seeding (spread of bacteria from the bloodstream to implant sites) (Trampuz and Zimmerli 2006) and is a much-feared complication of bone injury and surgery as the condition often becomes chronic and prevents bone from healing, leading to long-term pain and disability. The prevention of infections, including SSI, which may lead to osteomyelitis is particularly central to the care of all orthopaedic patients.

SSI is defined as:

> Infection occurring up to 30 days after surgery (or up to one year after surgery in patients receiving implants and affecting the incision or deep tissue at the operation site.
>
> *(Owens and Stoessal 2008)*

An estimated average of 2–5% of surgical patients develop SSI during their recovery and up to a year following orthopaedic implant surgery (NICE 2008). Most SSIs are caused by skin-derived bacteria, primarily *Staphylococcus aureus* (Dohmen 2008). Studies of SSI in orthopaedic patients report the incidence of serious deep infections associated with SSIs and highlight consequential increases in the length of hospital stay (Coello et al. 2005). For example, deep wound infection occurs in up to 3% of patients following hip fracture repair. Surveillance data focus on high-volume orthopaedic procedures such as arthroplasty and internal fixation of fractures (Morgan et al. 2005). Although rates are dropping each year, SSIs in this group remain a significant problem. In many countries surveillance of SSI rates following orthopaedic surgery for total hip replacement, total knee replacement, hemiarthroplasty and open reduction of long bone fracture is mandatory. Many patients are now discharged from hospital before the surgical wound has healed, so it is likely that the symptoms of SSI may not appear until after discharge from hospital. Following orthopaedic implant surgery, deep SSIs may take up to a year to manifest (Health Protection Agency 2008).

Numerous studies have examined the delayed healing of post-operative incisional orthopaedic wounds. Adogwa et al. (2014) compared the application of single-use negative-pressure wound therapy (sNPWT) to standard care after spinal surgery. Positive outcomes associated with sNPWT included a reduction in SSIs and wound dehiscence.

Furthermore, patients undergoing elective hip and knee arthroplasty and surgery after a hip fracture experienced fewer surgical site complications (SSCs) with sNPWT compared to standard dressings. SSCs include skin necrosis, wound dehiscence, hyperaemia, prolonged hospital stay and the need for surgical re-intervention (Masters et al. 2021; Helito et al. 2020; Karlakki et al. 2016; Nherera et al. 2017).

Sandell (2020) recommends prophylactic application of single-use disposable NPWT for high-risk patient groups undergoing joint arthroplasty.

Preventing SSI

The use of the most recent evidence-based guidelines for preventing HAIs is central to the prevention of SSI. This should focus on local and national guidance (Chapter 9). Specific measures for the prevention of SSI include:

- evidence-based preoperative preparation and perioperative care, including skin preparation and antibiotic prophylaxis
- aseptic non-touch technique when dressing or handing wounds and wound drains
- removing wound drains as soon as possible, preferably within 24 hours of surgery
- keeping wounds covered in the hospital environment and until the proliferation phase of healing is complete (Box 12.3) and tampering with the wound/dressing as little as possible
- ensuring the patient's general health status and tissue perfusion are optimised through good nutrition and hydration
- close post-operative assessment and surveillance of the wound for signs of infection until recovery is complete and immediate medical referral if infection is suspected.

A frequent change of dressings is a potential risk factor for SSI (Leaper 2000) as exogenous bacteria may contaminate the wound during the dressing procedure. The rate of miotic cell division and leucocyte activity (necessary for wound healing and bacterial defence) is increased under wound dressings which facilitate near to core body temperatures (Xia et al. 2000). Frequent cooling associated with changing the dressing should therefore be avoided as a means of reducing the risk of SSI.

Box 12.3   Evidence Digest: Wound Dressings to Prevent Wound SSI

Several studies have examined whether the choice of wound dressing impacts on the incidence of SSI after hip and knee surgery. Cosker et al. (2005) concluded that the incidence of SSI associated with adhesive fabric dressings or film plus fabric dressings was broadly similar. Ravenscroft et al. (2006), however, recorded a higher incidence of dressing failure (defined in part by the development of wound infection) with adhesive fabric dressings compared to hydrofibre and film. A similar trend in SSI reduction was noted when a Jubilee dressing (a primary, central hydro-fibre, overlaid with a thin hydrocolloid) was compared to an adhesive fabric dressing after arthroplasty of the hip and knee (Dillon et al. 2007). A reduction in peri-prosthetic joint infections was reported by Cai et al. (2014) when a post-operative dressing (comprising a hydro-fibre/silver hydro-fibre core and a hydrocolloid top layer) was compared to a standard dressing (sterile gauze and adhesive tape). Additional advantages are associated with this hydro-fibre/hydrocolloid dual component dressing. These include less post-operative skin blistering, a reduced number of dressing changes (Dillon et al. 2007) and increased patient satisfaction (showering permitted due to waterproof properties) (Springer et al. 2013).

Recognising SSI

There are two common approaches to diagnosing infection:

1) Assessment of the clinical symptoms of infection based on observation of the wound and the localised and systemic inflammatory response and generalised systemic patient symptoms.
2) The laboratory analysis of samples taken from the wound used to identify the type and amount of growth of organisms (microbial load) in the wound.

Clinical assessment findings are widely considered to be a reliable approach to identifying infection in most wounds (Serena et al. 2006) (Table 12.4). Damage to tissue causes an inflammatory reaction that is manifested as symptoms which provide potentially useful indicators of infection. There are four 'cardinal' signs of acute inflammation: redness, heat, swelling and pain. An important factor to consider is that, in deep SSIs, redness and heat at the base of the wound cannot be seen and may only manifest as pain. Hence any patient report of

Table 12.4 Signs of surgical site infection which should be considered as part of the clinical assessment.

Sign	Rationale
Wound site/ pain	Pain may reappear after the pain following injury or surgery has subsided. It may also last beyond that which would normally be expected for that injury or surgery.
Exudate	Excessive wound exudate, which does not settle, may be clear serous exudate or a purulent discharge. Discharge may also be dark brown if it arises from infection of a haematoma deep within the surgical site.
Foul odour	Indicates the presence of pathogenic microorganisms.
Wound breakdown	This may become apparent at the time of removal of sutures or clips and can be the result of an infected haematoma, which acts as a barrier to wound healing.
Systemic symptoms	The patient may feel generally unwell with flu-like symptoms such as aches, lethargy, pyrexia and hot or cold shivers, disturbed sleep and loss of appetite.

Source: Reproduced with permission from The Cochrane Collaboration.

increasing or unresolved pain must be taken seriously. The presence or drainage of pus is an additional sign of infection in some wounds where the causative organism is 'pyogenic' (pus-forming).

The use of 'film plus fabric' dressings and films (as retention dressings) does not permit clear visual assessment of the wound area for early signs of wound infection such as spreading erythema to be identified (Mansha et al. 2005). Additional signs of infection such as unexpected wound pain or tenderness, malodour, dehiscence, purulent discharge, localised swelling or heat in conjunction with microbiological analysis (Santy 2009) aid differentiation between the normal postoperative inflammatory response and that of inflammation due to infection.

A wound that exhibits clinical signs of infection may instigate sampling of the wound. Laboratory analysis of wound samples can provide the clinician with information about the microbial load within the wound. It cannot, however, differentiate between a colonised wound and an infected wound, so cannot diagnose infection. It can only confirm the presence of organisms in or around the wound and does not provide any information about whether this is having a detrimental effect on the host tissue (Sibbald et al. 2003). Hence, diagnosis of infection should be based on clinical signs. Wound sampling should only be considered in wounds not responding to chosen antibiotics.

Pressure Ulcers

Pressure ulcers (PUs, decubitus ulcers, bedsores, pressure sores/injuries) are localised areas of tissue damage that result from pressure or a combination of pressure and shear forces (European Pressure Ulcer Advisory Panel and National Pressure Ulcer Advisory Panel 2009). They usually occur over bony prominences, most commonly the sacrum and the heel bone, but can occur at any site that is subjected to pressure. Global incidence and prevalence surveys show that pressure ulcers remain a common problem. Prevalence rates are influenced by numerous factors, such as mortality, length of stay and the influx of admissions, which vary considerably, but can help measure the burden of the problem and help in decision-making regarding resource allocation. Incidence studies, which are based on the accumulation of new pressure ulcers, reflect the nosocomial (acquired in hospital/during care) problem and are particularly useful in determining patients at risk and allow inferences regarding the effect of preventive care measures (International Guidelines 2009). Some patient groups are at a higher risk than the general hospital population, including those who are critically ill, older adults (>65 years) and people who have reduced mobility, such as many orthopaedic patients.

It is difficult to determine the true cost of pressure-related tissue damage, but a high prevalence or incidence of pressure ulcers leads to human suffering, lost opportunity costs, use of extra resources and potential litigation. It is important that nurses act to reduce the number and severity of ulcers through the delivery of evidence-based care. The physical, social and psychological suffering experienced by patients with pressure ulcers is immense. Hopkins et al. (2006) used a phenomenological approach to explore the 'endless pain' and 'restricted life' that patients suffer. This distress is caused by (i) local factors such as pain, wound exudate and malodour, often leading to social isolation, (ii) delayed rehabilitation, which may result in economic hardship, and (iii) serious complications such as cellulitis, osteomyelitis, septicaemia, limb amputation and even death.

Classification of Pressure Ulcers

To improve written and verbal communication amongst practitioners the European Pressure Ulcer Advisory Panel and National Pressure Ulcer Advisory Panel (2009) scale is widely used to classify pressure ulcers. Ulcers are classified into four (six in the US version) categories depending on the depth of tissue damage:

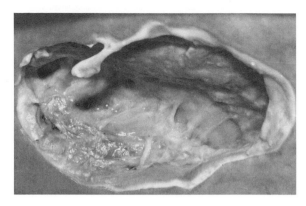

Figure 12.3 Pressure ulcer containing slough.

- The wound is assessed as category/stage I when there is observable erythema that is non-blanchable or persistent along with pain and raised tissue temperature.
- Category/stage II is denoted by partial thickness skin loss with a shallow, open, red/pink ulcer without slough or bruising. This stage might also present as a fluid-filled blister.
- Category/stage III presents as full thickness skin or tissue loss in which subcutaneous fat may be visible. The ulcer may, however, be either shallow or deep and there may also be slough, but not to any great depth (Figure 12.3).
- Category IV refers to deep ulcers in which there is full-thickness tissue loss in which there may be exposed bone, tendon or muscle. There may also be slough or eschar present within the wound along with undermining or tunnelling.

In the USA two further categories are often used. Unstageable/unclassified ulcers are those in which there is full-thickness skin or tissue loss but the depth is unknown as the wound may be obscured by slough and/or eschar. Suspected deep tissue injury is a further category referring to other wounds in which the depth is unknown. A localised area of purple or maroon but intact skin is recognised as denoting damage to the underlying tissue but the full depth of tissue damage cannot be ascertained.

A quick reference guide to this scale can be viewed and downloaded at http://www.npuap.org/wp-content/uploads/2012/02/Final_Quick_Prevention_for_web_2010.pdf, which offers the practitioner further advice and evidence-based rationale for use of the system.

Pressure Ulcer Formation

When an external load is applied to the skin, autoregulatory processes allow the internal capillary pressure to rise so that blood flow is reduced. It is believed that pressure damage occurs when the blood supply to the skin is occluded by an external perpendicular force which supersedes internal capillary closing pressure. Intense pressures of short duration are as injurious to tissues as lower pressures applied for a longer period. This demonstrates that to prevent pressure damage it is essential to reduce the intensity and duration of pressure by, for example, repositioning immobile patients and the use of pressure-redistributing support surfaces.

Other forces, such as friction and shear, can significantly decrease the tolerance of tissue to directly applied pressure. Extrinsic factors, such as moisture, friction and shear, impinge on the surface of the skin and intrinsic factors reduce the sensation or perception response mechanism or alter the structural constituents and perfusion of tissues. More than 200 contributing factors have been identified in the development of pressure ulcers.

Superficial Ulceration

It has been suggested that superficial pressure ulcers occur in one of two ways: (i) the epidermis is simply stripped away from the dermis, which typically occurs as a result of skin being abraded through, for example, repetitive rubbing or poor 'moving and handling' techniques (frictional forces), or (ii) shear forces distort and damage the microvasculature, which feeds the epidermal basal layer. The basal layer becomes ischaemic and sloughs off.

Deep Ulceration

There are two main ways in which deep tissue can suffer significant damage. A typical stage 4 pressure ulcer occurs when the fascia between fat and muscle is unable to block the pressure from damaging underlying muscle and bone (Black et al. 2007). This force directly occludes blood vessels, causing ischaemia. It may also affect arteries that penetrate into bone marrow, sometimes resulting in aseptic necrosis of underlying bone. Meanwhile the dermal capillaries remain largely unaffected, possibly because of other factors such as shear. Shear forces disrupt arterioles in the muscle but, since muscle is a well-vascularised tissue, the resulting haematoma is likely to be large and well beyond the capacity of the body to absorb. The lesion will track towards the skin surface. Tissue insult does not end when the pressures and forces are withdrawn, as rapid reperfusion may also contribute to injury.

Preventative Care

The detection of early or superficial tissue damage along with the instigation of appropriate and timely care can prevent or reverse the majority of impending pressure ulcers. Guidance for preventative care is enshrined in local, national and international guidelines that highlight that pressure ulcer prevention begins on admission with a baseline skin assessment to determine the presence or absence of pressure damage. This is followed by a holistic assessment to identify factors that may heighten susceptibility.

Risk assessment scales numerically rate a range of risk factors which are added together to indicate the likelihood of pressure damage. Many risk assessment scales, however, have not been tested for predictive ability and factors such as the client group and preventive care can affect sensitivity and specificity. It is important to use scales as a framework for assessment as opposed to the sole indicator of risk. The level of risk can change along with the patient's condition and it is vital that risk is reassessed at regular intervals. Most healthcare providers have a standard risk assessment format that is used by all staff and local guidelines often govern the frequency and triggers for this.

Following each assessment, a care plan must be tailored to address risk factors such as pressure, shear, friction, incontinence, pain and malnutrition with the goal of:

1) maintaining and improving tissue tolerance to pressure through evidence-based skin care and addressing malnutrition
2) protecting against the adverse effects of external mechanical forces.

Moisture (urine, faeces, perspiration and wound drainage) adversely affects skin in one of five ways:

1) It may make skin more susceptible to tissue damage by enhancing the frictional component of a shearing force (Sprigle 2000).
2) It can irritate and macerate skin, making it more prone to infections and rashes, resulting in superficial skin loss (Kotter and Halfens 2010).
3) Elevated humidity at the skin surface may cause discomfort and agitation, leading to abrasions (Clark 1996).
4) Many skin cleansers contain products that remove sebum and surface lipids, drying skin, rendering it vulnerable to water-soluble irritants and increasing friction (Gray et al. 2002).
5) Moisture may interact with chemical residues left on bed linen following the laundering process (Alberman 1992). resulting in chemical burn that leads to skin damage.

To combat these problems, clinical guidelines highlight the importance of:

- daily systematic skin assessments, paying attention to bony prominences
- the promotion of continence and immediate cleansing at time of soiling
- mild cleansing agents (pH 5.5) and judicious use of moisturisers that keep skin well hydrated
- minimising friction and shear forces through careful positioning, transferring and turning techniques.

Malnutrition, particularly protein-calorie malnutrition, increases an individual's risk of developing pressure ulcers. This point has been supported by Langer et al. (2003), who carried out a systematic review to (i) summarise the best available research and (ii) enable evidence-based guidance on the role of nutritional interventions in pressure ulcer prevention and treatment (Box 12.4 and Chapter 10).

Box 12.4 Evidence Digest: The Role of Nutritional Interventions in Pressure Ulcer Prevention and Treatment (Langer et al. 2003)

Only four studies met Langer et al.'s (2003) review inclusion criteria and for various reasons (methodological weaknesses of studies designed to detect the impact of nutritional interventions on pressure ulcer incidence) none of these were deemed to be sufficiently scientifically robust to detect the true impact of nutritional interventions on pressure ulcer incidence. Patient groups, interventions, outcome measurements and follow-up periods (ranging from 14 to 180 days) were too heterogeneous to allow for meta-analysis.

Despite these problems, it was noted that all of the studies that looked at the effect of mixed nutritional supplements in people recovering from hip fractures reported a lower incidence of pressure ulcers in the groups receiving dietary supplements. It was also noted that in the acute phase of a critical illness elderly people appeared to develop fewer pressure ulcers when given two daily supplement drinks. Other independent risk factors for pressure ulceration were also noted and included low serum albumin, a lower limb fracture, a Norton score <10 or a low Kuntzman score.

Given these findings and that collagen degradation occurs following injury and essential nutrients are required for collagen synthesis and stability during healing (Nixon 2001), it is reasonable to hypothesise that the skin of critically ill malnourished patients may be particularly vulnerable to the effects of pressure, shear and friction but this requires further investigation.

The adverse effects of external mechanical forces can be minimised in two ways:

1) Completely remove pressure (offload) from the pressure areas using manual repositioning techniques, devices such as pillows and splints and/or alternating mattresses.
2) Use a conforming support surface to distribute the body weight over a larger surface area (pressure reduction) and reduce the magnitude and/or duration of pressure between a patient and their support surface (the 'interface pressure') (McInnes et al. 2011).

Turning

The traditional 2-hourly turn originates from attempts to prevent pressure damage in a spinal injury unit (Clark 1998). While there appears to be very little scientific evidence to support its efficacy, research by Moore et al. (2011) indicates that 3-hourly repositioning using the 30° tilt reduced the incidence of pressure damage when compared to a 6-hourly turn. It is not always possible, however, to reposition patients if their underlying physiological condition is critical and unstable. One study that has examined this issue is considered in Box 12.5. Furthermore, 2-hourly repositioning can lead to sleep disruption, which can lengthen recovery, suppress immune function and predispose patients to infection (Carskadon and Dement 2005). Gillespie et al. (2012) note that whilst regular movement is important, unnecessary repositioning may cause increased discomfort for people with wounds, stiff joints, bony pain or contractures.

30° Tilting Regime

It has been argued that the 30° tilt is more effective in off-loading bony prominences than a 90° body turn (Figure 12.4). Each time the patient needs to be repositioned, they are gently rolled 20–30° medially or laterally from the starting point onto 'soft sites' (e.g. the side of the buttock) as opposed to bony prominences. Pillows are used to support the body and to act as space fillers. One corner of the pillow is placed under the ankle (to elevate the heel) and the rest of the pillow is moulded into any gaps made by the contour of the limb to create more uniform pressure loads. This should, in theory, reduce the pressure over any one area. Defloor (2000) used transcutaneous oximetry measurements to show the benefits of offloading bony prominences using the 30° tilt technique and Moore et al. (2011) showed that this reduced the incidence of pressure damage in elderly at-risk patients in comparison to standard care. The technique is not, however, suitable for all patients; it is contraindicated, for example, in patients with an acute spinal injury and may be contraindicated in patients following a hip arthroplasty due to the risk of iatrogenic injury and contractures.

Pillows

The benefits and risks associated with the use of pillows as a pressure-relieving device is under-researched. Heels which project beyond pillows are subject to zero pressure (Smith 1984), suggesting that carefully placed pillows (Figure 12.4c) can be a cost-effective way of offloading the heel. Smith, however, believed that pillows were

---

Box 12.5   Evidence Digest: Preventive Schemes to Assess the Effects of Turning (Defloor et al. 2005)

A study by Defloor et al. (2005) used a four arm experimental design (over a 4-week period) to compare four preventative schemes to assess the effects of turning with different intervals on the development of pressure ulcers. Subjects were recruited from 11 nursing homes caring for older people (*n* = 838). Of these:

- 65 patients were allocated to 2-hourly turns on a standard institutional mattress
- 65 patients were allocated to 3-hourly turns on a standard institutional mattress
- 67 patients were allocated to 4-hourly turns on a viscoelastic polyurethane foam mattress
- 65 patients were allocated to 6-hourly turns on a viscoelastic polyurethane foam mattress
- 576 patients were allocated to the standard care group.

Using logistic regression, the investigators found that the incidence of non-blanchable erythema was not significantly different between groups. However, the incidence of grade II and higher pressure ulcers was significantly less in the 4-hour interval group (3.0% compared with incidence figures in the other groups varying between 14.3% and 24.1%). The authors concluded that 4-hourly turns are a feasible preventive method in terms of effect, effort and cost. Interestingly, further data from this study presented by Vanderwee et al. (2005) indicated that 29.1% of the pressure ulcers were located at the heels. The authors concluded that elevating the heels from the mattress could have prevented these ulcers.

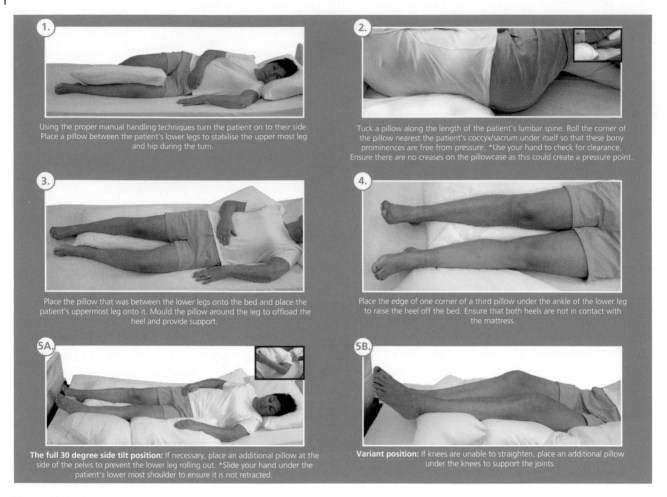

1. Using the proper manual handling techniques turn the patient on to their side. Place a pillow between the patient's lower legs to stabilise the upper most leg and hip during the turn.

2. Tuck a pillow along the length of the patient's lumbar spine. Roll the corner of the pillow nearest the patient's coccyx/sacrum under itself so that these bony prominences are free from pressure. *Use your hand to check for clearance. Ensure there are no creases on the pillowcase as this could create a pressure point.

3. Place the pillow that was between the lower legs onto the bed and place the patient's uppermost leg onto it. Mould the pillow around the leg to offload the heel and provide support.

4. Place the edge of one corner of a third pillow under the ankle of the lower leg to raise the heel off the bed. Ensure that both heels are not in contact with the mattress.

5A. The full 30 degree side tilt position: If necessary, place an additional pillow at the side of the pelvis to prevent the lower leg rolling out. *Slide your hand under the patient's lower most shoulder to ensure it is not retracted.

5B. Variant position: If knees are unable to straighten, place an additional pillow under the knees to support the joints.

Figure 12.4 Performing the 30° tilt. *Source:* This material is reproduced with permission from Northern Health and Social Care Trust, Northern Ireland.

unacceptable due to the increased risk of deep venous thrombosis and there are also concerns about the pressure which may be exerted over the Achilles tendon. Sigel et al. (1973) noted that a body tilt to a 10° foot-up position increased venous flow by 30%, suggesting that with a pillow in situ simply tilting the bed could offset any risk of deep venous thrombosis. In acutely ill bed-bound patients any potential risk of a venous thromboembolism would be minimised through the current standard treatment (Chapter 9). Concern that inappropriately placed pillows can lead to knee contractures can be overcome by placing pillows lengthways, i.e. from just below the crease of the knee to the ankle or using the pillow as a 'space-filler'. Both of these techniques should maximise the surface contact area and reduce pressure on all parts of the lower leg. In addition, bending the knee section of a profiling bed helps to reduce the risk that the knee will become hyperextended. Pillows are easily 'kicked' out of the safe position; heels may lie on the pillow rather than over the edge of the pillow and the heel area will be subject to pressure and tissue could become damaged (Donnelly 2005).

Collars

Cervical collar-related pressure ulcers remain relatively common. They commonly occur on the occiput, the chin and the shoulders. Risk factors include ICU admission ($P = 0.007$), mechanical ventilation ($P = 0.005$), the necessity for cervical MRI ($P \leq 0.001$) and time to cervical spine clearance ($P \leq 0.001$) (Ackland et al. 2007). Interestingly, the time to cervical spine clearance was the major indicator, with a 66% increase in risk of tissue damage for every 1 day increase in cervical collar time (Chapter 19). There are a number of actions which nurses can take to reduce the risk of pressure damage:

- change the patient from a rigid to a semi-rigid collar as soon as possible
- ensure the collar is fitted correctly and is the right size
- remove the collar every 4 hours for skin assessment and hygiene
- hair should be parted and hidden pressure points such as the occiput inspected for signs of redness or discolouration

- check the chin, mandible, ears, shoulders, sternum and laryngeal prominence for pressure damage
- wash and dry the skin carefully
- men should be shaved for comfort and to prevent skin irritation
- check the collar padding; this must be changed if it is wet or soiled
- if necessary adjust the pad so that no plastic touches the skin.

Heel Splints

Devices which completely offload the heel appear to be more effective than support surfaces in reducing the incidence of heel pressure ulcers. In a recent study (Donnelly et al. 2011), older patients with a fracture of the hip were randomly allocated to receive heel elevation plus use of a pressure-redistributing support surface or standard care (pressure-redistributing support surface alone). Findings indicated that subjects in the control group (heels down) were more likely than those in the intervention group (heel elevation) to suffer pressure damage. The challenge with current devices is that many patients find them uncomfortably warm and too heavy. Further consideration is given to safe care of casts and traction in Chapter 8.

Alternating Support Surfaces

Alternating pressure redistributing devices (mattresses replacements, overlays and cushions) contain a number of air-filled 'cells' that alternately inflate and deflate beneath the patient, mimicking normal body movement. As these cells inflate they generate high interface pressures, but because these are only sustained for a short period of time, the body is (arguably) able to withstand the pressure. As soon as the cells deflate, the hypoxic tissue is reperfused by the normal hyperaemic response. Allen et al. (1993) noted, however, that no studies have

shown that bony prominences such as the heel are completely offloaded and therefore they remain vulnerable to damage. As most immobilised patients experience reduced blood flow, alternating pressure may also have an effect on tissue perfusion, resulting in improved blood flow and facilitating the prevention of pressure ulcers.

Pressure-reducing Support Surfaces (Constant Low-pressure Devices)

Pressure-reducing support surfaces are designed to mould around the shape of the patient. They increase the amount of contact that the body has with the support surface, thus reducing the magnitude of interface pressures at any given anatomical location. Although many different types of pressure-reducing devices are available, a systematic review of the literature has been unable to determine which is most effective with regard to pressure ulcer prevention (McInnes et al. 2011). The review determined that higher specification foam mattresses offer more protection than standard hospital foam mattresses and that air-fluidised beds may improve pressure ulcer healing rates. Pressure-redistributing equipment presently used to prevent pressure ulcers has not been fully and reliably evaluated.

Management of Pressure Ulcers

Inevitably, most orthopaedic practitioners will continue to care for patients with pressure ulcers. Good fundamental care which includes nutritional support and hydration remains central to this. Without the pressure ulcer prevention measures discussed above no pressure ulcer will heal. Hence it is only when all possible prevention measures are in place that a focus on good wound management practice can be made with a view to healing the ulcer. Practitioners must make intelligent use of the wound management guidelines discussed in the first section of this chapter.

Further Reading

Bryant, R.A. and Nix, D.P. (ed.) (2011). *Acute and Chronic Wounds: Current Management Concepts*, 4e. St Louis: Mosby.

Dealey, C. (2012). *The Care of Wounds. A Guide for Nurses*, 4e. Oxford: Wiley Blackwell.

European Pressure Ulcer Advisory Panel and National Pressure Ulcer Advisory Panel (2009). *Treatment of*

Pressure Ulcers: Quick Reference Guide. National Pressure Ulcer Advisory Panel (online), Washington DC. http://www.npuap.org/wp-content/uploads/2012/02/Final_Quick_Prevention_for_web_2010.pdf (accessed 25 June 2022).

Flanagan, M. (2013). *Wound Healing and Skin Integrity. Principles and Practice*. Oxford: Wiley Blackwell.

References

Abuzakuk, T.M., Coward, P., Sheneva, Y. et al. (2006). The management of wounds following primary lower limb arthroplasty: a prospective, randomised study comparing hydrofibre and central pad dressings. *Int. Wound J.* 3 (2): 133–137.

Ackland, H.M., Cooper, J., Malham, G.M., and Kossmann, T. (2007). Cervical spine factors predicting cervical collar-related decubitus ulceration in major trauma patients. *Spine* 32 (4): 423–428.

Adogwa, O., Fatemi, P., Perez, E. et al. (2014). Negative pressure wound therapy reduces incidence of post-operative wound infection and dehiscence after long-segment thoracolumbar spinal fusion: a single institutional experience. *Spine J.* 14 (12): 2911–2917.

Aindow, D. and Butcher, M. (2005). Films or fabrics: is it time to reappraise postoperative dressings? *Bri. J. Nurs.* 14 (19): S15–S20.

Alberman, K. (1992). Is there any connection between laundering and the development of pressure sores? *J. Tis. Viabil.* 2 (2): 55–56.

Allen, V., Ryan, D.W., and Murray, A. (1993). Potential for bed sores due to high pressures: influence of body sites, body position, and mattress design. *Brit. J. Clin. Pract.* 47 (4): 195–197.

Ayliffe, G.A., Babb, J.R., and Taylor, L.J. (2001). *Hospital Acquired Infection. Principles and Prevention*, 3e. Arnold, London.

Bhattacharyya, M., Bradley, H., Holder, S., and Gerber, B. (2005). A prospective clinical audit of patient dressing choice for post-op arthroscopy wounds. *Wounds UK* 1 (1): 30–34.

Black, J., Baharestani, M., Cuddigan, J. et al. (2007). National pressure ulcer advisory panel's updated pressure ulcer staging system. *Urologic. Nurs.* 27 (2): 144–150.

Bryan, J. (2004). Moist wound healing: a concept that changed our practice. *J. Wound. Care.* 13 (6): 227–228.

Cai, J., Karman, J., Parvizi, J. et al. (2014). Aquacel surgical dressing reduces the rate of acute periprosthetic joint infection following Total joint arthroplasty: a case-control study. *J. Arthropl.* https://doi.org/10.1016/j.arth.2013.11.012.

Carskadon, M.A. and Dement, W.C. (2005). Normal human sleep: An overview. In: *Principles and Practice of Sleep Medicine*, 4e (ed. M.H. Kryger, T. Roth and W.C. Dement). Philadelphia: Elsevier Sanders.

Clark, M. (1996). The aetiology of superficial sacral pressure sores. In: *Proceedings of the 6th European Conference on Advances in Wound Management* (ed. D.L. Leaper, G.W. Cherry and C. Dealey), 167–170. Amsterdam: MacMillan Press.

Clark, M. (1998). Repositioning to prevent pressure sores – what is the evidence. *Nurs. Stand.* 13 (93): 58–64.

Clarke, J.V., Deakin, A.H., Dillon, J.M. et al. (2009). A prospective clinical audit of a new dressing design for lower limb arthroplasty wounds. *J. Wound. Care.* 18 (1): 5–11.

Coello, R., Charlett, A., Wilson, J. et al. (2005). Adverse impact of surgical site infections in English hospitals. *J. Hos. Infect.* 60 (2): 93–103.

Cooper, R. and Lawrence, J.C. (1996). The prevalence of bacteria and implications for infection control. *J. Wound. Care* 5 (6): 291–295.

Coulthard, P., Esposito, M., Worthington, H.V., et al. (2010) *Tissue adhesives for closure of surgical incisions. Cochrane Database of Systematic Reviews* **5** (Art. No.: CD004287). DOI: 10.1002/14651858.CD004287. pub3.

Cosker, T., Elsayed, S., Gupta, S. et al. (2005). Choice of dressing has a major impact on blistering and healing outcomes in orthopaedic patients. *J. Wound. Care* 14 (1): 27–29.

Cutting, K.F. and White, R.J. (2002). Maceration of the skin and wound bed 1: its nature and causes. *J. Wound. Care* 11 (7): 275–278.

Defloor, T. (2000). The effect of position and mattress on interface pressure. *App. Nurs. Res.* 13 (1): 2–11.

Defloor, T., De Bacquer, D., and Grypdonck, M.H. (2005). The effect of various combinations of turning and pressure reducing devices on the incidence of pressure ulcers. *Int. J. Nurs. Stud.* 42 (1): 37–46.

Department of Health (2006). *The Health Act 2006: Code of Practice for the Prevention and Control of Healthcare Associated Infection*. Department of Health, London.

Dillon, J.M., Clarke, J.V., Emmerson, S. and Kinninmonth, A.W.G. (2007). The Jubilee method: A novel, effective wound dressing following total hip and knee arthroplasty, Poster presentation, in *Proceedings of the American Academy of Orthopaedic Surgeons Annual Meeting*, San Diego, California.

Dohmen, P.M. (2008). Antibiotic resistance in common pathogens reinforces the need to minimise surgical site infections. *J. Hos. Infect.* 70 (S2): 15–20.

Donnelly, J. (2005). The Importance of a Pilot Study in Informing a Main Study Design, Poster Presentation, in *National Pressure Ulcer Advisory Panel 9th National Conference: Merging Missions*. Salt Lake City, USA. February 25–26.

Donnelly, J., Winder, J., Kernohan, W.G., and Stevenson, M. (2011). An RCT to determine the effect of a heel elevation device in pressure ulcer prevention post-hip fracture. *J. Wound. Care.* 20 (7) 309–312,: 314–318.

Doughty, D.B. and Defriese, B. (2007). Wound-healing physiology. In: *Acute and Chronic Wounds: Current*

Management Concepts, 3e (ed. R.A. Bryant and D.P. Nix). St Louis: Mosby.

European Pressure Ulcer Advisory Panel and National Pressure Ulcer Advisory Panel (2009). *Treatment of Pressure Ulcers: Quick Reference Guide*. National Pressure Ulcer Advisory Panel, Washington DC. http://www.npuap.org (accessed 25 June 2022).

European Wound Management Association (2005). *Identifying Criteria for Wound Infection*. Conference 15–17 September 2005, Stuttgart, Germany. Available via EWMA (conference2web.com) (accessed 25 June 2022).

Gaine, W.J., Ramamohan, N.A., Hussein, M.G. et al. (2000). Wound infection in hip and knee arthroplasty. *J. Bone Joint. Surg. (British)* 82-B (4): 561–565.

Gillespie, B.M., Chaboyer, W.P., McInnes, E. et al. (2012). Repositioning for pressure ulcer prevention in adults (protocol). *Cochr. Database. System. Rev.* 4: (Art. No.: CD009958). https://doi.org/10.1002/14651858.CD009958.pub2.

Gray, M., Ratliff, C., and Donovan, A. (2002). Perineal skin care for the incontinent patient. *Adv. Skin Wound Care* 15 (4): 170–175.

Gupta, S., Lee, S., and Moseley, L. (2002). Postoperative wound blistering: is there a link with dressing usage? *J. Wound. Care* 11 (7): 271–273.

Harle, S., Korhonen, A., Kettunen, J., and Seitsalo, S. (2005). A randomised clinical trial of two different wound dressing materials for hip replacement patients. *J. Orthopaed. Nurs.* 9 (4): 205–210.

Health Protection Agency (2008). *Protocol for Surveillance of Surgical Site Infection*. Version 3.4. Surgical Site Infection Surveillance Service. www.hpa.org.ukwebc/hpawebfile/hpaweb_c/1194947388966 (accessed 25 June 2022).

Helito, C., Sobrado, M., and Giglio, P. (2020). The use of negative-pressure wound therapy after total knee arthroplasty is effective for reducing complications and the need for reintervention. *BMC Musculoskel. Disord.* 21 (1): 490.

Holm, C., Petersen, J.S., Gronboek, F., and Gottrup, F. (1998). Effects of occlusive and conventional gauze dressings on incisional healing after abdominal operation. *Europ. J. Surg.* 164: 179–183.

Hopkins, A., Dealey, C., Bale, S. et al. (2006). Patient stories of living with a pressure ulcer. *J. Advan. Nurs.* 56 (4): 345–353.

International Guidelines (2009). *Pressure Ulcer Prevention: Prevalence and Incidence in Context. A Consensus Document*. MEP Ltd, London. http://www.woundsinternational.com/pdf/content_24.pdf (accessed 25 June 2022).

Jester, R., Russell, L., Fell, S. et al. (2000). A one hospital study of the effect of wound dressings and other related

factors on skin blistering following total hip and knee arthroplasty. *J. Orthopaed. Nurs.* 4 (2): 71–77.

Jones, V.J. (2006). The use of gauze: will it ever change? *Int. Wound. J.* 3 (2): 79–86.

Karlakki, S., Hamand, A., Whittall, C. et al. (2016). Incisional negative pressure wound therapy dressings in routine primary hip and knee arthroplasties. A randomised controlled trial. *Bone. Joint. Res.* 5: 328–337.

Kotter, J. and Halfens, R. (2010). Moisture lesions: inter-rater agreement and reliability. *J. Clin. Nurs.* 19: 716–720.

Knuutinen, A., Kokkonen, N., Risteli, J. et al. (2002). Smoking affects collagen synthesis and extracellular matrix turnover in human skin. *Bri. J. Dermatol.* 146: 588–594.

Langer, G., Knerr, A., Kuss, O. et al. (2003). Nutritional interventions for preventing and treating pressure ulcers. *Cochr. Database. Sys. Rev.* 4: (Art. No.: CD003216). https://doi.org/10.1002/14651858.CD003216.

Leaper, J. (2000). Wound infection. In: *Bailey and Love's Short Practice of Surgery*, 23e, 87–98. London: Arnold.

Lorenz, P. and Longaker, M.T. (2008). Wounds: biology, pathology and management. In: *Surgery: Basic Science and Clinical Evidence* (ed. J.A. Norton, P.S. Barrie, R.R. Bollinger, et al.), 191–205. New York: Springer.

Mansha, M., Sharif, K., Sharif, Z. et al. (2005). The impact of different methods of wound closure and dressing on the rate of wound infection in patients with fracture neck of femur. *J. Orthopaed. Nurs.* 9 (4): 195–198.

Masters, J., Cook, J., Achten, J., and Costa, M. (2021). A feasibility study of standard dressings versus negative-pressure wound therapy in the treatment of adult patients having surgical incisions for hip fractures: the WHISH randomized controlled trial. *Bone Joint. J.* 103-B (4): 755–761.

McInnes, E., Jammali-Blasi, A., Bell-Syer, S.E.M. et al. (2011). Support surfaces for pressure ulcer prevention. *Cochr. Database. Sys. Rev.* 4(Art. No.: CD001735). https://doi.org/10.1002/14651858.CD001735. pub4.

Moore, Z., Cowman, S., and Conroy, R.M. (2011). A randomised controlled clinical trial of repositioning, using the 30° tilt, for the prevention of pressure ulcers. *J. Clin. Nurs.* 20: 2633–2644.

Morgan, D.A. (2004). *Formulary of Wound Management Products. A Guide for Healthcare Staff*, 9e. Surrey: Euromed Communications Limited.

Morgan, M., Black, J., Bone, F. et al. (2005). Clinician-led surgical site infection surveillance of orthopaedic procedures: a UK multi-centre pilot study. *J. Hos. Infect.* 60 (3): 201–212.

NICE (2008). *Surgical Site Infection: Prevention and Treatment of Surgical Site Infection*. London: NICE.

Nherera, L., Trueman, P., and Karlakki, S. (2017). Cost-effectiveness analysis of single-use negative pressure wound therapy dressings to reduce surgical site complications (SSC) in routine primary hip and knee replacements. *Wound. Rep. Regen.* 25 (3): 474–482.

Nixon, J. (2001). The pathophysiology and aetiology of pressure ulcers. In: *The Prevention and Treatment of Pressure Ulcers*, 2e (ed. M.J. Morison), 17–36. Edinburgh: Mosby.

Owens, C.D. and Stoessel, K. (2008). Surgical site infections: epidemiology, microbiology and prevention. *J. Hos. Infect.* 70 (S2): 3–10.

Polatsch, D.B., Baskies, M.A., Hommen, J.P. et al. (2004). Tape blisters that develop after hip fracture surgery: a retrospective series and a review of the literature. *Am. J. Orthop.* 33 (9): 452–456.

Pudner, R. (2001). Postoperative dressings in wound management. *J. Comm. Nurs.* 15 (9): 33–37.

Ravenscroft, M., Harker, K., and Buch, K. (2006). A prospective, randomised, controlled trial comparing wound dressings used in hip and knee surgery: Aquacel® and Tegaderm™ versus Cutiplast™. *Ann. Royal. College. Surg. Eng.* 88 (1): 18–22.

Sandell, C. (2020). *Incisional management pathway using negative pressure wound therapy to reduce surgical site complication rates in elective orthopaedics, Poster presentation*, in European Wound Management Association virtual conference, 2020.

Santy, J. (2009). Recognising infection in wounds. *Nurs. Stand.* 23 (7): 53–54, 56, 58.

Serena, T., Robson, M.C., Cooper, D.M., and Ignatius, J. (2006). Lack of reliability of clinical/visual assessment of chronic wound infection: the incidence of biopsy-proven infection in venous leg ulcers. *Wounds* 18: 197–202.

Sibbald, R.G., Orsted, H., Schultz, G.S. et al. (2003). Preparing the wound bed 2003: focus on infection and inflammation. *Ostomy. Wound. Manag.* 49 (11): 24–51.

Sigel, B., Edlestein, A.L., Felix, R., and Memhardt, C.R. (1973). Compression of the deep venous system of the lower leg during inactive recumbence. *Arch. Surg.* 106: 38–43.

Smith, I. (1984). Heel aids. *Nurs. Times* 80 (36): 35–39.

Sprigle, S. (2000). Effects of forces and the selection of support surfaces. *Top. Geriat. Rehabilit.* 16 (2): 47–62.

Springer, B., Beaver, W., Griffin, W., et al. (2013). *The role of surgical dressings in total knee arthroplasty: A randomized clinical trial, Poster presentation*, in Annual Meeting of the American Association of Orthopaedic Surgeons, Chicago, March 2013.

Srinivasaiah, N., Dugdall, H., Barrett, S., and Drew, P. (2007). A point prevalence survey of wounds in the north-east of England. *J. Wound. Care* 16 (10): 413–419.

Trampuz, A. and Zimmerli, W. (2006). Diagnosis and treatment of infections associated with fracture fixation devices. *Injury* 37 (2 Suppl): S56–S59.

Vanderwee, K., Grypdonck, M.H.F., and Defloor, T. (2005). Effectiveness of an alternating pressure air mattress for the prevention of pressure ulcers. *Age and Ageing.* 34 (3): 261–267.

Voegeli, D. (2008). The effect of washing and drying practices on skin barrier function. *J. Wound. Ost. Cont. Nurs.* 35 (1): 84–90.

Winter, G.D. (1962). Formation of the scab and the rate of epithelialisation of superficial wounds in the skin of the young domestic pig. *Nature* 193: 293–294.

White, R. (2001). New developments in the use of dressings on surgical wounds. *Bri. J. Nurs.* 10 (6): S70.

Xia, Z., Sato, A., Hughes, M.A., and Cherry, G.W. (2000). Stimulation of fibroblast growth in-vitro by intermittent radiant warming. *Wound Repair. Regener.* 8 (2): 138–144.

Part III

Common Orthopaedic Conditions and their Care and Management

13

Key Conditions and Principles of Orthopaedic Management

Elaine Wylie[1] and Sonya Clarke[2]

[1] Craigavon Area Hospital, Craigavon, UK
[2] Queen's University Belfast, Belfast, UK

Introduction

This chapter provides an overview of the knowledge required to promote optimal care for patients presenting with common orthopaedic conditions in the young adult (and child when appropriate), adult and older person. Osteoarthritis (OA), sero-negative arthropathies, rheumatoid arthritis (RA), the metabolic condition osteoporosis, osteomyelitis, low back pain (LBP), scoliosis, spinal stenosis and intervertebral disc disease are considered. Each condition is discussed in relation to its definition, epidemiology, diagnosis, clinical presentation and management. This edition of the book includes Paget's disease, a second metabolic condition as an evidence digest. Although this chapter has a central nursing focus, it also considers the wider context of the 'specialist nurse' and multidisciplinary team (MDT). Management and care options will be explored with reference to best available evidence and national guidance. The final section of this chapter includes an overview of juvenile idiopathic arthritis (JIA).

Arthritis is often used as an umbrella term to refer to any disorder that affects the joints. Arthritis literally means joint inflammation, although joint inflammation is a symptom or sign rather than a specific diagnosis (National Institute of Arthritis, Musculoskeletal, and Skin Diseases 2022). Arthritis or musculoskeletal (MSK) diseases are widespread in the community with over 20 million people in the UK (around a third of the population) living with musculoskeletal conditions such as OA and LBP. They are more common among women, with 35% of women having an MSK condition compared to 28% of men. The symptoms caused by arthritis- and MSK-related conditions, for example pain and fatigue, result in a substantial reduction in an individual's quality of life. Versus Arthritis (2021), in their report *The State of Musculoskeletal Health*, found that musculoskeletal conditions account for up to one in three general practitioner (GP) consultations (Keavy 2020).

Osteoarthritis

The name 'osteoarthritis' comes from three Greek words meaning bone, joint and inflammation, and refers to a clinical disorder of joint pain accompanied by varying degrees of functional limitation and reduced quality of life. It is the most common degenerative joint disease, affecting more than 25% of the adult population (Di Chen et al. 2017). The most commonly affected peripheral joints are the knees, hips and small hand joints. Pathologically changes seen in an osteoarthritic joint are a progressive loss and destruction of articular cartilage, remodelling of adjacent bone, formation of osetophytes and variable degrees of inflammation of the synovium (Loeser et al. 2012).

Pathogenesis

Despite the disease being known for centuries, the exact pathogenic mechanisms of OA remain unclear. Initially, OA was considered an unavoidable age-related disease caused by biomechanical factors, i.e. 'wear-and-tear' (Yuchen et al. 2020). However, detailed examination revealed patient-specific variability in the clinical presentation and disease progression. Most cases of OA have a clear predisposing risk factor(s) such as genetics, trauma, ageing, obesity, chronic overload, gender, hormone profile and/or metabolic syndrome (Chaganti and Lane 2011). However, it should be noted that OA is not an inevitable consequence of these factors. In addition, the different risk factors may act together in the pathogenesis of OA. For example, in older adults with anterior cruciate ligament tear, OA develops faster than in younger adults (Roos et al. 1995).

It is now widely accepted that OA is a dynamic and complex process, involving inflammatory, mechanical and metabolic factors that result in the inability of the articular surface to serve its function of absorbing and distributing the mechanical load through the joint that ultimately leads to joint destruction (Griffin and Guilak 2005). Furthermore, it is now recognised that the disease is not restricted to the cartilage or subchondral bone; rather, it results from interplay among tissues of the osteochondral complex, including adipose and synovial tissue, as well as the ligaments, tendon and muscles that surround the joint (Loeser et al. 2012). The exact pathogenic mechanism(s) of OA are still unknown, (Geyer and Schönfeld 2018) and there are no current interventions to restore degraded cartilage or decelerate disease progression (Di Chen et al. 2017).

Signs and Symptoms

The main symptoms of OA are pain and stiffness. In the early stages, pain may be transient or even absent and progression is often slow. Pain is variable, with patients having good days and bad days with pain best at the start of the day or after rest and worst with joint use and at the end of the day. Severe OA can cause pain at rest and mobility, self-care and leisure. Morning stiffness or stiffness after a period of inactivity generally lasts less than 15–30 minutes. Pain is typically described as dull, aching or throbbing and localised to a specific region. Crepitus may be noticeable on movement due to roughened articular surfaces and the joint may be painful on palpation. Restricted movement can be caused by pain, joint capsule thickening or the presence of osteophytes.

Squaring of the first carpal metacarpal (CMC) joint may be evident in hand OA due to osteophyte formation. Changes often occur in the distal interphalangeal joints (Heberden's nodes) and at the proximal interphalangeal (PIP) joints (Bouchard's nodes). Once nodes have fully formed, pain and tenderness at the distal interphalangeal joints and PIP joints often improve but pain at the CMC joint will not improve. Hand OA can reduce grip strength, having significant implications for numerous functional activities and causing considerable frustration for patients who are no longer able to perform tasks with the same precision and strength (Hill et al. 2010).

Pain from OA of the hip is typically felt in the groin, although it can radiate down to the knee. This is often associated with reduced lower limb muscle strength due to lack of use. Patients commonly have an abnormal pattern of walking caused by weakness of the abductor muscles. OA of the foot commonly affects the first metatarsal phalangeal (MTP) joint and may result in a hallux rigidus or hallux valgus deformity. This, and associated deformities, can cause pain on walking or difficulty with finding appropriate footwear. Lack of comfortable footwear or diminished strength and fitness discourages many people from pursuing usual activities, such as shopping or going out walking.

Diagnosis

Diagnosis is based on clinical history and examination. The two most important diagnostic clues are the pattern of joint involvement and the presence or absence of fever, rash or other symptoms outside the joint. As part of the physical examination, the joint should be evaluated for swelling, limitations of range of movement, pain on movement and crepitus. There is no laboratory test that is specific for OA. Treatment is usually based on the results of diagnostic imaging. In patients with OA, X-rays may indicate narrowed joint spaces, abnormal density of the bone and presence of subacromial cysts or bony spurs. The patient's symptoms, however, do not always correlate with X-ray findings. It is important to exclude other medical conditions that may be present. Differential diagnoses may include pseudogout, bursitis, RA and reactive arthritis.

Management

Following a holistic assessment (see Figure 13.1), a management plan should be considered in relation to the person's quality of life, functional limitations and pain experience. It should aim to reduce pain and maintain or improve the individual's mobility and encourage self-management as this provides a greater sense of self-empowerment and reduces reliance on health services and pharmacological therapies. A range of options is available that can be used in multiple combinations to achieve maximum outcome for the individual.

Core treatments recommended in the National Institute for Health and Care Excellence (NICE) Clinical Guideline: Osteoarthritis: Care and Management (NICE 2014) include activity and exercise, recommendations for weight loss and access to information to aid self-management (refer to Figure 13.1).

Education, exercise and weight loss are mainstays in the management of OA and the promotion of general health (NICE 2014). Patient education about treatment objectives and the importance of changes in lifestyle, exercise, weight reduction and others should be focused on self-help and patient-driven treatments rather than on passive therapies delivered by health professionals.

Exercise is important in managing OA; it should be individualised and patient-centred, taking into account factors

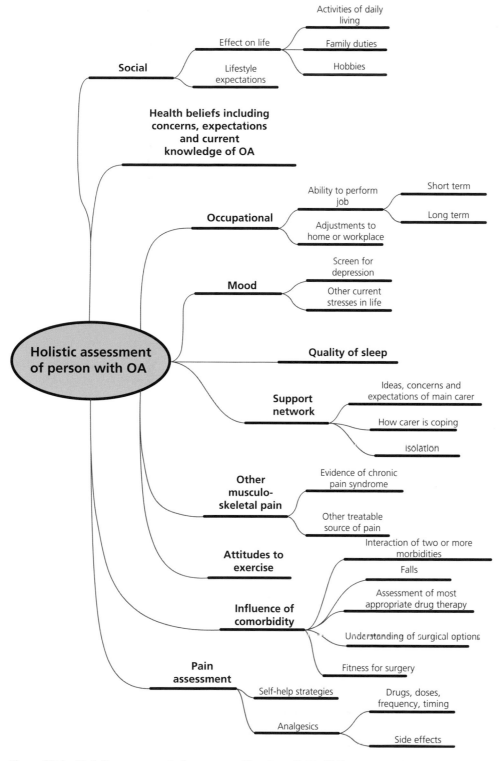

Figure 13.1 Holistic assessment of a person with osteoarthritis (OA).

such as age, comorbidity and overall morbidity. Research evaluating the effect of exercise for hip and knee OA has demonstrated improvement in pain, function and global assessment (Roddy and Doherty 2006). Group and home exercise are equally effective and patient preference should be considered. An exercise programme needs to be carefully tailored to individual needs and preferences, and should not hinder the person's ability and enthusiasm and, consequently, delay positive behavioural change. Hydrotherapy is also a useful adjunct to any exercise programme. Individuals experience an exacerbation of pain and stiffness after exercise, although most will not have any adverse reaction to controlled exercise (Hurley et al. 2007).

A reduction in weight transferred through joints, such as knees, hips and feet, may reduce the severity of the symptoms a person experiences. This may be achieved through the transfer of weight by using a walking stick or through sensible weight loss if the patient's body mass index is excessive. Patients should be encouraged to lose weight by eating healthily and adopting a sensible programme of exercise. However, this approach is difficult for many older people struggling with basic mobility or shopping and preparing meals. It is important to consider a holistic approach to OA and its effects on lifestyle and functional abilities before advocating strict regimes of diet and exercise. The use of insoles or knee braces can improve pain, stiffness and function in the knee, while hand splints can improve function in the hand and should be considered for those experiencing symptoms (NICE 2014). Referral to orthotics and occupational therapy services can provide assessment of biomechanical problems and appropriate orthoses to support painful joints and reduce joint pain.

Pharmacological Management

Medications helpful in the management of pain include simple analgesics, non-steroidal anti-inflammatory drugs (NSAIDs) and topical or oral opioids. Paracetamol is the first line of pharmacological pain management as it has few side effects. Paracetamol and topical NSAIDs can be used together to maximise pain relief, but if this is ineffective then changing to an oral NSAID should be considered, although side effects are more common. Around 10–20% of people who use oral NSAIDs experience dyspepsia and risk gastric complications, which are reduced when NSAIDs are used topically and these are now the first line of treatment (Zhang et al. 2010). Cox-2 selective anti-inflammatory drugs have reduced the incidence of gastric effects, but add to the risk of thrombus formation. They are also associated with a slight increase in risk of renal failure (Adam 2011). In summary, NSAIDs are effective for symptom relief in OA, but should be prescribed at the lowest effective dose for the shortest possible duration.

If paracetamol or topical NSAIDs are insufficient for pain relief for people with OA, then the addition of opioid analgesics should be considered (NICE 2014). Opioids can be very effective but their benefits can be outweighed by side effects: nausea, vomiting, dizziness and constipation. Even though the use of extended-release opioids in OA improves sleep, patients can be fearful about addiction.

Intra-articular corticosteroid injections should be considered as an adjunct to core treatments for the relief of moderate to severe pain in people with OA. Hyaluronic acid is not recommended for the management of OA (NICE 2014). Capsaicin, a topical cream based on chilli peppers, causes localised burning pain, but is then followed by pain relief and has been shown to alleviate mild to moderate pain caused by OA in the knee (Kosuwon et al. 2010) and should be recommended as an adjunct to core treatments for hand and knee OA (NICE 2014).

Transcutaneous electrical nerve stimulation (TENS) has shown to be helpful in relieving pain (Itoh et al. 2008), with anecdotal reports suggesting the application of heat or cold to joints to provide short-term pain relief. Heat can be applied by immersion in warm water, heat packs heated at home in the microwave, heat pads and wax. Cold is usually applied with an ice massage or by applying cold packs to the affected area. It is essential that a safe system for delivery be used to prevent any damage to the skin and surrounding tissues.

Most people with OA are managed in the primary care setting using conservative management options such as a combination of education, exercise and physiotherapy, weight loss and simple analgesia. Functional aids and orthotics may also be indicated. As symptoms worsen, the addition of anti-inflammatories and intra-articular steroids can be tried. However, if OA becomes severe with progressive limitation of functional and recreational activities, the opinion of an orthopaedic surgeon should be sought. Joint replacement is considered when conservative measures are unsuccessful and there is substantial impact on the person's quality of life (refer to Chapter 14 for elective care and arthroplasty of the hip, knee and shoulder).

Spondyloarthropathies

Spondyloarthropathies (SpA) are a group of common inflammatory rheumatic disorders characterised by axial and/or peripheral arthritis associated with enthesitis, dactylitis and potential extra-articular manifestations, such as uveitis and skin rash. These conditions share a common genetic predisposition, the HLA-B27 gene. Axial spondyloarthritis (AS) and psoriatic arthropathy are the two most common forms; Table 13.1 lists additional arthropathies.

Axial Spondyloarthritis

AS is a systemic, chronic inflammatory disease that affects the axial skeleton, causing inflammatory back pain, which can lead to structural and functional impairment There are 220 000 people in the UK with AS (NASS 2021).

Table 13.1 Other spondyloarthropathies.

Reactive arthritis	Usually manifests itself as arthritis 2–4 weeks following a urogenital or enteric infection, often in patients bearing the HLA-B27 antigen. The risk of developing reactive arthritis has been shown to occur up to 50 times higher in this population, as opposed to the HLA-B27-negative population following exposure to a preceding infection.
Inflammatory bowel disease	Associated arthritis is usually a peripheral, large joint, lower limb, asymmetric oligoarthritis. It accompanies inflammatory bowel disease in about 10% of patients and occasionally pre-dates the onset of IBD (Salvarani and Fries 2009).
Undifferentiated spondyloarthropathy or spondyloarthritis	This term is used to describe manifestations of spondyloarthritis in patients who do not meet criteria for any well-defined spondyloarthropathy. There is a female predominance of 1:3 and the clinical manifestations of this type of spondyloarthropathy are basically similar to all other spondyloarthropathies, with fewer extra-articular manifestations.

AS tends to present in the late teens to early 20s, with an average age of onset of 24. Around 95% of people are aged less than 45 years when their symptoms begin. It is an insidious disease and difficult to diagnose; patients have an average delay of 8 years from the onset of symptoms to diagnosis.

The aetiology of AS is not understood completely, but a strong genetic predisposition exists (van der Linden and van der Heijde 2000). A direct relationship between AS and the *HLA-B27* gene has been determined, but the precise role of *HLA-B27* in precipitating AS remains unknown.

AS is now seen as a continuum of disease, which can lead to AS. In patients with AS, inflammatory changes eventually affect the spinal and sacroiliac (SI) joints, leading to spinal fusion, reduced mobility and an increased risk of spinal fractures. It is now recognised that patients in earlier stages of disease do not have radiographic changes, but share similar symptoms and signs, family history and genetic risk factors, and can experience disability as severe as some patients with a confirmed diagnosis of AS (Rudwaleit et al. 2009). Patients in the early stage of disease are classified as having non-radiographic AS. Follow-up studies report that among patients diagnosed at this early stage, 6% develop AS after 5 years, 17% after 10 years and 26% after 15 years (Wang et al. 2016). Therefore, some patients may never develop

AS, while others may live with inflammatory back pain for a considerable time before developing AS.

Early diagnosis is important because early medical and physical therapy may improve functional outcome. The diagnosis of AS is generally made by combining the clinical criteria of inflammatory back pain and enthesitis or arthritis with radiologic findings. Laboratory investigations include C-reactive protein (CRP) and erythrocyte sedimentation rate (ESR), which may be mildly elevated. Rheumatoid factor (RF) and antinuclear tests are negative, with 95% of people with AS HLA-B27 positive. Although HLA-B27 is present in about 8% of the British population, most individuals will not have the condition, although there is a strong familial tendency in people with AS. X-rays are diagnostic only in established cases, with MRI imaging being a more helpful diagnostic tool.

A patient history that includes insidious onset of LBP, onset of symptoms before age 40 years, presence of symptoms for more than 3 months, symptoms worse in the morning or with inactivity and improvement of symptoms with exercise suggests AS (Passalent et al. 2010). It is important to differentiate between mechanical back pain, which in contrast often present with acute onset of pain and exacerbation of symptoms with activity, and radicular radiation of pain.

Symptoms of AS include those related to inflammatory back pain, peripheral enthesitis and arthritis, and extra-articular manifestations. Chronic pain and stiffness are the most common complaints of patients with AS. More than 70% of patients report daily pain and stiffness (O'Shea et al. 2010). Fatigue is another common complaint, occurring in approximately 65% of AS patients. Most patients report their fatigue to be moderately severe. Increased levels of fatigue are associated with increased pain and stiffness, and decreased functional capacity. Fever and weight loss may occur during periods of active disease.

Inflammatory back pain is the most common symptom and the first manifestation in approximately 75% of patients. The pain is typically dull and poorly localised to the gluteal and SI areas. Symptoms associated with inflammatory back pain include insidious onset occurring over months or years, generally with at least 3 months of symptoms before presentation. Most patients have mild chronic disease or intermittent flares with periods of remission. The pain often begins unilaterally and intermittently, and generally begins in the lumbosacral region (SI joints). However, as the disease progresses, it becomes more persistent and bilateral, and progresses more proximally, with ossification of the annulus fibrosus that results in fusion of the spine (bamboo spine).

Patients commonly experience morning stiffness lasting at least 30 minutes, improvement of symptoms with moderate physical activity and diffuse non-specific radiation of pain into both buttocks. Patients often experience stiffness and pain that awakens them in the early morning, a distinctive symptom not generally found in patients with mechanical back pain.

Peripheral enthesitis is the basic pathologic process, involving inflammation at the site of insertion of ligaments and tendons onto bone. This often progresses from erosion and osteitis to ossification, resulting in telltale radiological signs of periosteal new bone formation.

The following sites are commonly involved:

- Achilles tendon insertion
- insertion of the plantar fascia on the calcaneus or the metatarsal heads
- base of the fifth metatarsal head
- tibial tuberosity
- superior and inferior poles of the patella
- iliac crest.

Enthesopathic lesions tend to be quite painful (e.g. the plantar fascia when getting out of bed), especially in the morning. Some of the peripheral arthritis occurs at sites in which the major component is local enthesitis.

Joint involvement tends to occur most commonly in the hips, shoulders and joints of the chest wall, including the acromioclavicular and sternoclavicular joints, and often occurs in the first 10 years of disease. Involvement of the hips and shoulders may result in joint damage with radiographic changes. Other peripheral joints are involved less frequently and to a milder degree, usually as an asymmetric oligoarthritis predominantly involving the lower extremities. Involvement of the costovertebral and costotransverse joints can lead to decreased range of movement and restriction in respiration. Patients may complain of difficulty breathing or chest tightness.

Optimal treatment of AS requires a combination of non-pharmacological and pharmacological treatments. Non-pharmacological strategies involve mainly exercise therapies, education, lifestyle and behavioural changes, and self-management.

Non-pharmacological

There is a need for regular exercise in AS throughout the lifespan of the condition. The optimal intensity and format of this exercise remains unclear, but a combination of endurance and strength training is thought to be most effective (Regel et al. 2017). It is unlikely that there will be a single exercise regimen suitable for everyone with AS, so a more personalised approach is required, with the type and intensity of the exercise adapted to the patient's demographics, preferences, comorbidities and disease severity.

As for all chronic conditions, education is an important component of management and facilitates shared decision-making and self-management. Smoking cessation is encouraged as there an association with worse clinical and radiographic outcomes (Chung et al. 2012).

Pharmacological

NSAIDs remain the first-line drug treatment, in those without contra-indications, for symptoms in AS. The efficacy of NSAIDs for AS symptoms is established, with no significant differences between specific NSAID agents (Kroon et al. 2016).

Disease-modifying antirheumatic drugs (DMARDs) are drugs that work more slowly than NSAIDs but have the capability of modifying the progression of disease, e.g. sulfasalazine and methotrexate. These drugs have greater benefit in RA (see below). DMARDs do not have a beneficial effect on spinal disease. Some benefit may exist for arthritis of peripheral joints like the shoulders and hips.

Biologic treatments have revolutionised the treatment of axial spondylitis. There are five tumour necrosis factor (TNF) inhibitors, infliximab, etanercept, adalimumab, golimumab and certolizumab, which are shown to achieve partial or full remission of symptoms. Active infection (including latent or active tuberculosis, which should be treated before starting treatment), advanced heart failure, lupus, multiple sclerosis and cancer are contraindications for treatment with TNF inhibitors. Secukinumab, a monoclonal antibody to interleukin 17A, has also been shown to be effeective in the management of AS for those who are unable to use a TNF inhibitor (van der Heijde et al. 2017).

Surgical intervention for AS is more commonly used for the peripheral joints than for the spine. Osteoporosis can be a side effect of AS and lead to spinal fractures. The neck is the most common location for this fracture. Stabilisation of the spine is necessary to prevent damage to the spinal cord. Peripheral joints can be damaged to the degree of requiring a replacement. The hips and shoulders are the most commonly affected peripheral joints.

Psoriatic Arthritis

Psoriatic arthritis (PsA) is a chronic, inflammatory arthritis associated with the skin disorder psoriasis. Up to 30% of people with psoriasis may develop PsA over their lifetime; around 100 000 people have PsA in the UK (Ogdie et al. 2019). The risk of psoriatic arthritis increases with a family history of spondyloarthropathy or nail pitting and the onset usually occurs between 30 and 55 years of age, affecting men and women equally. PsA is considered a separate entity from RA because of the sero-negativity of RF and its tendency for asymmetrical involvement.

The exact aetiology has yet to be discovered. As with almost all autoimmune diseases, genetic, immunological and environmental factors are believed to play a part in the expression of PsA. It is an inflammatory disease that manifests in both articular and extra-articular features. Musculoskeletal manifestiations include peripheral arthritis, spondylitis, dactylitis (inflammation of the whole digit)

Table 13.2 Psoriatic arthritis treatment toolbox.

Therapy class	Therapies
Oral therapies	MTX, sulfasalazine, cyclosporine, leflunomide, apremilast
TNF inhibitors	Etanercept, infliximab, adalimumab, golimumab, certolizumab pegol
IL-12/23 inhibitor	Ustekinumab
IL-17A inhibitors	Secukinumab, ixekizumab
CTLA-4 Ig	Abatacept
JAK/STAT inhibitor	Tofacitinib
Symptomatic therapies	Nonsteroidal anti-inflammatory drugs, glucocorticoids, local glucocorticoid injections
Psoriasis therapies	Topical therapies, phototherapy, other oral therapies: retinoids IL-17R blocker, brodalumab IL-23 inhibitors guselkumab, tildrakizumab, rizankizumab
Non-pharmacological therapies	Physical therapy, occupational therapy, smoking cessation, weight loss, massage therapy, exercise

MTX, methotrexate; TNF, tumor necrosis factor; IL, interleukin; CTLA-4, cytotoxic T-lymphocyte-associated protein 4; JAK, janus kinase; STAT, signal transducer and activator of transcription.

and enthesitis (inflammation where tendon, ligament or joint capsule attach to a bone). Other features are fatigue, functional limitations, sleep disturbances, diminished work capacity and social participation (Orbai et al. 2017). Extra-articular features include uveitis and inflammatory bowel disease.

Diagnosis is made on history taking and clinical examination. There is no single blood test to diagnose PsA, but it is recognised that individuals affected are usually RF negative. Markers of inflammation may be elevated in active PsA.

PsA is a chronic condition and the aim of treatment is to achieve remission and slow down progression. The current treatment recommendations follow a step-up approach using conventional DMARDs and then biologic treatments, which are similar to other inflammatory arthritides (refer to Table 13.2 for the management of RA).

Rheumatoid Arthritis

RA is a complex, chronic inflammatory condition that has both articular and extra-articular effects. The most distinctive feature of RA is persistent symmetric polyarthritis that affects the hands and feet, though any joint lined by a synovial membrane may be involved. It is also characterised by its fluctuating disease pattern, with episodes of flares. Extra-articular involvement of organs such as the skin, heart, lungs and eyes can be significant.

RA is the most common inflammatory arthropathy and has the potential to cause a significant impact on quality of life. It has a prevalence of 1% in the population and it is estimated over 430 000 people in the UK have this condition (Versus Arthritis 2021). Although people of any age can be affected, the peak age range for onset is 30–50 years and women are affected two to four times more than men. RA has a significant impact on life and can affect roles, relationships and levels of independence as the disease progresses. Approximately one-third of people stop work because of RA within 2 years of its onset and this increases after that (Ledingham et al. 2017).

Although the pathogenesis of RA is still not fully understood, over the last 10 years the understanding of its underlying pathobiology has significantly increased. There is evidence that multiple different immunological and inflammatory pathways are involved, with descriptions of new cytokines, mediators and pathways that are assisting in understanding the pathology and developing new treatments. The search for a single trigger for RA is ongoing. It is hypothesised that an external trigger, e.g. cigarette smoking, infection or trauma, sets off an autoimmune reaction in genetically susceptible individuals, leading to synovial hypertrophy and chronic joint inflammation along with the potential for extra-articular manifestations.

RA is an autoimmune condition where pro-inflammatory cytokines are known to have an important role in causing chronic inflammation.

Abnormal production of numerous cytokines and other inflammatory mediators has been demonstrated in patients with RA, including the following:

- tumour necrosis factor alpha (TNF-α)
- interleukin (IL)-1
- IL 6
- IL-8.

Inflammation is the body's normal response to tissue injury, whether caused by bacteria, trauma, chemicals, heat or other phenomenon. Inflammation usually subsides when its task is completed, but maintenance of the inflammation in RA is thought to be caused by an abnormal autoimmune reaction.

The onset of clinical RA is preceded by a period of pre-rheumatoid arthritis (pre-RA). The development of pre-RA and its progression to established RA has been categorised into the following phases (Paul et al. 2017):

- Phase I: Interaction between genetic and environmental risk factors of RA

- Phase II: Production of RA autoantibodies, such as RF and anticyclic citrullinated peptide (anti-CCP)
- Phase III: Development of arthralgia or joint stiffness without any clinical evidence of arthritis
- Phase IV: Development of arthritis in one or two joints (i.e. early undifferentiated arthritis); if intermittent, the arthritis at this stage is termed palindromic rheumatism
- Phase V: Established RA

Not all individuals will progress through the full sequence of phases, and current research is investigating ways to identify patients who are at risk of progression and to delay or prevent RA in those patients (Deane and Holers 2021).

Inflammation of the synovial membrane surrounding the joint capsules and tendon sheaths is called synovitis. It causes synovial cell hyperplasia and endothelial cell activation, which can progress to uncontrolled inflammation, leading to destruction of various tissues, including cartilage, bone, tendons, ligaments and blood vessels. Although the articular structures are the primary sites involved in RA, other tissues are also affected.

The symptoms of inflammation are redness, pain, heat, swelling and possibly loss of function of the affected joint. The clinical presentation of RA is often pain, persistent synovitis and early-morning stiffness. Initial presentation is usually of symmetrical joint involvement with pain and inflammation of the metacarpal phalangeal (MCP), PIP and MTP joints, although this may progress to other joints. Affected joints are often described as stiff, as if trying to move them against a resistant force. There are also extra-articular features of RA and these include fever, weight loss, fatigue, anaemia, ocular problems (scleritis, episcleritis and keratoconjunctivitis sicca), cardiac (pericarditis, endocarditis, pulmonary pleural effusions and fibrosing alveolitis) and osteoporosis.

The American College of Rheumatology (ACR)/European League Against Rheumatism (EULAR) classification criteria 2010 for RA are designed to identify patients with unexplained inflammatory arthritis in at least one peripheral joint and a short duration of symptoms who would benefit from early therapeutic intervention. This is different from the 1987 ACR criteria, which lacked the sensitivity to detect early RA (Aletaha et al. 2010).

The ACR/EULAR classification system is a score-based algorithm for RA that incorporates the following four factors:

- joint involvement: swelling or tenderness on examination or the presence of synovitis, which may be confirmed on imaging studies
- serology test results: RF and/or anti-citrullinated protein antibody (ACPA)
- acute-phase reactant test results: CRP and/or ESR
- patient self-reporting of the duration of signs and symptoms.

The maximum number of points possible is 10. A classification of definitive RA requires a score of 6/10 or higher. Patients with a score lower than 6/10 should be reassessed over time. If patients already have erosive changes characteristic of RA, they meet the definition of RA, and application of this diagnostic algorithm is unnecessary.

NICE (2018a,b) recommends that people with suspected persistent synovitis be referred for specialist rheumatologist opinion with diagnosis based on clinical findings. Urgent referral should be made for patients who present with the small joints of the hands or feet affected, more than one joint affected and if there is a delay of 3 months or longer from the onset of symptoms.

A number of key blood tests assist in the diagnosis and monitoring of RA and fall into three categories: markers of inflammation, hematologic parameters and immunologic parameters. These include the following:

- ESR
- CRP level
- complete blood count (CBC)
- RF assay: RF is not specific for RA but is also present in other connective tissue diseases, infections and autoimmune disorders, as well as in 1–5% of healthy people. The presence of RF predicts radiographic progression of bone erosions, independent of disease activity (Aletaha et al. 2013).
- antinuclear antibody (ANA) assay: Although ANAs are present in approximately 40% of patients with RA, test results for antibodies to most nuclear antigen subsets are negative.
- anti-CCP.

Assays for anti-citrullinated protein antibody (ACPA, often tested as anti-CCP) are now being used clinically for diagnosing RA. ACPA-positive patients may have a more erosive RA disease course than ACPA-negative patients (Van Venrooji et al. 2011).

X-ray remains a useful investigation for monitoring joint deterioration where bone erosions clearly appear. The use of ultrasound scanning has become standard practice in assessing and measuring the degree of synovitis in joints and soft tissue. It can also ascertain early erosions and tendon ruptures (Kane et al. 2004).

Management

Management of inflammatory arthritis, i.e. RA and PsA, has advanced significantly over recent decades due to research and development in pharmacological treatments.

Early recognition of symptoms, diagnosis and rapid initiation of treatment are the key to reducing joint inflammation, preventing joint damage and therefore ensuring patients' independence. Treat to target is a key strategy recommended in the NICE (2018a,b) clinical guidelines on the management of RA in adults. This strategy involves treating active RA with the aim of achieving a target of remission or low disease activity if remission cannot be achieved, i.e. treat-to-target. Achieving the target may involve trying multiple conventional disease-modifying anti-rheumatic drugs and biological DMARDs with different mechanisms of action.

The first-line treatment for patients newly diagnosed with RA includes conventional DMARDs or a combination of DMARDs (one of which should be methotrexate) plus corticosteroids. Ideally treatment should be initiated within 3 months of symptom onset to prevent the development of erosions and deformities.

There are a number of different DMARDs with different modes of action, special precautions, indications, side effects and monitoring requirements. DMARDs can be used as monotherapy or in combination.

Methotrexate

Methotrexate is available as an oral or subcutaneous preparation. It is a once-weekly medication with the dose starting at 7.5 mg once weekly to a maximum dose of 25 mg weekly. Its mechanism of action is likely to involve T-cell suppression via its effects on purine and pyrimidine metabolism, but the mechanism is not fully understood (Cronstein 2005). Folic acid is co-prescribed with methotrexate to reduce the side effects associated with its use.

Sulphasalazine

Sulfasalazine is a prodrug that combines a salicylate and a sulfa antibiotic. The mechanism of action is not fully understood. It is usually commenced at 500 mg daily and increased weekly to a maximum tolerated dose of 2–3 g daily.

Leflunomide

This DMARD is frequently used when patients are intolerant to methotrexate or if methotrexate is contraindicated. Its mode of action is through inhibition of pyrimidine synthesis. It is an oral medication taken as 10–20 mg tablet daily.

Hydroxychloroquine

Hydroxychloroquine is generally considered a safe and well-tolerated DMARD, but is rarely used as monotherapy except in very mild disease. It is frequently used in combination with other DMARDs. This is an antimalarial compound that has been shown to suppress the immune system in a non-specific way. Dosing should be based on weight and the

Table 13.3 The Disease Activity Score (DAS28) for the assessment of rheumatoid arthritis disease activity.

DAS28 is a composite outcome measure that assesses:

- Patient global assessment using the visual analogue score from 0 (very good) to 10 (very bad)
  - Clinician assessment of 28 joints to count how many joints are tender and/or swollen
- Either an erythrocyte sedimentation rate or a C-reactive protein measurement

The results are combined to produce the DAS28 score, which correlates with the extent of disease activity:

- <2.6 disease remission
- 2.6–3.2 low disease activity
- 3.2–5.1 moderate disease activity
- >5.1 high disease activity

Royal College of Ophthalmologists recommends that the dosage does not exceed 6.5 mg/kg daily. This is because of the rare but potentially serious complication of retinal toxicity. Disease control is generally assessed using the Disease Activity Score (DAS28, see Table 13.3), which is a composite score that includes clinician-assessed tender and swollen joints, a visual analogue scale (VAS) and measurement of either ESR or CRP (both blood markers of inflammation). Treatment is titrated as per the DAS28 score. It is an important assessment tool for monitoring disease activity and should be used to determine whether an increase (including qualification for biological medications) or decrease of treatment is indicated.

Biologic Medications

The development of these targeted biological therapies has improved the management of patients with RA, offering a therapeutic option for moderate and active disease that is not controlled adequately by traditional DMARD therapies. There are number of biologic therapies licenced for use in RA all of which block pro-inflammatory cytokines, reducing inflammation, therefore symptoms and joint damage (see Table 13.4).

Janus Kinase Medications

Janus kinase (JAK) inhibitors are the newest class of drugs used to treat RA. Like biologic drugs, these are 'targeted' therapies, which work on the immune response. Unlike the biologics, they can be taken in tablet form, as they are small molecule therapies. These enzymes normally promote inflammation and autoimmunity (see Table 13.5).

The symptomatic management of RA consists primarily of NSAIDs and corticosteroids (Moura et al. 2018). NSAIDs are used in the acute phase response to reduce pain and

Table 13.4 Biologic therapies and licencing indications.

Drug name	Structure	Delivery	Indications
Abatacept	Reduced T-cell activity	IV infusion SC injection	RA
Adalimumab	mAb to TNF	SC injection	RA, PsA, AS
Anakinara	IL-1β inhibitor	SC injection	RA
Certolizumab Pegol	Pegylated antibody fragment to TNF	SC injection	RA
Etanercept	Soluble fusion TNF receptor	SC injection	RA, PsA, AS
Golimumab	mAb to TNF	SC injection	RA, PsA, AS
Infliximab	mAb to TNF	IV infusion	RA, PsA, AS
Ixekizumab	Binds to IL-17a	SC injection	PsA, AS
Rituximab	Depletes B cells	IV infusion	RA
Sarilimumab	IL-6 inhibitor	SC injection	
Secukinumab	Binds to IL-17a	SC injection	PsA, AS
Tocilizumab	mAb to IL-6 receptor	SC injection	RA

AS, axial spondyloarthritis; IL, interleukin; IV, intravenous; mAb, monoclonal antibody; PsA, psoriatic arthritis; RA, rheumatoid arthritis; SC, subcutaneous; TNF, tumour necrosis factor.

Table 13.5 Licensed indications for JAK inhibitors.

JAK inhibitor name	Indications
Tofacitinib	RA, PsA
Baricitinib	RA
Upadacitinib	RA, PsA, AS
Filgotinib	RA

AS, axial spondyloarthritis; PsA, psoriatic arthritis; RA, rheumatoid arthritis.

stiffness by decreasing inflammation However, the risk of harm should be considered as their use can lead to serious side effects such as bleeding, gastrointestinal ulceration, renal failure, heart failure, rashes, dizziness, confusion and seizures.

Corticosteroids have greater potency and efficacy than NSAIDs due to the complex mechanisms of their anti-inflammatory and immunosuppressive effects. Long-term side effects of steroids include weight gain, water retention, muscle weakness, diabetes and bone thinning. Thus, they have a short-term use and can be administered orally, intravenously and intramuscularly (Hua et al. 2020). Intra-articular steroids can be used for particularly swollen or painful joints. Side effects can be reduced by gradually tapering doses as a patient's condition improves. It is important to not abruptly discontinue corticosteroids as this can lead to suppression of the hypothalamic–pituitary–adrenal axis or flares of RA.

Non-pharmacological Management

Various non-pharmacological approaches to treating RA exist, the aim being to complement drug-based therapies. These include the following:

- exercise
- sleep
- diet
- weight loss
- management of comorbidities (e.g. cardiovascular risk, glycaemic control)
- smoking cessation.

As RA has a considerable psychosocial impact on the patient with reports of depression, low self-esteem and isolation, a multidisciplinary approach is recommended, including access to specialist physiotherapy, occupational therapy, podiatry and nurses (NICE 2018a,b).

Specialist physiotherapy aims to promote general fitness and exercise, as well as teaching specific exercises for joint flexibility, muscle strengthening and managing functional impairments. Hydrotherapy maybe offered. This can also help to control pain, and referral in the early stages of the disease can help prevent malalignment. Most patients also obtain relief from heat aids and some use TENS.

Specialist occupational therapy facilitates independence. Problems with hand function are evaluated and appropriate management advice given. Aids to assist with daily living may include gadgets to help with washing and dressing.

Specialist podiatrists provide advice with regard to footwear and foot care. The feet are often affected by RA, causing mechanical damage and pain. Insoles and suitable footwear can be discussed.

Specialist nurses are involved in monitoring and advising people about how to manage their disease to enable optimal physical, psychological and social functions. Important facets of the role include patient education, facilitating self-management of symptoms, support at diagnosis and throughout the disease process, drug counselling and monitoring, and the coordination of care within the MDT. The rheumatology nurse specialist can also provide telephone support and review. Psychological interventions, for example relaxation, stress management and cognitive coping skills, should also be offered to help adults with RA adjust to living with their condition.

Osteoporosis

Metabolic bone disease is the term used to describe a range of conditions inclusive of osteoporosis, Paget's disease, osteomalacia and osteogenesis imperfecta (OI) (see Chapter 23 for further information regarding OI) that affect the quality of bone and are characterised by pain, deformity and fracture. This chapter only discusses the most common of these, osteoporosis. The World Health Organisation (WHO 1994, p. 12) define osteoporosis as:

> a progressive systemic skeletal disease characterized by low bone mass and micro-architectural deterioration of bone tissue, with a consequent increase in bone fragility and susceptibility to fracture.

One in two women and one in five men over the age of 50 in the UK will fracture a bone mainly because of osteoporosis, with an estimated three million people in the UK alone suffering from the condition (www.nos.org.uk). Although fractures can occur in different parts of the body, the wrist, hip and spine are most commonly affected. Each year the numbers of people with osteoporosis in the UK rise as the population ages, resulting in over 70 000 hip fractures, 50 000 wrist fractures and 120 000 spinal fractures. Johnell and Kanis (2006) report the condition leading to nearly nine million fractures annually worldwide. Direct medical costs from fragility fractures to the UK healthcare economy were estimated at £1.8 billion in 2000, with the potential to increase to £2.2 billion by 2025,and with most of these costs relating to hip fracture care (see Chapters 18 and 19 for further exploration of fragility fractures relating to osteoporosis).

Prevention may not be totally attainable but the risk and severity can be reduced. For example, childhood through to young adulthood is the time to 'bank' good-quality bone through diet and weight-bearing activities as bone loses density with age. Consequently, as we age we are more at risk of a fragility fracture. From our mid-20s onwards, our bodies constantly repair and renew bone, with whole parts of our skeletons reproduced every 4–7 years. This process, known as bone remodelling, takes place on the bone's surface thanks to two sets of cells, osteoclasts and osteoblasts. Then from around the age of 40, the osteoclasts become more active and the osteoblasts less active; so more bone is removed and less is formed. This is known as age-related bone loss and can lead to osteoporosis, particularly for those whose bones pre-exist with low density. By the age of 60

approximately 15% of all women have osteoporosis and this figure increases to over 25% by the age of 80 (NICE 2008). Because of increased bone loss after the menopause in women and age-related bone loss in both women and men, the prevalence of osteoporosis increases markedly with age:

> . . .because of increased bone loss after the menopause in women, and age-related bone loss in both women and men, the prevalence of osteoporosis increases markedly with age, from 2% at 50 years to more than 25% at 80 years, 52% in women. As the longevity of the population increases, so will the incidence of osteoporosis and fragility fracture. (NICE 2012)

Education is therefore fundamental in the prevention and control of osteoporosis and in raising awareness, especially for primary and secondary prevention in post-menopausal women. The practitioner must identify what the patient knows already, identify risk factors, and inform of treatments and associated side effects of drug interventions. Box 13.1 provides examples of appropriate educational information.

Healthy bones have a shell of solid bone and an internal honeycombed network of spongy bone (see Chapter 4). When osteoporosis is present, bones lose a certain amount of both structures. This is caused by age-related bone loss but other risk factors also have an impact. Risk factors include (Tanna 2009):

- genetic: role in regulating bone, skeletal geometry and bone turnover density
- hormonal: post-menopausal women are at higher risk
- alcohol: heavy alcohol consumption is associated with reduction in bone density
- nutritional: important for bone health
- smoking: associated with increased risk of fracture
- corticosteroids: prolonged use is the most common cause of secondary osteoporosis
- physical inactivity/falls: low bone density
- low body weight/weight loss: associated with greater bone loss and increased risk of fracture.

Diagnosis

Osteoporosis is usually diagnosed from a bone scan post-fracture or at an osteoporosis clinic. The dual energy X-ray absorptiometry (DXA) scan is currently the most accurate and reliable means of assessing bone density and associated risk of fracture. It is a simple, painless procedure that routinely uses very low doses of radiation to scan the spine/hips, wrist or heel using *T* and *Z* scores as markers

---

Box 13.1   Patient Education on Osteoporosis

- Outline in simple terms what osteoporosis is
- Outline the causes and consequences of osteoporosis
- Emphasise how maintaining a healthy lifestyle can minimise the problem
- Explore patients' dietary habits, ensuring that they are eating meals that incorporate a wide variety of foods from the four main groups (fruit and vegetables, carbohydrates, dairy products and protein) for a natural way of providing minerals, vitamins and energy
- Identify the patient's knowledge of what foods contain calcium and their daily intake
- Emphasise that the minimal calcium intake should be 700 mg daily and in some cases 1000–12 000 mg a day and is vital for healthy bones, giving examples to achieve this intake
- Outline what foods are rich in calcium and that low-fat or fat-free dairy products often have more calcium than full-fat versions
- Discuss the importance of vitamin D to help the body absorb calcium: 15–20 minutes of sun exposure to the face and arms three or four times weekly during the summer should provide enough vitamin D for the year
- GP may prescribe a calcium and vitamin D supplement and or bisphosphonate, reinforce why it is important to comply with this and take as prescribed
- Identify if the patient smokes, explain how smoking impacts on the bone and construction and the need to avoid smoking
- Assess alcohol intake: risk factor if excessive (daily intake should be no more than 2–3 units daily for women), explain what a unit is
- Identify the degree of activity and exercise routine: outline the value of weight-bearing exercise, e.g. walking, swimming, golf
- Maintain a safe environment: raise awareness of the need to minimise the risk of falls, e.g. use of footwear, turn on the light at night to go to toilet
- Encourage questions and give accurate information
- Use available leaflets to illustrate and reinforce important points
- Ask some questions to check patient's understanding, record in notes

---

(Tanna 2009). The WHO (1994) criteria which generated the T score, implies the number of standard deviations (SD) which separate the patient from the mean value of a healthy young population. A Z score is the number of SDs that separates the patient from an age-matched health population. In reality, osteopenia (bone mineral density [BMD] lower than normal) has a T score between −1 and −2.5 SD, with osteoporosis has a T score of −2.5 SD or below and progressively more severe osteoporosis; a T score of −2.5 SD or below with one or more associated fractures.

Drug Treatments

Bisphosphonates are non-hormonal drugs that help maintain bone strength and reduce fracture rates. They inhibit osteoclast action and slow down the rate of bone resorption to maintain the patient's current BMD level and reduce the risk of fracture. The drugs have poor rates of absorption and potential gastrointestinal side effects, and compliance is reported to be poor. Guidance on taking the drug is fundamental to patient compliance and outcome; it should be swallowed on an empty stomach, with a glass of water, while standing, then the patient should remain upright and

fast for 30 minutes. The main drugs in this range are alendronic acid or alendronate (Fosamax), cyclical etidronate (Didronel PMO), ibandronate (Bonviva), risedronate (Actonel) and zoledronic acid (Aclasta). These have been shown to reduce the risk of fractures in the spine and, in some cases, the hip. NICE (2012) recommend Alendronate as a treatment option for the primary prevention of osteoporotic fragility fractures in the following groups:

- Women aged 70 years or older who have an independent clinical risk factor for fracture or an indicator of low BMD and who are confirmed to have osteoporosis. Women aged 75 years or older who have two or more independent clinical risk factors for fracture or indicators of low BMD. A DXA scan may not be required if the responsible clinician considers it to be clinically inappropriate or unfeasible.
- Women aged 65–69 years who have an independent clinical risk factor for fracture and who are confirmed to have osteoporosis.
- Post-menopausal women younger than 65 years who have an independent clinical risk factor for fracture (see below), at least one additional indicator of low BMD and are confirmed to have osteoporosis.

When the decision has been made to initiate treatment with Alendronate, the preparation prescribed should be chosen on the basis of the lowest acquisition cost available. Alternative therapies include:

- Hormone replacement therapy (HRT): oestrogen replacement for women at the menopause stage of their life, which helps maintain bone strength and reduces fracture rates.
- Selective oestrogen receptor modulator (SERM) drugs act in a similar way to oestrogen on the bone, helping to maintain bone strength and reduce fracture rates, especially in the spine.
- Testosterone therapy is testosterone replacement for men with low testosterone levels to help maintain bone strength, calcium and vitamin D.

Paget's Disease

Paget's disease is a metabolic condition that affects the normal repair and renewal process of bone. The Paget's Association (https://paget.org.uk), a national UK charity, report the disease to occur in any bone, often causing no symptoms and often diagnosed by chance. Symptoms include pain, deformity and fracture with either single or multiple bones affected and common sites being the spine, skull, pelvis and thigh (femur). The risk of developing Paget's disease increases with age and it is most commonly diagnosed in those over 50 years. It is the second most common metabolic bone disease after osteoporosis. Approximately 1% of people in the UK over the age of 55 years are thought to be affected. The condition is also common in other European countries such as France, Spain and Italy, and in people of European descent who have immigrated to other regions of the world, such as Australia, New Zealand, the USA and Canada (paget.org.uk/). Box 13.2 presents a recent clinical guideline for the diagnosis and management of the condition in adults.

Osteomyelitis

Osteomyelitis is an acute or chronic infection of bone and its structures. The most common organism responsible is *Staphylococcus aureus* (Lew and Waldvogel 2004). It is a progressive condition and associated inflammation leads to necrotic destruction of bone that can lead to an acute infection becoming chronic. It is relatively uncommon because bone is resistant to infection so it tends to occur in patients with significant risk factors such as diabetes that reduce their resistance or make their bone more vulnerable

---

Box 13.2   Evidence Digest: Paget's Disease

A clinical guideline for the diagnosis and management of Paget's disease of bone in adults was published in 2019 on behalf of the Paget's Association, the European Calcified Tissue Society (ECTS) and the International Osteoporosis Foundation (IOF). The guideline was reproduced from the work of Ralston et al. (2019). Six key questions form its basis. Based on these, a full literature search was performed, and the quality of the evidence was assessed using explicit criteria. The full document has unrestricted online access and it can be downloaded from https://paget.org.uk.

The following recommendations were highlighted by the Guideline Development Group as the most important.

1) Radionuclide bone scans, in addition to targeted radiographs, are recommended as a means of fully and accurately defining the extent of the metabolically active disease in patients with Paget's disease.
2) Serum total alkaline phosphatase (ALP) is recommended as a first-line biochemical screening test, in combination with liver function tests, for the presence of metabolically active Paget's disease.
3) Bisphosphonates are recommended for the treatment of bone pain associated with Paget's disease. Zoledronic acid is recommended as the bisphosphonate most likely to give a favourable pain response.
4) Treatment aimed at improving symptoms is recommended over a treat-to-target strategy aimed at normalising total ALP in Paget's disease.
5) Total hip or knee replacements are recommended for patients with Paget's disease who develop osteoarthritis for whom medical treatment is inadequate. There is insufficient information to recommend one type of surgical approach over another.

Source: With permission from Ralston et al. (2019).

---

through trauma or surgery. Its severity and progression can depend on the source of infection, the virulence of the organism involved and the general health of the patient (Brady et al. 2006). It is often a devastating problem for patients as it is very difficult to treat because of necrosis and disruption to the blood supply to bone which mean that systemic and local antibiotic therapy is unsuccessful. Many years of pain and disability are often the result, sometimes with suppurating sinus wounds. The prevention of osteomyelitis following injury and surgery is a major driver for good infection prevention and control practice throughout the patient's care journey. It is also one of the reasons that prophylactic antibiotic therapy is often given following open fracture and orthopaedic surgery. Gosselin et al. (2009) found antibiotics to reduce the incidence of early infections in open fractures of the limbs.

There are several different classifications of osteomyelitis depending on the source of infection. These are outlined in the following sections.

Endogenous (Haematogenous) Osteomyelitis

Endogenous osteomyelitis occurs when pathogens are carried in the blood from sites of infection elsewhere in the body, a process sometimes known as remote 'seeding'. The infection spreads from bone to adjacent soft tissues or remote infections such as urinary tract infection. The prevention of such infections is therefore central to orthopaedic care. This includes, for example, the avoidance of urinary catheterisation.

Endogenous osteomyelitis is more common in infants, children and older people. Before puberty bacteria can gain access to a child's bone, often accumulating in the metaphyseal region (growth area of the bone). The bacteria proliferate and trigger an initial inflammatory response. Once inflammation is initiated the small vessels in bone thrombose. The build-up of pressure in the bone causes the inflammatory exudate to move to the bone cortex separating the periosteum from underlying bone, resulting in a painful subperiosteal abscess. The white cells cannot remove the infected material, resulting in accumulation of infected and ischaemic tissue and the eventual necrosis of underlying bone tissue (sequestrum), which is radiologically visible. Lifting of the periosteum also stimulates an intense osteoblastic response and new bone is laid down partially or completely surrounding the infected bone (involucrum). Openings in the involucrum allow the exudate to escape into the surrounding tissues and ultimately the skin through a sinus tract.

Exogenous Osteomyelitis

Endogenous osteomyelitis is a key route of transmission. The infection enters through open fractures, penetrating wounds and surgical procedures.

Acute Osteomyelitis in Adults (Sudden Onset)

Acute osteomyelitis is usually haematogenous in origin but may be due to trauma in the femur, tibia humerus and thoracolumbar spine. Spinal osteomyelitis is more common in adults past middle age and can result in a spinal cord compression. Clinical presentation often includes (Chihara and Segreti 2010):

- a history of injury 2–3 months previously
- abrupt onset of high pyrexia
- generally feeling unwell
- restriction of movement of affected bone
- pain and tenderness, including on-bone palpation
- local signs of inflammation, including swelling, redness, heat and localised pain.

It is important that the symptoms are not confused with cellulitis, acute septic arthritis, acute rheumatism or a sickle cell crisis.

Investigations include:

- history and clinical examination
- blood counts
- microbiological culture of blood, wound swabs
- aspiration of material from the site of infection for microbiological analysis
- X-ray
- bone scan/CT/MRI.

Imaging will show soft-tissue swelling, narrowing or widening of joint spaces, bone destruction and periosteal reaction. Bone destruction, however, is not apparent until after 10–21 days of infection (Lew and Waldvogel 2004).

Treatment Options

Options include measures to support the limb or spine with a view to reducing pain. This might include traction, splintage or application of a cast. Intravenous antibiotic therapy is used initially and to cover any surgical period up to 2 weeks post-surgery. The switch to oral therapy may happen once the clinical condition stabilises and microbiology results suggest infection is resolved. Treatment for acute infection is usually for 4–6 weeks. Chronic infection is considered below. High doses of antibiotics are required to achieve suitable bone penetration in high enough concentrations in necrotic avascular bone (Lew and Waldvogel 2004).

Chronic Osteomyelitis (Slower Onset)

Chronic osteomyelitis is a severe, persistent and sometimes incapacitating infection of bone and bone marrow that is on the increase due to predisposing conditions such as diabetes mellitus and peripheral vascular disease (Hatzenbuehler and Pulling 2011). Aetiology includes inadequately treated acute osteomyelitis, post open fracture or surgery, infection with TB and syphilis, joint replacement/internal fixation of open fractures and contiguous spread from soft tissue infection. The inflammatory reaction to infection in bone continues over time, leading to sclerosis and deformity with the presence of sequestrum, involucrum, local bone loss and persistent drainage and/or sinus tract formation. The most common organisms are *Staphylococcus aureus*, *Streptococci*, *Pneumococci* and *Myobacterium tuberculosis* (Kneale and Davis 2005). Clinical presentation includes:

- previous history of acute infection/osteomyelitis
- chronic bone pain
- sinus formation and purulent drainage
- low-grade or absent pyrexia
- localised abscess, soft tissue infection or both if a sinus tract becomes obstructed
- persistently feeling unwell.

Treatment includes antibiotic therapy (IV/oral) for a minimum of 6–12 weeks. Surgery is almost always necessary with chronic osteomyelitis as necrotic and dead bone needs to be debrided. Management might also include Papineau technique/vacuum-assisted closure (VAC) (Archdeacon and Messerschmitt 2006) with flaps, antibiotic impregnated beads, bone grafting, soft tissue management and stabilisation. This may often involve the removal of previous metalwork and instability caused by bone damage or loss may require external fixation. Prognosis is dependent on the patient's general health status. Outcomes are improved if treatment is started 3–5 days after the onset of the infection.

Timely diagnosis and intervention in an otherwise well patient can lead to full recovery, although follow-up over several months is needed to monitor for relapse. The condition can have a psychological impact on the patient if recovery is slow and pain severe.

Back Pain

Back pain is a complex series of conditions with considerable variability in pathology and outcome. Most patients with new episodes recover within a few weeks but recurrence is common and individuals with chronic, long-standing back pain tend to show a more persistent course. Most back pain, fortunately, responds to a set of non-surgical interventions that facilitate a gradual return to normal activity for the patient. Patients need to be encouraged to move despite the presence of pain to aid recovery. Progressively intense range of movement and strengthening exercises offer improved stability of the lumbar spine under the guidance of a physiotherapist, while drugs facilitate increased movement and recommencement of normal activities. Drug regimens may include simple analgesics, NSAIDs and muscle relaxants, which can hasten a return to function. When back pain becomes chronic, additional health professionals may become involved. The chronic pain service is often pivotal in developing a personalised plan with a variety of approaches to manage the differing types of pain. For example, stronger opioids for escalating nociceptive type pain and additional medication for neuropathic pain and acupuncture, whilst psychology may better support a reduction in the patient's mood/depression with antidepressants and alternative interventions such as cognitive behavioural therapy as chronic pain does appear to increase the risk of depression in some patients.

LBP is the most common condition within the spectrum, with many people experiencing it at some point in their life. Most LBP episodes are mild and rarely disabling, with only a small proportion of individuals seeking intervention. LBP can impact on the person's quality of life due to reduced mobility and pain, and differential diagnosis is desirable to establish a probable cause, diagnosis and suitable treatments. A GP most often makes the referral to an orthopaedic consultant, which leads to a more in-depth history taking and physical examination using the 'look, feel and move' strategy in conjunction with radiological evidence, e.g. X-ray, MRI and CT, in an attempt to ascertain a diagnosis, which is not always attainable. Listening to the patient and family gives the practitioner the best opportunity to find the cause of LBP. Treatment and care need to consider the patients' individual needs and preferences. Good communication and the provision of information is central in facilitating patient involvement in their care. NICE (2009) offers specific guidance for the early management of LBP and this is summarised in Box 13.3.

In 70% of cases, LBP has no obvious aetiology or pathogenesis as most back pain is muscular or ligamentous in origin rather than skeletal. The soft tissue structures are located deep inside the body, so although radiography, including MRI and CT scans, can pinpoint anatomic anomalies in skeletal structures, such investigations cannot identify the specific causes of pain (Borenstein and Calin 2012). The presence of any of the 'red flags' (fever or weight loss, pain with recumbency, prolonged morning stiffness, acute fracture and viscerogenic pain related to a non-musculoskeletal organ system, e.g. genitourinary) might suggest systemic conditions (i.e. possible fracture, tumour or infection, cauda equina syndrome and spondyloarthropathy). Any red flag should be noted at the initial assessment, as they will influence the subsequent assessment and management of the patient.

Treatment should ideally involve an MDT approach to develop a patient-centred plan of care. A wide range of professionals can help the patient address challenges in both quality of life and the ability to undertake normal activities of daily living. Chronic back pain often leads to financial and relationship difficulties, which may lead to depression. Spinal surgery is considered in Chapter 14.

Box 13.3   Evidence Digest: Managing Low Back Pain and Sciatica (Adapted from NICE)

NICE Pathway (NICE 2021): Managing low back pain (LBP) and sciatica

This pathway is for people aged 16 and over with low back pain with or without sciatic. It provides advice and information, tailored to the person's needs and capabilities, to help them self-manage their low back pain with or without sciatica, at all steps of the treatment pathway. It promotes and facilitates a return to work or normal activities of daily living.

Quality standards include:

Self-management: Exercise

Consider a group exercise programme (biomechanical, aerobic, mind–body or a combination of approaches).

Pharmacological treatments: LBP

Consider NSAIDs, at the lowest effective dose for the shortest possible period of time, or weak opioids (with or without paracetamol) only if an NSAID is contraindicated, not tolerated or has been ineffective.

DO NOT offer paracetamol alone or offer routine opioids, selective serotonin reuptake inhibitors, serotonin–norepinephrine reuptake inhibitors or tricyclic antidepressants, gabapentinoids or antiepileptics for managing low back pain.

Pharmacological treatments: Sciatica

DO NOT offer gabapentinoids, other antiepileptics, oral corticosteroids or benzodiazepines as there is no overall evidence of benefit and there is evidence of harm. Do not offer opioids for managing chronic sciatica. If a person is already taking opioids, gabapentinoids or benzodiazepines for sciatica, explain the risks of continuing these medicines. As part of shared decision-making about whether to stop opioids, gabapentinoids or benzodiazepines for sciatica, discuss the problems associated with withdrawal with the person.

NB: If prescribing NSAIDs for LBP or sciatica take into account potential differences in gastrointestinal, liver and cardio-renal toxicity, and the person's risk factors, including age.

Scoliosis

The spine has gentle curves that develop as a child grows, but within such natural curves three key deformities can develop: scoliosis, kyphosis and lordosis. Only scoliosis, the type most commonly met by the practitioner, will be discussed here. Scoliosis refers to a side-to-side curvature of the spine that affects a small percentage of the population, approximately 2% in women and less than 0.5% of men. The condition has familial tendencies and the majority of scoliosis is idiopathic (of no known cause), usually starting in the early teens or pre-teens and gradually progressing in severity of the curvature as growth occurs. Once the rapid growth of puberty is over, mild curves often do not change whilst severe curves nearly always develop further. Although scoliosis can occur in children with cerebral palsy, muscular dystrophy, spina bifida and other miscellaneous conditions, most scoliosis is found in otherwise healthy young people, therefore parents should watch for the following signs of scoliosis beginning when their child is about 8 years of age, with any one sign warranting investigation:

- uneven shoulders
- prominent shoulder blade or shoulder blades
- uneven waist
- elevated hips
- leaning to one side.

Adult scoliosis may represent the progression of a condition that began in childhood and was not diagnosed or treated during growth. What might have started out as a slight or moderate curve could have progressed in the absence of treatment. If allowed to progress, in severe cases adult scoliosis can lead to chronic severe back pain, deformity and difficulty in breathing.

Cobb's angle is the measurement used for the evaluation of curves in scoliosis on an AP radiographic image of the spine using a protractor. A line is drawn along the superior end plate of the superior end vertebra involved in the curve and a second line drawn along the inferior end plate of the inferior end vertebra. If the end plates are indistinct, the line may be drawn through the pedicles. The angle between these two lines (or lines drawn perpendicular to them) is measured as the Cobb angle. Shaw et al. (2012) reported on the use of smart phone technology to offer an equivalent Cobb measurement tool equal to the manual protractor. In S-shaped scoliosis, where there are two contiguous curves, the lower end vertebra of the upper curve will represent the upper end vertebra of the lower curve. Because the Cobb angle reflects curvature only in a single plane and fails to account for vertebral rotation, it may not accurately demonstrate the severity of three-dimensional spinal deformities. As a rule, a Cobb angle of 10° is regarded as the minimum angulation to define scoliosis.

Treatment options include the following:

- Doing nothing, which may be reasonable depending on the age of the person and the predicted outcome. Doing nothing in the teen years, however, may be disastrous.
- Bracing has been shown to be an effective method to prevent curves from getting more progressive. However, this treatment is reserved for children and young people in whom a rapid increase in the curve needs to be thwarted. A brace worn 16 or more hours per day has been shown to be effective in preventing 90% or more of the curves from getting worse. Unfortunately, a brace worn 23 hours per day and worn properly does not guarantee that the curve will not continue to increase. Yet, in curves that are mild, i.e. between 20° and 35°, a brace may be quite effective. However, bracing cannot 'hold' curves greater than 40°. The brace may feel hot, hard and uncomfortable, and although it normally cannot be seen under the clothes, it can make a young person more self-conscious about their body image (http://www.scoliosisrx.com).
- For those who already have a significant curve and deformity, surgery can reduce the curve and significantly reduce the deformity.

Surgery is usually offered to teen and pre-teens who already have a curve of around 40° or more. Surgery can commence around 40° while there are many excellent surgeons who defer to 45° or 50°. In the adult, the reasons for surgery include increasing discomfort or pain with an increasing curve. For many women the combination of a deformity in the hip line and the increasing discomfort make surgery a reasonable option. Others note the increasing deformity in the chest coupled with an increase in the rib hump. However, for those people surgery can (not always and certainly not guaranteed) reduce the deformity and the discomfort or pain.

Common surgical intervention includes anterior and posterior spinal fusion (PSF). Posterior spinal infusion with spinal instrumentation (Matusz et al. 2005) has been the mainstay of surgical treatment since the late 1960s. Thoracoscopic anterior instrumentation is an alternative as instead of a long open thoracotomy to obtain exposure of the anterior spine, small incisions are made to allow the introduction of a thoracoscope and working instruments. The advantages are less postoperative pain in the chest wall, better long-term cosmetics and equal release when compared to open discectomy plus alternative growth rod instrumentation (Ember and Noordeen 2005).

Spinal Stenosis

Spinal stenosis refers to narrowing of the central spinal canal. Although narrowing does not always result in nerve compression, it can create pressure on the nerves, often resulting in pain or numbness in the region impacted by the compressed nerve or nerves. There are many causes, including tumours, congenital defects, physical injury and bone disease. However, the most prevalent causes are the ageing effects of intervertebral disc degeneration, bone overgrowth and ligament thickening. Lumbar and cervical areas are most commonly affected and both lead to significant pain, disability and impact on quality of life. Lumbar spinal stenosis has become the most common indication for spinal decompression surgery in older patients.

Intervertebral Disc Disease

Age-related changes in the intervertebral disc can lead to degeneration and increased likelihood of a clinical problem. A prolapsed intervertebral disc (often termed a 'slipped disc') commonly occurs in the lumbar and cervical areas, which have more mobility, which puts the discs at high risk of damage (Smith 2005). The primary symptom is pain of varying severity and frequency. Depending on the site of the disc prolapse and the nerve involvement, the patient will typically have intense radicular (nerve root) pain. The pressure that the disc puts on the nerve roots often causes neurological symptoms in addition to the pain, with some patients developing motor weakness.

The management of back pain is usually treated conservatively, initially with MDT involvement and discussion with patients regarding realistic options (Murray 2011). Medication, exercises and/or a local steroid injection via epidural may benefit patients. Surgery is indicated if the following indicators are present:

- unrelenting leg pain
- neural damage
- cauda equina syndrome.

A central disc prolapse constitutes a medical emergency and an immediate MRI scan is required. Decompression within 24 hours of the onset of symptoms is needed as the disc presses on the cauda equina, causing the following motor and sensory problems:

- loss of perianal sensation, known as saddle anaesthesia
- bilateral motor weakness in the legs
- sphincter disturbance to the bowel and bladder.

Juvenile Idiopathic Arthritis: An Outline

NICE (2015) define JIA as 'an inflammation of the joints that begins in people under 16 years of age where the cause or trigger is uncertain or unknown (idiopathic). JIA lasts for at least six weeks and causes pain, stiffness and swelling of the affected joints'. It can also cause stress and negative emotions for the child and young person (CYP), affecting their health and wellbeing and may impact their education. It is a chronic condition and the most common type of arthritis in CYP. It can also affect the eyes, bones, mouth/jaw, neck, ankles/feet, skin, lungs, heart, digestive tract, reproductive organs, and weight loss/gain (Juvenile Idiopathic Arthritis Foundation 2021).

Types of JIA

NICE (2015) identify several different forms of JIA, characterised by the number of affected joints or associated features:

- Oligoarticular: begins by affecting four or fewer joints, but by after 6 months, or longer, five or more joints become affected.
- Polyarticular: five or more joints are affected.
- Enthesitis associated with JIA relates to swelling of tendons at the point of insertion into bones, i.e. these insertion points are known as enthesitis.
- Psoriatic: associated with psoriasis and flaky skin condition.

Diagnosis

JIA is diagnosed using an array of diagnostic approaches, medical history, physical examination and laboratory tests (Juvenile Idiopathic Arthritis Foundation 2021) alongside differential diagnosis.

Differential diagnosis of JIA can include:

- septic arthritis
- post-infective/reactive arthritis
- systemic lupus erythematosus
- acute lymphoblastic leukaemia
- trauma
- joint hypermobility
- fibromyalgia
- complex regional pain syndrome
- osteomyelitis
- bone tumour
- inflammatory bowel disease
- Henoch-Schönlein purpura or other vasculitis
- rheumatic fever.

(Adapted from the Royal Australian College of General Practitioners (RACGP). Clinical guideline for the diagnosis and management of juvenile idiopathic arthritis, 2009. Available at www.racgp.org.au/guidelines/musculoskeletal diseases).

Treatment

There is no cure for JIA, the aim is remission. The Juvenile Idiopathic Arthritis Foundation (2021) reports that the goals of JIA treatment are to:

- slow down or stop inflammation
- relieve symptoms, control pain and improve quality of life
- prevent joint and organ damage
- preserve joint function and mobility
- reduce long-term health effects
- achieve remission (little or no disease activity or symptoms).

A well-rounded plan includes medication, complementary therapies and healthy lifestyle habits.

- Medications: JIA commonly follows a stepped approach that begins with an NSAID, followed by corticosteroids and a DMARD such as methotrexate. If an adequate response is not achieved with methotrexate, one of several biologic DMARDs may be offered (NICE 2018a,b). The reviewed NICE guidance was moved to the static list in 2018 due to no change: the biologic DMARDs abatacept (Orencia), adalimumab (Humira), etanercept (Enbrel) and tocilizumab (RoActemra) are recommended as possible treatments for people with polyarticular JIA. Adalimumab and etanercept are also recommended as possible treatments for people with enthesitis-related JIA. Etanercept is recommended as a possible treatment for people with psoriatic JIA (NICE 2018a,b).
- Multidisciplinary care: The aim is to develop an individualised plan for affected children and young people as it gives the best chance of meeting their medical, psychological and educational needs (Whitehead 2010).
- Self-care: Certain habits can help manage the disease and relieve symptoms, for example healthy eating, hot and cold treatments, mind–body therapies, balancing activity with rest and topical treatments.

Summary

All key orthopaedic conditions discussed here continue to challenge patients and the nurse practitioners who care for them. With significant development of professional roles and increasing autonomy for nurses along with heightened engagement in evidence-based practice and national guidance such as that from NICE, the way in which care is delivered can ensure optimum outcomes whether treatment is conservative, pharmacological or surgical.

Further Reading

Coates, L., Corp, N., van der Windt, D. et al. (2021). GRAPPA treatment recommendations: an update from the 2020 GRAPPA Annual Meeting. *J. Rheumatol.* https://doi.org/10.3899.jrheum.201681.

Hamilton, L., Barkham, N., Bhalla, A. et al. (2017, 2017). BSR and BHPR guideline for the treatment of axial spondyloarthritis (including ankylosing spondylitis) with biologics. *Rheumatology* 56: 313–316.

Hertz, K. and Santy-Tomlinson, J. (ed.) (2018). *Fragility Fracture Nursing: Holistic Care and Management of the Orthogeriatric Patient* [Open Access]. Cham (CH): Springer PMID: 31314236. https://pubmed.ncbi.nlm.nih.gov/31314236.

National Institute for Health and Care Excellence (2020) *Osteoarthritis: care and management.* Clinical Guidance NG 177.

National Institute for Health and Care Excellence (2018) *Rheumatoid Arthritis in Adults.* Clinical Guidance NG 100.

Smolen, J., Landewé, R.B.M., Bijlsma, J.W.J. et al. (2020). EULAR recommendations for the management of rheumatoid arthritis with synthetic and biological disease-modifying antirheumatic drugs: 2019 update. *Ann. Rheum. Dis.* 79 (6): 685–699.

References

Adam, W.R. (2011). Non-steroidal anti-inflammatory drugs and the risks of acute renal failure: number needed to harm. *Nephrology* 16 (2): 154–155.

Aletaha, D., Neogi, T., Silman, A.J. et al. (2010). Rheumatoid arthritis: classification criteria: an American College of Rheumatology/European League Against Rheumatism Collaborative Initiative. *Arthritis Rheum.* 62 (9): 2569–2581.

Aletaha, D., Alasti, F., and Smolen, J.S. (2013). Rheumatoid factor determines structural progression of rheumatoid arthritis dependent and independent of disease activity. *Ann. Rheum. Dis.* 72 (6): 875–880.

Archdeacon, M.T. and Messerschmitt, P. (2006). Modern Papineau technique with vacuum-assisted closure. *J. Orthop. Trauma* 20 (2): 134–137. https://doi.org/10.1097/01.bot.0000184147.82824.7c. PMID: 16462567.

Borenstein, D. and Calin, A. (2012). *Fast Facts: Low Back Pain*, 2e. Oxford: Health Press.

Brady, R.A., Leid, J.G., Costerton, J.W., and Shirtliff, M.E. (2006). Osteomyelitis: clinical overview and mechanisms of infection. *Clin. Microbiol. Newsl.* 28 (9): 65–72.

Chaganti, R.K. and Lane, N.E. (2011). Risk factors for incident osteoarthritis of the hip and knee. *Curr. Rev. Musculoskelet. Med.* 4: 99–104.

Cronstein, B.N. (2005). Low-dose methotrexate: A mainstay in the treatment of rheumatoid arthritis. *Pharmacol. Rev.* 57 (2): 163–172.

Di Chen, D., Shen, J., Zhao, W. et al. (2017). Osteoarthritis: toward a comprehensive understanding of pathological mechanism. *Bone Res.* 5: 16044.

Chihara, S. and Segreti, J. (2010). Osteomyelitis. *Dis. Mon.* 56 (1): 66.

Chung, H.Y., Machado, P., van der Heijde, D. et al. (2012). Smokers in early axial spondyloarthritis have earlier disease onset, more disease activity, inflammation and damage, and poorer function and health-related quality of life: results from the DESIR cohort. *Ann. Rheum. Dis.* 71: 809–816.

Deane, K.D. and Holers, V.M. (2021). Rheumatoid arthritis pathogenesis, prediction and prevention: an emerging paradigm shift. *Arthritis Rheumatol.* 73 (2): 181–193.

Ember, T. and Noordeen, H. (2005). Growth rod spinal instrumentation to control progressive early onset scoliosis. *Spinal J.* 5 (340): S125.

Geyer, M. and Schönfeld, C.J.C.R.R. (2018). Novel insights into the pathogenesis of osteoarthritis. *Curr. Rheumatol. Rep.* 14: 98–107.

Gosselin, R., Roberts, I., and Gillespie, W. (2009). Antibiotics for preventing infection in open limb fractures. *Cochrane Database Syst. Rev.* (1): CD003764. https://doi.org/10.1002/14651858.CD003764.pub2.

Griffin, T.M. and Guilak, F. (2005). The role of mechanical loading in the onset and progression of osteoarthritis. *Exerc. Sport Sci. Rev.* 33: 195–200.

van der Heijde, D., Ramiro, S., Landewé, R. et al. (2017). Recommendations for axial spondyloarthritis. *Ann. Rheum. Dis.* 76 (6): 978–991.

Hatzenbuehler, J., and Pulling, T.J. (2011). Diagnosis and management of osteomyelitis. *Am. Fam. Phys.* 84 (9): 1027–1033. PMID: 22046943.

Hill, S., Dziedzi, K., and Ong, B. (2010). The functional and psychological impact of hand osteoarthritis. *Chronic Illn.* 6 (2): 101–110.

Hua, C., Buttgereit, F., and Combe, B. (2020). Glucocorticoids in rheumatoid arthritis: current status and future studies. *RMD Open* e000536. https://doi.org/10.1136/rmdopen-2017-000536.

Hurley, M.V., Walsh, N.E., Mitchell, H.L. et al. (2007). Clinical effectiveness of a rehabilitation program integrating exercise, self-management, and active coping strategies for chronic knee pain: a cluster randomized trial. *Arthritis Rheum.* 57 (7): 1211–1219.

Itoh, K., Hirota, S., Katsumi, Y. et al. (2008). A pilot study on using acupuncture and transcutaneous electrical nerve stimulation (TENS) to treat knee osteoarthritis. *Chin. Med.* 3: 2.

Johnell, O. and Kanis, J.A. (2006). An estimate of the worldwide prevalence and disability associated with osteoporotic fractures. *Osteoporos. Int.* 17: 1726–1733.

Juvenile Idiopathic Arthritis Foundation (2021) Available at https://www.arthritis.org/diseases/juvenile-idiopathic-arthritis (accessed 24 June 2021).

Kane, D., Grassi, W., Sturrock, R., and Balint, P.V. (2004). Musculoskeletal ultrasound – a state of the art review in rheumatology. Part 2: Clinical indications for the musculoskeletal ultrasound in rheumatology. *Rheumatology* 43 (7): 829–838.

Keavy, R. (2020). The prevalence of musculoskeletal presentations in general practice: an epidemiological study. *Br. J. Gen. Pract.* 70 (Suppl 1): bjgp20X711497.

Kneale, J. and Davis, P. (ed.) (2005). *Orthopaedic and Trauma Nursing*, 2e. Edinburgh: Churchill Livingstone.

Kosuwon, W., Sirichatiwapee, W., Wisanuyotin, T. et al. (2010). Efficacy of symptomatic control of knee osteoarthritis with 0.0125% of capsaicin versus placebo. *J. Med. Assoc. Thai.* 93 (10): 1188–1195.

Kroon, F.P.B., van der Burg, L.R.A., Ramiro, S. et al. (2016). Nonsteroidal antiinflammatory drugs for axial spondyloarthritis: a Cochrane review. *J. Rheumatol.* 43: 607–617.

Ledingham, J., Snowden, N., and Ide, Z. (2017). Diagnosis and early management of inflammatory arthritis. *Br. Med. J.* 358: j3248.

Lew, D.P. and Waldvogel, F.A. (2004). Osteomyelitis. *Lancet* 364: 369–379.

van der Linden, S. and van der Heijde, D. (2000). Clinical aspects, outcome assessment, and management of ankylosing spondylitis and postenteric reactive arthritis. *Curr. Opin. Rheumatol.* 12 (4): 263–268.

Loeser, R.F., Goldring, S.R., Scanzello, C.R., and Goldring, M.B. (2012). Osteoarthritis: a disease of the joint as an organ. *Arthritis Rheum.* 64: 1697–1707.

Matusz, D., Perez, O., Pateder, D. et al. (2005). Posterior only vs. combined anterior and posterior approaches to lumbar scoliosis in adults: a radiological comparison. *Spinal J.* 5 (120): S162.

Moura, M.D.G., Lopes, L.C., Silva, M. et al. (2018). Use of steroid and nonsteroidal anti-inflammatories in the treatment of rheumatoid arthritis: systematic review protocol. *Medicine* 97 (41): e12658.

Murray, M.M. (2011). Reflections on the development of nurse-led back pain triage clinics in the UK. *Int. J. Orthop. Trauma Nursing* 15 (3): 113–120.

National Ankylosing Spondyloarthritis Society (2021) *Facts and Figures*. https://nass.co.uk/about-as/ as-facts-and-figures/.

National Institute of Arthritis, Musculoskeletal, and Skin Diseases (2022) *What is Arthritis & What Causes it?* National Institute of Arthritis, Musculoskeletal and Skin Diseases http://nih.gov. January 2022.

NICE (2014). *Clinical Guideline: Osteoarthritis: Care and Management*. London: NICE.

NICE (2008). *Alendronate, Etidronate, Risedronate, Raloxifene and Strontium Ranelate for the Primary Prevention of Osteoporatic Fragility Fractures in Postmenopausal Women*. TA160. London: NICE.

NICE (2009). *Low Back Pain: Early Management of Persistent Non-specific Low Back Pain*. CG88. London: NICE.

NICE (2012). *Osteoporosis: Assessing the Risk of Fragility Fracture*. GC146. London: NICE.

NICE (2015) *Abatacept, adalimumab, etanercept and tocilizumab for treating juvenile idiopathic arthritis*. TA373. NICE, London.

NICE (2018a) *Abatacept, adalimumab, etanercept and tocilizumab for treating juvenile idiopathic arthritis*. Review of TA373. NICE, London.

NICE (2018b) *Rheumatoid Arthritis in Adults: Management*. NG100. NICE, London.

NICE (2021) *Low Back Pain and Sciatica*. Pathway last updated 12 November 2021. http://pathways.nice.org.uk/pathways/low-back-pain-and-sciatica.

Ogdie, A., Langan, S., Love, T. et al. (2019). Prevalence and treatment patterns on psoriatic arthritis in the UK. *Rheumatology* 52 (3): 568–575.

Orbai, A., de Wit, M., Mease, P. et al. (2017). International patient and physician consensus on a psoriatic arthritis core outcome set of clinical trials. *Ann. Rheum. Dis.* 76: 673–680.

O'Shea, F.D., Boyle, E. et al. (2010). Inflammatory and degenerative sacroiliac joint disease in a primary back pain cohort. *Arthriris Care Res.* 62 (4): 447–454.

Passalent, L., Soever, L., O'Shea, F., and Inman, R. (2010). Exercise in ankylosing spondylitis: discrepancies between recommendations and reality. *J. Rheumatol.* 37 (4): 835–841.

Paul, B.J., Kandy, H.I., and Krishnan, V. (2017). Pre-rheumatoid arthritis and its prevention. *Eur. J. Rheumatol.* 4 (2): 161–165.

Ralston, S.H., Corral-Gudino, L., Cooper, C. et al. (2019). Diagnosis and management of Paget's disease of bone in adults. *J. Bone Miner. Res.* 34: 579–604.

Regel, A., Sepriano, A., Baraliakos, X. et al. (2017). Efficacy and safety of non-pharmacological and non-biological pharmacological treatment: a systematic literature review informing the 2016 update of the ASAS/EULAR recommendations for the management of axial spondyloarthritis. *RMD Open* 3: e000397.

Roddy, E. and Doherty, M. (2006). Changing life-styles and osteoarthritis: what is the evidence? *Best Pract. Res. Clin. Rheumatol.* 20: 81–97.

Roos, H., Adalberth, T., Dahlberg, L., and Lohmander, L.S. (1995). Osteoarthritis of the knee after injury to the anterior cruciate ligament or meniscus: the influence of time and age. *Osteoarthritis. Cartilage J.* 3: 261–267.

Rudwaleit, M., van der Heijde, D., Landewé, R. et al. (2009). The development of Assessment of SpondyloArthritis international Society classification criteria for axial spondyloarthritis (part II): validation and final selection. *Ann. Rheum. Dis.* 68 (6): 777–783. https://doi.org/10.1136/ard.2009.108233. Epub 2009 Mar 17. Erratum in: Ann. Rheum. Dis. 2019 Jun;78(6): e59. PMID: 19297344.

Salvarani, C., and Fries, W. (2009). Clinical features and epidemiology of spondyloarthritides associated with inflammatory bowel disease. *World J. Gastroenterol.* 15 (20): 2449–2455.

Shaw, M., Adam, C.J., Izatt, M.T. et al. (2012). Use of the iPhone for Cobb angle measurement in scoliosis. *Eur. Spine J.* 21 (6): 1062–1068.

Smith, M. (2005). Care of patients with spinal conditions and injuries. In: *Orthopaedic and Trauma Nursing* (ed. J. Kneale and P. Davis) Chapter 18. London: Churchill Livingstone.

Tanna, N. (2009). Osteoporosis and fragility fractures: identifying those at risk and raising public awareness. *Nurs. Times* 105 (38): 28–31.

The Royal Australian College of General Practitioners. (2009). Clinical guideline for the diagnosis and management of early rheumatoid arthritis. Available at www.racgp.org.au/guidelines/rheumatoidarthritis.

Van Venrooji, W.J., van Beers, J.J., and Pruijn, G.J. (2011). Anti-CCP antibodies: the past, the present and the future. *Nat. Rev. Rheumatol.* 7 (7): 391–398.

Versus Arthritis (2021) *The State of Musculoskeletal Health 2021*. Versus Arthritis Report.

Wang, R., Gabriel, S.E., and Ward, M.M. (2016). Progression of patients and non radiographic axial spondyloarthritis to ankylosing spondylitis: a population based cohort study. *Arthritis Rheumatol.* 68: 1415–1421.

Whitehead, B. (2010). Juvenile idiopathic arthritis. *Aust. Fam. Physician* 39 (9): 630–636.

WHO (1994). *Assessment of Fracture Risk and its Application to Screening for Postmenopausal Women.* Geneva: WHO.

Yuchen, H., Zhong, L., Alexander, P.G. et al. (2020). Pathogenesis of osteoarthritis: risk factors, regulatory pathways in chondrocytes, and experimental models. *Biology* 9 (8): –194.

Zhang, W., Nuki, G., Moskowita, R.W. et al. (2010). OARSI recommendations for the management of hip and knee osteoarthritis. Part III: Changes in evidence following systematic cumulative update of research published through. *Osteoarthr. Cartil.* 18 (4): 476–499.

14

Elective Orthopaedic Surgery

Rebecca Jester[1], Sandra Flynn[2], and Mary Drozd[3]

[1] Royal College of Surgeons, Ireland, and Medical University, Manama, Bahrain
[2] University of Chester, Chester, UK
[3] Aston University, Birmingham, UK

Introduction

The aim of this chapter is to provide an overview of the evidence base for the practice of orthopaedic elective surgical care. Planned, or elective, surgery deals with a broad range of musculoskeletal conditions. Elective surgery is a major life event for patients, and they have high expectations of a successful operation and recovery. Orthopaedic practitioners and the wider multiprofessional team both in primary and secondary care settings have a shared commitment to deliver high-quality, person-centred care. They play a key role in ensuring that patients are fully prepared for surgery and that they are supported during the pre-operative, intra-operative and post-operative domains of care.

Principles of Care

The focus of care provision and the key care principles of elective surgery are firmly rooted in the ethos of safe and high-quality service delivery. In the late 1990s the Danish surgeon Henrik Kehlet hypothesised that multimodal interventions could moderate the stress caused by surgical trauma and complications, resulting in accelerated recovery after surgery and reduction in morbidity and length of stay (Kehlet 1997). Consequently, the model of accelerated or enhanced recovery pathways (ERPs) of care was introduced in 1997.

Enhanced recovery employs a coordinated multimodal and multiprofessional evidence-based approach across the pre-operative, intra-operative and post-operative domains of care to optimise the patient's physiological and psychological state (Kaye et al. 2019; NICE 2020a, p. 6). ERPs or enhanced recovery after surgery (ERAS) aim to improve outcomes, optimise patient experience and thereby assist the transition to baseline activity level and functional status after surgery. The enhanced recovery approach is a flexible model of teamwork that adapts and evolves alongside improving technologies and treatments in healthcare (Taurchini et al. 2018). The principles of enhanced recovery are that it:

- unifies the organisation of both evidenced-based care and clinical management
- involves patients, carers and families in the design and management of their own care and recovery
- focuses on minimally invasive surgical procedures, effective pain management strategies and the administration of nutrition and fluids to promote timely post-operative recovery
- helps patients, where possible, to maintain a daily routine that closely resembles their life at home (NHS England 2021).

Communication

Communication is a vital tool for the delivery of safe and quality care, and is a key priority for the multidisciplinary team. Effective communication helps to develop partnerships between service providers and service users. Patients must be kept informed about their treatment and be involved in decisions about their care.

Good communication helps to manage patient expectations and make the care pathway less stressful, helping to promote a sense of control so the patient is more able to participate in the recovery process.

Shared Decision Making

Shared decision making has become a prominent feature in the drive to achieve good healthcare outcomes and at its core is the fundamental legal and ethical principle of consent (GMC 2020). The patient has the right to be involved in decisions and choices about their care, medical treatment and interventions. Shared decision making is an ongoing process and involves clinicians working with their patients to ensure they are empowered to reach a decision about the treatment and care they want (Tonelli and Sullivan 2019; GMC 2020).

Respect for the patient as a person and understanding their preferences, personal circumstances, beliefs, values and goals is important in shared decision making. This includes respecting the choice to refuse or withdraw from treatment and care options (GMC 2020).

In England, the National Health Service (NHS) is moving away from a 'one size fits all' approach across health and care systems to implement a comprehensive model of personalised care by 2023/2024 so that people have 'control and choice over the way their care is planned and delivered' (NHS England 2019, p. 6). This shift in power will be embedded in a system that is committed to health promotion and improved health, wellbeing outcomes and experiences through people engagement. Importantly this service model aims to ensure that people have a wider range of options, better support and properly coordinated care at the right time in the optimal care setting (NHS England 2019).

Education Information and Support

Education and the provision of information are key to ensuring that patients are fully prepared both physically and psychologically throughout the surgical care pathway (Buus et al. 2021). In recent years this process has evolved to ensure that patients have an interactive involvement in their preparation for surgery and recovery stages.

The joint school or hip and knee school is a significant educational component of enhanced recovery programmes and is embedded in orthopaedic care pathways (O'Reilly et al. 2018). It provides patients with key information delivered directly or online by healthcare professionals including doctors, nurses, anaesthetists, physiotherapists and occupational therapists. Information leaflets and online films are available to patients and their carers which cover the entire patient journey, including members of the multidisciplinary team and their roles.

Prehabilitation, the process of optimising the physical fitness, functional capacity and mental status of a patient prior to surgery, is a key component of enhanced recovery aimed at enhancing post-operative recovery and outcomes, including length of stay, post-operative pain and complications (Molenaar et al. 2019; Punnoose et al. 2019) (see Chapter 6 for further information).

At a face-to-face joint school patients can meet with the team in person and be involved in question-and-answer sessions. Many joint schools invite previous patients along to provide a subjective experience of the journey. The joint school team and delivery of sessions will vary by hospital, although the principles of joint school remain comparable.

Joint school plays an important role in the ERP, providing information on the goals of joint replacement surgery and how patients can take an active part in their own recovery. Every patient and every operation is unique, but joint school can help to improve and optimise health prior to surgery through good standards of pre-operative education, such as the provision of personalised instructions relating to:

- comorbidities
- benefits and risks
- medications and supplements
- eating a healthy well-balanced diet
- smoking and alcohol cessation
- low-impact exercise such as walking or swimming
- preparing the home for discharge, including equipment and adaptation needs
- oral hygiene and dental evaluation
- skin advice prior to admission, including developing a rash or infection, any cuts, grazes or open wounds and who to contact
- footcare
- reducing infection prior to surgery, such as what to do if diagnosed with a urinary tract infection
- organising support, including shopping and housework
- what to bring with you into hospital
- transport home.

Social Support

Social support is an alliance between people and networks that can provide substantial emotional, informational and financial assistance during stressful life events (Brembo et al. 2017; Wylde et al. 2019). Navigating orthopaedic surgical pathways can place an emotional burden on patients. Strong social support together with material resources are key factors in reducing stress and can have a positive effect on health status, behaviour and patient-reported outcomes across the continuum of musculoskeletal care (Wu et al. 2018; Wylde et al. 2019).

Patients are encouraged to bring a family member, carer or friend along to joint school. Involving and encouraging family member or carer participation can play a significant role in reinforcing the principles of enhanced recovery by helping to instil confidence prior to admission and following discharge from hospital, and providing a means of support when the patient is no longer in direct contact with members of their healthcare team. Some hospitals provide peer-support groups where patients can meet and chat with others who have had similar surgery.

Information concerning advice and who to contact should be provided to all patients during every stage of their care pathway and on discharge from hospital.

Following discharge from hospital patients may receive support from face-to-face, virtual or telephone clinic sources. Support and advice can be provided by dedicated contact points or non-urgent helplines at the unit or hospital where surgery will or has taken place.

Some helplines provide 24-hour cover and others are available Monday–Friday during daytime hours. Calls are monitored by experienced healthcare professionals who can provide help with patient queries and concerns about their recent surgery. They can undertake an initial assessment to help decide on the best course of action and whether any further assessment or urgent review is required.

In recent years multiplatform messenger apps have been used to help patients receive timely expert help and advice from healthcare professionals prior to admission and following discharge from hospital. Messaging service technology allows chat groups to be set up where patients can stay in touch and benefit from professional and peer support, keeping them better informed and engaged (Day et al. 2018; Campbell et al. 2019).

Patients who have lived experience of similar conditions, treatments and procedures are able to interact socially to offer emotional support and practical help, and to share knowledge and support one another to better understand their condition, recovery and self-management. These services are effective in helping to detect and reduce complications following surgery, reduce readmission rates to hospital, and improve outcomes and patient satisfaction (Hallfors et al. 2018; Luo et al. 2019; Zheng et al. 2019; Zhang et al. 2021).

More recent initiatives involve the development of websites for pre-operative educational purposes. It is important that any website used for educational purposes is user-friendly, easy to navigate and meets the need of the user. This is an important consideration as effective patient education improves patient psychological and physical wellbeing. Patient satisfaction indicators with educational websites are similar when compared to the more traditional paper-based information material (Dayucos et al. 2019).

Similar support can be offered through face-to-face sessions and video teleconferencing services.

Peer support is an expanding field of study and has been extensively researched in mental health. Evidence suggests further research is required to explore the benefits of peer support for patients with physical health conditions (Grant et al. 2021).

Telemedicine and Virtual Clinics

Telemedicine and virtual clinics have been established in trauma and orthopaedics for several years albeit in a limited capacity. However, the recent Covid-19 pandemic has accelerated the development and adoption of virtual clinics (Kamecka et al. 2021; Pradhan et al. 2021). They are a cost-effective means of efficiently addressing wait times for out-patient clinic appointments (Gupta et al. 2017) and are acceptable to clinicians and patient users where previous clinical examination has been undertaken or is considered unnecessary (Kruse et al. 2017; Pradhan et al. 2021).

The use of telemedicine technology has been evaluated in terms of cost reduction, patient satisfaction, reliability and quality and as an effective alternative to the traditional face-to-face clinics (Gilbert et al. 2020; El Ashmawy et al. 2021).

The value of face-to-face consultation and the personal interaction this affords remains highly valued by patients (Parkes et al. 2019).

Common Types of Orthopaedic Surgery

The decision to undertake surgery may have taken place after many months or years of conservative measures such as physiotherapy and various medications prior to agreeing to elective surgical intervention. Much orthopaedic surgery is conducted for joint arthropathies such as osteoarthritis (Chapter 13) and bone, joint and soft tissue deformities and conditions. While there are many types of orthopaedic surgery, the elective orthopaedic procedures discussed in this chapter will focus on the principles of care following surgery and on the most commonly performed procedures: joint replacement surgery and spinal decompression.

Arthroplasty or Total Joint Replacement

Arthroplasty refers to the surgical refashioning of a joint. It aims to relieve pain and to retain or restore movement, is considered to be one of the most successful operations in orthopaedic surgery and is well established. Arthroplasty surgery has become available for almost every joint, with the hip and knee being the joint most frequently replaced. People are living longer and consequently the incidence of osteoarthritis is increasing. It is a debilitating condition that negatively affects quality of life. The aim of arthroplasty is to resolve pain and disability by removing diseased components of joints and replacing them with dynamically stable material such as metal, plastic or ceramics. Over many years replacement of most joints has become possible, but the most commonly performed surgeries are total hip replacement (THR) and total knee replacement (TKR). Shoulder, elbow and ankle replacements are undertaken less frequently and further information can be found on the National Joint Registry (NJR) website (www.njrcentre.org.uk).

It is anticipated that a hip or knee replacement should last for at least 15 years. The NJR provides a central database for hip, knee, elbow, shoulder and ankle replacements for statistics related to patient outcomes and complications. Annual reports enable sharing of important data and clinical evidence with clinicians, helping surgeons to choose the best implants for their patients as well as understand joint replacement survivorship (how long a device lasts before it needs replacing or modifying). The NJR collects details of hip, knee, ankle and shoulder replacements done in England, Wales, Northern Ireland and the Isle of Man. Thousands of these joint replacement operations take place in the UK every year and the NJR collects and monitors information on them to improve clinical standards and benefit patients, clinicians and the orthopaedic sector as a whole.

Different types of arthroplasties include the following:

- *Excision arthroplasty*: The bone surfaces are removed and the space between them is allowed to fill with fibrous tissues. It is the simplest and sometimes most satisfactory arthroplasty but leaves an unstable joint. An excision arthroplasty of the hip is called a Girdlestone's procedure. It is most often used as a salvage procedure for a failed THR. The patient's leg will be shorter as a result of this surgery.
- *Replacement hemiarthroplasty*: Only one surface of the joint is replaced with an artificial material such as metal and this is used for some patients with a hip fracture (Chapter 19).
- *Arthroplasty or total joint replacement* (TJR): Usually performed to relieve pain, improve function and reduce the degree of disability for a patient suffering with a degenerative, inflammatory or traumatic condition. TJR is the surgical treatment of choice when conservative treatments are not successful in managing the pain

(NICE 2020b). Articular bone ends are replaced by prosthetic implants. Prostheses are made from a variety of materials, including:
- stainless steel
- chrome/cobalt
- titanium alloy
- high-density polyethylene.
- Prostheses can either be cemented or uncemented into position. In the case of THR, total hip prostheses include metal-on-metal, ceramic-on-ceramic and metal-on-ceramic in the hope that they have the potential to improve outcomes for longer periods of time, but their efficacy currently remains uncertain (Pivec et al. 2012).

Total Hip Replacement Surgery

A THR is one of the most commonly performed elective orthopaedic procedures. Its primary functions are to treat hip pain and disability caused by diseases such as osteoarthritis or rheumatoid arthritis. It is occasionally performed for patients with a hip fracture (NICE 2011/2017) (see Chapter 19).

THR surgery involves the dislocation of the hip joint so that the femoral head and any damaged cartilage in the acetabulum can be removed. This is achieved through a 20–30 cm surgical incision allowing dissection of soft tissue, muscle and joint capsule. Incisions may be lateral, antero-lateral or posterior. A lateral or antero-lateral approach preserves the posterior part of the joint capsule, thus reducing the risk of posterior dislocation of the prosthesis post-operatively. These approaches necessitate the splitting of the abductor muscles, which can lead to an increased incidence of post-operative limp and muscle weakness. A posterior approach weakens the posterior joint capsule with a greater risk of dislocation, but the abductor muscles are not split. However, it is now recognised that lateral approaches for THR are associated with worse outcomes, including more deaths and revisions, than the antero-lateral or posterior approaches (NJR 2021).

Minimally invasive THR aims to avoid damage to the muscles and tendons around the hip joint (NICE 2010a). A single or double incision of 10 cm or less in length is made. Division of muscles is less extensive than in standard approaches and specially designed retractors and customised instruments are used. However, longer-term results of surgery using a smaller incision are not yet available and there are concerns about increased prosthesis malpositioning and transient lateral femoral cutaneous nerve palsy due to reduced visibility of the joint during surgery.

Regardless of surgical technique, the joint is prepared and the prosthesis inserted in a similar way. After removal of the femoral head the femur is prepared by reaming a hole down its medullary canal so that the femoral component can be fitted; this may be cemented in place or be cementless (press-fit). The acetabular socket is prepared to receive the cup in which the femoral component rotates; this may also be cemented or cementless. The surgeon aims to achieve equal leg length but on occasions there is a leg length discrepancy, either a shorter or longer operated leg, because of the extent of bone loss due to disease or because of the need to ensure a stable joint. Patients should be made aware of this possibility prior to surgery. After insertion of the femoral and acetabular components the hip joint is then put through the full range of movement to test for stability before the joint capsule and overlying muscles are sewn up.

The NJR (2021) includes four distinctive categories of hip arthroplasy:

1) type of hip replacement, i.e. THR and hip resurfacings (the NJR does not currently collect data on hip hemiarthroplasty)
2) fixation of the replacement, i.e. cemented, uncemented, hybrid and reverse hybrid
3) bearing surfaces of the hip replacement
4) size of femoral head/internal diameter of the acetabular bearing.

Hip Resurfacing

Hip resurfacing involves the resurfacing of the femoral head with a titanium shell. A long incision, often longer than a traditional THR incision, is required because although the hip is dislocated to expose the femoral head, this is not removed but rather smoothed to fit the shell on top so it is not as easy to visualise the acetabulum, which is reamed and fitted with a metal cup. This procedure is used for younger patients with osteoarthritis who may need a THR in the future as it aims to reduce pain, restore function and delay the need for a THR for some years. Clinicians may be more likely to offer resurfacing arthroplasty to men than to women because higher revision rates have been observed in women, which may be associated with women tending to have smaller hips (NICE 2014). Hip resurfacing and large diameter metal-on-metal (MoM) THR reduce the risk of dislocation because the contact area between the components is greater. They also have less debris due to wear.

There were concerns that the metal debris from MoM hip replacements may cause elevated metal ions systemically leading to metal toxicity and possibly cancer, though the evidence is not conclusive. The fears have led to a decline in the use of MoM prostheses, especially in women of childbearing years as there some evidence that metal ions can cross the placenta. The Medicines and Healthcare products Regulatory Agency (MHRA) (2017) in consultation with its independent MoM Expert Advisory Group, has continued to monitor the performance of MoM hip joint articulations for the occurrence of soft tissue reaction associated with these devices. The majority of patients with MoM hip replacements currently have well-functioning hips. However, it has been recognised that some patients will develop progressive soft tissue reactions to the wear debris associated with MoM articulations. Furthermore, clinical orthopaedic experts have also observed that soft tissue necrosis may occur in both asymptomatic and symptomatic patients, and believe early detection of these events should give a better revision outcome should this become necessary. There is no agreed threshold value for whole-blood metal levels that either predicts outcome or mandates revision and decisions to revise are influenced by patient factors, blood metal levels, imaging findings, and implant type and position. Other patient-specific factors may need to be considered when interpreting results for blood metal levels (MHRA 2017).

Revision of THR

The THR may need revision after 15 years due to aseptic loosening of the prosthetic joint and/or cement cracking, although for many patients the prosthesis may last much longer. Occasionally a revision is needed earlier due to infection or aseptic loosening of the prosthesis causing pain and discomfort. Complications that may lead to THR revision surgery include prosthesis instability, dislocation, aseptic loosening, osteolysis (bone reabsorption), infection and prosthesis failure (NICE 2014).

Revision surgery is more complex than the primary THR and is usually performed by specialist surgeons. The procedure involves opening the joint, removing the prosthetic components and any bone cement followed by a reconstruction of the joint using new prosthetic components. Bone grafting may be indicated. For an infected prosthesis surgery is conducted in two stages. The first stage is removal of the infected prosthesis and treatment with antibiotics, usually intravenously. Once it has been established that the infection has been eradicated the second stage is carried out: insertion of the new prosthesis.

Specific post-operative nursing care after THR or hip resurfacing is related to reducing the risk of dislocation, mobilisation and psychological recovery. The prevalence of dislocation varies but is around 4% (Smith et al. 2012). It tends to occur either in the first 3 months, due to component malposition or abductor deficiency, or many years post-operatively secondary to prosthesis wear. A triangular-shaped abduction wedge, often known as a Charnley wedge, is used in some centres to prevent abnormal hip movements for the first few days after surgery. To reduce the risk of dislocation patients are taught:

- not to flex their hip joint more than 90°
- to avoid excessive adduction of the leg
- to avoid twisting on the leg when turning.

Patients are often advised to sleep on their back for the first 6 weeks and are provided with a raise for their bed and chair as well as a raised toilet seat to prevent hip flexion greater than 90°. There is some evidence to suggest that such precautions may not be necessary and that patients should be allowed more freedom of movement, especially following an anterior or anterolateral surgical approach (Restrepo et al. 2011; Barnsley et al. 2015).

Within enhanced recovery programmes early mobilisation is encouraged and in some centres the physiotherapists will get the patient out of bed in the recovery room. The point at which a patient is mobilised is tailored to the individual and influenced by additional factors such as spinal anaesthesia and pain management modality. The majority of patients are allowed to fully weight-bear immediately, although if there is any potential instability a period of 6–12 weeks non- or partial-weight bearing may be required. Patients initially mobilise with a walking frame or sticks for up to 6 weeks, although in some centres patients may stop using them earlier. Physiotherapy is rarely needed after discharge from acute care, but postoperative exercises should be performed by patients up to three times per day for at least 6 weeks.

THR surgery is a major life event and preoperative education should have prepared patients for the extended recovery period, which may be 3–6 months. This may need reinforcing after surgery as patients experience the reality of initial restricted mobility and discomfort from the surgery.

Total Knee Replacement Surgery

The most common indication for TKR is osteoarthritis of the knee joint.

The knee is made up of three compartments: medial, lateral and patellofemoral. When a TKR is implanted, the medial and lateral compartments are always replaced, and the patella may be resurfaced. If a single compartment is replaced then the term unicompartmental is applied to the procedure. The medial, lateral or patellofemoral compartments can all be replaced independently, if clinically appropriate. Medial and lateral unicompartmental knee replacements are also referred to as medial or lateral unicondylar knee replacements. The term multicompartmental knee replacement is used to indicate the combination of more than one unicompartmental knee replacement (NJR 2021).

The NJR (2021) highlights that knee replacements can be defined by the number and type of compartments replaced, the fixation of the components (cemented, uncemented or hybrid), level of constraint, the mobility of the bearing, whether the implants are of a modular design and the presence or absence of a patella in the primary knee replacement.

The most commonly used incision is midline with a medial parapatellar approach, with the patella and extensor mechanism everted to gain access to the joint. The mini-incision TKR involves an incision 10–12 cm long over the knee, compared with the conventional TKR, which requires an incision 20–30 cm long. The same prostheses are inserted using specially designed instruments (NICE 2010b). The tibial plateau and the distal femoral joint surfaces are resected and holes are then drilled in the bones so that the prostheses can be inserted. The tibial joint surface is replaced by a polyethylene bearing, usually attached to a metal base prosthesis and the distal femur with a metal prosthesis. Any arthritis on the patella surface may be removed and a plastic component, like a button, inserted although this is not always performed. The patella is then flipped back into position and the incision closed. As with THR, aseptic loosening of the knee prosthesis may require revision surgery after 10–15 years or earlier due to infection.

For some individuals only part of the knee may be affected by arthritis and a partial or unicompartmental knee replacement may be indicated. This can be performed for younger patients who do not wish to undergo a more invasive TKR. However, there is a risk that the patient may develop arthritic changes in the remaining aspects of the knee, requiring a conversion to a TKR. Another reason for revision of unicondylar knee replacements is loosening of the prosthesis.

If only the patella is damaged, an operation called a patellofemoral replacement or patellofemoral joint arthroplasty can be performed. This is a simpler operation with a faster recovery time. However, the long-term results are still unclear and it is not suitable for most people with osteoarthritis.

NICE (2020b) recommend that patients undergoing a TKR should have patella resurfacing. Current practice varies, with resurfacing carried out in around 35–40% of knee replacements. This recommendation can be expected to increase the number of knee replacement operations with patella resurfacing. There may be an initial increase in costs because of more costly hospital stays for resurfacing, but this is expected to be more than offset by reduced numbers of hospital readmissions in the long term. NICE (2020b) looked at three options: resurfacing, no resurfacing and selective resurfacing. There was not enough clinical evidence to indicate whether any of the options was more beneficial than the others. However, strong economic evidence showed that resurfacing is cost-effective compared with no resurfacing over a 10-year time horizon because of reduced hospital readmissions. Because of the lack of clinical evidence, the committee also made a recommendation for research on selective resurfacing in knee replacement.

After TKR or unicondylar knee replacement it is important that the knee joint is mobilised so that flexion and extension can be maximised. For the majority of patients this can be achieved with exercises supervised by physiotherapy and nursing staff. The evidence suggests that there is little advantage of using a continuous passive movement (CPM) machine to improve the range of movement and functional outcomes, or reduce adverse events or length of hospital stay (Yang et al. 2019).

Patients can normally fully weight-bear immediately after surgery unless there is any instability in the joint, which may necessitate a period of partial weight-bearing and/or the wearing of a removable splint. The use of crutches or a stick for the first 4–6 weeks may be helpful in providing support, although not all centres advocate this. Full recovery can take up to 2 years as scar tissue heals and muscles are restored by exercise. A very small number of people will continue to have some pain after 2 years (NHS 2019).

Other Types of Knee Surgery

Other types of knee surgery may be undertaken prior to a knee replacement:

- *Arthroscopic washout and debridement*: A tiny telescope called an arthroscope is inserted into the knee, which is then washed out with saline to clear any debris such as loose bone or cartilage (NICE 2007).
- *Osteotomy*: The surgeon cuts the tibia and realigns it so that the patient's weight is no longer carried by the damaged part of the knee.
- *Mosaicplasty*: a keyhole operation that involves transferring plugs of hard cartilage, together with some underlying bone from another part of the knee, to repair the damaged surface (NICE 2018a).

Shoulder Arthroplasty

A shoulder replacement is indicated for patients with a painful shoulder and destruction of the glenohumeral joint. Glenohumeral arthroplasty is performed for degenerative joint disease such as rheumatoid arthritis or other inflammatory arthropathy, osteoarthritis or fractures of the proximal humerus. Other reasons may be avascular necrosis of the humeral head, mal or non-union of a proximal humeral fracture and chronic deficiency of the rotator cuff (NICE 2010b, 2020b). The procedure can be successful at reducing the pain from arthritis, but due to the complexity of the shoulder joint, function and mobility are not as successful as for THR or TKR at this time.

There are different types of shoulder replacement surgery. A total shoulder replacement (TSR) involves replacing the arthritic joint surfaces with a humeral component consisting of a metal ball with a stem fixed into the humerus and a plastic glenoid component. The humeral component may be cemented or uncemented; the glenoid component is generally cemented. A shoulder hemiarthroplasty consists of a stemmed humeral component articulating on the natural glenoid cavity and is suitable for patients with a healthy glenoid cavity. Surface replacement arthroplasty in the form of a small metal cap placed over the humeral head is less invasive and can be used for patients with earlier stages of shoulder joint degeneration. The aim of shoulder resurfacing arthroplasty is to replace only the damaged joint surfaces, with minimal bone resection. A reverse TSR is used for patients who have a torn rotator cuff, severe arthritis and a torn rotator cuff, or a previous failed TSR. The metal ball is attached to the glenoid cavity and the plastic socket to the humerus. This allows the patient to move the arm using the deltoid muscle rather than the torn rotator cuff. However, although reverse TSR was originally designed for people with a rotator cuff tear, it is being used more widely for people with no rotator cuff tear to obviate the need for early revision surgery after rotator cuff failure (NICE 2020b). Further research is needed to compare reverse TSR with conventional TSR.

There is evidence to suggest that conventional TSR provides more overall benefit than humeral hemiarthroplasty, although TSR is limited to people with adequate glenoid bone because this is necessary for conventional TSR to be considered. For people without adequate glenoid bone, another solution, such as reverse shoulder replacement or other surgery, is needed (NICE 2020b).

Shoulder replacements can be defined by the type and subtype of replacement (NJR 2021). The four main types of replacement are:

1) proximal humeral hemiarthroplasty
2) conventional TSR
3) reverse polarity TSR
4) interpositional arthroplasty.

There are three main subtypes based on variations on the humeral side of the joint:

1) resurfacing, i.e. putting a new metal surface over the existing humeral head
2) stemless, i.e. removing the humeral head and putting on a new head with an anchoring device that does not project beyond the metaphysis of the proximal humerus

Table 14.1 Recommendations for all types of surgery

Communication	Make sure patients are informed about the type of tests they need and why
	Ensure the results of any pre-operative tests undertaken in primary care are included when referral for surgical consultation is made
Existing medicines	Consider any medicines patients are taking when considering offering any pre-operative test
Pregnancy tests	Ascertain in a sensitive manner if women of childbearing age may be pregnant
	With the woman's consent carry out a pregnancy test if there is any doubt about whether she is pregnant
	Make sure women who could possibly be pregnant or who are pregnant are aware of the risks of the anaesthetic and the procedure to the foetus
Sickle cell disease or sickle cell trait tests	Do not routinely offer testing for sickle cell disease or sickle cell trait before surgery
	If the patient has sickle cell disease and their disease is managed by a specialist sickle cell service, liaise with this team before surgery
HbA1c testing for people without diagnosed diabetes	Do not routinely offer HbA1c testing before surgery to people without diagnosed diabetes
HbA1c testing for people with diabetes	People with diabetes should have their most recent HbA1c test results included in their referral information from primary care
	Offer HbA1c testing to people with diabetes having surgery if they have not been tested in the last 3 months
Urine tests	Do not routinely offer urine dipstick tests before surgery
Chest X-ray	Do not routinely offer chest X-ray before surgery
Echocardiogram	Do not routinely offer echocardiogram, consider resting echocardiogram if patient has heart murmur or cardiac symptoms
	Before ordering the resting echocardiogram, do ECG and discuss the findings with an anaesthetist

Source: adapted from NICE (2016).

Table 14.2 Example of investigations required for patient ASA Grade 3 undergoing total knee replacement (major surgery)

Test	Investigations
ECG	Required
Full blood count	Required
Haemostasis: prothrombin time, INR	Consider in people with chronic liver disease
	If people taking anticoagulants need modification of their treatment regimen, make an individualised plan in line with local guidance
	If clotting status needs to be tested before surgery (depending on local guidance) use point-of-care testing
Kidney function	Required
Lung function/ arterial blood gases	Seek advice from a senior anaesthetist as soon as possible after assessment for people who are ASA grade 3 or 4 due to known or suspected respiratory disease
Urine test	Microscopy and culture of midstream urine sample before surgery

Source: adapted from NICE (2016).

the procedure itself and post-operative expectations, care and rehabilitation. The knowledge gained can affect the perception of patients' preparedness for surgery and their ability to control post-operative pain, which therefore improves a patient's overall stay (Kearney et al. 2011).

Education can be delivered via one-to-one instruction, group sessions, printed information (i.e. booklet, pamphlet, information sheet), learning package, audio-visual presentation and lectures or a combination of these methods (Stern and Lockwood 2005). Some surgeons now offer structured online courses regarding surgery, whilst other patients choose their own online searches (Kearney et al 2011). With recent technological initiatives, surgical teams need to cater for the change in trend and provide information via differing media to assess the effectiveness of this teaching tool. Involvement of the multidisciplinary team (MDT) enables each member of the team to contribute to the patient's care and prevents duplication.

Furthermore, it is important to commence discussions with the patient and their family about discharge planning early in the journey during joint school/pre-operative assessment. This is discussed later in the chapter.

Admission

Patients are usually admitted on the day of surgery unless there is significant medical history and high anaesthetic risk; Admission nursing assessment should focus on the

more effective than post-admission teaching in terms of patients' knowledge and retention (Stern and Lockwood 2005). The aim is to provide the foundations for effective decision making enabling informed consent, information regarding patient's overall health status and nursing care plans are based on mutually established realistic, patient-centred, measurable, clear and concise goals. The admission process requires nurses with specialised knowledge in orthopaedics to ensure that the patient is safely prepared for the operation, provide support and reaffirm information about their surgery and post-operative care previously provided during the pre-operative assessment/joint school phase of their journey.

Skin Preparation

Tartari et al. (2017) highlight that healthcare workers should encourage patients to take an active participatory role throughout the surgical journey as this may have an influence on the prevention of surgical site infections (SSIs). Their expert panel review suggests that shaving is strongly discouraged prior to surgery and patients should be advised not to remove hair at the site of the planned incision when at home. The hair removal procedure has been performed historically because it is thought that the presence of hair can interfere with the exposure of the incision, the suturing of the incision and the application of adhesive wound dressings (Tanner et al. 2011). Nonetheless, hair does not need to be removed pre-operatively unless the hair in or around the incision site interferes with the operation. While the data for the timing of hair removal are less convincing, usually hair removal should be done as close to the time of the operation as possible. The preferred method of hair removal is to use an electric clipper with a single-use head on the day of surgery (Niel-Weise et al. 2005; Tanner et al. 2011; NICE 2020c). A razor can irritate the skin and lead to micro lesions, which can result in microorganisms colonising the affected skin and this can significantly increase the risk of post-operative infection. While depilating creams are comparable to clippers in regard to post-operative wound infections, some patients may experience skin irritation and the procedure seems less practical and requires additional cleaning with water afterwards (Niel-Weise et al. 2005; Tanner et al. 2011). Patients should be encouraged to ensure their skin is clean before surgery and they should shower or bathe (full body) with soap on the day before or on the day of surgery (NICE 2020c). The rationale behind whole-body bathing or showering before surgery is to make the skin as clean as possible by removing the transient flora and some resident flora. Showering with an antiseptic reduces the amount of bacteria found on the skin but the effect on SSIs in the scientific evidence remains inconclusive (Webster and Osborne 2015). There is no specific recommendation favouring one antiseptic agent over another and some products may cause hypersensitivity or skin irritation for specific patients. There are no benefits for using body wipes or disposable disinfectant washcloths as compared to showering with an unmedicated bar soap that have been reported in the evidence for the prevention of SSI. Also, there is no specific recommendation in terms of optimal timing for showering prior to surgery, the total amount of soap or antiseptic application (Veiga et al. 2009; Webster and Osborne 2015).

Fasting

The principle of fasting from fluids and solids prior to surgery is to reduce the risk of vomiting and aspiration of stomach contents at the induction of general anaesthetic (GA) (Khoyratty et al. 2010). Patients are rarely aware of the rationale for fasting, so this should be included in pre-operative education to reduce anxiety. This is considered in more detail in Chapter 10. It is important that patients are not fasted for excessive periods to avoid dehydration and to minimise post-operative nausea and vomiting (PONV). Patients should be encouraged to drink clear fluids up to 2 hours prior to their surgery (NICE 2020a).

Premedication

Premedications were traditionally given to reduce pre-operative anxiety and/or reduce PONV, but there has been limited evidence to support the effectiveness of this practice and many healthcare organisations no longer routinely prescribe premedications. A Cochrane systematic review (Smith and Pittaway 2002) found that premedication did not improve the length of stay and the sedated patient may require closer attention for safety and closer monitoring while awaiting surgery. The Joanna Briggs Institute (2010) note an absence of clear research findings surrounding the use of anxiolytic premedication in adult patients undergoing day surgery under general anaesthetic, so this should be based on clinical judgement. A randomised controlled trial by Xie et al. (2020) of 240 patients undergoing hip and knee replacement compared premedication regimens of dexamethasone (10 mg) before anaesthesia induction or dexamethasone (10 mg) before anaesthesia induction as well as oral mosapride (5 mg) before and after surgery, and reported that those receiving oral mosapride had reduced incidence of PONV, especially post-operative nausea, during 6–12 hours post-operatively.

Patients should take their routine medications prior to surgery unless otherwise advised by the anaesthetist, and surgeons should ask that anticoagulant medications such as warfarin, aspirin and clopidogrel be stopped for at least 5 days prior to surgery and sometimes replaced with LMWH dependent on the patient's medical history and risk of thromboembolism (Chapter 9). Patients taking a vitamin K antagonist may require peri-operative anticoagulation bridging therapy, but this needs to be balanced against risk of bleeding.

Consent

Informed consent is legally required and should be obtained prior to all nursing and medical procedures (Cohn and Larson 2007). Patients must have full understanding of the procedure, the risks and any alternatives that are available, and have made the decision of their own free will, without coercion and are legally able to make the decision. In many orthopaedic centres procedure-specific consent forms are utilised. Obese/morbidly obese patients undergoing major orthopaedic surgery such as hip and knee replacement are potentially at increased risk of intra-operative and post-operative complications and should receive specific information regarding this to ensure their consent is fully informed (Jester and Rodney 2021).

Communication is a particularly important component of the consent process, especially for people with a learning/intellectual disability or other cognitive impairment. There should be adequate time available for discussion with the person with a learning disability, their family, carers, local advocacy group managers and/or best interest assessors prior to consent being obtained. Information needs to be provided in an accessible and comprehensible manner, such as with the use of pictorial aids to ensure that the person with a learning disability has sufficient information on which to base their decision to be involved in any procedure (Drozd et al. 2021).

The Mental Capacity Act (2005) directs that all reasonable steps are taken to support capacity and states that 'A person is not to be treated as unable to make a decision unless all practicable steps to help him to do so have been taken without success' (Mental Capacity Act 2005, p. 1). The Mental Capacity Act (2005) Code of Practice (The Stationary Office 2007) informs that the assessment of capacity is a two-stage test.

Stage 1: The diagnostic approach asks the following: 1. Does the person have an impairment or disturbance of the functioning of the mind or brain? This can include people with a learning disability.

Stage 2: The decision-making process. Assessment using the following criteria which confirms if a person had the capacity to make a decision themselves if the answer to these statements was yes:

- They understand the information about the decision that needs to be made.
- They can retain the information for long enough to make a decision.
- They can weigh up the pros and cons of the options available to them and understand the long-term implications of the decision.
- They can communicate their decision to you.

(British Institute of Learning Disabilities 2009).

Safety Checklist

The World Health Organization (WHO) revised its surgical safety checklist in 2009 and this is advocated as best practice in the NICE (2020a) guideline for peri-operative care in adults. In addition to the WHO Surgical Safety Checklist NICE (2020a) recommend adding steps to minise risk of preventable events reported locally or nationally, The Surgical Safety Checklist (WHO 2009) is intended for use by clinicians to improve the safety of operations and reduce unnecessary surgical deaths and complications. The safety checks begin on the ward and once the checklist and documentation are complete, the patient is transferred to the operating department where the peri-operative phase commences. See Box 14.1 and Figure 14.1.

Box 14.1 Evidence Summary: Improving Clinical Outcomes through Implementation of the WHO Surgical Safety Checklist (Haynes et al. 2009)

Reproduced with permission from the Massachusetts Medical Society.

This large-scale study was conducted in eight hospitals in eight cities (including London, UK), representing a variety of economic circumstances and diverse patient populations. The hospitals participated in the WHO's Safe Surgery Saves Lives programme and implemented a 19-item checklist designed to improve team communication and consistency of care. It was hypothesised that this would reduce complications and deaths relating to surgery.

The study prospectively studied pre-intervention and post-intervention periods at the participating sites. The checklist was introduced via lectures, written materials or written guidance. Patients were followed up prospectively until discharge or for 30 days, whichever came first, for death and complications such as myocardial infarction, wound infection or sepsis. A total of 3733 patients were enrolled during the baseline period and 3955 patients after the post-implementation phase. There were no significant differences between the patients in the two phases of the study. The in-hospital death rate was shown to decrease from 1.5 to 0.8% and serious complications from 11 to 7% after introduction of the checklist. The overall rates of SSI and unplanned reoperation also declined significantly.

The authors acknowledged that the combined effects of team building and cultural changes may also have played a part in the positive results, rather than the checklist on its own.

SIGN IN (to be read out loud)

Before induction on anaesthesia
Has the patient confirmed his/her identity, site, procedure and consent? ☐ Yes **Is the surgical site marked?** ☐ Yes/not applicable **Is the anaesthesia machine and medication check complete?** ☐ Yes **Does the patient have a:** **Known allergy?** ☐ No ☐ Yes **Difficult airway/aspiration risk?** ☐ No ☐ Yes, and equipment/assistance available **Risk of >500 ml blood loss (7 ml/kg in children)?** ☐ No ☐ Yes, and adequate IV access/fluids planned

TIME OUT (to be read out load)

Before start of surgical intervention for example, skin incision
Have all team members introduced themselves by name and role? ☐ Yes **Surgeon, Anaesthetist and Registered Practitioner verbally confirm:** ☐ What is the patient's name? ☐ What procedure, site and position are planned? **Anticipated critical events** **Surgeon:** ☐ How much blood loss is anticipated? ☐ Are there are specific equipment requirements or special investigations? ☐ Are there any critical or unexpected steps you want the team to know about? **Anaesthetist:** ☐ Are there any patient specific concerns? ☐ What is the patient's ASA grade? ☐ What monitoring equipment and other specific levels of support are required, for example blood? **Nurse/ODP:** ☐ Has the sterility of the instrumentation been confirmed (including indicator results)? ☐ Are there are equipment issues or concerns? **Has the surgical site infection (SSI) bundle been undertaken?** ☐ Yes/not applicable ○ Antibiotic prophylaxis within the last 60 minutes ○ Patient warming ○ Hair removal ○ Glycaemic control **Has VTE prophylaxis been undertaken?** ☐ Yes/not applicable **Is essential imaging displayed?** ☐ Yes/not applicable

SIGN OUT (to be read out loud)

Before any member of the team leaves the operating room
Registered Practitioner verbally confirms with the team: ☐ Has the name of the procedure been recorded? ☐ Has it been confirmed that instruments, swabs and sharp counts are complete (or not applicable)? ☐ Have the specimens been labeled (including patient name)? ☐ Have any equipment problems been identified that need to be addressed? **Surgeon, Anaesthetist and Registered Practitioner:** ☐ What are the key concerns for recovery and management of this patient?

PATIENT DETAILS
Last name: First name: Date of birth: NHS Number*: Procedure: *If the NHS Number is not immediately available, a temporary number should be used until it is

Name:
Signature of
Registered Practitioner:

Name:
Signature of
Registered Practitioner:

Figure 14.1 Surgical checklist.

Peri-operative Care

Peri-operative care refers to the practice of patient-centred, multidisciplinary and integrated clinical care for patients from contemplation of surgery until full recovery (Royal College of Anaesthetists 2022). Good peri-operative care aims to improve patient experience and satisfaction. It should also facilitate safe and effective return to home/ work and quality of life, and reduce the cost of healthcare through improving value.

The care of patients in the operating theatre, from arrival in the anaesthetic room to leaving the recovery area, requires staff who are skilled and knowledgeable in both orthopaedic and theatre care. While dealing predominantly with surgery requiring inpatient care, the principles are also applicable to day case orthopaedic surgery.

Anaesthetic Preparation

The approach to anaesthesia is carefully planned by the anaesthetic team prior to surgery, taking into consideration the patient's general health status. The anaesthetic options should be fully discussed with the patient, encouraging them to ask questions about the various options and their related benefits and risks to facilitate shared decision making. Anaesthesia allows surgery to take place by rendering the patient insensible to pain and sensation, together with loss of consciousness if a general anaesthetic is used (Woodhead and Wicker 2005). Depending on the type of surgery and the patient characteristics, anaesthesia may be:

- local: only the immediate area is anaesthetised, e.g. a block to allow carpal tunnel surgery to be performed
- regional: axillary block for hand or forearm surgery (Wing Wai and Irwin 2012) or spinal anaesthetic for lower limb surgery (Royal College of Anaesthetists 2008)
- general: the patient is unconscious for the operation. This can be used for all operative procedures in patients who are fit for general anaesthesia.

For pain relief an epidural anaesthetic or a nerve block may be used in addition to a spinal or general anaesthetic, for example a femoral nerve block for analgesia in THR surgery (see Chapter 11 for more detail).

Intra-operative Period

Along with general surgical considerations, effective operating department procedures include ensuring the correct positioning of the patient to allow surgical and anaesthetic access while at the same time maintaining patient dignity and managing risk from harm, for example shoulder surgery patients can be positioned in an upright/beach chair or supine position (Dutta 2011), resulting in different pressure points. The maintenance of patient safety, temperature, correct patient moving/handling and infection control measures must also be considered. The NICE (2020a) peri-operative care in adults guidelines recommend cardiac output monitoring intra-operatively for all patients undergoing major or complex surgery and consideration of intravenous crystalloid for intra-operative fluid maintenance. Patients undergoing major orthopaedic surgery and/or are at risk of deep vein thrombosis (DVT)/pulmonary embolism (PE) may have anti-embolic stockings in situ in the intra-operative period. The nurse has an important role in ensuring the patient is accurately measured for anti-embolic stockings

There is a plethora of roles within the operating theatre which vary according to the way in which operating department practice has developed locally and nationally. Advanced roles in the operating department now include practitioners who have received additional training and education and may assist with retaining retractors, dissecting soft tissue/bone, preparing ligament grafts, placing intraoperative drains, closing wounds and safely transferring the patient from operating table to bed post-surgery (Jones et al. 2012). All practitioners who work within the sterile field need to attend not only to the technical aspects of surgery but also to non-technical skills (Mitchell et al. 2011), including situation awareness (watching and anticipating the next stage of the procedure), communication (verbal and non-verbal cues), teamwork (coordinating activities), task management and coping with stress and fatigue (their own and other members of the team). An important consideration for patients having regional anaesthesia is communication during the surgery as they have two overarching needs: wanting to have control (knowledge) and trust in staff (Bergman et al. 2012)

Recovery

After surgery patients should be fully conscious and clinically stable before they return to the ward or are discharged. NICE (2020a) recommend that immediate post-operative care is provided in a specialist recovery area (a high-dependency unit, a post-anaesthesia care unit or an intensive care unit) for people with a high risk of complications or mortality. Transfer of the patient from the operating theatre to the recovery room is an important consideration as transfers from one surface to another involve risk such as dislocation of a hip prosthesis following joint arthroplasty, and appropriate equipment such as abduction wedges or pillows may need to be in place to maintain the correct position. The recovery staff will assume responsibility for the patient and care for them according to a model such as ABCDE (Hatfield and Tronson 2009):

- A airway
- B breathing
- C circulation
- D drips, drains and drugs
- E extras.

Extra considerations may include elevation of a limb and care of a cast or a back slab (Chapter 8). Peripheral neurovascular observations are necessary following limb surgery and where casts/traction are being used (Chapters 8 and 9).

Recovery occurs in stages and can be characterised as Stages 1–3 (Hatfield and Tronson 2009):

Stage 1: Patients have just left the theatre and are expected to stay in the recovery room for 1 hour following general anaesthesia and half an hour after local anaesthesia. Vital signs, nausea/pain, conscious level and output from drains or bleeding from wound sites should be monitored and any abnormalities reported to the anaesthetist and/or surgeon. Operations performed under tourniquet, such as limb surgery, may result in up to 1 litre of blood loss in the recovery room, requiring careful monitoring along with checking of vacuum drains. Thirty minutes should elapse before the last dose of opioid analgesia and discharge from the recovery room.

Stage 2: Relates to transfer of patients to the ward once vital signs are stable, the patient is conscious, pain is controlled and there is no excessive wound drainage or bleeding. Transfer should take place with portable suction, oxygen and other emergency equipment available. Some elective orthopaedic patients will be transferred to the intensive care unit (ICU) for extended Stage 1 recovery. A review of 22 000 primary and revision THR patients found that 130 were admitted to ICU and that independent risk factors were smoking, cemented arthroplasty, general anaesthesia, allogeneic transfusion, higher C-reactive protein, lower haemoglobin level, higher body mass index and older age (AbdelSalam et al. 2012). Whatever the transfer destination, it is important that the receiving staff have a comprehensive handover, including operation performed, surgeon's instructions and intra-operative details such as blood loss, anaesthetic type, condition in recovery and checking of the wound dressing, drains and any other drains or infusions by the receiving staff (Woodhead and Wicker 2005).

Stage 3: Discharge home and longer-term follow-up. For day-case procedures this happens when vital signs have been stable for at least 1 hour, pain is adequately controlled, there is an absence of nausea/vomiting and the patient is able to drink, eat and pass urine.

Post-operative Care

When it is safe to transfer the patient from the specialist recovery area to the ward environment careful monitoring and observation are essential to promptly identify any deterioration or complications. Effective post-operative care involves:

- monitoring of clinical observations in accordance with policy and appropriately recorded onto early warning score/NEWS charts (Chapter 16)
- assessment of neurovascular status bilaterally (Chapter 9)
- management of pain (Chapter 11)
- monitoring of input (oral and IV)/output (vomitus, urinary and blood loss) via fluid balance chart, especially in the first 24 hours (Chapter 10)
- assessment and management of wound/dressings/drains (Chapter 12)
- encouraging deep breathing exercises and initiating chest physiotherapy if required to prevent chest infection
- encouraging leg exercises to reduce risk of DVT and administering VTE prophylaxis (Chapter 9)
- initiating mobilisation and rehabilitation.
- keeping the patient up to date regarding their progress, provision of information and checking of patients' understanding.

Patients should be encouraged to be active partners in their postoperative care via shared decision making.

ERPs emphasise the need for early mobilisation and commencement of exercises. To facilitate this patients' pain must be assessed and managed effectively both at rest and on movement.

Blood Replacement

Blood loss during orthopaedic surgery is unavoidable, particularly during major procedures such as THR, and transfusion is sometimes required. There has been a move towards minimising the use of transfusions whenever possible due to issues of cost, supply, increasing the length of stay and risk of serious complications leading to mortality. Serious hazards of transfusion (SHOT) definitions were updated in 2022 and include:

incorrect blood component transfused
avoidable transfusion (patient transfused but not clinically justified)
delayed transfusion (patient required transfusion, but the decision/transfusion was delayed)
under or over transfusion
haemolytic transfusion reactions, acute and delayed.

If the decision to transfuse is made this should whenever possible be discussed with the patient and their consent obtained. The principles of right blood/right patient should be adopted and careful monitoring of the patient during and following transfusion carried out to promptly identify reactions.

There are currently three techniques available for transfusing blood within the orthopaedic setting:

- allogeneic: blood from an unrelated donor
- cell salvage: collecting blood from the patient during surgery for transfusion during or after surgery
- peri-operative autologous donation (PAD): collection of the patient's own blood prior to surgery for transfusion if required (Carless et al. 2010).

Allogeneic blood transfusion in elective orthopaedic surgery is risky and best avoided. PAD is justified in patients who have developed immune responses because of repeated transfusions or in situations where there is doubt about the safety of the blood supply. It is also believed to reduce the need for transfusions of donor blood and is safer than receiving an allogeneic transfusion (Henry et al. 2001; Carless et al. 2010). A Cochrane review suggested that cell salvage reduces the need for allogeneic red cell transfusion and did not appear to impact adversely on clinical outcomes (Carless et al. 2010). Many alternative strategies are currently being employed to reduce the number of transfusions required, including anti-fibrinolytic compounds such as aminocaproic acid and tranexamic acid. Tranexamic acid is an antifibrinolytic agent that effectively blocks this fibrinolytic activity, causing a marked reduction in postoperative bleeding (Sepah et al. 2011).

Discharge Planning/Rehabilitation

The aim of discharge planning is to reduce hospital length of stay, prevent unplanned readmissions and improve the coordination of services following discharge from hospital using a discharge plan tailored to the individual patient (Shepperd et al. 2010). Addressing the physical, psychological and social needs of the patient (and their partner or carer) pre-operatively enables discharge to be considered early in the care process with any referrals to MDT or other agencies made early to prevent delays in discharge.

The benefits of early discharge from acute hospital care are indisputable and nurses are in the key position of coordinating discharges in collaboration with the patient, family and MDT. Planning commences in the pre-operative phase as delayed discharges and prolonged hospitalisation can place the patient at additional health risks and there are financial and efficiency implications for the service. Good practice requires units to develop standards, protocols and audit tools to monitor the quality of discharges (Royal College of Nursing 2013). Information recorded at the ward round should make clear the thinking around the clinical decisions

and include clinical criteria for discharge (Royal College of Physicians 2021). Nurse-led discharge should be undertaken by appropriately trained members of the team who have been deemed competent. Those undertaking this extended role should have completed a competency-based educational programme and been assessed by a senior member of staff. See Chapter 6 for further information related to rehabilitation. Intensive rehabilitation during the acute phase of hospital admission achieves better outcomes for patients when delivered 7 days a week (British Orthopaedic Association 2015).

The criteria for a safe discharge from hospital to home are listed in Box 14.2.

Box 14.2   Criteria for Discharge from Hospital to Home

- Vital signs are stable and comparable to those on admission.
- Correct orientation as to time, place and person or comparable to that on admission.
- Adequate pain control and provision of a supply of oral analgesia to take home.
- Patient or carer understands how to use all medications supplied and has been given written information about these, including specific instructions regarding prescribed analgesia, antiemetics, anticoagulants or antibiotics.
- Patient is able to dress and walk where appropriate.
- Minimal nausea, vomiting or dizziness.
- Minimal bleeding.
- Understands wound care and when the patient is able to bathe or shower.
- Arrangements made for wound dressing renewal and suture removal (if appropriate).
- Patient has passed urine if at high risk of retention.
- Check patient is not constipated prior to discharge.
- Patient has a responsible adult to take them home.
- Transport home should be by private car or taxi; public transport is not normally appropriate.
- Patient has a named carer to take responsibility for the next 24 hours.
- Written and verbal instructions given about postoperative care.
- Knows when to come back for follow-up (if appropriate).
- Speciality specific emergency contact number supplied for information or in an emergency (must not be an answer phone).
- General practitioner letter should be given to the patient/carer or posted/emailed depending on unit policy.

Box 14.3   Procedure-specific Information Prior to Discharge Home

- X-rays reviewed by surgical team confirming correct placement of prosthesis.
- Safe mobility using appropriate aids to a level dependent on surgery and physiotherapy goals achieved.
- Explain when to resume normal activities, including return to work, sexual activities and exercise.
- Provide information regarding recovery at home, both verbal and written or web-based if available and appropriate.
- Explain what 'normal' symptoms may be expected and their duration.
- Explain what symptoms may indicate a problem and what to do if they occur.
- Explain the arrangements for follow-up (telephone and/or outpatient).
- Home environment should be suitable for the patient following the procedure/surgery undertaken and equipment in place prior to the time of discharge if possible.
- Patient/carer/support network arrangements made for taking time off work or arranging care of children and pets to reduce initial stress during recovery period.

It is good practice whenever possible to include the patient's identified carer in all pre-discharge assessment and information giving. Nursing staff must ensure that they assess both the patient and their carer's understanding of their ongoing care responsibilities through structured questioning. Written documentation of this process is required. Box 14.3 lists some procedure-specific information.

Patient Education/Health Promotion

Patients are expected to continue care at home unless they are discharged to a rehabilitation unit, residential, nursing or care home.

It is important that patients are advised to:

- continue taking regular analgesics as prescribed to help control pain and help with exercises and mobility
- eat a healthy well-balanced diet and stay hydrated (1.5–2 litres of water daily unless otherwise advised)
- continue exercises and progress mobility, although timescales will differ for everyone.

Recovery can be affected by age, general fitness and comorbidities.

Other issues include:

- Hip replacement dislocation precautions: avoid bending >90°, avoid adduction (crossing operative leg over midline), avoid internal/external rotation or twisting.
- Knee replacement: elevate the leg and apply ice to knee to relieve swelling. Kneeling can be problematic and it is advised to kneel on a pillow.
- Driving a car usually around 6 weeks post-surgery and able to perform an emergency stop with operated leg. This time frame will vary according to the type of car, e.g. automatic or manual. Patients should establish with their orthopaedic team when it is safe to drive after surgery. Failure to do so may invalidate their car insurance.
- Inform dentist of prosthetic joint as antibiotic cover is required for any procedures lasting >30 minutes due to risk of bacterial infection.
- Air travel should be avoided within 4 weeks of surgery because of an increased risk of DVT. Patients should consult their surgeon for advice.
- Metal detectors have varying levels of sensitivity and can alarm; a medical alert card or letter indicating an artificial joint can be provided by the hospital or surgical team.
- Details of implant size and type is provided to NJR with the patient's consent.

There are some significant problems that may arise and require urgent treatment. Patients and carers should be aware of these and the importance of seeking medical advice immediately:

- It is common to have a low-grade fever after surgery. Increased pain with activity and on rest, a high fever, redness swelling, tenderness or drainage from the wound may indicate an infection.
- Swelling is normal for the first 3–6 months after surgery, but severe lower limb pain accompanied by tenderness and swelling should be reported due to increased risk of DVT.
- Sudden onset of chest pain, localised chest pain accompanied by coughing or shortness of breath may be signs of a PE.

Summary

Elective orthopaedic surgery encompasses a range of procedures from day-case surgery such as knee arthroscopy to joint replacements requiring in-patient stay. However, the principles of care remain the same. Patients benefit from surgery if they are involved in the decision to operate and are fully prepared for what will happen to them along the patient pathway. Orthopaedic nurses can play a key role in ensuring systems are in place, such as joint schools, to allow this preparation to occur. Fitness for surgery and anaesthesia also need to be established and can be achieved through nurse-led pre-operative assessment. Orthopaedic theatre staff require skills and knowledge not only in perioperative nursing but also in orthopaedic care if they are to

play a full part in maximising the benefits of surgery for the patient. Key orthopaedic principles such as correct moving and handling, and early detection of potential complications such as peripheral neurovascular deficit are vital skills for theatre staff. In the recovery phase of elective orthopaedic surgery patients require skilled care from orthopaedic nurses who are knowledgeable about the normal recovery pathway and can act if any abnormalities occur.

Further Reading and Resources

Association of Anaesthetists (2019) *Guidelines for day case surgery offer information and guidance on day care and short stay surgery*. https://anaesthetists.org/Home/Resources-publications/Guidelines/Day-case-surgery.

Blandford, C. and Dunstan, E. (2020). *Day Case Hip & Knee Replacement*, 2e. British Association of Day Surgery.

British Association of Day Surgery publish an annual *Directory of Procedures* which provides aspirational benchmarks for day surgery (including outpatient surgery). https://daysurgeryuk.net/en/home.

Jester, R., Santy-Tomlinson, J., and Rogers, J. (2021). *Oxford Handbook of Trauma and Orthopaedic Nursing*, 2e. Oxford: Oxford University Press.

Model Hospital is a free digital tool which enables trusts to compare their productivity and identify opportunities to improvise. The database contains published Getting It

Right First Time and British Assiciation of Day Surgery day-case metrics across an array of specialties. http://www.model.nhs.uk.

NHS websites for resources on hip and knee replacements. www.nhs.uk.

NICE guidelines. www.nice.org.uk www.nice.org.uk/guidance/conditions-and-diseases/musculoskeletal-conditions (accessed 27 January 2022).

Royal College of Anaesthetists (2020) *Guidelines for the Provision of Anaesthesia Services for Day Surgery*. www.rcoa.ac.uk/gpas/chapter-6#.

Serious Hazards of Transfusion (2022) *SHOT definitions Version 7*. https://www.shotuk.org/?msclkid=46fde558a79211ec9e41f57b6cd9dce0 (accessed 19 March 2022).

Versus Arthritis website. www.versusarthritis.org.

References

AbdelSalam, H., Restrepo, C., Tarity, T.D. et al. (2012). Predictors of intensive care unit admission after total joint arthroplasty. *The Journal of Arthroplasty* 27 (5): 720–725.

ASA (2020) *Physical Status Classification System Committee of Oversight: Economics* (Approved by the ASA House of Delegates on October 15, 2014, and last amended on December 13, 2020). American Society of Anesthesiologists Physical Status Classification System. asahq.org (accessed 20 March 2022).

Barnsley, L., Barnsley, L., and Page, R. (2015). Are hip precautions necessary post total hip arthroplasty? A systematic review. *Geriatric Orthopaedic Surgery and Rehabilitation* 6 (3): 230–235.

Bergman, M., Stenudd, M., and Engström, A. (2012). The experience of being awake during orthopaedic surgery under regional anaesthesia. *International Journal of Orthopaedic and Trauma Nursing* 16 (2): 88–96.

Brembo, E.A., Kapstad, H., Van Dulmen, S., and Eide, H. (2017). Role of self-efficacy and social support in

short-term recovery after total hip replacement: a prospective cohort study. *Health and Quality of Life Outcomes* 15 (68): https://doi.org/10.1186/s12955-017-0649-1.

British Institute of Learning Disabilities (2009) *Brief Guide to the Mental Capacity Act 2005. Implications for people with learning disabilities*. www.scie.org.uk/files/mca/directory/bild-mca.pdf?res=true (accessed 26 January 2022).

British Orthopaedic Association (2015) *A national review of adult elective orthopaedic services in England: Getting it right first time*. British Orthopaedic Association, London.

Buus, A., Hejlsen, O.K., Dorisdatter Bjornes, C., and Laugesen, B. (2021). Experiences of pre-and postoperative information among patients undergoing knee arthroplasty: a systematic review and narrative synthesis. *Disability and Rehabilitation* 43 (2): 150–162. https://doi.org/10.1080/09638288.2019.1615997.

Campbell, K.J., Louie, P.K., Bohl, D.D. et al. (2019). A novel, automated text-messaging system is effective in patients undergoing total joint arthroplasty. *The Journal of Bone and Joint Surgery*. 101 (2): 145–151.

Carless, P.A., Henry, D.A., Moxey, A.J. et al. (2010). Cell salvage for minimising perioperative allogeneic blood transfusion. *Cochrane Database of Systematic Reviews* (4): CD001888. https://doi.org/10.1002/14651858.CD001888.pub4.

Cohn, E. and Larson, E. (2007). Improving participant comprehension in the informed consent process. *Journal of Nursing Scholarship* 39 (3): 273–280.

Day, M.A., Anthony, C.A., Bedard, N.A. et al. (2018). Increasing perioperative communication with automated mobile phone messaging in total joint arthroplasty. *The Journal of Arthroplasty* 33 (1): 19–24.

Dayucos, A., French, L.A., Kelemen, A. et al. (2019). Creation and evaluation of a preoperative education website for hip and knee replacement patients-a pilot study. *Medicina* 55 (32): https://doi.org/10.3390/medicina55020032.

Deyo, R.A. and Mirza, S.K. (2006). Trends and variations in the use of spine surgery. *Clinical Orthopaedics and Related Research* 443: 139–146.

Drozd, M., Chadwick, D., and Jester, R. (2021). The voices of people with an intellectual disability and a carer about orthopaedic and trauma hospital care in the UK: an interpretative phenomenological study. *International Journal of Orthopaedic and Trauma Nursing* https://doi.org/10.1016/j.ijotn.2020.100831.

Dutta, A.K. (2011). Positioning in upper-extremity surgery. *Operative Techniques in Sports Medicine* 19 (4): 231–237.

El Ashmawy, A.H., Dowson, K., El-Bakoury, A. et al. (2021). Effectiveness, patient satisfaction, and cost reduction of virtual joint replacement clinic follow-up of hip and knee arthroplasty. *The Journal of Arthroplasty* 36 (3): 816–822. https://doi.org/10.1016/j.arth.2020.08.019.

General Medical Council (2020) *Shared Decision Making is Key to Good Patient Care*. https://www.gmc-uk.org/news-archive/shared-decision-making-is-key-to-good-patient-care-gmc-guidance.

Gilbert, A.W., Billany, J.C.T., Adam, R. et al. (2020). Rapid implementation of virtual clinics due to COVID-19: report and early evaluation of a quality improvement initiative. *BMJ Open Quality* 9: e000985. https://doi.org/10.1136/bmjoq-2020-000985.

Grant, E., Johnson, L., Prodromidis, A., and Giannoudis, P.V. (2021). The impact of peer support on patient outcomes in adults with physical health conditions: a scoping review. *Cureus* 13 (8): e17442. https://doi.org/10.7759/cureus.17442.

Gupta, S., Jones, G., and Shah, S. (2017). Optimising orthopaedic follow-up care through a virtual clinic. *International Journal of Orthopaedic and Trauma Nursing* 28: 37–39.

Hallfors, E., Saku, S.A., Makinen, T.J., and Madanat, R. (2018). A consultation phone service or patients with total joint arthroplasty may reduce unnecessary emergency department visits. *The Journal of Arthroplasty* 33 (3): 650–654. https://doi.org/10.1016/j.arth.2017.10.040.

Hatfield, A. and Tronson, M. (2009). *The Complete Recovery Room Book*. Oxford: Oxford University Press.

Haynes, A.B., Weiser, T.G., Berry, W.R. et al. (2009). A surgical safety checklist to reduce morbidity and mortality in a global population. *The New England Journal of Medicine* 360 (5): 491–499.

Henry, D.A., Carless, P.A., Moxey, A.J. et al. (2001). Preoperative autologous donation for minimising perioperative allogeneic blood transfusion. *Cochrane Database of Systematic Reviews* (4): CD003602. https://doi.org/10.1002/14651858.CD003602.

Jester, R. and Rodney, A. (2021). The relationship between obesity and primary total knee replacement: a scoping review of the literature. *International Journal of Orthopaedic and Trauma Nursing* https://doi.org/10.1016/j.ijotn.2021.100850. Published online 16/2/2021.

Joanna Briggs Institute (2010) *Day Surgery (Adults): Premedication for Anxiety*. Evidence Summaries. Available via day surgery guidelines. Evidence search. Joanna Briggs Institute/NICE (accessed 19 March 2022).

Jones, A., Arshad, H., and Nolan, J. (2012). Surgical care practitioner practice: one team's journey explored. *Journal of Perioperative Practice* 22 (1): 19–23.

Kamecka, K., Rybarczyk-Szwajkowska, A., Staszewska, A. et al. (2021). Process of posthospital care involving telemedicine solutions for patients after total hip arthroplasty. *International Journal of Environmental Research and Public Health* 18 (10135): https://doi.org/10.3390/ijerph181910135.

Kaye, A.D., Urman, R.D., Cornett, E.M. et al. (2019). Enhanced recovery pathways in orthopaedic surgery. *Journal of Anaesthesiology Clinical Pharmacology* 35: S35–S39.

Kearney, M., Jennrich, M.K., Lyons, S. et al. (2011). Effects of preoperative education on patients outcomes after joint replacement surgery. *Orthopaedic Nursing* 30 (6): 391–396.

Kehlet, H. (1997). Multimodal approach to control postoperative pathophysiology and rehabilitation. *British Journal of Anaesthesia* 78 (5): 606–617.

Khoyratty, S., Modi, B.N., and Ravichandran, D. (2010). Preoperative starvation in elective general surgery. *Journal of Perioperative Practice* 20 (3): 100–102.

Kruse, C.S., Krowski, N., Rodriguez, B. et al. (2017). Telehealth and patient satisfaction: a systematic review and narrative analysis. *BMJ Open* 7 (8): 1, e016242.–12.

Lam, W.W.-K., Loke, A.Y., and Wong, C.-K. (2020). Personal and physical factors affecting the decision of patients to opt for spinal surgery: a case-control study. *International Journal of Orthopaedic and Trauma Nursing* 37: 1, 100753.–7.

Luo, J., Dong, X., and Hu, J. (2019). Effect of nursing intervention via a chatting tool on the rehabilitation of patients after total hip arthroplasty. *Journal of Orthopaedic Surgery and Research* 14: 417.

Lurie, J.D., Spratt, K.F., Blood, E.A. et al. (2011). Effects of viewing an evidence-based video decision aid on patients' treatment preferences for spine surgery. *Spine* 36 (18): 1501.

Mental Capacity Act (2005) www.legislation.gov.uk/ ukpga/2005/9/pdfs/ukpga_20050009_en.pdf (accessed 26 January 2022).

MHRA (2017) *All metal-on-metal (MoM) hip replacements: updated advice for follow-up of patients.* Medicines and Healthcare products Regulatory Agency. https://www.gov. uk/drug-device-alerts/all-metal-on-metal-mom-hip- replacements-updated-advice-for-follow-up-of-patients (accessed 20 March 2022).

Mitchell, L., Flin, R., Yule, S. et al. (2011). Thinking ahead of the patient. *International Journal of Nursing Studies* 48 (7): 818–828.

Molenaar, C.J.L., Papen-Botterhuis, N.E., Herrle, F., and Slooter, G.D. (2019). Prehabilitation, making patients fit for surgery-a new frontier in perioperative care. *Innovative Surgical Sciences* 4 (4): 132–138. https://doi.org/10.1515/ iss-2019-0017.

NHS (2018) *Lumbar decompression surgery.* https://www.nhs. uk/conditions/lumbar-decompression- surgery/#:~:text=Lumbar%20decompression%20 surgery%20is%20a,the%20nerves%20in%20the%20spine (accessed 12 February 2022).

NHS England (2019) *Universal Personalised Care: Implementing the Comprehensive Model.* www.england.nhs. uk/personalisedcare/comrehensive-model-of-care (accessed 10 January 2022).

NHS England (2021) *Online Library of Quality Service Improvement and Redesign tools: Enhanced Recovery.* https://www.england.nhs.uk/wp-content/ uploads/2021/03/qsir-enhanced-recovery.pdf.

NJR (2021) *18th Annual Report.* National Joint Registry for England and Wales. https://reports.njrcentre.org.uk/ Portals/0/PDFdownloads/NJR%2018th%20Annual%20 Report%202021.pdf (accessed 26 January 22).

NICE (2007). *Arthroscopic Knee Washout, with or without Debridement, for the Treatment of Osteoarthritis.* London: NICE.

NICE (2010a). *Minimally Invasive Total Hip Replacement.* London: NICE.

NICE (2010b). *Shoulder Resurfacing Arthroplasty.* London: NICE.

NICE (2011) (updated 2017). *Hip Fracture Management.* London: NICE.

NICE (2014). *Total Hip Replacement and Resurfacing Arthroplasty for End-Stage Arthritis of the Hip (Review of Technology Appraisal Guidance 2 and 44) G304.* London: NICE.

NICE (2016). *Routine Preoperative Tests for Elective Surgery.* London: NICE. www.nice.org.uk/guidance/ ng45ullguideline.pdf (accessed 24 January 2022).

NICE (2018a). *Mosaicplasty for Symptomatic Articular Cartilage Defects of the Knee.* London: NICE.

NICE (2018b). *Venous Thromboembolism in over 16s: Reducing the Risk of Hospital-Acquired Deep Vein Thrombosis or Pulmonary Embolism.* London: NICE.

NICE (2020a) *Perioperative care in adults [B]. Evidence review for enhanced recovery programmes.* www.nice.org.uk/ guidance/ng180/evidence/b-enhanced-recovery- programmes-pdf-8833151055 (accessed 23 November 2021).

NICE (2020b). *Joint Replacement (Primary): Hip, Knee and Shoulder.* London: NICE.

NICE (2020c). *Surgical Site Infections: Prevention and Treatment.* London: NICE.

Niel-Weise, B.S., Wille, J.C., and van den Broek, P.J. (2005). Hair removal policies in clean surgery: systematic review of randomized, controlled trials. *Infection Control and Hospital Epidemiology* 26: 923–928.

O'Reilly, M., Mohamed, K., Foy, D., and Shheehan, E. (2018). Educational impact of joint replacement school for patients undergoing hip and knee arthroplasty: a prospective cohort study. *International Orthopaedics* 42 (12): 2745–2754. https://doi.org/10.1007/s00264-018-4039-z.

Parkes, R.J., Palmer, J., Wingham, J., and Williams, D.H. (2019). Is virtual clinic follow-up of hip and knee joint replacement acceptable to patients and clinicians? A sequential mixed methods evaluation. *BMJ Open Quality* 8: e000502. https://doi.org/10.1136/bmjoq-2018-000502.

Pivec, R., Johnson, A.J., Mears, S.C., and Mont, M.A. (2012). Hip arthroplasty. *The Lancet* 380 (9855): 1768–1777.

Pradhan, R., Peeters, W., Boutong, S. et al. (2021). Virtual phone clinics in orthopaedics: evaluation of clinical application and sustainability. *BMJ Open Quality* 10 (4): e001349. https://doi.org/10.1136/bmjoq-2021-001349.

Punnoose, A., Weiss, O., Khanduja, V., and Rushton, A.B. (2019). Effectiveness of prehabilitation for patients undergoing orthopaedic surgery: protocol for a systematic review and meta-analysis. *BMJ Open* 9: e031119. https:// doi.org/10.1136/bmjopen-2019-031119.

Restrepo, C., Mortazavi, S.M., Brothers, J. et al. (2011). Hip dislocation: Are hip precautions necessary in anterior approaches? *Clinical Orthopaedics and Related Research* 469 (2): 417–422.

Royal College of Anaesthetists (2008) *Anaesthetic Choices for Hip or Knee Replacement.* Royal College of Anaesthetists, London.

Royal College of Anaesthetists (2022) *Guidelines for the Provision of Anaesthesia Services for the Perioperative Care of Elective and Urgent Care Patients*. Royal College of Anaesthetists, London.

Royal College of Nursing (2013) *Day Surgery Information: Discharge Planning*. Sheet 4. Royal College of Nursing, London.

Royal College of Physicians (2021) *Modern Ward Rounds. Executive summary and recommendations*. Royal College of Physicians, London.

Sepah, Y.J., Umer, M., Ahmad, T. et al. (2011). Use of tranexamic acid is a cost effective method in preventing blood loss during and after total knee replacement. *Journal of Orthopaedic Surgery and Research* 6: 22.

Shepperd, S., McClaran, J., Phillips, C.O. et al. (2010). Discharge planning from hospital to home. *Cochrane Database of Systematic Reviews* (1) See update 2013: CD000313. https://doi.org/10.1002/14651858.CD000313.pub4.

SHOT Team (2022) SHOT definitions version 7. https://www.shotuk.org/?msclkid=46fde558a79211ec9e41f57b6cd9dce0 (accessed 19 March 2022).

Smith, A.F. and Pittaway, A.J. (2002). Premedication for anxiety in adult day surgery. *Cochrane Database of Systematic Reviews* (3). See update Walker, K.J. and Smith, A.F. Premedication for anxiety in adult day surgery. *Cochrane Database of Systematic Reviews* 2009, 4 (Art. No.: CD002192). https://doi.org/10.1002/14651858. CD002192.pub2.

Smith, A.J., Dieppe, P., Vernon, K. et al. (2012). Failure rates of stemmed mental-on-metal hip replacements: analysis of data from the National Joint Registry of England and Wales. *The Lancet* 379 (9822): 1199–1204.

Stern, C. and Lockwood, C. (2005). Knowledge retention from preoperative patient information. *International Journal of Evidence-Based Health Care* 3 (3): 45–63.

Tanner, J., Norrie, P., and Melen, K. (2011). Preoperative hair removal to reduce surgical site infection. *Cochrane Database of Systematic Reviews* CD004122. https://doi.org/10.1002/14651858.CD004122.pub4.

Tartari, E., Weterings, V., Gastmeier, P. et al. (2017). Patient engagement with surgical site infection prevention: an expert panel perspective. *Antimicrobial Resistance and Infection Control* 6: 45. https://doi.org/10.1186/s13756-017-0202-3.

Taurchini, M., Del Naja, C., and Tancredi, A. (2018). Enhanced recovery after surgery: a patient centered process. *Journal of Visulaized Surgery* 4 (40): https://doi.org/10.21037/jovs.2018.0.

The Stationery Office (2007) *The Mental Capacity Act 2005 Code of Practice 2007*. The Stationery Office, London. https://assets.publishing.service.gov.uk/government/uploads/system/uploads/attachment_data/file/497253/Mental-capacity-act-code-of-practice.pdf (accessed 26 January 2022).

Tonelli, M.R. and Sullivan, M.D. (2019). Person-centred shared decision making. *Journal of Evaluation in Clinical Practice* 25 (6): 1057–1062. https://doi.org/10.1111/jep.13260.

Veiga, D.F., Damasceno, C.A.V., Veiga-Filho, J. et al. (2009). Randomized controlled trial of the effectiveness of chlorhexidine showers before elective plastic surgical procedures. *Infection Control and Hospital Epidemiology* 30: 77–79.

Webster, J. and Osborne, S. (2015). Preoperative bathing or showering with skin antiseptics to prevent surgical site infection. *Cochrane Database of Systematic Reviews* (2): CD004985. https://doi.org/10.1002/14651858.CD004985.pub5. 45.

WHO (2009) *Implementation Manual WHO Surgical Safety Checklist 2009*. World Health Organization. Implementation manual WHO surgical safety checklist 2009 (acccessed 19 March 2022).

Wing Wai, C.L. and Irwin, M.G. (2012). Regional blocks in orthopaedics. *Anaesthesia and Intensive Care Medicine* 13 (3): 89–93.

Woodhead, K. and Wicker, P. (2005). *A Textbook of Perioperative Care*. Edinburgh: Elsevier.

Wu, K.T., Lee, P.S., Chou, W.Y. et al. (2018). Relationship between the social support and self-efficacy for function ability in patients undergoing primary hip replacement. *Journal of Orthopaedic Surgery and Research* 13 (150): https://doi.org/10.1186/s13018-018-0857-3.

Wylde, V., Kunutsor, S.K., Lenguerrand, E. et al. (2019). Association of social support with patient-reported outcomes after joint replacement: a systematic review and meta-analysis. *The Lancet Rheumatology* 13 (19): 30050–30055. https://doi.org/10.1016/S2665-9913(19)30050-5.

Xie, J., Cai, Y., Ma, J. et al. (2020). Oral mosapride can provide additional antiemetic efficacy following total joint arthroplasty under general anesthesia: a randomized, double-blinded clinical trial. *BMC Anesthesiology* 20: 297. https://doi.org/10.1186/s12871-020-01214-4.

Yang, X., Li, G.H., Wang, H.J., and Wang, C.Y. (2019). Continuous passive motion after total knee arthroplasty: a systematic review and meta-analysis of associated effects on clinical outcomes. *Archives of Physical Medicine and Rehabilitation* https://doi.org/10.1016/j.apmr.2019.02.001.

Zhang, X., Chen, X., Kourkoumelis, N. et al. (2021). A social media-promoted educational community of joint replacement patients using the WeChat app: survey study. *JMIR mHealth and uHealth* 9 (3): e18763. https://doi.org/10.2196/18763.

Zheng, Q.Y., Geng, L., Ni, M. et al. (2019). Modern instant messaging platform for postoperative follow-up of patients after total joint arthroplasty may reduce re-admission rate. *Journal of Orthopaedic Surgery and Research* 14 (464): https://doi.org/10.1186/s13018-019-1407-3.

15

Musculoskeletal Oncology over the Lifespan

Helen Stradling

Sarcoma UK, London, UK

Introduction

Sarcoma is a rare form of cancer that affects all age groups and all parts of the body. There are approximately 5300 new diagnoses in the UK each year and these account for approximately 1.4% of all cancer diagnoses (Sarcoma UK 2020). Sarcoma affects the connective tissue of the body, including bone, muscle, nerve, fat and blood vessel cells. A sarcoma is often described as either 'bone', 'soft tissue' or gastrointestinal stromal tumour. Sarcoma that usually affects bone can be found extraskeletally and conversely sarcoma that primarily affects soft tissue can also be found in bone. Sarcoma is a primary cancer, which originates from one of the cells of connective tissue. Bone cancer can also be metastatic in instances where a primary cancer, for example lung or breast, has spread to the bone. This is treated very differently to sarcoma and so practitioners need to be aware of the differences.

Bone sarcoma is more prevalent in younger age groups whereas soft tissue sarcoma is more likely in older age, although this does not make either exclusive to these age groups and there is currently no definitive evidence to show any reason for this. Sarcoma has a slightly higher incidence in males than females but the reason for this is also unclear. The importance of a prompt diagnosis cannot be overstated as this has a direct effect on prognosis, especially if the delay leads to the patient presenting with metastatic disease. The signs and symptoms of sarcoma can be as simple as a non-painful soft tissue swelling or as severe as a pathological fracture of bone. Figure 15.1 shows a soft tissue sarcoma of the upper arm. Figure 15.2 shows a pathological fracture of the distal femur.

Patients do not tend to become systemically unwell with sarcoma at an early stage and this can be a deterrent to diagnosis as a painful limb could have many differential diagnoses, of which sarcoma does not rank highly in the minds of many practitioners. It is suggested that a general practitioner will only encounter an average of one or two sarcoma diagnoses in their career. It is important for practitioners to not only be aware of sarcoma, but to have a knowledge base that will support them well when coming into contact with these patients and their families. Due to the less common nature of this cancer type is it unlikely that a person newly diagnosed with sarcoma would have heard of it before or know of someone who has been given the diagnosis previously. It is estimated that 75% of people in the UK do not know, or are unsure, of what sarcoma is (Sarcoma UK 2020). This can make the diagnosis even more daunting than a diagnosis of a more common cancer type. For them to be cared for by a practitioner who is also unaware of the implications of their diagnosis and treatment can lead to a very disjointed, misinformed care pathway in which the patient and family feel unsupported.

The majority of sarcoma will be treated surgically in an orthopaedic setting but, due to the fact that sarcoma can be diagnosed in any anatomical site, practitioners could come into contact with sarcoma in any setting. It is therefore of paramount importance for sarcoma education to be included in orthopaedic as well as oncology texts.

Bone Sarcoma

Bone sarcoma often occurs in the younger age group under the age of 30 years, but not exclusively. There is one type of bone cancer, chondrosarcoma, which originates from cartilage cells, that has greater prevalence in the older age range of 50 years plus, and chordoma which originates from the notochord likewise. The two most common types

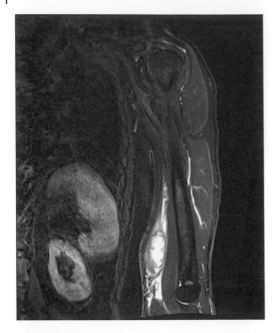

Figure 15.1 MRI scan showing soft tissue sarcoma of the upper arm.

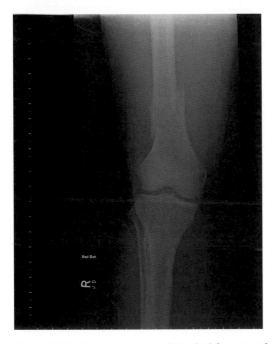

Figure 15.2 X-ray showing pathological fracture of the distal femur.

of bone sarcoma in the younger population are Ewing's sarcoma and osteosarcoma. Bone sarcoma can occur in any skeletal bone but remains more prevalent in the long bones of the limbs and the pelvis. It often occurs around joints, which may be a reason for it being misdiagnosed as the differential diagnoses can be seen as a more likely diagnosis.

Signs and Symptoms

The most common symptom of bone sarcoma is pain in the affected area. This pain can be more of an issue at night and can wake a person from their sleep due to its intensity. In some cases the bone tumour can break through the cortex of the bone involved and invade soft tissue, resulting in a noticeable soft tissue mass unlike tumours, which are contained within bone. Bone tumours can also weaken bone and this can lead to the first symptom presenting as a pathological fracture. Although pathological fractures are associated with older patients, they can occur in patients of all ages with bone tumours. Although the majority of patients with a primary bone sarcoma do not feel systemically unwell, patients with Ewing's sarcoma can suffer from fever and a general malaise.

Diagnosis

Bone sarcoma cannot always be detected on X-ray and therefore the need for further investigation where bone pain cannot be explained is very important. Diagnosis of bone sarcoma should never be given without a proven histological diagnosis. This ensures the type of sarcoma is established and the correct treatment regimen is administered from the outset. It is vital that the diagnosis is made correctly in the first instance to reduce delays in treatment and therefore to improve outcomes. Any patient with a suspected bone sarcoma should be referred to a specialist centre. In 2015 the National Institute for Health Care Excellence (NICE) published quality standards to ensure that all patients with sarcoma are informed about sarcoma, receive timely and appropriate advice, and can access relevant services. Specialist centres ensure that patients are cared for by clinicians and specialist staff who regularly care for patients and families with this rare group of cancers. Any lesion that is suspicious of a primary malignant bone tumour should have a biopsy in a specialist centre (Gerrand et al. 2016). The biopsy can be undertaken in a number of ways: either under image guidance, be it ultrasound, fluoroscopy or computed tomography (CT), or as an open procedure in the operating theatre (the preferred option for children). The decision relating to how the biopsy should be performed will be discussed within the specialist multidisciplinary team (MDT) and will depend on the size, location and suspected histological subtype of the tumour. Biopsies need to be undertaken by specialists and it is important to ensure the biopsy tract can be removed as part of the surgical plan. Caution is needed for patients who are taking anticoagulation therapy as this may lead to a delay in the biopsy whilst the medication is temporarily withdrawn in order for clotting assessment to

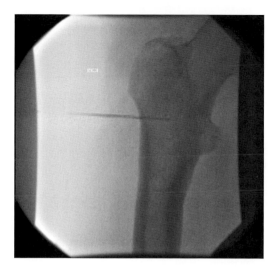

Figure 15.3 Fluoroscopic guided biopsy of a chondrosarcoma of the distal humerus.

be made. Figure 15.3 shows a fluoroscopic guided biopsy of a chondrosarcoma of the right femur.

Impact of Delayed Diagnosis

Delays in diagnosis of bone sarcoma are common in all parts of the pathway mainly due to lack of awareness of the potential for a malignant diagnosis (Grimer et al. 2010). The longer a patient has to wait for a diagnosis, especially with high-grade bone sarcoma, the more likely it will be that they may have metastases at diagnosis. This is a factor in a poorer prognosis, and it is therefore vital to gain a diagnosis and, in most cases, commence treatment as soon as possible. Lawrenz et al. (2020) stated that a review of over 2100 patients with localised, high-grade primary bone sarcoma showed that a delay of 10 days between diagnosis and initiation of treatment had no effect on overall survival, allowing patients to receive a second opinion or referral to a higher volume specialist sarcoma centre, and this is important for healthcare practitioners to be aware of when counselling patients. See Box 15.1 for a discussion of the evidence underpinning early diagnosis.

Staging

Staging of sarcoma should be undertaken once a definite diagnosis has been given. Staging should include a CT scan or a positron emission tomography (PET) scan; these give the treating clinician information relating to whether metastatic disease is present. This is important when deciding on the treatment plan for patients, for example it would be less likely for a surgeon to offer an amputation as a surgical option if the patient already has lung metastases.

Box 15.1   **Evidence Digest**
Study of sarcoma size at presentation (Grimer 2006)   This study looked at a total of 1460 patients who had been diagnosed with sarcoma and who had received 3 years of post-operative follow-up. The patients had been cared for at one hospital and the aim of the study was to look at whether the size of sarcoma at presentation had a bearing on the patient's outcome. The NICE (2005) guidelines for sarcoma state that any patient with a soft tissue mass of over 5 cm should be referred to a sarcoma specialist and the mass presumed to be a sarcoma until proven otherwise. The study took the size of sarcoma at time of diagnosis and this information was gained from the medical notes of all the patients. It showed that the mean size of soft tissue sarcoma at presentation was 10 cm, which is double the recommended size for referral. Bone sarcoma had an average of 11.3 cm and there seemed to be little difference, with changes in patient age or type of sarcoma diagnosis. The detection of metastatic disease at presentation had a direct link to the size of sarcoma at diagnosis. The prognosis for all patients without metastatic disease worsened with the increase in the size of the tumour. The outcome of the study was to increase the awareness of sarcoma to try to reduce the size of these tumours at diagnosis. The hope is that with smaller tumours being diagnosed the patient's overall outcomes and prognoses will improve.

Treatments

The treatment for a sarcoma will depend on the histological diagnosis of each lesion. Treatments, including surgery, chemotherapy and radiotherapy, are options that will be determined by the results of histology. Some patients receive surgery alone, where others may need to have a combination of surgery, chemotherapy and radiotherapy.

Surgery can vary considerably for both bone and soft tissue sarcoma removal. For soft tissue sarcoma it can be as simple as wide local excision of the lesion or there could be extensive excision of the tumour and surrounding soft tissue that necessitates subsequent plastic surgery reconstruction. For bone sarcoma, the surgery can be as straightforward as an excision of a bone tumour with no reconstruction needed, to surgery including amputation of a limb or limb lengthening using external fixation and bone transport (Chapter 8). Surgery for bone sarcoma of a limb now focuses much more on limb salvage, whereas in the past amputation would have been the preferred surgical option. Limb salvage is the preferred choice due to the advances in limb salvage surgery. This includes the improvement of the type of prostheses that are available to be used and also the new techniques available to orthopaedic surgeons, for example bone transport. Orthopaedic nurses are therefore very involved in the surgical care of bone sarcoma patients. Children now have the option of a non-invasive growing prosthesis, which enables lengthening of the prosthesis as a day case non-operative procedure rather than having to undergo a number of operations to extend the prosthesis, which was the previous method. Patients with chordoma of the sacrum may require a total sacrectomy; this can be very invasive surgery, which can lead to the loss of nerves, potentially leaving the patient incontinent and in need of stoma reconstruction. Surgery with a curative intent aims to be much more radical than surgery for a palliative intent. The surgery for sarcoma should be discussed with the patient, who should be supported by the MDT.

Radiotherapy for primary bone sarcoma is usually undertaken on a daily basis, Monday–Friday for a period of up to 6 weeks.

Chemotherapy for primary bone sarcoma will also depend on the histological diagnosis but can be given in the day-care setting or as an inpatient for up to 4–5 days depending on the treatment regimen. This means that the length of treatment for primary bone sarcoma can last as long as 9–12 months. This is a factor that needs to be taken into account when the patients are of an age where they are at school, attending university or in the early stages of employment. A number of the chemotherapy agents used to treat bone sarcoma can cause infertility. This is an issue for teenagers and young adults and needs to be discussed in detail with them. Healthcare professionals caring for sarcoma patients whose fertility could be affected by their treatment should prioritise their referral to fertility specialists prior to commencing treatment (Lopategui et al. 2017). The type of chemotherapy used is extremely toxic and the team need to ensure that patients are fit enough to tolerate it. Many centres do not offer high-dose chemotherapy to patients over the age of 40. Due to the toxic nature of the treatments used, patients over the age of 40 will have the option of high-dose chemotherapy discussed with them on an individual basis. From experience, many people over the age of 40 who do start high-dose chemotherapy are unable to finish the course of treatment due to the high incidence of side effects, which become intolerable for them.

The types of treatments used will be discussed in more detail with each subtype of sarcoma and also in the evidence digest. The most common types of bone sarcoma will now be further explored. See Box 15.2 for a discussion of clinical practice guidelines.

Box 15.2 Evidence Digest

Clinical practice guidelines: Bone sarcomas: UK guidelines for the management of bone sarcomas (Gerrand et al. 2016)

Soft tissue sarcomas: UK guidelines for the management of soft tissue sarcomas (Dangoor et al. 2016)

A number of leading specialists have worked together to produce European guidelines for the diagnosis, treatment and follow-up of these tumours.

The guidelines clearly define the pathway that any patients with suspected sarcoma should follow, including:

- referral to a specialist sarcoma service
- biopsy to ONLY be undertaken by a member of the specialist sarcoma MDT
- treatment plans to be discussed by the sarcoma MDT and decided on an individual basis
- follow-up to include regular scanning for disease recurrence and metastatic disease.

These guidelines are intended to ensure the early diagnosis and correct treatment for sarcoma patients. It is, however, identified that all patients should be taken on an individual basis when it comes to treatment planning, taking into account size, grade and location of tumour, along with age and comorbidities of the patient and the presence or not of metastatic disease.

Osteosarcoma

Osteosarcoma is a disease that is still not fully understood. It was first described in 1805 by French surgeon Alexis Boyer, who found that these lesions were a very different type of disease to other bone lesions (Peltier 1993). Osteosarcoma is the most common type of bone sarcoma and in the UK, for example, it accounts for approximately 131 new diagnoses each year (National Cancer Intelligence Network 2012). Osteosarcoma has its highest incidence between the ages of 5 and 20 years. It is very uncommon in the under-5s, although not unreported, and increases in incidence with age throughout the teenage years. It has a higher incidence in males than females, although there is no apparent reason for this.

Osteosarcoma becomes a life-threatening condition once metastatic disease is present. Once a diagnosis of osteosarcoma has been made the need for staging scans, usually CT scan of the chest or PET CT, is of paramount importance. Metastatic disease can be undetectable very early on in the disease process but it is reported that approximately 80% of patients with a high-grade osteosarcoma diagnosis will

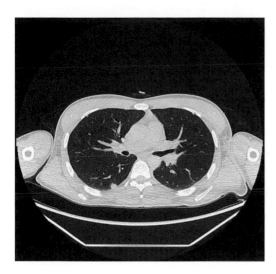

Figure 15.4 CT scan of the chest showing metastatic osteosarcoma.

present with metastatic disease (Kim and Helman 2010). Figure 15.4 shows metastatic chest disease of a 32-year-old osteosarcoma patient.

Treatment for osteosarcoma depends, as with all sarcomas, on the histological subtype. A low-grade parosteal osteosarcoma can be treated with surgery alone to remove the tumour. A high-grade osteosarcoma of bone is treated with a combination of chemotherapy and surgery. The chemotherapy is given neo-adjuvantly and again adjuvantly depending on response rate. The chemotherapy regime used most often is methotrexate, doxorubicin, and cisplatinum (MAP) chemotherapy strategy, a combination of doxorubicin, cisplatin and methotrexate. Although there is still no worldwide census on the best chemotherapy regimens for osteosarcoma, a review by Anninga et al. (2011) shows that drug regimens using three drugs, such as MAP, are the most effective. This chapter does not expand on MAP as this is an orthopaedic text and it is hoped to focus the nurse on the orthopaedic treatments for these patients. Links for the chemotherapy treatments are included for further reading.

When caring for patients in the orthopaedic setting who have received chemotherapy as part of their treatment it is important to be aware of the side effects, which may affect their health. Surgery is usually planned in the window between chemotherapy cycles to take advantage of reduced risk from the side effects. Neutropenic sepsis is the most important side effect to be considered and is due to cytotoxic chemotherapy agents causing myelosuppression and immunosuppression. If neutropenic sepsis occurs it can be life-threatening and all cancer centres have guidelines for practitioners to follow when this is suspected. Patients require intravenous antibiotics

within a certain timescale and this has been described as 'door to needle in 60 minutes'. Signs to look for are:

- temperature of >38 °C
- flu-like symptoms
- dehydration.

If these occur an urgent blood test is required to assess the patient's neutrophil count. An absolute neutrophil count (ANC) of $<1.0 \times 10^9/l$ is diagnostic of neutropenia.

Nausea and vomiting are side effects of chemotherapy which can often be avoided with the use of antiemetic agents. Unfortunately, hair loss is a side effect that cannot be avoided in most cases as the drugs affect rapidly dividing cells such as the hair.

In 2011 NICE licenced the use of mifamutide (Mepact) in the treatment of patients with fully resected, non-metastatic osteosarcoma between the ages of 2 and 30 years. Mepact is an immunomodulator and is the first real advance in drug treatment for osteosarcoma in 20 years. Its precise mode of working in osteosarcoma is not known but it is thought to cause white blood cells to release chemicals that kill the cancer cells. It is used alongside conventional surgery and chemotherapy. The drug is given as an IV infusion over 1 hour, twice a week for the first 12 weeks and once a week for the following 24 weeks. It is a very expensive treatment option but has been shown to produce an increase in overall survival (Kager et al. 2010).

Ewing's Sarcoma

Ewing's sarcoma was first described in 1921 by James R Ewing, who noted that the histology in a bone tumour that had been thought to be an osteosarcoma looked different in that it had 'round cells' which looked like blood vessels and initially he termed it 'endothelioma of bone'. He first discussed a patient who was thought to have osteosarcoma of bone, who for some reason had not received the usual treatment of surgery at that time but had been treated with other modalities, including radiation. Osteosarcoma was known to not be radiosensitive and so when his patient had a complete response to the radiation treatment, Ewing knew that he was dealing with something different. Unfortunately, the patient then went on to have a recurrence of the tumour and it was decided that biopsy was required to settle the conundrum. It was here that Ewing found the different histological appearances and a little while later James Codman termed it Ewing's sarcoma. Surgery and radiotherapy were the only treatments used to treat Ewing's sarcoma until the 1960s, when it was found to be responsive to certain chemotherapy agents

(Samuels and Howe 1967; Cupps et al. 1969). In the 1980s the genetic diagnosis of Ewing's sarcoma became possible with the identification of the chromosomal translocation between chromosomes 22 and 11, t (11;22). This defect can be found only in Ewing's cancer cells, is not inherited and is found in approximately 90% of Ewing's sarcomas. This has helped with the histological diagnosis and subsequent treatment.

As with osteosarcoma, patients diagnosed with Ewing's sarcoma have systemic staging undertaken prior to commencement of treatments. Ewing's can be treated successfully with chemotherapy and radiotherapy, but in certain cases surgery is also part of the treatment regime. Chemotherapy for Ewing's sarcoma has been streamlined over the years. All patients are now treated with the vincristine, doxorubicin, cyclophosphamide, ifosfamide and etoposide (VDC/IE) protocol which includes induction of treatment for 18 weeks on 3 weekly cycles. Consolidation of treatment is then decided on the results from the local treatment of either surgery, radiotherapy or a combination of the two, and will be following a discussion at the sarcoma multidisciplinary team meeting (MDT). Again, due to the nature of the toxicity of the drugs, patients require echocardiogram and ethylenediaminetetraacetic acid (EDTA) creatinine clearance tests prior to the commencement of the regime. As discussed in the osteosarcoma section, patients who are having these toxic drug regimens need to have attention paid to their general health to diagnose any potential problems as soon as they occur.

Chondrosarcoma

Chondrosarcoma is a bone sarcoma which tends to affect those in the older age group but, as with all sarcomas, it is seen in all ages. The chance of being diagnosed with a chondrosarcoma increases with age and has no known definite cause. Chondrosarcoma is most common in the humerus and distal femur, and has only a slightly higher incidence in males than females. Chondrosarcoma accounts for approximately 25% of malignant bone tumours and has a diverse behaviour pattern from the low-grade local tumour to the highgrade metastasising tumour (Flemming and Murphey 2000). Chondrosarcoma arises from the cartilage cells and certain conditions increase the chance of benign bone tumours differentiating into a chondrosarcoma, including enchondroma, osteochondroma, multiple exostosis, Ollier's disease and Malfucci's syndrome (Unni and Inwards 2010). Patients with a diagnosis of chondrosarcoma require full staging

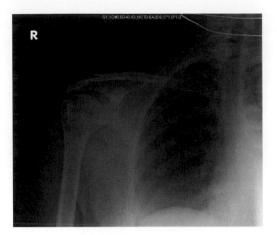

Figure 15.5 X-ray showing chondrosarcoma of the proximal humerus.

as with all sarcoma patients and this is usually in the form of a bone scan and CT scan of the chest. The majority of chondrosarcoma are low-grade localised tumours that require only surgical excision. This can be anything from a curettage and cementation to an endoprosthetic replacement. Figure 15.5 is an X-ray showing chondrosarcoma of the proximal humerus.

Patients receiving surgery for excision of chondrosarcoma are cared for very similarly to any orthopaedic patient, but it needs to be remembered that they have been given a cancer diagnosis and therefore will require psychological support. Very few patients have a diagnosis of dedifferentiated chondrosarcoma, and they will need to discuss their treatment options with an experienced sarcoma oncologist who may or may not offer chemotherapy as a treatment option depending on the extent of disease and the patient's age. Most chondrosarcoma are resistant to radiotherapy treatment and so this is not a preferred treatment option.

Other bone sarcoma diagnoses are less common and are beyond the scope of this chapter but need to be assessed and treated on an individual basis.

Soft Tissue Sarcoma

Soft tissue sarcoma is more common than bone sarcoma, accounting for 88% of all sarcoma diagnoses (Sarcoma UK 2020), and it can affect all age groups and all anatomical sites of the body. There are many more subtypes of soft tissue sarcoma than bone sarcoma. From clinical experience liposarcoma and leiomyosarcoma appear to be the most common subtypes and the thigh appears to be the most common anatomical site.

Signs and Symptoms

Soft tissue sarcomas usually present as a soft tissue mass which can be either painful or pain-free and can cause symptoms or be asymptomatic. The fact that the signs and symptoms can vary so drastically could also be a reason for them to be misdiagnosed. Soft tissue sarcomas are often difficult to locate on plain X-ray but ultrasound and magnetic resonance imaging (MRI) are much more useful to describe the size, site and positioning of the tumour in relation to other anatomical structures. As with bone sarcoma, patients do not usually become systemically unwell.

Diagnosis

As with bone sarcoma the guidance for the pathway to diagnosis of a soft tissue sarcoma is very clearly set out, and anyone with a suspected sarcoma should be referred to a sarcoma specialist centre for diagnostic tests (Dangoor et al. 2016). MRI can show suspicious features of a soft tissue mass but again the histological diagnosis is crucial to treatment decisions. Suspected soft tissue sarcoma is mainly biopsied under ultrasound guidance, although in some cases the soft tissue biopsies are undertaken by clinicians in the outpatient clinic setting. Again, consideration and caution may need to be taken for patients receiving anticoagulation therapy. Grimer (2006) undertook a study which showed that the size of soft tissue sarcoma at diagnosis has an impact on prognosis. This study reviewed the cases of over 3000 patients who had been diagnosed with soft tissue sarcoma over a 20-year time period. It was shown that the average size of soft tissue sarcoma at diagnosis was 10.7 cm and this had not significantly reduced in the last 20 years. It also showed that the size of tumour at diagnosis had a direct effect on whether the patient could receive limb salvage surgery against amputation, and the incidence of metastatic disease at presentation. The UK guidance on sarcoma is currently that any soft tissue mass of 5 cm or over should be treated as a soft tissue sarcoma until proven otherwise (National Institute of Clinical Excellence 2005).

Treatments

As with bone sarcoma, the treatments offered to soft tissue sarcoma patients also depend on the histological subtype. The main treatment options for soft tissue sarcoma without metastatic disease are surgery and radiotherapy. Chemotherapy is usually used more when the disease is metastatic.

The most common subtypes of soft tissue sarcoma will now be considered in more detail.

Liposarcoma

Liposarcoma is the most common type of soft tissue sarcoma in adults. It was first described in the 1860s as a malignant tumour of fat by Rudolph Virchow. Liposarcoma can arise in any part of the body and is currently subtyped as follows:

- well differentiated
- dedifferentiated
- myxoid
- round cell
- pleomorphic.

The most common sites of presentation are as follows:

- well-differentiated liposarcoma tends to arise in the limb and retroperitoneum
- myxoid and/or round cell as well as pleomorphic arise in the limbs
- dedifferentiated liposarcoma mainly arises in the retroperitoneum.

Liposarcoma is more common in the older population, is rare in children (Vocks et al. 2000) and has a slightly higher incidence in males than females. Figure 15.6 shows an MRI scan of liposarcoma of the thigh.

The presentation of liposarcoma, as with most soft tissue sarcoma, usually includes:

- soft tissue swelling
- pain
- reduced range of movement
- numbness.

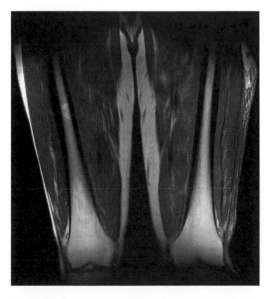

Figure 15.6 MRI scan of liposarcoma of the thigh.

However, patients with liposarcoma of the retroperitoneal cavity often complain of:

- abdominal pain
- weight loss
- nausea
- vomiting.

The treatment for liposarcoma is usually surgical excision, although radiotherapy is now being used more frequently as a neo-adjuvant treatment for myxoid liposarcoma of the limb and trunk. It allows less radiation to be used than in the adjuvant setting and clinically does not appear to cause any adverse complications for surgery. Chemotherapy is not routinely used for liposarcoma in the primary diagnosis setting but can be used in the presentation of high-grade tumours and metastatic liposarcoma (Dalal et al. 2008). This would be discussed with each individual patient after presentation at a specialist sarcoma MDT.

Synovial Sarcoma

Synovial sarcoma is another common type of soft tissue sarcoma and is more prevalent in younger age groups, especially within the first two decades of life (Vargas 2012). Synovial sarcoma does not, as its name suggests, arise in synovial joints but is named due to its similarity of cells to those of primitive synoviocytes. The most common anatomical sites for these tumours are around the knee but they can also be found often in the hands and feet. Synovial sarcoma has a specific chromosomal translocation which makes its diagnosis more specific as this is present in 90% of confirmed cases. The chromosomal translocation occurs at t(X;18) (p11.2;q11.2) (Knösel et al. 2010). This means that the X18 chromosome is affected and the p11:q11 are the points on the chromosome where the translocation takes place. Surgery is the main treatment option in this group of tumours. Although there have been discussions relating to the use of neo-adjuvant chemotherapy, it has been shown to date that this does not increase overall survival and so it remains controversial (Vargas 2012).

As with all tumour removal surgery the ultimate aim is to gain local control and therefore a wide local excision is recommended; an excision margin of 1–3 cm is appropriate. The ability to gain this much clearance during surgery will depend on the location of the tumour and radiotherapy may be used adjuvantly if there is concern about clear margins. Synovial sarcoma has a high incidence of metastatic spread (Stefanovski et al. 2002) and patients with this disease should have very careful follow-up, as with all sarcoma patients.

Leiomyosarcoma

Leiomyosarcoma is a soft tissue sarcoma that originates in smooth muscle cells and can appear at any site of the body. For the purpose of this text, leiomyosarcoma of the trunk and limbs will be the focus, but these tumours are common gynaecological tumours. Leiomyosarcoma tends to arise most commonly in adults and is one of the few soft tissue sarcomas that is more common in women, possibly related to the fact that they are most common in the gynaecological setting (Shah et al. 2005). Leiomyosarcoma accounts for approximately 10% of all soft tissue sarcomas (Schwartz 2007). Those that arise within venous walls have a poorer prognosis due to their ability to spread through the venous system, leading to a higher incidence of metastatic disease. In the limb, leiomyosarcoma is most commonly treated with surgery to remove the tumour, the extent depending on its location, size and the patient's general health. Radiotherapy and chemotherapy can be used in the treatment of high-grade tumours and metastatic disease, and this would be discussed with each individual patient as required following discussion at the sarcoma MDT.

Malignant Peripheral Nerve Sheath Tumour

Malignant peripheral nerve sheath tumours (MPNSTs) arise from peripheral nerves or cells related to nerve sheath, for example Schwann cells, perineural cells or fibroblasts. The term MPNST is now used to cover tumours that were previously named malignant schwannoma, neurofibrosarcoma and neurogenic sarcoma (Weiss and Goldburn 2001). MPNST is most commonly seen in adults, but has been noted in babies as young as 11 months (Ellison et al. 2005). It is seen most commonly in conjunction with large peripheral nerves such as the sacral nerve, brachial plexus and sacral plexus.

Treatment for MPNST is again surgically focused. The completion of surgery gaining wide (negative) margins is the intended outcome as this has been shown to reduce the likelihood of recurrence and metastatic disease (Geller and Gerbhardt 2006). The use of radiotherapy and chemotherapy in this tumour type is also controversial and needs to be discussed with each patient on an individual basis to weigh up the potential benefits against potential costs in terms of side effects, which may be long-term.

Epithelioid Sarcoma

Epithelioid sarcoma is the most common sarcoma of the hand and is a disease that is often found in the younger age group. These tumours are aggressive in nature and although they tend to be slow growing, they are known to often cause ulceration (Schwartz 2007). Epithelioid sarcoma often spreads along tendon sheaths and to lymph nodes associated with a high rate of recurrence and metastatic disease. It is suggested that an aggressive wide local excision should be used in the first instance (Schwartz 2007). Due to the aggressive nature of this disease, radiotherapy is often used in the neo-adjuvant setting and chemotherapy is used on an individual basis.

Rhabdomyosarcoma

Rhabdomyosarcoma accounts for approximately 20% of all soft tissue sarcoma. The embryonal and alveolar types are common in children and are the most common sarcoma in children, whereas the pleomorphic type affects adults. A clear histological definition of rhabdomyosarcoma was available in 1946 when these tumours were found to have a distinct morphology of rhabdomyoblasts (Stout 1946). Due to the nature of this disease and its occurrence in children, the treatment consists of a combination of surgery, radiotherapy and chemotherapy. The survival rate for childhood rhabdomyosaorcma is currently 70% at 5 years (Children with Cancer UK 2021). In patients with metastatic disease, however, the survival rate has not really improved, with a disease-free survival rate at 5 years of only 30% (Oberlin et al. 2008).

Metastatic Bone Disease

Metastatic bone tumours are becoming more common now that treatments for cancer are improving. These tumours occur when a primary cancer of another origin spreads to bone. The most common of these are breast, lung, renal and prostate, and they usually present with the following symptoms:

- pain in affected bone
- loss of mobility
- very often pathological fracture.

Figure 15.7 shows metastatic renal cell carcinoma of the proximal humerus.

If these tumours are solitary, they can be treated successfully with surgery and adjuvant treatment as deemed necessary by the oncologist treating their primary cancer site. It is important for the orthopaedic surgeon planning to operate on these patients to discuss their prognosis with the relevant oncologist. It would be more appropriate to offer an endoprosthetic replacement to a patient who had a relatively good prognosis than to someone who may only have weeks or months to live. This can sometimes be a very difficult decision to make so honest discussion relating to

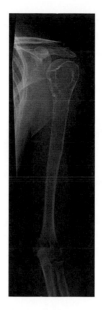

Figure 15.7 Metastatic renal cell carcinoma of the proximal humerus.

prognosis with all of the parties involved, including the patient and family, is key to ensuing the surgery is in the best interest of the patient.

Patients who are inpatients in the orthopaedic setting for surgery for metastatic bone disease often have more complex needs due to their primary cancer diagnosis, especially if they are still receiving oncology treatments. To have links to the patient's specialist nurse/keyworker and oncology teams during this time will enable the practitioner caring for them to discuss any needs that may arise which are oncological rather than orthopaedic. The following provides good practice recommendations for the management of metastatic bone disease: http://www.boos.org.uk/wp-content/uploads/2016/03/BOOS-MBD-2016-BOA.pdf.

Clinical Trials

Clinical trials for sarcoma take place in various centres. The location of these depends on the nature of the trial and the services needed to undertake the clinical trial. Bone sarcoma, due to its rarity, does not have a large number of trials open at any one time and it is the responsibility of the lead clinician to ensure the patient and family are aware of any clinical trials which they may be eligible to enter, even if it means they will receive their treatment in a different treatment centre. The problem with clinical trials in this group of patients is the fact that the number of patients diagnosed each year is low and therefore recruitment into clinical trials is small. The importance of clinical trials cannot be reiterated enough in a disease process where the development of treatments is slow to progress. Clinical trials relating to specific genetic mutations within the tumours is now becoming more widespread, which can only be positive for sarcoma patients as this will open up access to more clinical trials than those previously for disease-specific purposes only.

Nursing and Psychological Care

The nursing care of patients who have a diagnosis of primary sarcoma will depend very much on the treatments they receive. Surgery is usually undertaken in an orthopaedic setting under the care of an orthopaedic surgeon but frequently in collaboration with a plastic surgeon. The plastic surgery component of sarcoma treatment allows reconstruction of defects following the initial tumour removal. This is often done at the time of initial surgery but can also be undertaken at a later date if necessary. The age of the patient will also determine if the surgery is undertaken within the paediatric or adult setting. Depending on the nature of the surgery performed, patients can have a short hospital stay, for example for a straightforward excision of bone/soft tissue tumour, or a longer hospital stay for amputation, complex endoprosthetic replacement or limb lengthening with Ilizarov technology. Patients receiving chemotherapy will usually do so as an inpatient and within the oncology setting. Orthopaedic practitioners need to be aware of the common side effects of chemotherapy treatments, especially when surgery is an integral part of the treatment regimen and often within a very tight timescale between chemotherapy cycles.

Psychological support for patients and families with cancer is of paramount importance (Macmillan Cancer Support 2011) and 'efficacious, timely and acceptable psychological interventions are a necessary component of comprehensive cancer care' (Hulbert-Williams et al. 2018). The diagnosis of cancer in itself is frightening, but when you are then given a diagnosis that you have probably never heard of, or known anyone with the same, it can be even more challenging. The Internet is a growing resource for information and can be very useful but can also be extremely confusing and frightening for patients and their families. If a patient searches 'sarcoma' the result will be several million hits and the information available is not always in a format that meets the patient's needs. It is therefore important for appropriate information to be given regarding the disease as well as a treatment plan in a carefully considered and timely fashion with specialist nursing support. Sarcoma support groups are also available for patients and their families, although this is a personal choice and not all patients are happy to take part. General psychological support for cancer patients is available in cancer centres, but this service is not always easily accessible so specialist nurses and other sarcoma professionals are crucial to the provision of the appropriate psychological support of sarcoma patients. Charities also provide psychological support and information in the form of helplines, and Sarcoma UK provides a freephone support line for anyone affected by sarcoma.

The Role of Specialist Nursing

Specialist nursing in cancer care has been found to be of great benefit to both patients and families (National Cancer Action Team 2010). These roles allow a continuity of care to patients at a time when they may feel very 'out of control' following a cancer diagnosis. The roles are mainly supportive and advisory, but some of them include hands-on care also, especially in a chemotherapy setting. Specialist nursing roles can be health service funded or funded by cancer charities, for example Macmillan Cancer Support or Marie Curie in the UK. See Box 15.3 for discussion of the value of specialist roles.

These roles enable the patient and their family access to:

- specialist support prior to diagnosis
- specialist support and information at the time of diagnosis and throughout the treatment pathway
- a 'constant' in the huge number of different health professionals that they encounter throughout their journey
- a point of support that can refer the patient and family onto other services as required, including benefits advice, and dietician and palliative care.

Sarcoma Follow-up

Sarcoma follow-up, as with most cancer follow-up regimes, is a regular process of having scans and X-rays undertaken to assess for recurrent/metastatic disease and a clinical examination. The following shows a typical follow-up pathway for patients who have had surgery and/or radiotherapy for sarcoma:

- Two-week following surgery histology and wound check review.
- Three-month follow-up with baseline MRI and chest X-ray and clinical examination.
- Three-monthly reviews up to year 2 with chest X-ray and clinical examination at each appointment.
- Six-monthly reviews up to year 5 with chest X-ray and clinical examination at each appointment.
- Annual review with chest X-ray and clinical examination at each appointment up to year 10.

Box 15.3   Evidence Digest

The patient's perspective: a patient narrative written by a sarcoma patient who had access to specialist nurses

'In October 2010 I was diagnosed with a sarcoma in my left calf, a very rare cancerous tumour which was high grade and aggressive. I was immediately faced with the likelihood that I was about to undergo surgery which could result in part amputation of my left leg. Upon visiting the [hospital where my treatment would take place] beforehand, my family and I met Sarah, a specialist Macmillan Nurse. We were all touched by Sarah's incredibly positive, sensitive nature straight away, and we knew that we were in good hands. She gave us her contact details during the first meeting and told us to contact her with any query or problem, at any time.

Sarah, together with Jane (Sarah's colleague), provided a high level of support during the process of diagnosis, hospital admittance and after care. Whenever we were in need of advice and help in any way, Sarah and Jane would always reply to our calls or emails and gave 110% to resolve every issue every time. Their help and guidance helped to speed up my recovery after surgery and radiotherapy.

Following the dedication and world-class expertise of everyone in the Sarcoma Unit, we are now living life normally again. Thankfully, my leg is completely intact, after undergoing five hours of intensive surgery last October, although I was told afterwards that the margins were very narrow. I have now carefully resumed my favourite sport of mountain biking.

My family and I have felt so fortunate to have such a compassionate and professional team to support us with my fight against this cruel and indiscriminate illness. We would like to thank Sarah, Jane and everybody in the [hospital] for everything that they have done for us, and for their continued care'. James (age 37)

Note: Names have been changed to protect confidentiality.

Patients who are receiving, or have received, chemotherapy may have a slightly increased rate of follow-up. If at any point during the follow-up plan the patient should have signs of recurrent or metastatic disease, they should automatically have an MRI/CT scan and if disease is confirmed they would be treated accordingly. Patients with high-grade disease at presentation are more likely to go on to develop disease recurrence or metastatic disease, but this cannot be ruled out for any sarcoma patient, hence the need for regular follow-up.

A diagnosis of recurrent or metastatic disease can be as devastating for a patient and family as their original diagnosis was. The support needed by them can be much more intense than previously and professionals may find that patients given a subsequent diagnosis become even more anxious. Treatment for recurrent or metastatic disease is decided on an individual basis, taking into account the amount of disease present, its anatomical site and the age of the patient. It is in the metastatic setting that more chemotherapy may be used than in the initial primary treatment, especially for soft tissue sarcoma, and this will be discussed on an individual basis. In some cases, the specialist teams will need to discuss with some patients and families that treatment is no longer an option, and this is where specialist palliative care teams are involved to ensure the patient and family receive the supportive care they require.

Palliative Care

Palliative care for sarcoma patients will be needed when there is no cure for the disease and patients begin to suffer symptoms. The input from palliative care providers is crucial to ensure end-of-life care needs are met. Often, palliative care services are happy to be contacted prior to the patient needing any input so that contact can be made and the start of a relationship can be sought. Palliative care can be undertaken in a number of settings:

- In the hospital setting palliative care can be provided by the ward staff with or without input from specialist hospital palliative care nurses. This sometimes has to be undertaken when a patient deteriorates very quickly and it becomes very difficult to transfer them to a hospice or home.
- In the hospice setting palliative care is undertaken by specialist palliative care staff in a more relaxed, appropriate setting.
- At home palliative care can be undertaken by family with support from community staff, both general and specialist palliative care.

Hospices can very often provide support prior to any interventional palliative care input being needed. This can include relaxation treatments, music therapy and other services. It is important to discuss with patients and families the value of the services that hospices can provide. Some find it very difficult to attend a hospice for supportive care as they feel they 'only go to a hospice to die'. It is therefore essential to explain the nature of the services that can be provided which other NHS settings are unable to offer.

The preferred place of palliative care should be the decision of the patient and family. When patients have had to travel a large distance to have their sarcoma treatment it is often more appropriate for them to receive palliative care in a setting which is closer to home. This allows them to have visits from all family and friends who may not be able to travel. It also allows patients and families to move away from what may have been a time of very intense treatment.

Summary

It will now be obvious that sarcoma care is not straightforward. The need for definite histological diagnosis is key to ensuring patients receive the correct treatments for their disease, be it surgery, radiotherapy, chemotherapy or a combination of all three. Due to the fact that sarcoma can affect all age groups and all anatomical sites, the need for knowledge about this disease in the general orthopaedic community is high. Care of these patients has to be within the realms of a specialist MDT and be undertaken by specialist teams who are experienced in sarcoma care (Dangoor et al. 2016; Gerrand et al. 2016). The importance of early diagnosis cannot be stressed enough. Prognosis depends

very much on a diagnosis that is made before metastatic disease has a chance to present. Hopefully by raising awareness of this disease everyone can work towards a common goal of earlier diagnosis.

Practitioners working in the specialty of orthopaedics will inevitably care for sarcoma patients or suspected sarcoma patients during their working time. It is important to remember that even though this is a less common disease there are health professionals specialising in sarcoma who are happy to share their knowledge to help raise awareness and make the patient pathway a smooth and informed one. See Box 15.4 for further online resources to find out more about sarcoma care and musculoskeletal oncology.

Box 15.4   Sarcoma-related Websites

http://www.sarcoma.org.uk (accessed 7 June 2021)
http://www.bcrt.org.uk (accessed 4 June 2021)
https://www.macmillan.org.uk/cancer-information-and-support/bone-cancer (accessed 7 June 2021)
https://www.macmillan.org.uk/cancer-information-and-support/soft-tissue-sarcoma (accessed 7 June 2021)
http://www.boos.org.uk/wp-content/uploads/2016/03/BOOS-MBD-2016-BOA.pdf (accessed 7 June 2021)

Further Reading

Anninga, J.K., Gelderblom, H., Fiocco, M. et al. (2011). Chemotherapeutic adjuvant treatment for osteosarcoma: where do we stand? *Eur. J. Cancer* 47 (16): 2431–2445.

Dancsok, A., Asleh-Aburaya, K., and Nielsen, T. (2017). Advances in sarcoma diagnosis and treatment. *Oncotarget* 8 (4): 7068–7093. https://www.ncbi.nlm.nih.gov/pmc/articles/PMC5351692 (accessed 4 June 2021).

Fauske, L., Lorem, G., Grov, E., and Bondevik, H. (2015). Changes in the body image of bone sarcoma survivors following surgical treatment – a qualitative study. *J. Surg. Oncol.* https://onlinelibrary.wiley.com/doi/full/10.1002/jso.24138 (accessed 7 June 2021).

Grimer, R.J., Mottard, S., and Briggs, T. (2010). Focus on earlier diagnosis of bone and soft-tissue tumours. *J. Bone Joint Surg.* 92-B (11): 1489–1492. http://www.bjj.boneandjoint.org.uk/content/92-B/11/1489, Abstract (accessed 13 July 2012).

NICE (2006). *Improving outcomes guidance for people with sarcoma.* National Institute of Clinical Excellence. http://www.nice.org.uk/nicemedia/live/10903/28934/28934.pdf (accessed 24 April 2014).

NICE (2015). *Sarcoma Quality Standard (QS78).* https://www.nice.org.uk/guidance/qs78 (accessed 9 June 2021).

References

Anninga, J.K., Gelderblom, H., Fiocco, M. et al. (2011). Chemotherapeutic adjuvant treatment for osteosarcoma: where do we stand? *Eur. J. Cancer* 47 (16): 2431–2445.

Children with Cancer UK (2021) *What is rhabdomyosarcoma (RMS)?* https://www.childrenwithcancer.org.uk/childhood-cancer-info/cancer-types/rhabdomyosarcoma (accessed 7 June 2021).

Cupps, R.E., Ahmann, D.L., and Soule, E.H. (1969). Treatment of pulmonary metastatic disease with radiation therapy and adjuvant actinomycin D. Preliminary observations. *Cancer* 24 (4): 719–723.

Dalal, K.M., Antonescu, C.R., and Singer, S. (2008). Diagnosis and management of lipomatous tumors. *J. Surg. Oncol.* 97 (4): 298–313.

Dangoor, A., Seddon, B., Gerrand, C. et al. (2016). UK guidelines for the management of soft tissue sarocmas. *Clin. Sarcoma Res.* https://clinicalsarcomaresearch. biomedcentral.com/articles/10.1186/s13569-016-0060-4 (accessed 4 June 2021).

Ellison, D.A., Parham, D.M., and Jackson, R.J. (2005). Malignant triton tumor presenting as a rectal mass in an 11-month-old. *Pediatr. Dev. Pathol.* 8 (2): 235–239.

Flemming, D.J. and Murphey, M.D. (2000). Enchondroma and chondrosarcoma. *Semin. Musculoskelet. Radiol.* 4 (1): 59–71.

Geller, D. and Gerbhardt, M. (2006) *Malignant Peripheral Nerve Sheath Tumours (MPNST)*. http://sarcomahelp.org/ mpnst.html (accessed 12 October 2012).

Gerrand, C., Athanasou, N., Brennan, B., et al., on behalf of the British Sarocma Group. UK guidelines for the management of bone sarcomas. *Clincial Sarcoma Research.* https://clinicalsarcomaresearch.biomedcentral.com/ articles/10.1186/s13569-016-0047-1 (accessed 4 June 2021).

Grimer, R. (2006). Size matters for sarcoma. *Ann. R. Coll. Surg. Engl.* 88 (6): 519–524.

Grimer, R.J., Mottard, S., and Briggs, T. (2010). Focus on earlier diagnosis of bone and soft-tissue tumours. *J. Bone Joint Surg.* 92 (11): 1489–1492.

Hulbert-Williams, J., Beatty, L., and Dhillon, H. (2018). Psychological support for patients with cancer: evidence review and suggestions for future directions. *Curr. Opin. Support. Palliat. Care* 12 (3): 276–292.

Kager, L., Potschger, U., and Bielack, S. (2010). Review of mifamurtide in patients with osteosarcoma. *Ther. Clin. Risk Manag.* http://www.ncbi.nlm.nih.gov/pmc/articles/ PMC2893760 (accessed 12 September 2012).

Kim, S.Y. and Helman, L.J. (2010). Strategies to explore new approaches in the investigation and treatment of osteosarcoma. *Cancer Treat. Res.* 152: 517–528.

Knösel, T., Heretsch, S., Altendorf-Hofmann, A. et al. (2010). TLE1 is a robust diagnostic biomarker for synovial sarcomas and correlates with t(X;18): analysis of 319 cases. *Eur. J. Cancer* 46 (6): 1170–1176.

Lawrenz, J., Featherall, J., Curtis, G. et al. (2020). Time to treatment initiation and survival in adult localised high grade bone sarcoma. *Sarcoma* https://www.hindawi.com/ journals/sarcoma/2020/2984043 (accessed 4 June 2021).

Lopategui, D., Yechieli, R., and Ramasamy, R. (2017). Oncofertility in sarcoma patients. *Transl. Androl. Urol.* https://www.ncbi.nlm.nih.gov/pmc/articles/PMC5673827 (accessed 4 June 2021).

Macmillan Cancer Support (2011) *Psychological and emotional support provided by Macmillan Professionals: An evidence review.* http://www.macmillan.org.uk/ Documents/AboutUs/Commissioners/PsychologicalandE motionalSupportProvidedbyMacmillanProfessionalsEvide nceReviewJuly2011.pdf (accessed 23 July 2012).

National Cancer Action Team (2010) *Quality in Nursing Excellence in Cancer Care: The Contribution of the Clinical Nurse Specialist.* http://www.ncat.nhs.uk/sites/default/ files/Excellence%20in%20Cancer%20Care.pdf (accessed 17 August 2012).

National Cancer Intelligence Network (2012) *Bone Sarcomas: Incidence and Survival Rates in England.* http://www.ncin. org.uk/publications/data_briefings/bone_sarcomas_ incidence_and_survival.aspx (accessed 13 July 2012).

NICE (2005) *Referral Guidelines for Suspected Cancer.* http:// www.nice.org.uk/nicemedia/pdf/CG027quickrefguide.pdf (accessed 15 August 2012).

Oberlin, O., Rey, A., Lyden, E. et al. (2008). Prognostic factors in metastatic rhabdomyosarcomas: results of a pooled analysis from United States and European cooperative groups. *J. Clin. Oncol.* 26 (14): 2384–2389.

Peltier, L.F. (1993). *Orthopedics: A History and Iconography.* San Francisco: Norman Publishing.

Samuels, M.L. and Howe, C.D. (1967). Cyclophosphamide in the management of Ewing's sarcoma. *Cancer* 20 (6): 961–966.

Sarcoma UK (2020) http://www.sarcoma.org.uk/about-sarcoma/understanding-sarcoma-0 (accessed 4 June 2021).

Schwartz, H. (2007). *Orthopaedic Knowledge Update: Musculoskeletal Tumors 2.* Rosemont, IL: American Academy of Orthopaedic Surgeons.

Shah, H., Bhurgri, Y., and Pervez, S. (2005). Malignant smooth muscle tumours of soft tissue – a demographic and clinicopathological study at a tertiary care hospital. *J. Pak. Med. Assoc.* 55 (4): 138–143.

Stefanovski, P.D., Bidoli, E., De Paoli, A. et al. (2002). Prognostic factors in soft tissue sarcomas: a study of 359 patients. *Eur. J. Surg. Oncol.* 28: 153–164.

Stout, A.P. (1946). Rhabdomyosarcoma of the skeletal muscles. *Ann. Surg.* 123: 447–472.

Unni, K.K. and Inwards, C.Y. (2010). *Dahlin's Bone Tumours*, 2e. Philadelphia: Lippincott Williams and Wilkins.

Vargas, B. (2012) *Synovial Cell Sarcoma.* http://emedicine. medscape.com/article/1257131-overview (accessed 8 August 2012).

Vocks, E., Worret, W.I., and Burgdorf, W.H. (2000). Myxoid liposarcoma in a 12-year-old girl. *Pediatr. Dermatol.* 17 (2): 129–132.

Weiss, S.W. and Goldburn, J.R. (ed.) (2001). *Enzinger and Weiss's Soft Tissue Tumors*, 4e. St Louis: Mosby.

Part IV

Musculoskeletal Trauma Care

16

Principles of Trauma Care

Fiona Heaney[1], Yvonne Conway[2], and Stefanie Cormack[3]

[1] *Galway University Hospitals, Galway, Ireland*
[2] *Department of Nursing, Health Sciences and Integrated Care, Atlantic Technological University (Mayo), Castlebar, Ireland*
Atlantic Technological University (Mayo), Castlebar, Ireland
[3] *University of Wolverhampton, UK*

Introduction

Trauma is a major cause of death and disability worldwide, and is the primary cause of mortality in the first four decades of life (Henning et al. 2011; World Health Organization [WHO] 2014). Those who survive physical trauma are often left with significant long-term or permanent life-changing disabilities resulting particularly from head, spine and limb-threatening injuries. It is now recognised that trauma has a bimodal age distribution, with the first peak occurring in those under 20 and a second peak occurring in those over 65. In the United States, trauma is the leading cause of death in young adults and accounts for 10% of deaths in all men and women. It is the biggest killer of people aged below 45 years in the UK and in those people that survive a traumatic injury a large number will have permanent disabilities (National Institute for Health and Care Excellence [NICE] 2016a). The Trauma Audit Research Network (TARN), a trauma registry with data submitted from all hospitals in England, Wales, Northern Ireland and the Republic of Ireland, suggests that the typical major trauma patient has changed from being young and male to being older with a lower degree of male prevalence. Older major trauma patients have a similar injury severity and distribution of injury to younger patients and brain injury is the most common cause of death. The TARN network in its report on trauma and older people found that 56% of older patients had significant injuries due to falls of less than 2 metres (Dixon et al. 2020) and it was also the mechanism of injury associated with the highest morbidity (National Office of Clinical Audit 2020). Reports suggest that management of the patient sustaining trauma is often suboptimal (NCEPOD 2007).

This chapter will discuss the priorities of care in the assessment, management and treatment of individuals suffering musculoskeletal trauma whilst considering the impact of injury to other tissue besides bone on care needs. In emergency and initial care of the patient following trauma the practitioner works as part of a multidisciplinary team with the aim of preserving life and preventing death, and then with the aim of preventing complications and facilitating recovery and prevention of disability.

Pre-hospital Care

Timely pre-hospital systematic management of the trauma patient can have a major impact on overall outcome and care. There is some evidence to suggest that systems that provide for early involvement of physicians at the scene may result in better patient survival rates, but better audit tools and data are required to support this hypothesis (Hepple et al. 2019). The primary destination for many of these patients should be a major trauma centre (MTC), although sometimes the patient's condition may need to be stabilised with urgent clinical issues addressed first in a local emergency department (ED) (NICE 2016a).

Management at the scene and during transfer to hospital consists of (Soloman et al. 2005):

- maintenance of airway
- protection of the spine
- ensuring and supporting ventilation and perfusion
- controlling bleeding
- initiating IV and fluid replacement, and managing shock
- pain management

- immobilisation of fractures and soft tissue injury
- safe transfer to hospital.

Pre-hospital documentation records must be given to staff at the receiving unit as soon as possible and should reflect the (<C>ABCDE) approach to care: catastrophic haemorrhage, airway with spinal protection, breathing, circulation, disability (neurological), exposure, and environment (NICE 2016b). Control of catastrophic haemorrhage is now recommended as the first stage of assessment and resuscitation of a critically injured person.

Mechanism of Injury

Traumatic injury results from the transfer of energy from the environment to human tissue. It can be subdivided into blunt and penetrating trauma. Penetrating trauma involves tissue directly affected by an object which enters tissue, while blunt trauma may affect other tissue further away from the site of impact during energy transfer. Assessment of the patient following blunt trauma can be more difficult as the extent of the injury may not be externally obvious at first. Understanding the potential effects of the mechanism of injury is useful in patient triage as well as in predicting morbidity and mortality (Haider et al. 2009), although there is some uncertainty about validity (Boyle et al. 2008). The mechanism of injury can have a predictive value for diagnosing a subsequent injury. For example, the classic presentation of a patient who fell from a height and sustained bilateral calcaneal fractures should also instigate investigation for vertebral injury as this type of mechanism often involves a transfer of energy/trauma to the spine. Although the mechanism of injury can raise suspicion as to the presence of certain injuries, Richards (2005) warns that the presence of other injuries cannot predict the presence of spinal injury or vice versa and that each patient requires an individual full examination as soon as possible after the injuring event.

Primary Survey

On arrival at the ED trauma patients are assessed and treated based on the advanced trauma life support (ATLS) protocol (American College of Surgeons 2018). This offers a globally standardised approach to trauma resuscitation that is understood by the whole team and enables a focus on the life-threatening aspects of injury as a priority rather than the injury that is most obvious. This means that musculoskeletal injury may not be an early priority. The primary survey is performed by the emergency/trauma care team simultaneously with resuscitation and consists of the following (mnemonic ABCDE):

- Airway maintenance with restriction of cervical spine motion
- Breathing and ventilation
- Circulation with haemorrhage control
- Disability (assessment of neurologic status)
- Exposure/Environmental control.

The primary survey should be repeated whenever there is a change in the patients' status. It is followed by a more definitive secondary survey where a head-to-toe examination is performed to identify all injuries and formulate a plan of care.

Airway with Spinal Precautions

Airway management is one of the core priorities in caring for trauma patients. It has been suggested that loss of a patent airway is second only to complete cardiopulmonary arrest as the most significant cause of death following trauma (WHO 2004). The airway is the gateway to the chain of oxygen delivery (Figure 16.1) without which all other links in the chain will fail, leading to organ dysfunction and death.

Assessment of the airway involves observing for causes of obstruction such as foreign bodies, tongue, teeth, oedema, blood and other secretions. Obstructions should be cautiously removed and excess secretions controlled by suctioning. A 'blind sweep' should never be performed to remove a foreign body as it may push the obstruction further down the pharynx. The simplest method of assessing a patient's airway is to ask them 'Are you OK?'. A logical response in a normal voice indicates the patient not only has a patent airway, but also that the brain is adequately perfused with oxygen. In the unconscious patient, the airway can be maintained by insertion of an oropharyngeal airway (Figure 16.2).

An intact gag reflex indicates that the patient can maintain their own airway and the insertion of an airway device could lead to vomiting, cervical movement or raised intracranial pressure and must be avoided. Potential threats to the airway should also be assessed such as the presence of fractures, soft tissue injuries and burns. Establish a definitive airway if there is any doubt about the patient's ability to maintain it.

The victim of trauma is at risk for spinal injury and it should be assumed based on the mechanism of trauma that a spinal injury is present. During interventions aimed at establishing a definitive airway care should be taken to avoid excessive movement of the spine. Spinal immobilisation is maintained by placing the patient on a spinal board with immobilisation of the cervical region using sandbags or a 'head hugger' until any potential spinal injury can be

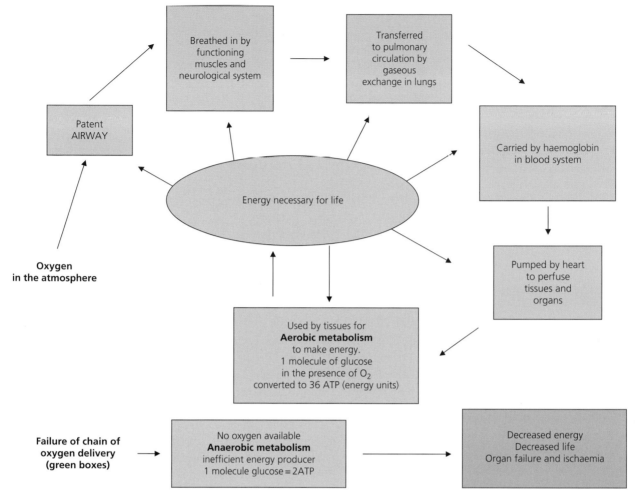

Figure 16.1 The chain of O$_2$ delivery.

Figure 16.2 Insertion of a Guedal airway.

1. Select correct size: When you place the airway against the patient's cheek with the flange parallel to front teeth, the tip of the oropharyngeal airway should reach no further than the angle of the jaw.	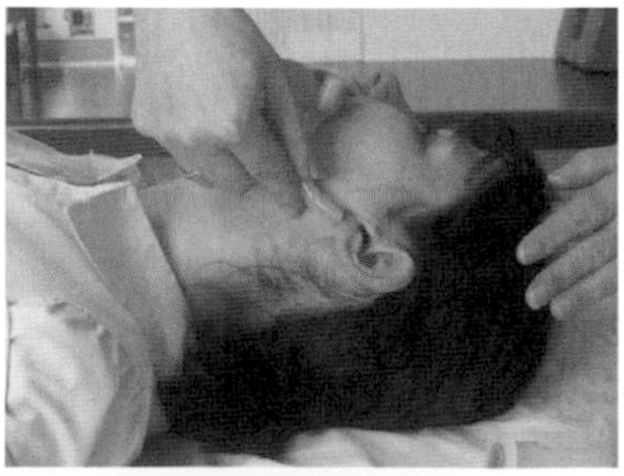
2. Open the patient's mouth and insert the airway upside down with the curvature towards the tongue. 3. When the airway reaches the back of the tongue, rotate the device 180 degrees	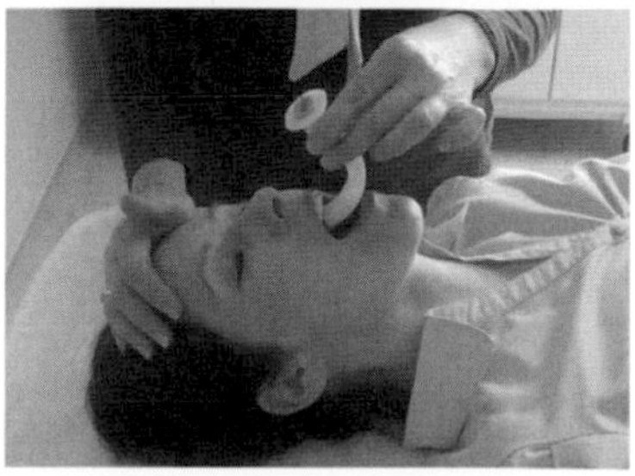

Head tilt/chin lift One hand is placed over patient's forehead and firm backward pressure is applied with the palm to tilt the head back. Fingers of the other hand are placed under the bony portion of the lower jaw near the chin to bring the chin forward	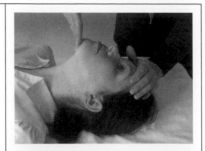
Jaw thrust (where spinal injury suspected) Place the four fingers of both hands on each side of the lower jaw. Once in place, the jaws are tilted upward making sure that the head and neck remain in position.	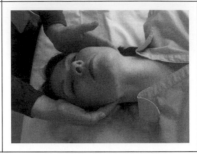

Figure 16.3 Maintaining an airway.

ruled out. The head tilt/chin lift and jaw thrust positions are the standard manoeuvres for maintaining a patent airway (Figure 16.3). Frequent reassessment of the airway is required, and a surgical intervention may be necessary if intubation is not successful.

Breathing

The patient should be assessed for the presence of injuries that may impede breathing. These include those that would affect the muscular act of breathing such as injuries to the lungs, chest wall and diaphragm along with those impeding the neurological response such as brain and spinal nerve injuries. Significant potential chest injuries in the trauma patient include the following:

- *Tension pneumothorax* occurs when a pleural tear allows air into the pleural cavity during inspiration but prevents it from exiting on expiration. Emergency treatment involves the insertion of a large-bore cannula into the pleural cavity to allow the air to escape, followed by a chest drain.
- *Open pneumothorax* occurs when there is a significant wound to the chest wall that allows air to move freely into the pleural cavity. Treatment involves insertion of a chest drain.
- *Haemothorax* occurs when a laceration leads to accumulation of blood in the pleural cavity, leading to compression of the lung and impaired breathing. Treatment involves draining the pleural cavity of blood, although this is done cautiously in the case of a massive haemothorax as rapid blood loss may lead to circulatory collapse.

- *Flail chest* occurs when more than one rib is fractured at multiple sites and seriously affects breathing. Emergency treatment involves intubation and ventilation.
- *Cardiac tamponade*: A wound that penetrates the heart results in bleeding into the pericardial sac. This reduces the volume of blood entering the ventricles prior to systole, which reduces cardiac output and affects the delivery of oxygen and perfusion of tissues and vital organs. Emergency treatment consists of removing the blood from the pericardial sac by pericardiocentesis or thoracotomy.
- *Tracheal or bronchial injuries* are uncommon but must be diagnosed and managed immediately as they are life-threatening. They are injuries that occur between the cricoid cartilage and right and left main-stem tracheal bifurcation (Altinok and Can 2014).

Nursing/clinical assessment involves a full set of vital signs, paying particular attention to respiration. Observing the thoracic region for bruising and lacerations can help identify the presence of soft tissue injury. Supplemental oxygen (SO) should be administered to patients with injuries and, if not intubated, should be administered via a mask-reservoir device to achieve optimal oxygenation. However, careful consideration needs to be given to those patients that have an oxygen saturation >97% on room air as an exploratory study suggests SO administration may lead to an increase in incidence of in-hospital mortality and acute respiratory distress syndrome (Christensen et al. 2021). In all trauma patients, the goal is to achieve an inspired oxygen concentration of 100% (Gwinnutt and Driscoll 2003). Treatment of trauma patients with significant chest injuries often involves the insertion of a chest drain. Hence, practitioners should be competent in the care of the patient with a chest drain.

Circulation

Clinical signs of haemorrhage may be detected by changes in the level of consciousness, skin perfusion, pulse and blood pressure. Control of bleeding is the first priority by application of direct pressure where possible at the site of bleeding using pressure bandages/dressings or by application of a tourniquet in the case of uncontrolled arterial bleeding (Rossaint et al. 2010). Recent ATLS guidelines have increased emphasis on additional skills in the management of local haemorrhage control, including wound packing and tourniquet application, and transfusion of blood components as a key intervention (ATLS 2018). Perfusion of vital organs and tissues with oxygenated blood is dependent on blood volume and rapid replacement of lost volume is crucial in preventing a break in the chain of oxygen delivery (Figure 16.1). In addition to blood seepage from wounds and other injuries, loss of extracellular fluid from wounds involving a large surface area of the body (e.g. degloving injuries and large abrasions) should be considered when estimating volume loss. Assessment must involve observing the patient's colour, temperature, capillary refill and degree of diaphoresis (sweating). The rate and quality of the pulse should be determined manually. IV access should be obtained, chosen fluids administered and wounds dressed to control bleeding. A randomised controlled trial suggests tranexamic acid should be administered pre-hospital or within 3 hours of injury as it improves survival rates (CRASH-2 Collaborators, et al. 2010). Inadequate resuscitation of major haemorrhage is an important cause of avoidable death and aggressive replacement of fluids with definitive bleeding control is required.

Disability

The AVPU score (Box 16.1) can be used to perform a brief assessment of an individual's level of consciousness. AVPU is commonly used pre-hospital and in the initial

Box 16.1	The AVPU System

A Alert
V Only responding to verbal stimulus
P Only responding to painful stimuli
U Unresponsive to any stimulus

assessment as it can be performed quickly. It should be followed up with a more detailed Glasgow Coma Scale assessment if the AVPU score is below A (Romanelli and Farrell 2021) (Box 16.1). Blood glucose should always be checked in the unconscious patient as hypoglycaemia may be responsible for the loss of consciousness as aerobic metabolism in the neurological system is reliant on sufficient levels of glucose in addition to oxygen (Figure 16.1).

Exposure/Environment Control

To make a comprehensive assessment it is imperative that all clothing be removed from trauma patients whilst making every effort to maintain dignity and privacy. Wet clothing can have the added effect of reducing body temperature. Clothing is often removed with the use of scissors to ensure minimal movement of patients with suspected spinal injury. If alert, the patient's permission should be sought and the practitioner must be mindful of preserving the individual's dignity and the rapid loss of body heat related to exposure. To prevent sudden hypotension some garments may be left on the patient with gross hypovolaemia until adequate fluid resuscitation is ensured (Gwinnutt and Driscoll 2003) as clothing can provide pressure. Hypothermia is a lethal complication of trauma and the trauma patient should be kept warm with the administration of warmed crystalloid fluids and blankets (ATLS 2018).

Secondary Survey

The secondary survey is performed by the team after the primary survey has been completed and any immediate threats to life have been treated. A head-to-toe assessment is performed to determine any undiagnosed injuries or fractures.

Haemorrhage Control and Acute Coagulopathy

Uncontrolled post-traumatic bleeding is one of the leading causes of potentially preventable death in trauma patients, so much so that the ABC approach to trauma may be changed to CABC to take account of catastrophic haemorrhage control as the initial priority (Henning et al. 2011; NICE 2016a). Significant blood loss is affected by both direct injury and trauma related coagulopathy. Early identification of the bleeding source with timely efforts to minimise bleeding, restore tissue perfusion and achieve haemodynamic stability are key in the management of patients with massive bleeding (Rossaint et al. 2010). The coagulation process in haemorrhaging

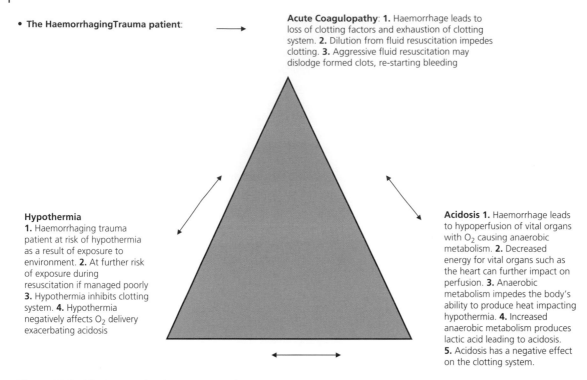

- The HaemorrhagingTrauma patient:

Acute Coagulopathy: 1. Haemorrhage leads to loss of clotting factors and exhaustion of clotting system. **2.** Dilution from fluid resuscitation impedes clotting. **3.** Aggressive fluid resuscitation may dislodge formed clots, re-starting bleeding

Hypothermia
1. Haemorrhaging trauma patient at risk of hypothermia as a result of exposure to environment. **2.** At further risk of exposure during resuscitation if managed poorly **3.** Hypothermia inhibits clotting system. **4.** Hypothermia negatively affects O_2 delivery exacerbating acidosis

Acidosis 1. Haemorrhage leads to hypoperfusion of vital organs with O_2 causing anaerobic metabolism. **2.** Decreased energy for vital organs such as the heart can further impact on perfusion. **3.** Anaerobic metabolism impedes the body's ability to produce heat impacting hypothermia. **4.** Increased anaerobic metabolism produces lactic acid leading to acidosis. **5.** Acidosis has a negative effect on the clotting system.

Figure 16.4   The haemorrhaging trauma patient.

patients is adversely affected by exhaustion of the coagulation system, dilution from fluid resuscitation and physical factors such as acidosis and hypothermia that further compromise coagulation function (Spahn and Ganter 2010). The changes in coagulopathy in conjunction with hypothermia and acidosis are interlinked and have been termed the 'lethal triad' (Figure 16.4). Updated European guidelines (Maegele 2021) on the management of major bleeding and coagulopathy following trauma emphasise the treatment required at the scene, i.e. manual compression, tourniquet use and (non-) commercial pelvic slings followed by rapid transfer to a trauma centre. Coagulation monitoring and support are to be initiated immediately on arrival to hospital, with surgical control of bleeding being the mainstay of treatment in conjunction with blood product transfusion and early administration of tranexamic acid. The haemorrhaging patient is at an acute risk for development of hypovolaemic shock and death is most likely to occur within the first 3 hours of hospital admission (Vulliamy et al. 2019). For more information on the physiology and management of shock, consult Chapter 9.

Wound Management

Controlling bleeding is the primary concern in the initial management of an acute wound. Inspection and exploration of a wound in a well-lit environment can help facilitate identification and management of the source of bleeding. Early transfer to surgery for haemorrhage control has been associated with increased survival (Rossaint et al. 2010).

The key messages from the latest European guidelines on management of major bleeding and coagulopathy following trauma (Spahn et al. 2019) are as follows:

- Traumatically injured patients should be transported quickly and treated by a specialised trauma centre whenever possible.
- Measures to monitor and support coagulation should be initiated as early as possible and used to guide a goal-directed treatment strategy.
- A damage-control approach to surgical intervention should guide patient management.
- Coagulation support and thromboprophylactic strategies should consider trauma patients who have been pre-treated with anticoagulants or platelet inhibitors.
- Local adherence to a multidisciplinary, evidence-based treatment protocol should serve as the basis of patient management and undergo regular quality assessment.

Box 16.2 considers best practice in the management of acute traumatic wounds.

In the UK, many hospital trusts have published their own evidence-based guidelines to aid medical and

---

Box 16.2   Evidence Digest

Acute wound management: revisiting the approach to assessment, irrigation, and closure considerations (Nicks et al. 2010)

An evidence-based approach must be adopted in the assessment and management of acute traumatic wounds. The objectives are to attain a functional closure, decrease risk for infection and minimise scar formation. Although every wound must be assessed and managed individually, Nicks et al.'s (2010) systematic review of the evidence gives the following general recommendations:

- Assessment of the wound, including location, length, width, depth, tissue type, neurovascular and functional status, of surrounding structures, presence of debris and contaminants, and range of motion.
- Patient assessment, including history of injury, infection/contamination risk, medication history and allergies, tetanus cover and comorbidities that may affect wound healing.
- Assessment and management of wound pain through topical, local or regional anaesthesia.
- Decontamination of the wound, including brushing off any dry chemicals prior to irrigation.
- Cleansing of the wound through application of a compress, irrigation or soaking as appropriate.
- All wound surfaces should be irrigated, paying particular attention to flaps and wound edges.
- Avoid unnecessary and excessive irrigation of clean wounds in highly vascularised areas.
- Wounds appearing dry, gangrenous and/or ischaemic are non-healable due to ischemia.
- Debridement may be necessary to remove devitalised tissue.

- In the absence of intrinsic, extrinsic or mechanical damage acute wounds may be debrided and closed immediately.
- Heavily contaminated wounds may need delayed primary closure to decrease infection risk.
- Wounds that are left to heal by secondary intention need follow-up assessment and possible secondary debridement.
- Dependent on wound severity, all patients with an unknown vaccination history or who have received fewer than three doses should receive a tetanus diphtheria vaccine (Td).
- Inadequately vaccinated patients (excluding those with a clean, minor wound) should also receive tetanus immune globulin (TIG).
- Patients who have received three or more tetanus vaccines prior to the injury only need Td vaccination if their previous dose was:
  – >10 years ago for clean, minor wounds
  – >5 years ago for other wounds.
- The need for antibiotic therapy is determined by wound type and method of closure, patient characteristics and infection risk.
- The best predictive factors for wound infection are wound location, wound age, depth, configuration, contamination and patient age.
- Antibiotic therapy should be considered for patients at heightened risk, such as those with prosthetic joints, on corticosteroids, at risk of endocarditis or that are immunocompromised.
- A dressing that provides a warm, moist healing environment is recommended.

---

nursing clinicians. In 2018, the Irish Health Service Executive (HSE) developed national wound management guidelines, which provide a comprehensive review, and best practice recommendations to support clinicians in providing evidence-based wound care (Health Service Executive 2018). This detailed document provides excellent information to guide clinical decision making and is divided into sections according to wound type and situation:

- general wound care
- diabetic foot ulcers
- pressure ulcers
- leg ulcers
- palliative wound care
- education.

At the time of publication, there are no recent systematic reviews of best practice in the management of acute wounds. However, the Nicks (2010) review cited within the guidelines still has relevance for today's practice.

Spinal Precautions

Spinal precautions is a term used to describe strict immobilisation of the spine. Wherever a spinal injury is diagnosed or suspected the whole spine should be immobilised. Spinal immobilisation signifies the maintenance of spinal alignment, which should take into account the normal alignment of the individual's spine and pre-existing conditions such as ankylosing spondylitis. Although a mainstay of trauma care for decades, more recent systematic reviews have highlighted the lack of high-quality studies and evidence for spinal immobilisation (Oteir et al. 2015; Hood and Considine 2015; Maschmann et al. 2019). Cervical immobilisation can be attained by application of a cervical collar and a 'head-hugger' or sandbags. The use of spinal immobilisation devices may be difficult in agitated and distressed people, including children, and they could become counterproductive. In cases like this, consider letting the patient find a position where they are comfortable with manual inline stabilisation (NICE 2016b). A Cochrane review (Kwan et al. 2009) raised concern that cervical spine immobilisation may be associated with a higher morbidity and mortality than non-immobilisation and highlighted the paucity of evidence on the effectiveness of spinal immobilisation strategies. Some studies suggest patients with penetrating trauma and no obvious neurological deficits do not require spinal immobilisation (Kreinest et al. 2016; Feller et al. 2021). The literature suggests a move towards more selective approaches with provision for decision making by clinicians and pre-hospital providers on the use of immobilisation rather than a blanket approach. In light of the continuing debate and lack of consensus there is a clear need for large prospective studies to determine the impact of prehospital spinal immobilisation on patient outcomes as well as identification of the subgroups most or least likely to benefit. Current UK NICE Guidelines are summarised in Box 16.3.

Cervical collars are designed to restrict neck flexion, extension, lateral tilt and rotation, and do not restrict axial loading. In choosing a collar for a patient, it is important to follow manufacturers' instructions regarding sizing to ensure a proper fit. The patient's chin should rest centrally on the chin rest and not slide down inside or protrude out over the chin rest. The collar is designed to fit snugly and not constrict the patient's ability to breathe, cough, swallow or vomit (Webber-Jones et al. 2002). Once the collar is fitted the patient should be regularly assessed to ensure the following:

- The collar fits the patient correctly.
- Neurological status is assessed before and after any interventions involving changing the collar.
- Skin care is performed at least daily. When the collar is removed to perform skin care manual in-line stabilisation of the patient's head and neck should be ensured by adopting the correct head hold. One part of the collar is removed at a time and the back of the patient's head can be inspected during the log roll. *Always follow the immobilisation directions documented in the patient's chart.*
- The skin is assessed for evidence of breakdown, particularly the occiput, chin, ears, mandible ridge, shoulders, sternum and laryngeal prominence.
- The collar itself should be cleaned daily and inside padding changed/cleaned as per manufacturers' instructions.

Box 16.3 NICE Guidelines for Spinal Injury Assessment and Initial Management (NICE 2016b)

1) Carry out or maintain full in-line spinal immobilisation if:
   - a high-risk factor for cervical spine injury is identified and indicated by the Canadian C-spine rule
   - a low-risk factor for cervical spine injury is identified and indicated by the Canadian C-spine rule and the person is unable to actively rotate their neck 45° left and right
   - indicated by one or more of the following factors
     - age 65 years or older and reported pain in the thoracic or lumbosacral spine
     - dangerous mechanism of injury (fall from a height of greater than 3 metres, axial load to the head or base of the spine, for example falls landing on feet or buttocks, high-speed motor vehicle collision, rollover motor accident, lap-belt restraint only, ejection from a motor vehicle, accident involving motorised recreational vehicles, bicycle collision, horse-riding accidents)
     - pre-existing spinal pathology or known or at risk of osteoporosis, for example steroid use
     - suspected spinal fracture in another region of the spine
     - abnormal neurological symptoms (paraesthesia or weakness or numbness)
   - on examination:
     - abnormal neurological signs (motor or sensory deficit)
     - new deformity or bony midline tenderness (on palpation)
     - bony midline tenderness (on percussion)
     - midline or spinal pain (on coughing)
     - on mobilisation (sit, stand, step, assess walking): pain or abnormal neurological symptoms (stop if this occurs).

2) Do not carry out or maintain full in-line immobilisation in people if:
   - they have low-risk factors for cervical spine injury as identified and indicated by the Canadian C-spine rule, are pain free and are able to actively rotate their neck 45° left and right
   - they do not have any of the factors listed above in 1.

Patients wearing cervical collars may be at increased risk of developing collar-related pressure ulcers. A multidisciplinary approach to care, early identification of at-risk patients, utilisation of cervical spine clearance protocols, nursing education and routine nursing care with the use of pressure-relieving devices such as air mattresses were found to be effective strategies to preventing cervical collar-related pressure ulcers (Lacey et al. 2019). The use of pressure-relieving devices such as air mattresses should always first be approved with the primary physician.

It is important thoracic and lumbar spine immobilisation can be achieved by placing the patient on a spinal board for transfer and on a firm mattress surface. However, the National Association of Emergency Medical Services Physicians and the American College of Surgeons Committee on Trauma recommend judicious use of spinal backboards for transporting patients so that the benefits outweigh the potential risks of pressure ulcers, respiratory compromise and pain (White et al. 2014). Access to the patient's posterior surface can be achieved by performing a log roll. A log roll is a manual handling procedure whereby a patient is rolled from lying on one aspect of the body to lying on another, whilst maintaining correct vertebral alignment. It may be required for inserting or removing a spinal board, examination, providing specific nursing care or for the purpose of relieving pressure (Harrison 2000). A guide to performing a safe log roll is provided in Figure 16.5.

Neurological assessment should take into account any motor or sensory deficits that may indicate a spinal cord injury. On arrival in the ED, patients are assessed for their risk of spinal injury. Decision-making tools such as the NEXUS score (Hoffman et al. 2000) and Canadian C-spine rule (Stiell et al. 2001) can assist in determining which patients can be cleared from suspected cervical spine injury without imaging. These scores apply to conscious patients and a difficulty arises when attempts are made to clear the spine of an unconscious patient. Richards (2005) suggests that decision-making tools with the aid of imaging technology also have a place in diagnosing spinal clearance of unconscious patients and recommends extending the computerised tomography (CT) of the brain to include the cervical spine in at-risk unconscious trauma patients.

Musculoskeletal Assessment

All limbs and joints are palpated and examined for signs of fracture, soft tissue injury or neurovascular compromise. It is important that a baseline neurovascular assessment is performed to determine limb perfusion and motor and sensory function. Any deficit or change in neurovascular status

needs further medical consultation and investigation. Affected limbs may be manipulated and splinted to maintain optimal alignment and stability. Open limb fractures should be managed prior to attending to closed fractures as there is an increased risk of chronic infection if treatment is delayed. See Chapter 7 for guidance on performing a thorough musculoskeletal assessment.

Severe Injury and Polytrauma

Once the primary and secondary surveys have taken place there is a need to plan the definitive care of any skeletal injuries. The existence of more than one injury (be it skeletal, soft tissue or organ) indicates, however, that not only has the patient sustained significant high-energy trauma, but that there is a greater likelihood of an extreme physiological response to tissue damage which can result in severe life-threatening complications, such as extreme inflammatory responses, metabolic dysfunction, severe immunosuppressive responses and coagulopathy (clotting disorders), which can lead to multiorgan failure and potential death (Keel and Trentz 2005). It is essential, therefore, that all injuries are identified at the time of the secondary survey so that their existence can be included as part of the overall management plan. The severity of these injuries is sometimes assessed using a trauma scoring system designed to help practitioners to identify care and management priorities and to ascertain risks to life. Such scoring systems can be useful when there is an isolated injury, but tend to be less accurate where more than one injury is involved. They categorise injuries of the respiratory, cardiovascular, nervous systems, abdomen, extremities and skin as minor to critical and take into account any existing complications. Their main purpose is to provide an alert for the need for prompt assessment and treatment as well as a way of prioritising injuries (Pape et al. 2010).

Multiple trauma (often termed polytrauma) can include, in addition to skeletal injury, injuries to the head, face, neck, spine, chest, trunk and abdomen and their underlying organs and structures, including major blood vessels and nerves, along with severe traumatic skin wounds. The physiological assault of a complex pattern of injury often requires care in an intensive/critical care unit where the patient's condition can be carefully monitored from a respiratory and cardiovascular perspective, and mechanical ventilation and other therapies can be provided.

Injuries to the pelvis, head and spine are those injuries which are the most likely to lead to death. Hence, these are often the focus of emergency care and in the period immediately after resuscitation and stabilisation, and following

Wherever the injury suggests the possibility of spinal injury, the whole spine should be immobilized during any transfers between surfaces (Harrisson, 2000)

Preparation

1. Ensure all equipment required is at hand considering the reason for rolling the patient.
2. Ensure the availability of the correct number of staff. As a rule a minimum of five people is required (Harrisson 2000), more may be required depending on the size of the patient and manual handling assessment. This consists of team leader, three assistants and the remaining person to insert a spinal board or provide required nursing care. The team leader is the most experienced person.
3. The area must be free from clutter and the head of the bed should be removed.
4. The bed should be adjusted to the height of the leader who is in control of the cervical region. Ensure the brakes are on.
5. Wash hands as per local policy.

Performing the roll

6. The leader approaches the patient in the patient's line of vision, explains the procedure and gains verbal consent.
7. The patient's motor and sensory function is assessed and recorded by the team leader.
8. If a cervical collar is in situ, do not remove it for the log rolling procedure.
9. The leader takes position at the head of the bed and takes control of the patient's head.
10. Traction should never be applied.
11. If head blocks are in situ, the leader places a hand on the lateral aspects of the block.
12. As an assistant removes a block, the leader replaces their hand on the side of the patient's head and carefully slides hands one at a time into the head-hold position.
13. The assistant staff assume position: The tallest at the patient's shoulders, the next at the patient's hips and the other at the patient's legs. The patient's arms are placed across their chest.

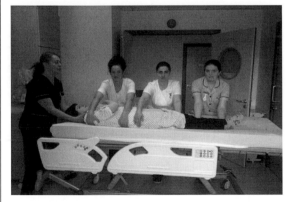

14. The command for rolling the patient is given. For example **"ready, steady, roll"**. When the command for **"roll"** is issued the patient is rolled in a smooth controlled manner, as a unit, towards the assistants.

15. As the patient is rolled towards staff, their weight is transferred from the front to the back leg while remaining forward facing.

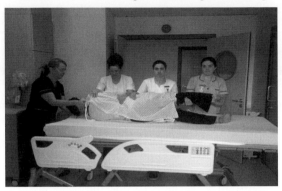

16. The staff and patient remain in this position until the appropriate nursing care or examination is complete.
17. The leader monitors patient alignment continually to keep the spine in line. In a healthy patient without pre-existing spinal disease, spinal alignment implies that the patient's nose should be in line with his/her umbilicus. If the patient has evidence of pre-existing spinal disease such as ankylosing spondylitis, keeping the spine in line implies that the **spine should be kept in the line that is normal for the patient before the injury (Wardrope et al., 2004).** Difficulties may arise when maintaining spinal alignment in children, due to the disproportionate size of the child's head compared to their body. Therefore, before rolling the child back into the supine position ensure an appropriate level of padding is placed in situ below the level of the child's shoulders (Harrison, 2000). An appropriate sized neck roll should be inserted to support the cervical curve and a thin pad positioned beneath the occiput to relieve pressure (Harrison, 2000).
18. The patient is returned onto their back as follows: The leader issues the command to roll back as in step 14.
19. As the patient is rolled away from staff, their weight is transferred from the back to the front leg while remaining face forward.
20. On return to the supine position, the team members must remain in position until released by the leader, who first ensures that torso, pelvis and legs are in alignment.
21. As the blocks are being replaced the leader carefully slides hands out from position, one at a time.
22. The team leader re-examines and records the patient's motor and sensory function. It is crucial that the same person undertakes both pre-and post-transfer examinations (Harrisson, 2000). Any changes in sensory/ motor function should be reported to a senior member of the medical staff and documented clearly.
23. Wash hands as per hospital policy.
24. Document care as appropriate.

Figure 16.5 Performing a safe log roll.

admission. Where there are several injuries and where there is no reason to suspect vascular damage (with potential for severe bleeding) the principles of damage control orthopaedics are usually employed. This acknowledges a need to focus on stabilising those injuries most likely to threaten life before undertaking definitive final orthopaedic surgery to stabilise limb fractures, for example. This often, initially, involves temporary splintage or external fixation of long bone fractures of the limbs and conservative management of major wounds until such time as other injuries are stabilised and the patient is physiologically able to cope with major orthopaedic surgery (McRae and Esser 2008). This provides specific challenges for the care of the patient in both the critical care and ward settings.

Pelvic Fractures

The pelvis is a large bowl-shaped ring made up of several bony components and strong ligaments that provides protection for the pelvic organs and transfers weight from the upper to lower body. As such, it is an extremely stable structure, requiring significant trauma to disrupt it. Most commonly, the pelvic ring suffers major injury through the crushing of the lower abdomen. Examples of mechanisms of injury include a motor vehicle or industrial accident or disasters such as earthquakes and blasts where parts of buildings trap victims. A significant amount of force is needed to disrupt the pelvic ring and this can result in two significant effects:

1) the mechanism of injury involved significant force: this warns the clinical team that any resultant injury to the area is likely to be severe
2) there is potential for severe damage to structures contained within the pelvis, such as major blood vessels and nerves, the bladder, urethra, bowel and genitalia.

Because the pelvis forms a ring, it is often the case that crushing it involves breaking it in two places (either by bony fracture or disruption to ligaments and joints) and may also involve severe disruption of the ligaments that contribute to pelvic stability at the symphysis pubis and sacroiliac joints. This can result in an unstable injury in which two parts of the pelvis become capable of moving separately, potentially resulting in further severe damage to the structures within the pelvis. Bleeding from damaged major blood vessels within or around the pelvis is a major cause of death in the trauma patient and requires careful fluid replacement and haemodynamic stabilisation. This bleeding may not always be obvious at first as the retroperitoneum has the capacity to hold up to 4 litres of blood in the adult. Therefore, careful assessment and monitoring of all vital signs is paramount as hypotension may be a late sign in diagnosing haemorrhage. The individual's normal blood pressure and previous diagnosis of hypertension should be considered in this assessment. In patients with severely displaced pelvic fractures or where blood loss from pelvis fractures is suspected, application of a pelvic binder, sheet or temporary external fixation is a priority (Chapter 8). Signs of injury to the bladder and urethra must be carefully observed, including assessment of urinary output and any signs of blood at the urethral meatus. Any suspicion of urethral trauma suggests urethral catheterisation is contraindicated and a supra-pubic catheter should be inserted. Injury to

the bowel is also a concern and observation should include an assessment for the presence of any lower abdominal pain, distension and absence of bowel sounds.

Minimally displaced stable fractures of the pelvic ring can often be treated conservatively. These can be very painful and the patient requires careful support and pain management while healing and remobilisation commence gradually.

Head Injury

Skeletal trauma is often associated with head injury – a major cause of death and long-term disability following traumatic injury – which may be associated with other skeletal and soft tissue injuries. Head injury is defined as (Scottish Intercollegiate Guidelines Network 2009, p. 2):

> a history of a blow to the head or the presence of a scalp wound or those with evidence of altered consciousness after relevant injury.

The level of consciousness according to the Glasgow Coma Scale (GCS) (Box 16.4) is usually used to categorise the severity of a head injury as follows (Scottish Intercollegiate Guidelines Network 2009):

- mild 13–15
- moderate 9–12
- severe <8.

Box 16.4 The Glasgow Coma Scale Reproduced with permission from Elsevier (Teasdale and Jennett 1974)

Eyes open	
Spontaneously	4
To speech	3
To pain	2
None	1
Best verbal response	
Orientated	5
Confused	4
Inappropriate words	3
Incomprehensible sounds	2
None	1
Best motor response	
Obey commands	6
Localise pain	5
Withdraw to pain	4
Decorticate	3
Decerebrate	2
No response	1

Injury is usually the result of blunt trauma to the head and includes injury to the skull and may or may not include injury to the brain. Fractures of the skull can include both closed and compound fractures and are usually linear or depressed. Depressed fractures are most likely to cause associated brain injury due to damage caused by the bone being pushed in towards the brain.

There are a number of different types of brain injury with potential intracranial complications that might lead to death or disability:

- contusion or bruising of brain tissue
- cerebral laceration
- focal injuries localised to specific areas
- intracerebral haemorrhage
- vascular damage, including:
  - extradural haematoma
  - subdural haematoma.

Minor head injury (e.g. GCS > 13) requires careful observation using the GCS and identification of any deteriorating parameters. Apparent minor head injury can lead to significant cerebral damage and physical effects, and it is therefore essential that the practitioner recognises any need for immediate medical attention. Frequent neurological observation using the GCS is essential in all patients who meet the definition of head injury defined above until the patient is deemed stable neurologically. It is essential that the GCS is recorded clearly and it is recommended that the three individual components of the scale (eye-opening, verbal response and motor responses) are described separately in all verbal and written communications and records so that the information always accompanies the total score. NICE (2007b) also recommend that in all head-injured patients it is essential that pain is managed effectively (especially if there are other skeletal injuries) as unmanaged pain can lead to a rise in intracranial pressure and increased risk of haemorrhage.

Detecting early neurological deterioration can expedite neurosurgical interventions that can prevent permanent disability or death from the deteriorating brain injury. Although the majority of head injuries are minor, they can be associated with other skeletal injuries or other trauma and the mechanism of injury may mean that in some hospitalised trauma patients severe head injury is more likely. It may also be masked by a focus on other more obvious injuries in the early stages of management of the multiply injured patient.

The following are indications of significant brain injury (NICE 2007b) and should instigate medical referral and urgent CT scan of the brain:

- GCS < 13 when first assessed in the ED
- GCS < 15 when assessed in the ED 2 hours after injury

- suspected open or depressed skull fracture
- sign of fracture at skull base (blood in the ear, 'panda' eyes/periorbital ecchymosis, cerebrospinal fluid leakage from ears or nose, Battle's sign/bruising over the mastoid process)
- post-traumatic seizure
- focal neurological deficit
- more than one episode of vomiting
- increased amnesia of events more than 30 minutes before trauma.

In addition it is recommended that a neurosurgeon is involved if the patient is on a non-neurosurgical unit if any of the following occur:

- persistent coma
- unexplained confusion for more than 4 hours
- deterioration in GCS (especially in motor response)
- progressive focal neurological signs
- seizure without full recovery.

Careful frequent assessment and recording of these parameters can detect the patient in need of intervention and the practitioner is central to this.

Major Wounds, Crush Injuries and Traumatic Amputations

Injury can be associated with major wounds due to both blunt and sharp trauma. Mechanisms of injury that involve the 'crushing' of a part of the body between two hard surfaces occur most commonly in motor vehicle and industrial accidents as well as in incidents where blasts, collapsed buildings or multiple passenger transport systems are involved. Underlying tissues are compressed and surrounding tissue and organs may be severely damaged. An underlying fracture associated with significant tissue damage presents a major challenge to the trauma team for four main reasons:

1) A high possibility of severe infection, not only of damaged soft tissue, but of underlying skeletal tissue (see Chapter 17 for further discussion the management of compound fractures).
2) Damage to the blood vessels supplying tissue, leading to ischaemia and necrosis of tissue and a risk of anaerobic infection.
3) Such severe damage to neurovascular structures that the limb (or part of a limb) has no viable circulation and damage is so severe that amputation is the only possible course of action. In some incidents, the limb or part of limb may have been traumatically amputated at the time of the injury. In this instance, it is important to consider the care of the severed body part when attending to

wound care, taking into account X-rays, ischaemic time and asepsis.

4) The physiological impact of a large amount of tissue damage may result in a patient who is critically ill as discussed above.

Patients with significant wounds may require resuscitation and need careful monitoring for signs of vascular instability and sepsis along with judicious intravenous hydration and pain management. Significant wounds require meticulous asepsis and their management needs to be considered using a team approach, which involves orthopaedic trauma surgery as well as plastic surgery teams. The decision to amputate or salvage an injured limb is based on multiple factors such as location of injured part, age and pre-existing conditions, type of injury, ischaemic time and presence of infection, and generally a consensus from two experts is required prior to amputation. Scoring systems can be helpful in making the decision between primary amputation and limb salvage (Shanmuganthan 2008). Long-term care focuses on rehabilitation (Chapter 6) and wound care (Chapter 12), paying particular attention to debridement of devitalised tissue, shaping of the stump, psychological care, pain assessment and relief of phantom sensations, and promoting optimal function and mobility.

Rhabdomyolysis

Skeletal injury, particularly where significant soft tissue and muscle is involved, can release the contents of muscle cells into the circulation, releasing the muscle protein myoglobin into the bloodstream. This can result in a relatively uncommon but serious condition known as crush syndrome or rhabdomyolysis. Because of the size and toxicity of the myoglobulin, it can affect the glomerular filtration rate of the kidney and result in acute renal failure. The patient becomes seriously ill. Although rhabdomyolysis may be largely without symptoms, the practitioner should assess renal function by observing the volume of urine output as well as for red or 'cola' coloured urine; the patient may also complain of generalised muscle pain and weakness. Any concerns should be immediately reported to medical staff. Diagnosis is confirmed by detecting the level of muscle enzymes in the blood and treatment centres on flushing the myoglobulin out of the system through dialysis. Rhabdomyolysis can often coincide with compartment syndrome (Chapter 9) and a high suspicion of its development should be maintained when caring for patients following crush injuries.

Monitoring, Deterioration and Early-warning Scores

Patients with severe or multiple injury can be physiologically unstable for several days or weeks following admission and even following transfer from the intensive care setting to a general hospital trauma ward. It is essential therefore that the patient's physiological status is carefully monitored until complete stability is assured. Even some weeks after the injury and subsequent surgery patients remain at risk of significant complications (see Chapter 9 for further discussion of these).

A common and widely recommended approach to monitoring patients following injury is the use of an early-warning score (EWS) with the aim of detecting clinical deterioration in the patient as early as possible so that active measures can be taken to prevent further deterioration and intensive care unit admission. This recognises the link between physiological observations and adverse clinical outcomes. A variety of different EWS methods are in use internationally depending on local policy, but the principles remain the same. EWSs involve calculating a score derived from regular observations of the following parameters:

- mental response
- pulse rate
- blood pressure
- respiratory rate
- temperature
- urinary output.

Of these, respiratory rate is considered to be the most important in identifying a change in the patient's condition and some systems do not include urinary output, although there are numerous reasons why this should be included in standard monitoring practice. Careful and frequent (as often as every 30 minutes if the practitioner has reason to suspect the patient may be at risk of deterioration) recordings are made on a specialised chart which enables the practitioner to identify any changes immediately. The score will often have a threshold of deterioration in the physiological parameters at which the practitioner needs to take action. This action initially involves seeking immediate medical attention, referral to a senior medical practitioner if necessary and possible referral to the intensive/critical care team. Many hospitals now provide an intensive care outreach service or similar where ward staff can seek the support of a critical care practitioner in monitoring the patient, making decisions and identifying action needed. Research is increasingly indicating that EWSs are an effective way to recognise the deteriorating patient in need of intervention, with potential to decrease the number of patients who require emergency resuscitation, and some are now being developed for specific populations such as children.

Early-warning Scores and the Deteriorating Patient

The ability to identify a deteriorating patient and act appropriately is fundamental to quality orthopaedic nursing care in all settings, especially in the trauma setting. Odell et al. (2009) suggest that inexperience, lack of skill and excessive workloads greatly impede the ward nurse's ability to detect and manage these patients. The use of EWSs, also known as patient at risk scores (PARSs) or modified early-warning scores (MEWSs), has become increasingly popular for the identification and monitoring of critically ill patients, with their use being recommended in the care of all patients admitted to an acute hospital setting (NICE 2007a). In the UK EWSs are commonly used for the assessment of ill patients (Rees 2003) and the more recently developed National Early Warning Score 2 (NEWS2) is currently used across 100% of ambulance trusts and 76% of acute trusts (NICE 2020). Ireland was the first country to adopt a national early-warning system (Health Service Executive 2018). A software-based national EWS system has recently been developed in the United Kingdom and is recommended for use in all acute hospitals (NICE 2020). This technology moves from a paper-based assessment to integrative software systems that output the score, freeing up staff resources and time to care.

EWSs are calculated from simple physiological parameters that are routinely monitored at the patients' bedside (Figure 16.6). Depending on the observations made, the patient is given a score which helps quantify their health status and risk for critical illness. This score highlights the need for clinical intervention and/or admission to an intensive care facility. It is anticipated that EWSs taking into account all physiological parameters can more readily identify deteriorating patients than waiting for more obvious changes such as a marked drop in systolic blood pressure, which is often a pre-terminal event (Rees 2003). Once the patient's score indicates they are at risk for further deterioration or a critical event, a response system is enacted depending on the individual hospital's policy. In general, a score of 3 indicates the need for a medical review. Box 16.5 considers the evidence base for EWS.

The use of EWSs in conjunction with clinical judgement has been found to be more effective at identifying patients at risk of adverse clinical outcomes than clinical judgement alone in pre-hospital admitted patients (Fullerton et al. 2012). There have been many advances and expansions on the role of the orthopaedic nurse. Nursing decision making and intuition are linked to clinical experience and are thought to improve over time as the nurse progresses to expert level (Banning 2007). It is often the nurses' intuitive judgement that alerts them to deterioration in patient condition and vital signs are then performed to confirm these findings (Odell et al. 2009). Conversely, Thompson et al. (2007) suggest that clinical experience is not a predictor of high-quality decision making in recognising patients at risk of a critical event, with nurses overestimating the need to intervene, and recommend a more structured approach. EWSs are designed as an assistive tool in identifying the critically ill or deteriorating patient, but they should not overrule clinical judgement, with many institutions recommending an escalation of care regardless of score if the nurse is concerned (Health Service Executive 2018).

Once a patient is identified as at risk for a critical incident, fast intervention and review are imperative. Some nurses may find it hard to articulate their clinical concerns about a patient to their medical colleagues, resulting in a delayed response and acknowledgement of the gravity of these concerns, which can be frustrating for both parties (Odell et al. 2009). In the same manner, junior nurses may lack the confidence to alert senior medics to their concerns. EWSs afford nurses the means to insist on a medical review and to refer upwards to more senior clinicians, as indicated by the patient's EWS (Rees 2003), assisting them in their role as patient advocates.

A set of vital signs usually includes the patient's temperature, pulse, respirations, blood pressure and, more recently, oxygen saturations. It is a core tool in performing a nursing assessment routinely as part of a patient's care and more often dependent on the individual's condition and treatment (e.g. performed more regularly in post-operative care). In the ritual of performing vital signs, their importance can sometimes be overlooked and they are a task that is often delegated to student nurses or healthcare assistants. Many healthcare institutions have abandoned vital signs monitors in preference for the traditional sphygmomanometers and nursing assessments of look, listen and feel, believing that it encourages a more accurate assessment of patient condition (Raynor 2010).

Respirations

Respiratory rate is the most important observation for assessing a patient's clinical status, yet it is often the one that is least recorded (Parkes 2011). When assessing respirations, consider rate, rhythm and depth. The rhythm indicates the pattern of breaths a minute. Ventilation can be monitored using end tidal carbon dioxide ($ETCO_2$) levels using colorimetry, capnometry or capnography, a non-invasive monitoring technique that negatively correlates with lactate and is an early predictor of shock in trauma patients (Stone et al. 2017). One of the most common breathing abnormalities, Cheyne strokes, involves a pattern of breaths followed by apnoeic episodes. Abnormalities of depth are mainly hypopnea and hyperpnoea. Hypopnea involves shallow respirations usually indicative of impending respiratory failure (Massey and

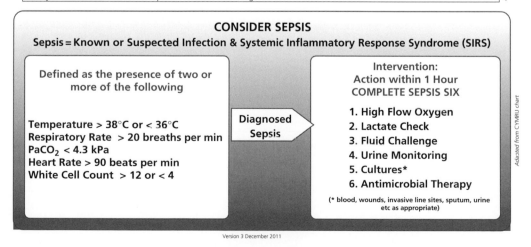

Figure 16.6 Example of an early warning score assessment sheet. *Source:* Reproduced with permission from the Irish Health Service Executive (2018).

Feidhmeannacht na Seirbhíse Sláinte Health Service Executive	Early Warning Score System	Patient Name: Date of Birth: Healthcare Record No: *Addressograph*
	0 1 2 3	
	Consultant:	

Ward:

	Frequency of observations		
Year	**Date**		
ABCDE Assessment	**Time**		

AB

RESPIRATORY DISTRESS

Consider:
- Airway
- Hypoxia
- Acidosis

Intervention:
- Immediate medical review
- ABCDE assessment
- Give Oxygen to target: 90% in COPD patients, 96% or more in all other patients
- Request CXR & ABG
- Airway Obstruction: activate Emergency Response System
- Respiratory Acidosis: Consider early non-invasive ventilation

Respiratory Rate (breaths per minute):
≥25	≥25
21-24	21-24
12-20	12-20
9-11	9-11
≤8	≤8

Respiration Score

SpO₂ %:
≥96	≥96
94-95	94-95
92-93	92-93
≤91	≤91

SpO₂

Room Air — RA

F₁O₂ or% L/min — % or L/min

F₁O₂ Score

C

HYPERTENSION

Consider:
- Pain
- Hypercapnia

Intervention:
- Immediate medical review
- 12-lead ECG

HYPOTENSION

Consider:
- Bleeding
- Myocardial Infarction
- Sepsis

Intervention:
- Immediate medical review
- Check BP manually
- 12-lead ECG
- If no heart failure, stat IV fluids - 500ml
- If no improvement after 20 ml/kg: immediate review by doctor
- Systolic BP ≤ 90: consider activating ERS

Systolic BP ≥ 200: Doctor to review

Blood Pressure (mmHg): 250, 240, 230, 220, 210, 200, 190, 180, 170, 160, 150, 140, 130, 120, 110, 100, 90, 80, 70, 60, 50, 40

BP Score

TACHYCARDIA

Consider:
- Seagull Sign**
- Loss of conciousness
- Myocardial ischaemia on ECG
- Heart failure. If YES- consider activating ERS

Intervention:
- Immediate medical review
- ACLS Algorithm as appropriate

BRADYCARDIA

Consider:
- Electrolyte Disturbance
- Drug Side-effect
- Complete Heart Block

Intervention:
- Immediate medical review
- 12-lead ECG
- Telemetry
- Heart Rate ≤ 40: consider activating ERS
- Document irregular Heart Rate

Heart Rate (beats per minute): 180, 170, 160, 150, 140, 130, 120, 110, 100, 90, 80, 70, 60, 50, 40, 30

Heart Rate ≤ 40: Immediate medical review

Heart Rate Score

D

NEUROLOGICAL DETERIORATION

Consider:
- Hypoglycaemia
- Acute brain injury
- Pupil response

Intervention:
- Immediate medical review
- Capillary glucose
- Sudden fall in level of consciousness: consider activating ERS

AVPU:
Alert (A)	(A)
Voice (V)	(V)
Pain (P)	(P)
Unresponsive (U)	(U)

AVPU Score

Temperature (°C): 39.0, 38.5, 38.0, 37.5, 37.0, 36.5, 36.0, 35.5, 35.0, 34.5

E

PYREXIA OR HYPOTHERMIA

Consider:
- Sepsis

Intervention:
- Immediate medical review
- C-Reactive protein
- Two or more sepsis indicators present
- Commence SEPSIS SIX Regimen

Temp Score

Total EWS	
Blood Glucose	
Bowel Movement	
Weight (kg)	
Initials	

Urine Output: If there are concerns about urine output (< 0.5 ml/kg/hr), contact Doctor for review

Figure 16.6   (Continued)

National Early Warning Score Key (ViEWS)

SCORE	3	2	1	0	1	2	3
Respiratory Rate (bpm)	≤ 8		9 - 1	12 - 20		21 - 24	≥ 25
SpO₂ (%)	≤ 91	92 - 93	94 - 35	≥ 96			
Inspired O₂ (F₁O₂)				Air			Any O₂
Systolic BP (mmHg)	≤ 90	91 - 100	101 - 110	111 - 249	≥ 250		
Heart Rate (BPM)	≤ 90	≤ 40	41 - 50	51 - 90	91 - 110	111 - 130	≥ 131
AVPU/CNS Response				Alert (A)			Voice (V), Pain (P), Unresponsive (U)
Temp (°C)	≤ 35.0	35.1 - 36.0		36.1 - 38.0	38.1 - 39.0	≥ 39.1	

Note: Where systolic blood pressure is ≥ 200 mmHg, request Doctor to review.

This Section is for reference only. Where Glasgow Coma Score is required, please use separate sheet.

Please use this space for additional monitoring charts, e.g. Pain Score Chart

Glasgow Coma Scale

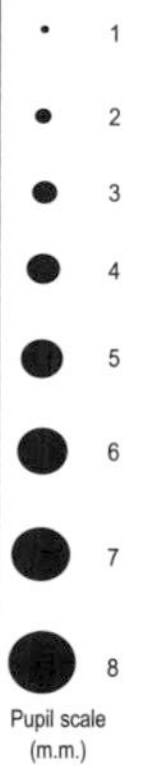

		Date:					
		Time:					
			G				
			C				
			S				
		Spontaneously	4				
Eyes open		To Speech	3		Eyes closed		
C		To Pain	2		by swelling		
C		None	1		= C		
M	Best verbal response	Orientated	5				
A		Confused	4		Endotracheal		
S		Inappropriate words	3		tube or		
C		Incomprehensible sounds	2		tracheostomy		
		None	1		=T		
A	Best motor response	Obey commands	6		Usually record		
L		Localize Pain	5		the		
E		Flexion to Pain	4		best arm		
		Abnormal Flexion	3		response		
		Extension to Pain	2				
		No Response	1				
		Total G.C.S.					
PUPILS	right	Size			+ reacts		
		Reaction			− no reaction		
	left	Size			C eyes closed		
		Reaction					
L		Normal power			Record		
I	A	Mild weakness			right (R)		
M	R	Severe weakness			and left (L)		
B	M	Spastic flexion			separately if		
M	S	Extension			there is a		
O		No response			difference		
V		Normal power			between the		
E	L	Mild weakness			two sides		
M	E	Severe weakness					
E	G	Extension					
N	S	No response					
T							
							Initials

With kind permission of Beaumont Hospital

Pupil scale (m.m.)
1
2
3
4
5
6
7
8

** **Seagull Sign: This is when the Heart Rate is above the Systolic Blood Pressure**

Note: The National Early Warning Score has adopted the VitalPAC™ Early Warning Score (ViEWS) parameters.
Acknowledgements: A modified version of the CQUCDKLI Vital Signs Record was reproduced with permission from its developers. Support and advice was provided by the Health Directorate, ACT Government, Australia.

Figure 16.6 (Continued)

Box 16.5   Evidence Digest: The Evidence for EWSs to Date

In 1997 Morgan et al. (1997) first reported the use of an EWS in the detection of seriously ill deteriorating patients (Morgan et al. 1997) and their use on both medical and surgical wards is now well established (Fullerton et al. 2012). Several studies suggest that the presence of critically abnormal vital signs can be a good predictor of patient deterioration and mortality risk (Bleyer et al. 2011; Fullerton et al. 2012; Garcea et al. 2010). This implies that monitoring and rapid response to abnormal vital signs may positively influence mortality rates. Although there has been a mass acceptance of EWS use, they have yet to be rigorously validated. A Cochrane review suggested there was minimal evidence to support the adoption of EWSs in the identification and management of critically ill patients (McGaughy et al. 2007), but there does appear to be strong evidence for the ability of EWSs to predict death and cardiac arrest within 48 hours, although its impact on positive patient outcomes requires greater research (Smith et al. 2014; Fu, Li- Heng et al. 2020). EWSs and critical care outreach teams are often introduced concurrently, and it may be difficult to solely assess the impact of EWSs on patient outcomes, when in fact the effectiveness of EWSs relies heavily on the escalation plan and response to an abnormal score (Downey et al. 2017). Downey's systematic review suggests that EWSs are an effective tool in predicting and improving patient outcomes, although inaccurate scorings and responses may undermine potential benefits and they can never replace clinical judgement. A more recent systematic review suggests that methodological weaknesses in studies examining the validation of EWSs were at risk of bias, which could result in scoring systems that perform poorly in clinical practice, and recommendations are provided to address these issues for future practice and research (Gerry et al. 2020).

A recent meta-analysis examined the prognostic accuracy of using the NEWS2 for predicting clinical deterioration in COVID 19 patients and found it had moderate sensitivity and specificity, where a score of 5 should activate a rapid response (Zhang et al. 2021).

Meredith 2010). Hyperpnoea is characterised by rapid and deep respirations (Kussmals) indicative of the body's compensatory mechanism. Hyperventilation occurs in the effort to dispose of excess carbon dioxide (Massey and Meredith 2010). The normal respiratory rate for an adult is 14–20 breaths a minute. The rate is assessed by observing the chest wall (rise and fall) for a full minute. Bradypnoea indicates a respiratory rate <8 breaths a minute and is seen in depression of the respiratory centre, for example a narcotic overdose. Tachypnoea indicates a respiratory rate >20 breaths a minute and can indicate either a drop in arterial blood oxygen saturation or compensation in the presence of metabolic acidosis. Rates above 27 breaths a minute are an important predictor of cardiac arrest (Smith et al. 2011). Some reasons for tachypnoea in the orthopaedic patient include:

- fat embolism
- pulmonary embolism
- respiratory tract infection
- airway trauma/obstruction
- haemothorax/pneumothorax
- sepsis
- haemorrhage
- rhabdomyolysis
- pulmonary oedema
- pneumonia

- bone metastases-related hypercalcaemia
- cervical/thoracic spinal cord injury.

Oxygen Saturation

Pulse oximetry (SpO_2) indicates a patient's arterial oxygenation levels and, in conjunction with respiratory rate, can give a clearer clinical picture of pulmonary status. A pulse oximetry reading of 95% or above indicates adequate peripheral arterial oxygenation ($PaO_2 > 70$ mmHg or 9.3 kPa) (ATLS 2018). However, it is important not to be too reliant on oxygen saturation as there can be falling oxygen delivery despite normal arterial oxygen saturation; metabolic acidosis can increase the respiratory rate even though the arterial oxygen saturation may be normal. Hence, a normal SpO_2 does not rule out acute respiratory distress. In addition, pulse oximetry can be affected by other variables, such as movement, the presence of unusual haemoglobin varieties, a cold environment, poor perfusion, arrhythmias and the presence of nail varnish (ACT Health 2007). Some reasons for decreased oxygen saturations in the orthopaedic patient include:

- fat embolism
- pulmonary embolism
- respiratory tract infection

- airway trauma/obstruction
- haemothorax pneumothorax
- sepsis
- hypovolaemia
- rhabdomyolysis
- pulmonary oedema
- pneumonia.

Temperature

A raised temperature often indicates the presence of infection. However, sepsis should also be considered in a patient with a 'normal' temperature. Septic patients often present as hypothermic as an overwhelmed immune system may lack the ability to generate a response. For more information on septic shock, see Chapter 9. Some reasons for altered temperature in the orthopaedic patient include:

- infection or sepsis
- exposure
- autonomic dysreflexia (refer to Chapter 20).

Pulse

The heart rate is an important aspect of the chain of oxygen delivery (Figure 16.1). In simple terms, when there is a deficiency in oxygen delivery, the heart beats faster to try and compensate. Cardiac output is the amount of blood pumped out by each ventricle in 1 minute. Cardiac output is dependent on the heart rate and stroke volume, which is the amount of blood pumped out by a ventricle with each contraction. When the blood volume is decreased or heart muscle damaged, the stroke volume is decreased and the heart rate is increased in an effort to maintain cardiac output (tachycardia). Some common reasons for tachycardia in an orthopaedic patient include:

- hypovolaemia
- sepsis
- fat embolism
- pulmonary embolism
- electrolyte imbalance
- substance abuse.

Blood Pressure

blood pressure = cardiac output × peripheral resistance

Systolic blood pressure (SBP) is a strong sign in terms of reflecting blood loss and trauma severity. An initial SBP in the range of 90–110 mmHg in a trauma patient may be indicative of hypoperfusion and is associated with poor patient outcome (Kassavin et al. 2011) A decrease in blood pressure suggests a decrease in cardiac output and may result in delayed or insufficient oxygenation of tissues. EWSs focus on systolic measurement and hypotension, as a falling blood pressure is a key indicator of a critical event. This is not to say that a hypertensive patient does not warrant review, and clinical judgement should be used at all times.

Common causes of hypertension in the orthopaedic patient include:

- pain
- autonomic dysreflexia
- bone metastases-related hypercalcaemia.

Common causes of hypotension in the orthopaedic patient include:

- hypovolaemia
- sepsis
- cardiogenic shock
- neurogenic shock
- dehydration.

The patient in spinal shock or with a spinal cord injury will have a lower pulse rate and blood pressure due to unopposed vagal nerve activity (Chapter 19).

Mental Status

A depressed level of consciousness or sudden onset of confusion is a clear sign of a deteriorating patient and may be as a result of intracranial disease, inadequate oxygen delivery or metabolic abnormalities (e.g. hypoglycaemia). The patient with a head injury or sudden altered consciousness level requires more in-depth monitoring than that provided by EWSs such as the GCS. Some reasons for a depressed level of consciousness in the orthopaedic patient include:

- head trauma/injury
- cerebrovascular disease/haemorrhage
- encephalitis
- delirium
- hypoglycaemia
- electrolyte imbalances
- substance abuse
- hypoxia related (e.g. fat embolism, pulmonary embolism, sepsis).

Urinary Output

Urinary output is not routinely recorded as part of an EWS but some institutions have adopted it as a sixth parameter where patients are catheterised. A decreased urine output is an indicator of patient deterioration and is often one of the earliest signs of decline. The expected output for an adult is >0.5 ml/kg/h. For example, a patient weighing 60 kg should produce 30 ml/h. Some reasons for a low urinary output in the orthopaedic patient include:

- dehydration
- hypovolaemia
- shock

- urinary obstruction/trauma
- renal failure
- low output, cola-coloured urine, consider rhabdomyolysis.

Summary

Significant traumatic injury can be life-threatening. Care systems are in place that are designed to prevent death at each stage of care. Knowledge of the effects of trauma and careful assessment and observation of the patient following trauma is the main feature of successful care and of preventing and recognising life-threatening deterioration and the potential for significant life-changing disability.

Further Reading

Duncan, N.S. and Moran, C. (2009). Initial resuscitation of the trauma victim. *Orthop. Trauma* 24 (1): 1–8.

Gwinnutt, C.L. and Driscoll, P.A. (ed.) (2003). *Trauma Resuscitation: The Team Approach*. London: Taylor and Francis.

NCEPOD (2007) *Trauma: Who Cares? A Report of the National Confidential Enquiry Into Patient Outcome and Death*. www.ncepod.org.uk/2007report2/Downloads/SIP_report.pdf (accessed 1 August 2012).

O'Shea, R.A. (2005). *Principles and Practice of Trauma Nursing*. Edinburgh: Churchill Livingstone.

Skinner, D.V. and Driscoll, P.A. (2013). *ABC of Major Trauma*, 4e. Oxford: Wiley Blackwell.

References

ACT Health (2007) *Early Recognition of the Deteriorating Patient Program*. http://health.act.gov.au/professionals/general-information/compass/login/adult-program (accessed 1 July 2012).

Altinok, T. and Can, A. (2014). Management of tracheobronchial injuries. *Eurasian J. Med.* 46 (3): 209–215. https://doi.org/10.5152/eajm.2014.42 (accessed December 2021).

American College of Surgeons (2018) *ATLS 10th Edition Student Course Manual*. https://learning.facs.org/system/files/ATLS%2010th%20Edition%20Student%20Manual_0.pdf (accessed December 2021).

Banning, M. (2007). A review of clinical decision making: models and current research. *J. Clin. Nurs.* 17 (2): 187–195.

Bleyer, A.J., Vidya, S., Russel, G.B. et al. (2011). Longitudinal analysis of one million vital signs in patients in an academic medical center. *Resuscitation* 82 (11): 1387–1392.

Boyle, M.J., Smith, E.C., and Archer, F. (2008). Is mechanism of injury alone a useful predictor of major trauma? *Int. J. Care Inj.* 39 (9): 986–992.

Christensen, M.A., Steinmetz, J., Velmahos, G., and Rasmussen, L.S. (2021). Supplemental oxygen therapy in trauma patients: an Exxploratory registry-based study. *ACTA Anaesthesiol. Scand.* 65 (7): 967–978.

CRASH-2 Collaborators, Shakur, H., Roberts, I. et al. (2010). Effects of tranexamic acid on death, vascular occlusive events, and blood transfusion in trauma patients with significant haemorrhage (CRASH-2): a randomised, placebo-controlled trial. *Lancet* 376: 23–32.

Dixon, J.R., Lecky, F., Bouamra, O. et al. (2020). Age and the distribution of major injury across a national trauma system. *Age Ageing* 49 (2): 218–226.

Downey, C.L., Tahir, W., Randell, R. et al. (2017). Strengths and limitations of early warning scores: a systematic review and narrative synthesis. *Int. J. Nurs. Stud.* 76:

106–119. https://doi.org/10.1016/j.ijnurstu.2017.09.003. Epub 2017 Sep 13. PMID: 28950188.

Feller, R., Furin, M., Alloush, A., and Reynolds, C. (2021). EMS immobilization techniques. In: *StatPearls*. Treasure Island, FL: StatPearls Publishing PMID: 29083568.

Fullerton, J.N., Price, C.L., Silvey, N.E. et al. (2012). Is the modified early warning score (MEWS) superior to clinical judgment in detecting critical illness in the pre-hospital environment? *Resuscitation* 83 (5): 557–562.

Garcea, G., Ganga, R., Neal, C.P. et al. (2010). Preoperative early warning scores can predict in-hospital mortality and critical care admission following emergency surgery. *J. Surg. Res.* 159: 729–734.

Gerry, S., Birks, J., Kirtley, S. et al. (ed.) (2020). Early warning scores for detectin deteriorsation in adult hospital patients: systematic review and critical appraisal of methodology. *Br. Med. J.* 369: m1501.

Gwinnutt, C.L. and Driscoll, P.A. (ed.) (2003). *Trauma Resuscitation: The Team Approach*. London: Taylor and Francis.

Haider, A.H., Chang, D.C., Haut, E.R. et al. (2009). Mechanism of injury predicts patient mortality and impairment after blunt trauma. *J. Surg. Res.* 153 (1): 138–142.

Harrison, P. (2000). *Managing Spinal Injury: Critical Care*. London: Spinal Injuries Association.

Health Service Executive (2018). *National Wound Management Guidelines*. Dublin: Office of Nursing and Midwifery Services Director.

Heng, L.F., Schwartz, J., Moy, A. et al. (2020). Development and validation of early warning score system: A systematic literature review. *Biomed. Inform.* 105: 103410.

Henning, J., Woods, K., and Howley, M. (2011). Management of major trauma. *Anaesthesia Intensive Care Med.* 12 (9): 383–386.

Hepple, D.J., Durrand, J.W., Bouamra, O., and Godfrey, P. (2019). Impact of a physician-led pre-hospital critical care team on outcomes after major trauma. *Anaesthesia* 74 (4): 473–479.

Hoffman, J.R., Mower, W.R., Wolfson, A.B. et al. (2000). Validity of a set of clinical criteria to rule out injury to the cervical spine in patients with blunt trauma. National Emergency X-radiography Utilization Study Group. *N. Engl. J. Med.* 343 (2): 94–99.

Hood, N. and Considine, J. (2015). Spinal immobilisaton in pre-hospital and emergency care: a systematic review of the literature. *Australas. Emerg. Nurs. J.* 18 (3): 118–137. https://doi.org/10.1016/j.aenj.2015.03.003. Epub 2015 Jun 4. PMID: 26051883.

Irish Health Service Executive (2011). *National Policy and Procedure for the Use of the Modified Early Warning Score System to Recognise and Respond to Clinical Deterioration*. Dublin: Health and Safety Executive.

Kassavin, D., Kuo, Y., and Ahmed, N. (2011). Initial systolic blood pressure and ongoing internal bleeding following torso trauma. *J. Emerg. Trauma Shock* 1: 37–41.

Keel, M. and Trentz, O. (2005). Pathophysiology of polytrauma. *Injury* 36 (6): 691–709.

Kreinest, M., Gliwitzky, B., Schüler, S. et al. (2016). Development of a new emergency medicine spinal immobilization protocol for trauma patients and a test of applicability by German emergency care providers. *Scand. J. Trauma Resusc. Emerg. Med.* 24: 71. https://doi.org/10.1186/s13049-016-0267-7.

Kwan, I., Bunn, F., and Roberts, I. on behalf of the WHO Pre-Hospital Trauma Care Steering Committee(2009). Spinal immobilisation for trauma patients. *Cochrane Database Syst. Rev.* 2: (Art. No.: CD002803). https://doi.org/10.1002/14651858.CD002803.

Lacey, L., Palokas, M., and Walker, J. (2019). Preventative interventions, protocols or guidelines for trauma patients at risk of cervical collar-related pressure ulcers: a scoping review. *JBI Database System Rev. Implement. Rep.* 17 (12): 2452–2475. https://doi.org/10.11124/JBISRIR-2017-003872. PMID: 31464850.

Maegele, M. (2021). The European perspective on the management of acute major hemorrhage and coagulopathy after trauma: summary of the 2019 updated European guideline. *J. Clin. Med.* 10 (2): 362. https://doi.org/10.3390/jcm10020362.

Maschmann, C., Jeppesen, E., Rubin, M.A., and Barfod, C. (2019). New clinical guidelines on the spinal stabilisation of adult trauma patients – consensus and evidence based. *Scand. J. Trauma Resusc. Emerg. Med.* 27: 77.

Massey, D. and Meredith, T. (2010). Respiratory assessment 1: why do it and how to do it? *Br. J. Card. Nurs.* 5 (11): 537–541.

McGaughy, J., Alderdice, F., Fowler, R. et al. (2007). Outreach and early warning systems (EWS) for the prevention of intensive care admission and death of critically ill adult patients on general hospital wards. *Cochrane Database Syst. Rev.* 3, (Art No.:CD005529). doi: https://doi.org/10.1002/14651858.CD005529.PUB.2.

McRae, R. and Esser, M. (2008). *Practical Fracture Treatment*, 5e. Edinburgh: Churchill Livingstone.

Morgan, R.J., Williams, F., and Wright, M.M. (1997). An early warning scoring system for detecting developing critical illness. *Clin. Intensive Care* 8: 100.

National Office of Clinical Audit (2020). *Major Trauma Audit National Report 2018*. Dublin: National Office of Clinical Audit.

NCEPOD (2007) *Trauma: Who Cares? A Report of the National Confidential Enquiry Into Patient Outcome and Death*. www.ncepod.org.uk/2007report2/Downloads/SIP_report.pdf (accessed 1 August 2012).

NICE (2007a). *Head Injury. Triage, Assessment, Investigation and Early Management of Head Injury in Infants, Children and Adults. CG56*. London: NICE www.nice.org.uk/nicemedia/pdf/CG56QuickRedGuide.pdf (accessed 22 April 2014).

NICE (2007b). *Acutely Ill Patients in Hospital: Recognition of and Response to Acute Illness in Adults in Hospital*. London: NICE.

NICE (2016a). *Major trauma: assessment and initial managment*. NG 39. www.nice.org.uk/guidance/ng39/resources/major-trauma-assessment-and-initial-management-pdf-1837400761285 (accessed December 2021).

NICE (2016b) *Spinal Injury Assessment and Initial Management*. www.nice.org.uk/guidance/ng41/resources (accessed 13 January 2021).

NICE (2020). *National early warning score systems that alert to deteriorating adult patients*. www.nice.org.uk/advice/mib205/resources/national-early-warning-score-systems-that-alert-to-deteriorating-adult-patients-in-hospital-pdf-2285965392761797.

Nicks, B.A., Ayello, E.A., Woo, K. et al. (2010). Acute wound management: revisiting the approach to assessment, irrigation, and closure considerations. *Int. J. Emerg. Med.* 3 (4): 399–407.

Odell, M., Victor, C., and Oliver, D. (2009). Nurses' role in detecting deterioration in ward patients: systematic literature review. *J. Adv. Nurs.* 65 (10): 1992–2006.

Oteir, A.O., Smith, K., Stoelwinder, J.U. et al. (2015). Should suspected cervical spinal cord injury be immobilised?: a systematic review. *Injury* 46 (4): 528–535. https://doi.org/10.1016/j.injury.2014.12.032.

Pape, H., Pietzman, A.B., Schwab, C.W., and Giannoudis, P.V. (ed.) (2010). *Damage Control Management in the Polytrauma Patient*. New York: Springer.

Parkes, R. (2011). Rate of respiration: the forgotten vital sign. *Emerg. Nurse* 19 (2): 12–17.

Raynor, F.K. (2010). Trust brings back manual checks of vital signs to enhance patient safety. *Nurs. Stand.* 24 (30): 8.

Rees, J.E. (2003). Early warning scores. *Update in Anaesthesia* 17 (10): 30–33.

Richards, P.J. (2005). Cervical spine clearance: a review. *Int. J. Care Inj.* 36 (2): 248–269.

Romanelli, D. and Farrell, M.W. (2021) *AVPU Score* (updated 5 April 2022), in StatPearls. StatPearls Publishing, Treasure Island, FL. https://www.ncbi.nlm.nih.gov/books/NBK538431 (accessed December 2021).

Rossaint, R., Bouillon, B., Cerny, V. et al. (2010). Management of bleeding following major trauma: an updated European guideline. *Crit. Care* 14 (2): 1–29.

Scottish Intercollegiate Guidelines Network (2009). *Early Management of Patients with a Head Injury*, vol. 110. National Clinical Guideline www.sign.ac.uk/pdf/sign110.pdf (accessed 3 January 2013).

Shanmuganthan, R. (2008). The utility of scores in the decision to salvage or amputate in severely injured limbs. *Indian J. Orthop.* 42 (4): 368–376.

Smith, I., Mackay, J., and Fahrid, N. (2011). Respiratory rate measurement: a comparison of methods. *Br. J. Health. Asst.* 5 (11): 18–23.

Smith, M.E.B., Chipvaro, J.C., O'Neil, M. et al. (ed.) (2014). *Early Warning System Scores*. Washington, DC: Department of Veterans Affairs (US) https://www.ncbi.nlm.nih.gov/books/NBK259024/.

Soloman, L., Warwick, D.J., and Nayagam, S. (2005). Management of major injuries. In: *Apleys Concise System of Orthopaedics and Fractures*, 3e (ed. L. Soloman, D.J. Warwick and S. Nayagam), 257–265. London: Hodder Arnold.

Spahn, D.R. and Ganter, M.T. (2010). Towards early individual goal-directed coagulation management in trauma patients. *Br. J. Anaesth.* 105 (2): 103–105.

Spahn, D.R., Bouillon, B., Cerny, V. et al. (2019). The European guideline on management of major bleeding and coagulopathy following trauma, fifth edition. *Crit. Care* 23: 98.

Stiell, I.G., Wells, A.G., Vandemheen, K.L. et al. (2001). The Canadian C-spine rule for radiography in alert and stable trauma patients. *J. Am. Med. Assoc.* 286 (15): 1841–1848.

Stone, M.E. Jr., Kalata, S., Liveris, A. et al. (2017). End-tidal CO_2 on admission is associated with hemorrhagic shock and predicts the need for massive transfusion as defined by the critical administration threshold: a pilot study. *Injury* 48 (1): 51–57. www.tarn.ac.uk/content/downloads/19/5.%20Published%20reports%202021.pdf (accessed December 2021.

Teasdale, G. and Jennett, B. (1974). Assessment of coma and impaired consciousness. A practical scale. *Lancet* 2 (7872): 81–84.

Thompson, C., Bucknall, T., Estabrookes, C.A. et al. (2007). Nurses' critical event risk assessments: a judgment analysis. *J. Clin. Nurs.* 18: 601–612.

Vulliamy, P., Thaventhiran, A.J., and Davenport, R.A. (2019). What's new for trauma haemorrhage management? *Br.*

J. Hosp. Med. 80 (5): 268–273. https://doi.org/10.12968/hmed.2019.80.5.268.

Wardrope, J., Ravichandran, G., and Locker, T. (2004). Risk assessment for spinal injury after trauma. *BMJ* 328: 721–723.

Webber-Jones, J.E., Thomas, C.A., and Bordeaux, R.A. (2002). The management and prevention of rigid cervical collar complications. *Orthop. Nurs.* 21 (4): 19–25.

White, C.C. et al. (2014). EMS spinal precautions and the use of the long backboard – resource document to the position statement of the National Association of EMS physicians and the American College of Surgeons Committee on

trauma. *Prehosp. Emerg. Care* 18 (2): 306–314. PMID: 24559236.

WHO (2004). *Guidelines for Essential Trauma Care*. Geneva: World Health Organization.

WHO (2014). *Injuries and Violence: The Facts, 2014*. Geneva: World Health Organization.

Zhang, K., Zhang, X., Ding, W., et al. (2021). *The Prognostic Accuracy of National Early Warning Score 2 on Predicting Clinical Deterioration for Patients With COVID-19: A Systematic Review and Meta-Analysis*. https://www.frontiersin.org/article/10.3389/fmed.2021.699880.

17

Principles of Fracture Management

Julie Craig[1], Sonya Clarke[2], and Pamela Moore[1,3]

[1] *Belfast Health and Social Care Trust, UK*
[2] *Queen's University Belfast, Belfast, UK*
[3] *Nursing Development Lead, Belfast Health and Social Care Trust, Belfast, UK*

Introduction

Resulting from a variety of mechanisms of injury, fractures form the bulk of orthopaedic work in the trauma setting. The care of patients with fractures demands an understanding of how injury affects bone and the surrounding soft tissue and how the process of bone repair can be facilitated through effective management and care. In spite of the relatively severe forces required to fracture a bone, skeletal injuries are extremely common and are a major reason for attending the emergency department. Fracture clinics are often the largest and busiest outpatient settings in any acute general hospital and sustaining a fracture is a common reason for admission to hospital. The incidence of fracture in the general population in England, as one example, has been estimated to be as high as 3.6 fractures per 100 people per year. This represents a significant public health burden and significant cost to society (Donaldson et al. 2008). The highest incidence of fracture is found in young males from 16 to 24 years of age, often due to high-energy trauma and frequently involving long bones. Conversely, those aged 65 or older primarily suffer a fracture due to falls, following which the most common injuries include those occurring as fragility fractures in the wrist, proximal femur, proximal humerus, vertebrae and pelvis/pubic rami as these sites are most often affected by osteoporosis. See Chapter 16 for further general information about the care and management of the patient following polytrauma, i.e. multiple injuries sustained in high-energy mechanisms. The present chapter mainly focuses on the principles of fracture management and care in the adult, although many such principles can be applied to the care of the child and young adult. Chapters 24 and 25 specifically consider fractures in the infant child and young person.

Causes and Types of Fractures

Fractures involve a loss of continuity in the substance of bone. They are usually the result of different types and magnitude of blunt force. The force required to result in a fracture of the shaft of femur in a healthy person aged 25, for example, is significant and is also considerably greater than that needed to result in the fracture of a hip in the older person with osteoporotic bone. An assessment and understanding of the mechanism of injury can provide essential information that can assist with differential diagnosis and subsequent management of fractures. This can also help identify non-accidental injury in vulnerable patients such as children (Chapter 21), and those with complex physical disabilities or cognitive impairment. Injuries out of keeping with the described mechanism of injury should arouse suspicions, either of the potential for non-accidental injury or the potential for pathological fractures resulting from local or generalised bone weakness such as tumours or metabolic bone diseases.

Five blunt forces commonly result in fracture: shearing, compression, bending, torsion and tension.

Shearing

Shearing occurs when one end of a bone is motionless while the other end is bowed or bent. When a shearing force is applied, a transverse or linear fracture occurs in which one section of bone moves away from the other. This is often the result of a person attempting to stop themselves falling by putting out a hand to save themselves, known as a fall on an outstretched hand (FOOSH). Shearing forces are also created by a direct blow from a large object and can be significant in injures to the epiphyseal plate in children and young adults.

Compression

Compression is a force that pushes inward from the end of a bone. This often causes crushing or fragmentation of the bone (comminution). This type of force is most often applied to the skull or vertebral bodies. This mechanism is also common in fragility fractures of osteoporotic bone or vertebral body fractures in patients who fall from a height, where the force is transmitted up through their spine.

Bending

Bending is the most common type of force. The force is delivered at an angle, rather than along the axis of the bone. The direction of the displaced distal portion of the bone often reflects the direction of the force that has created the fracture. One such fracture caused by a bending force is a 'night stick' fracture of the ulna, occurring when a person holds out their arms in self-defence and the impact causes inward displacement of the bone, although such a direct blow can also occur in falling against the edge of a hard surface such as a bench.

Torsion

Torsion involves twisting forces: one end of the bone is held motionless while the other end is twisted, often resulting in a spiral fracture. This can occur in sporting injuries such as football and skiing. In children and babies, spiral fractures can be the result of non-accidental injury, but can also result from twisting of a limb during a fall while one end is held stationary, e.g. falling from a seat while their foot is caught in it.

Tension

Tension is a force that pulls on the long axis of a bone, which may cause a fracture, but more often causes dislocation of the joint. When the force is strong enough, a section of healthy bone may be pulled away by a ligament under tension; this is known as an avulsion fracture.

Describing Fractures

Fractures are described according to several criteria, often in combination:

- the anatomical site of the fracture, e.g. intertrochanteric (proximal femur), mid-shaft (diaphyseal femur), supracondylar (distal femur) and any articular surface involvement
- whether the fracture is undisplaced or displaced

- the direction of displacement of the bone, e.g. either translation or angulation (either of which can occur in more than one direction)
- the severity of the fracture, e.g. simple, complex, comminuted (several fragments)
- the pattern of the fracture, e.g. oblique, transverse, spiral
- the classification of the fracture, if applicable for management or prognosis, e.g. the Garden classification of intracapsular hip fractures, the Weber classification of distal fibular fractures
- special features of the fracture, e.g. open (compound) or closed, incomplete (or greenstick).

Some fractures are also named after the doctor who first described them, for example Colles' fracture of the wrist. However, caution should be used when applying eponymous terms to fractures, as most fracture types do not fit any eponymous fracture description and the use of some terms may have become ambiguous. Figure 17.1 shows a few examples of types of fractures.

The mechanism of injury determines the fracture pattern. Sudden or direct trauma, for example, typically results in a complete fracture in adults with an oblique/transverse pattern. In children, this can sometimes result in an incomplete fracture such as a buckle fracture or greenstick fracture (Chapter 24). Indirect forces away from fracture site often produce a spiral pattern. Repetitive force on a bone causes mechanical strain and fatigue, resulting in a stress fracture.

It is important for the nurse/practitioner to understand the terms used to describe fractures and orthopaedic terminology as this is the language that is used in team discussions when planning and reviewing fracture management options.

Fracture Repair

The process of fracture repair is a remarkable physiological process that results in a healed structure that, providing the conditions are right, will be as mechanically sound post-healing as prior to the fracture. It is essential that the practitioner has an understanding of the physiology of fracture healing and the stages and events in the bone healing process as this has a bearing on the management options.

The process of bone healing can be broken down into several phases (Figure 17.2), but usually occurs in a seamless sequence of events. The timing of these events will vary according to the nature of the bone fractured, the type of fracture and other factors such as blood supply and the state of health of the patient. Fracture healing times are shortest in young children with incomplete fractures, sometimes as little as 2 or 3 weeks. A long bone fracture (e.g. femur or tibia) in a healthy adult takes on average 12 weeks to heal,

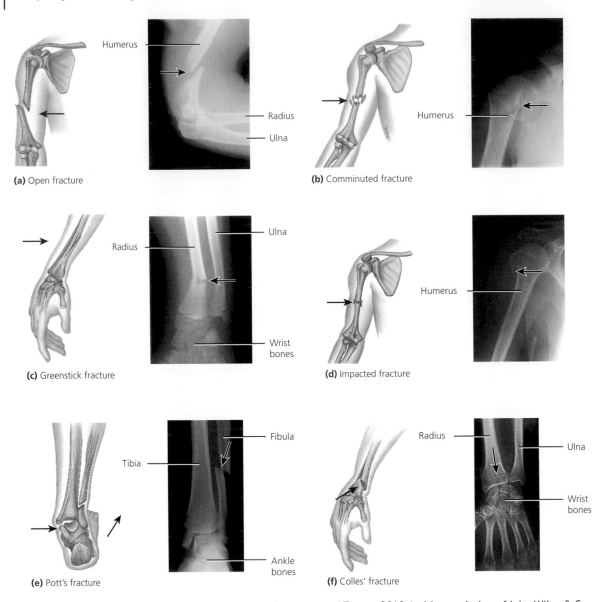

Figure 17.1 Examples of types of fractures. *Source:* Kuntzman and Tortora 2010 / with permission of John Wiley & Sons.

but this time is extended considerably in patients with concurrent medical conditions. Some bones have a poorer blood supply and this has a significant impact on healing. While some factors affecting bone healing are intrinsic to the patient, such as their age, general medical health or the presence of diabetes, efforts should be made to minimise modifiable risk factors that could impair bone healing, such as smoking, the use of non-steroidal anti-inflammatory drugs (NSAIDs) and malnutrition.

Haematoma and Inflammation

In the early weeks following injury, fracture healing is much like that of any other tissue. Bone is highly vascularised and as

it breaks, bleeding occurs from damaged capillaries and vessels. Providing clotting and haemostatic mechanisms are working effectively, a haematoma rapidly forms between the two bone ends and/or amongst the fragments. This haematoma is essential in the healing process that follows and it quickly becomes vascularised by new blood vessels. The injury to the bone and surrounding tissue results in an initial acute inflammatory response, which stimulates the migration of macrophages to the site of injury. These are central in the phagocytosis of the haematoma and necrotic tissue debris. Disturbance of this inflammatory process can adversely affect healing, therefore medications that interfere with this process, such as steroids, NSAIDs and immunosuppressants, can impair bone healing.

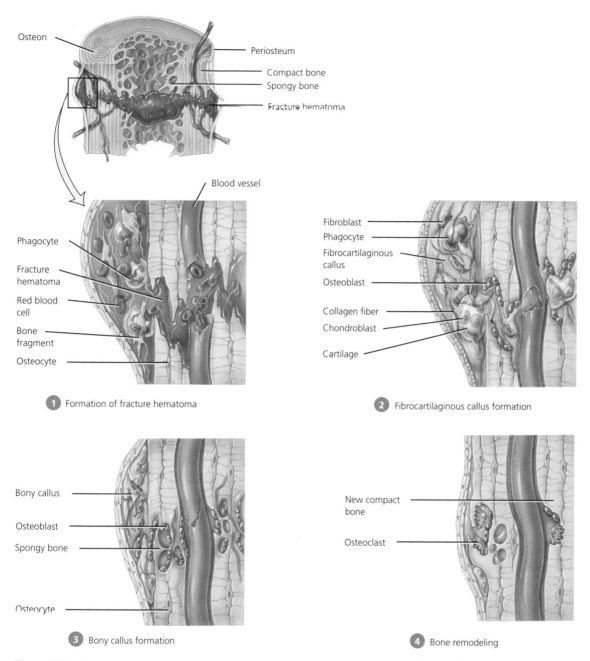

Figure 17.2 The process of fracture repair. *Source:* Kuntzman and Tortora 2010 / with permission of John Wiley & Sons.

There are two types of specialised cells that are central to bone healing:

Osteoblasts: lay down new bone matrices
Osteoclasts: resorb bone, enabling bone remodelling to take place.

Granulation

Gradually collagen fibres are laid down within the haematoma as it is absorbed by the macrophages. Mineral salts, including calcium, are deposited within the new framework. During the first few weeks after the fracture, the haematoma is invaded by macrophages and osteoclasts, and the sharp bone edges are removed (Dandy and Edwards 2009).

Primary Callus (Soft Callus)

Cells begin to proliferate and lay down new woven bone with collagen arranged in short bundles of fibres. This stage relies greatly on a good blood supply to the fracture site.

A cuff of woven bone gradually forms, initially under the periosteum and at the ends of the bone. This stage lacks the lamellar arrangement of mature bone and yet has little strength (Woolf 2000).

Bridging Callus (Hard Callus)

Gradually the gap between the bone ends is bridged by the formation of mineralised callus. The number of weeks required for this process varies between different fractures and different fracture patterns.

Remodelling

Once union has taken place and load bearing has begun to occur, the bone is gradually reshaped and smoothed through a process of resorption. This can take up to a year. This process enables any minor displacement of bone to be rectified as the bone develops a structure that reflects the mechanical forces placed upon it. For this reason, fracture healing is greatly enhanced by weight-bearing (axial loading) once bridging callus has formed and this is considered when making treatment decisions.

Primary and Secondary Bone Healing

The bone healing process described above is referred to as secondary bone healing and involves the production of callus. Primary bone healing is a bone healing process that occurs in many open reduction and internal fixation operations, where the bone ends are directly opposed and held with screws and/or a plate. In this process, no callus develops, as the osteoclasts and osteoblasts, respectively, continue their normal processed or removing (as 'cutting cones') and laying down bone, resulting in new bone crossing the fracture. As a result, callus may not be visible during the healing of bones after open reduction and internal fixation (e.g. plating). However, intramedullary nailing procedures still rely on callus formation.

Assessment and Emergency Care

A full holistic assessment of the patient is an essential part of providing care for patients with fractures rather than focusing entirely on the suspected fracture. In addition to the general care and management of the multiply injured patient described in Chapter 16, there are a number of specific considerations in relation to the patient with a fracture in the first hours following the injury.

A full history that includes the mechanism of injury should comprise:

- description of events
- time since injury

- pain and inability to weight-bear or use the affected limb/area since the time of injury.

Clinical assessment of the patient and injury should include:

- observation for swelling
- observation for visible deformity of the limb
- assessment for localised tenderness
- assessment for any associated numbness or paraesthesia
- assessment for any signs of compromised blood supply
- observation for any wounds over or close to the fracture site
- assessment of other possible sites of injury sustained at the time of the incident.

The main symptom of fracture is pain. Often this makes the patient seek treatment within minutes or hours after the initial injury. Overall, this pain is severe but there are some types of fractures (e.g. undisplaced stable ankle fractures) that produce less pain and may lead the patient to delay seeking treatment. Effective pain management should be provided, as discussed in Chapter 11, prior to any detailed assessment of the injury. Other symptoms include swelling and reduced mobility of the affected limb/joint. There may also be a tendency to protect the limb due to tenderness and discomfort over the affected area and the patient will be reluctant to allow the practitioner to touch the limb. Loss of power, deformity of the limb and irregularity of the contour of the limb may also be noted. Crepitus (bony grating) may be also heard or felt and movement at the fracture site may have been noted by the patient at the time of injury, but during examination this should not be tested for as movement at the fracture site should be avoided.

All patients with a suspected fracture require a radiographic examination. X-ray images taken from two or more angles provide the team with a detailed view of the fracture that can be used in planning treatment. A number of decision rules are in use in the emergency department to help the practitioner decide if a patient requires an X-ray. The most common of these are the Ottawa Ankle Rules (Stiell et al. 1994) and Ottawa Knee Rules (Stiell et al. 1997), which provide assessment criteria that have been shown by research to be predictive of fracture or otherwise and help to reduce the number of unnecessary X-rays.

While assessment and definitive treatment planning is taking place, care needs to focus on ensuring minimum mobility at the fracture site to reduce pain and blood loss (particularly in long bone fractures). The limb or body part should be carefully but firmly splinted to prevent undue movement of the fracture while the patient is being moved and assessed. No attempt should be made to change the position of the limb or manipulate the fracture at this time, except for under senior advice, such as in cases of gross deformity or new vascular compromise distal to the fracture. The type of splinting used will vary according to the site of the fracture. In upper limb injuries, a sling can often be used to support the arm. If an unstable pelvic fracture is suspected, a pelvic binder can be applied to reduce the volume of the pelvic cavity and potentially slow the loss of blood into this area. Pelvic binders are readily available to ambulance teams or a makeshift alternative may be achieved by wrapping a folded sheet around the proximal femurs. Direct pressure should be applied to any sites of active haemorrhage. Suspected spinal fractures are initially immobilised using a spinal board, along with 'sandbags' (or head blocks) placed either side of the head, a cervical spine collar and forehead tape to immobilise the neck. Splints and immobilising devices should only be applied temporarily until a full assessment can be conducted. The neurovascular status of the limb should be assessed and recorded/documented prior to and following application of any splint (Chapter 9).

An important consideration in the initial management of fractures at the scene of injury, during transfer and in early hospital management is the management of pain. Pain can vary but is often very severe and increased by any movement. In spite of this, pain management can often be neglected both at the scene of the injury and during emergency management (Chapter 11). Pre-hospital care practitioners are increasingly able to administer both systemic and regional analgesia at the scene and it is important that good pain assessment and analgesia practise be maintained throughout the early stages of care to facilitate patient comfort and reduce anxiety whilst assessment and planning take place. In the case of lower limb fractures, femoral nerve blocks are increasingly used. The advantages of this approach include better facilitation of assessment with less pain, faster and more effective pain relief, and avoidance of the complications of systemic analgesics (Black et al. 2012), which can be particularly important in the older person with a fracture.

The use of NSAIDs remains controversial and they are often avoided by orthopaedic surgeons because of their possible influence on bone healing. This view stems from multiple studies, in particular animal studies, that show delayed bone healing or non-unions associated with NSAID exposure. This does, however, mean that an important group of analgesics is not generally available for this group of patients and so other options must be considered carefully. A systematic review by Marquez-Lara et al. (2016) highlights the great variability in the interpretation of the literature addressing the impact of NSAIDs on bone healing. The review reported a lack of consensus regarding the safety of NSAIDs following orthopaedic procedures. The first author of this chapter, an orthopaedic doctor, does recognise that for some patients the use of NSAIDs may be unavoidable, but where other analgesics can be used, this should be discussed with their treating doctor. Non-union is a serious problem, causing prolonged pain and often requiring surgery, so while other medications are available it is usually taking an unnecessary risk to use NSAIDs in preference over alternatives.

The Complications of Fractures

The care of patients with fractures should take into account the fact that injuries can be associated with complications and a significant physiological response to trauma. The complications of fractures are seen more often in severe fractures of long bones and the bones of the axial skeleton such as the pelvis, spine, head and chest wall, as these are usually associated with high-impact mechanisms of injury. These injuries are frequently combined with other injuries such as multiple fractures and significant injury to soft tissue and visceral organs. The main complications of fractures include (see Chapter 9 for further detail):

- *haemorrhage*: blood loss from a closed fracture of the midshaft of the femur can, for example, amount to up to 1 litre, and blood loss from a severe 'open book' fracture of the pelvis can be up to 3 litres (McRae and Esser 2008), amounting to life-threatening haemorrhage and shock
- *fat embolism* and fat embolism syndrome, especially in fractures of the shaft of femur
- *compartment syndrome* and other types of neurovascular injury
- *infection*, especially in open fractures, which can lead to osteomyelitis
- *complications arising from immobility*, e.g. venous thromboembolism, pressure ulcers (Chapter 12), chest infection, urinary tract infection, muscle wasting, constipation
- *complications arising from surgery*, e.g. haemorrhage and shock, haematoma, wound infection (Chapter 12), wound dehiscence.

Complications of fractures can be categorised in several ways, including timescale, area of effect and underlying reasons:

- *damage to soft tissue structures*, e.g. risk of nerve injury, vascular injury (and bleeding, which can be potentially life-threatening in femoral and pelvic fractures) or compartment syndrome
- *problems with bone healing*, e.g. delayed union (slow bone healing), non-union (failure of bone healing) and malunion (bone healing in a poor position)

- *problems related mainly to the recovery of soft tissues and localised immobility*, e.g. the potential for ongoing pain or restricted movement in the affected area
- *problems related to general immobility*, i.e. the inability to sit up and mobilise as usual, e.g. deep venous thrombosis/pulmonary embolism, pressure ulcers, chest infections, urinary tract infection, muscle wasting, constipation
- *problems related to specific fractures*, e.g. soft tissue infection or osteomyelitis in open fractures, fat embolism, avascular necrosis, osteoarthritic change, myositis ossificans, heterotopic ossification
- *problems related to surgery*, e.g. wound-healing problems, blood loss, infection and osteomyelitis, periprosthetic fractures close to the operative site (either intra-operatively or in future), procedure failure or the need for reoperation, risks of anaesthesia such as cardiorespiratory problems, risks related to the specific procedures such as dislocation of prosthetic joint replacements.

It should be noted that many of the risks associated with non-operative management of fractures remain possible despite surgery. Surgery itself may pose potential risks such as infection or wound problems so it is only considered worthwhile if it offers a substantial improvement to other potential problems that may be more detrimental to the patient. For example, surgery does not eliminate the risk of non-union, but in some fractures surgery makes non-union much less likely, therefore justifying the other potential surgical risks.

Management of Fractures

The primary goals of fracture management are to achieve fracture healing without deformity and to restore function so that the patient can resume normal daily life (McRae and Esser 2008). The key principles of fracture management involve four steps:

- *resuscitation*, if needed
- *reduction* (achievement of an acceptable)
- *immobilisation* (maintenance of an acceptable bone position)
- *rehabilitation* (restoration of use of the affected area).

Resuscitation

Resuscitation of the patient following trauma is always a priority and is considered in detail in Chapter 16. Fracture and associated soft tissue trauma can cause considerable bleeding and potential shock. First aid is fundamental when there is high suspicion of fracture, and immobilisation of the fracture is pivotal in preventing haemorrhage and further injury.

Reduction

This is the restoration of an acceptable anatomical position of the bone. For some fractures, and for some patients, exact restoration of the anatomical position is not required because adequate function will still be maintained even with a degree of change in position (as in humeral shaft fractures) or due to the natural remodelling process (as occurs in children's fractures). For fractures where there is no displacement, no reduction is required. If needed, reduction is achieved by either closed reduction or open reduction.

Closed reduction is often called manipulation and refers to movement of the bone into an improved position without opening the soft tissues overlying the fracture site itself. This usually involves movement of the bone or joints adjacent to the fracture site, and can be performed under local anaesthetic, regional block, strong analgesic control, conscious sedation or general anaesthesia, depending on the site of the fracture and the degree of muscle relaxation required. Facilities, staff and expertise must be adequate for the chosen method of anaesthetic or analgesic, and the risks and benefits of each option for individual patients should be considered.

Closed reduction is commonly used for reduction of fractures such as wrist and ankle fractures and is a common emergency department procedure. Closed reduction under general anaesthesia can also be performed in the operating theatre, where the muscle relaxation of general anaesthesia can make reduction easier.

Closed reduction under general anaesthesia in the operating theatre is also used in long bone fractures such as tibial and femoral shaft fractures in preparation for intramedullary nailing. Avoidance of surgically opening the soft tissue envelope around such fractures is preferable to minimise disruption to the blood supply to the fracture site.

Open reduction involves a surgical procedure to open the soft tissues overlying the fracture so that the bone can be seen and fragments repositioned. Open reduction is generally reserved for fractures where closed reduction attempts do not achieve adequate reduction. This is more common for highly comminuted or intra-articular fractures, where adequate position is difficult to restore without directly viewing the bone.

Immobilisation

Fractures can present as displaced or undisplaced. When a satisfactory position of the bone is achieved, the bone should be immobilised to maintain this position. Fractures which are undisplaced at the time of injury do not require reduction as their position by definition is already satisfactory.

At the time of injury, the force that a bone is subjected to (e.g. when it impacts the ground in a fall) will either cause a bone to displace or create a risk of the bone displacing in that direction in the first few weeks, most commonly in the first week or two. Undisplaced fractures are usually more stable than displaced fractures and less likely to change position (i.e. lose reduction), but the risk still exists and should be minimised. The aim for undisplaced fractures is therefore to maintain their position. This may be achieved by different methods depending on the site of the injury. For example, undisplaced ankle fractures, which remain undisplaced during weight-bearing X-rays, may be suitable for treatment in a removable walking boot. In the case of an undisplaced tibial fracture, this may be treated in cast as long as no displacement occurs in the initial weeks of its treatment. However, some fractures need additional support to ensure that displacement does not occur due to the forces applying to that bone. In the case of undisplaced distal radius fractures, application of a cast (such as a short arm plaster of Paris) can maintain the position of the bone, but the chance of loss of position is further reduced by applying moulding to the cast. The process of moulding is that of applying pressure to the outside of the cast while the cast material (e.g. plaster of Paris) is still soft, so that an impression is made in the cast material as if to prevent the bone from slipping out of position (As most wrist fractures are prone to displacing dorsally and radially, pressure is applied to the dorsal and radial sides of the cast over the distal fragment of the bone to prevent it from slipping in that direction). Some bones are subject to such great muscle forces that even if they sustain an undisplaced fracture they may still require surgical stabilisation, such as undisplaced intracapsular hip fractures.

For fractures that are displaced, reduction is required, but the risk of loss of reduction is also greater as significantly displaced fractures more likely to be unstable. For most displaced fractures with X-ray confirmation, an initial closed reduction should be considered if there is the potential for either the position to be returned to normal or to reduce deformity, which can cause tension on the surrounding skin, soft tissues and neurovascular structures. In the case of most displaced fractures, such as ankle or wrist fractures, after closed reduction (i.e. under local anaesthesia or conscious sedation) is performed, a moulded cast would be applied to maintain the achieved position. This combination of achieving the correct position of the bone and maintaining that position is often described as manipulation under sedation (MUS) and cast. Moulding a cast can add some further

improvement in fracture position (as if the manipulation is being done through the cast), but only small amount of position change in the fracture can be achieved this way.

Fractures that do not achieve adequate position by closed reduction under local anaesthetic or sedation (based on X-rays after manipulation and application of the moulded cast) may be considered for closed reduction under general anaesthetic, also called manipulation under anaesthetic (MUA), in an operating theatre. For fractures in adults necessitating MUA, this usually signifies either a difficulty in reduction or a higher level of instability, therefore a moulded cast is often insufficient for definitive stabilisation of such an injury. In some wrist fractures that can achieve a correct position by MUA, the position can then be maintained using percutaneous wires (known as Kirschner wires or K-wires). For this reason, achieving reduction and maintaining the reduction go hand-in-hand, as in MUA and K-wiring. It should be noted that the reduction (i.e. restoration of the position of the bone) is generally achieved prior to the insertion of these metal wires, rather than being achieved by the insertion of the wires. Insertion of metalwork while the bone is in an inadequate position only keeps the bone in that inadequate position. Percutaneous wires are normally left protruding from the skin to allow easy removal after a few weeks of bone healing.

Among long bone fractures such as the femur and tibia, intramedullary nailing is usually performed after closed reduction under anaesthetic, with X-ray guidance. In this way, relatively small incisions are made far from the fracture site for the insertion of the nail into the medullary canal of the bone and securing it at each end.

For fractures that cannot be adequately reduced by closed reduction methods, open reduction is usually required. After the bone has been surgically exposed, internal fixation is most commonly performed with metalwork such as plates and screws to maintain the bone's position. The abbreviation ORIF is routinely used for open reduction and internal fixation, but it signifies the two-step process of achieving adequate position (open reduction) and maintaining the position (internal fixation). Wrist and ankle fractures are among the most common fractures that require ORIF, and a variety of specially designed plates are available for these and fractures of other specific bones.

In essence, the process of fracture management is to ensure that the position of the bone is restored and then maintained. As such, you have to get the position right and then make it stay there. It then becomes clear that if an attempt to restore the position is unsuccessful, another option to get it right must be tried, and so it continues until an acceptable position is achieved. Only then should the bone be held in that position with measures such as a cast or metalwork. The only exception to this rule is that when a closed reduction is done, a cast normally needs to be applied before X-ray confirmation of the position is available (unless this is done in an operating theatre where an image intensifier X-ray machine is commonly available). Craig's[1] system of fracture management describes a simplified process of progressing through potential options for fractures in Table 17.1, and its specific application to wrist fractures is described in Table 17.2.

It is a common misconception that insertion of metalwork corrects the position of the bone, as in most cases the position of the bone is achieved by an open or closed reduction technique prior to the insertion of metal, and the metalwork only serves as a temporary device to maintain the position until the bone heals to its original strength. Most forms of internal fixation metalwork become redundant once the bone has healed and regained its original strength, but internal fixation implants are seldom removed due to

the risk of surgical complications such as neurovascular injury in during removal.

For some fracture types, even open reduction and internal fixation would yield a poor result. This may be due to the risk of poor healing or avascular necrosis due to poor blood supply (as may occur in displaced intracapsular hip fractures or some proximal humeral fractures) or due to the fracture being unreconstructable (as may occur in highly comminuted radial head fractures or distal humeral fractures). In these cases, joint replacement may be considered, either as hemiarthroplasty (replacement of one of the two surfaces or the joint) or total joint replacement (replacing both the surfaces of the joint). However, few joints are suitable for replacement as an option for fracture management due to limited functional outcomes. In other cases of unreconstructable joints, such as in some finger fractures, arthrodesis (joint fusion) can be considered to provide a joint that is stable but without movement.

Table 17.1 Craig's system for fracture management.

Fracture position	Pain relief	Reduce	Maintain
Undisplaced	As per local policy, e.g. nitrous oxide	N/A	Cast (e.g. moulded cast for wrist and ankle fracture, long leg cast for undisplaced tibial fracture) or brace (e.g. humeral brace for humeral shaft fracture, various spinal orthotic braces for spinal fracture)
Displaced	As per local policy, e.g. sedation/local anaesthetic/block	Closed reduction	Cast or brace (as above, as definitive treatment or temporary measure to avoid soft tissue/nerve/blood vessel damage pending surgery)
	General anaesthetic	Closed reduction	Percutaneous fixation (e.g. K-wires wrist fracture, some hand fractures excluding scaphoid, some unstable paediatric fracture) or intramedullary nail (e.g. lower limb shaft fracture) or external fixation (standard external fixator, usually as temporary stabilisation, if severe soft tissue damage, e.g. open fractures, fine-wire circular frame external fixation, e.g. Ilizarov frame, as definitive treatment for some complex lower limb fracture)
	General anaesthetic	Open reduction	Internal fixation (e.g. plates/screws, often locking plates in osteoporotic fractures, e.g. proximal humerus)
	General anaesthetic	Replacement or salvage procedures	For unreconstructable intra-articular/periarticular fracture: replacement (e.g. shoulder hemiarthroplasty, radial head replacement) or salvage procedures (e.g. finger joint arthrodesis)

Table 17.2 Craig's system for fracture management in wrist fractures.

Fracture pattern	Pain control	Reduce	Maintain
Undisplaced	e.g. nitrous oxide	N/A	Moulded short arm cast
Displaced	Sedation or block	Closed reduction (manipulation under sedation)	Moulded short arm cast
	General anaesthetic	Closed reduction (manipulation under anaesthetic)	Percutaneous wires (K-wires)
	General anaesthetic	Open reduction	Internal fixation

For most fractures, the degree of displacement correlates with the degree to which the structures that maintain normal bone position have been damaged and therefore the degree of instability of the fracture site. This structural damage can relate to broken bones or to the rupture of ligaments, which normally maintain the position, and alignment of bones around joints. In ankle fractures, the distal tibia and fibula form the 'mortise' in which the upper aspect of the talus is held to form the ankle joint, but several ligaments maintain the alignment of these bones, therefore damage to ligaments or bones can result in subluxation or dislocation of the ankle. Due to the undulating surfaces of the tibial plafond (the load-bearing surface of the distal tibia) and the top of the talus, even a tiny amount of displacement of the talus can cause mismatching of these two bony surfaces, resulting in rapid degeneration.

Ankle fractures can include a number of ligamentous injuries and fractures to the distal tibia (either in the load-bearing surface of the plafond or the medial malleolus which forms the medial edge of the ankle joint) and the distal fibula. The distal fibula is of particular importance in preventing the talus from subluxing laterally, as is the most likely direction of displacement based on the biomechanical forces of the muscles around the ankle. The distal fibula is held in place by the tibio-fibular syndesmosis, a strong ligament complex between the distal fibula and distal tibia, which can itself be damaged at the time of ankle injury. Damage to this ligament is increasingly common with more proximal levels of distal fibular fractures, with fibular fractures more proximal to the ankle joint having an increased chance of syndesmosis damage and failure of the fibula to prevent talar shift (subluxing of the talus). As a result, fibular fractures are often described by the Weber classification (1972) (sometimes called the Danis–Weber

classification). In the Weber classification, Weber A distal fibular fractures are distal to the level of the tibial plafond (with minimal risk of syndesmosis injury), Weber B distal fibular fractures are at the level of the syndesmosis (with around a 50% chance of syndesmosis injury) and Weber C distal fibular fractures are proximal to the syndesmosis (usually involving substantial syndesmosis injury) (Weber 1972).

The Lauge–Hanson (1950) classification of ankle fractures describes a number of patterns of ankle fractures based on the direction that the foot moves in relation to the lower leg. Each injury pattern involves a stepwise accumulation of sites of injury around the ankle, ranging from relatively minor ligamentous tears to circumferential disruption of the ankle joint. It can be imagined as the twisting of the foot causing a sequence of damage to ligaments or bones that spirals around the ankle, with increasing damage, increasing instability and increasing potential for subluxation or dislocation as this progresses.

Some common themes run through all the injury patterns of the Lauge–Hanson classification. Four areas of the ankle are of key importance. As a rule of thumb, ankle fractures with substantial injuries to two or more of these areas usually imply instability, with a likelihood of talar shift and a need for surgical stabilisation, as described in Table 17.3. These areas are:

1) the medial malleolus or the medial ankle ligaments (the deltoid ligament)
2) the lateral malleolus (i.e. the distal fibula) or lateral ligamentous complex
3) the posterior malleolus (i.e. the posterior edge of the distal tibial plafond)
4) the syndesmosis ligament.

Table 17.3 Craig's system for fracture management in ankle fractures.

Fracture pattern	Pain control	Reduce	Maintain
Undisplaced and stable	e.g. nitrous oxide	N/A	Short leg cast or removable walking boot
Displaced (or undisplaced unstable[a])	Sedation or block	Closed reduction (manipulation under sedation)	Moulded short leg cast as temporising measure until surgery or if surgery contra-indicated (not percutanaeous wires)
	General anaesthetic	Closed reduction (manipulation under anaesthetic)	Percutaneous wires (K-wires)
	General anaesthetic	Open reduction	Internal fixation

Note that posterior malleolar fractures and Weber C distal fibular fractures are seldom in isolation. Weber B distal fibular fractures need specific consideration of stability, e.g. stress/weight-bearing X-rays.

[a] Consider instability if two of the following four areas are injured:
1) the medial malleolus or the medial ankle ligaments (the deltoid ligament)
2) the lateral malleolus (i.e. the distal fibula) or lateral ligamentous complex
3) the posterior malleolus (i.e. the posterior edge of the distal tibial plafond)
4) the syndesmosis ligament.

Isolated injuries to the medial malleolus, lateral ligaments or lateral malleolus (without associated syndesmosis injury) are generally stable and can often be treated non-surgically, with early weight-bearing. Bimalleolar ankle fractures (i.e. fractures of medial and lateral malleoli) and trimalleolar fractures (i.e. fractures of medial, lateral and posterior malleoli) are unstable and generally require surgical fixation. Injuries to the posterior malleolus or syndesmosis ligament injuries are seldom seen in isolation, but are usually associated with other sites of injury as listed above and therefore usually require surgery. As described above, distal fibular fractures may be associated with syndesmosis injuries (in the case of some Weber B fractures and practically all Weber C fractures). The presence of talar shift on X-ray implies instability and a strong chance that surgery will be required. In cases of Weber B distal fibular fractures (without other bony injury) where there is uncertainty about the integrity of the syndesmosis, stress views of the ankle, such as weight-bearing ankle X-rays, may be used. If the latter demonstrates talar shift, this indicates instability due to ligamentous injury elsewhere. Conversely, the absence of talar shift implies a stable injury.

For stable undisplaced injuries that do not suffer from talar shift on weight-bearing, many can be treated non-operatively with early weight-bearing in either a cast or a removable boot.

Closed reduction and application of a moulded short leg cast (with moulding pressure applied to the lateral side of the cast over the distal fibula) should be used in the emergency department setting to achieve adequate reduction of any ankle fracture displaying talar shift. Options for sedation are similar to those described for wrist fractures (i.e. MUS and cast). This should be performed promptly to minimise soft tissue damage and blistering, which results from soft tissue stretching around a deformed ankle.

As described earlier for wrist fractures, the purpose of surgical fixation is to achieve open reduction and maintain this position by the insertion of metalwork. Medial malleolar fractures may require either screws or a small plate to maintain their position. Distal fibular fractures are usually stabilised with plates and screws, although alternative fixation methods (such as fibular intramedullary nails) are now available, particularly for patients with compromised skin. The syndesmosis should be assessed intraoperatively and if the ankle joint subluxes under stressing, the syndesmosis should be supported with one or more screws from the fibular into the tibia or with other specific high-strength suture materials. Percutaneous wires are usually not strong enough to withstand the displacing forces of the muscles around the ankle unless used as part of a fine wire circular frame, which is generally reserved for more complex fractures such as those involving comminution of the articular surface (pilon fractures) or open fractures where the metalwork is kept away from the area of contamination.

Rehabilitation

Following a significant period of immobilisation, joints become stiff and muscles are weakened by lack of use, even if the patient exercised the joints which were not immobilised. The patient will need to gradually re-engage with movement of the limb, joints and muscles as strength and flexibility gradually improve. This process will depend on a number of factors, including the severity of the injury, the adequacy of their analgesia, the medical and general fitness of the patient, and their motivation to reach their rehabilitation potential (see Chapter 7 for further discussion of the principles of rehabilitation). This often requires a period of outpatient physiotherapy. Some patients may have residual disability following rehabilitation.

Facilitating Fracture Healing

An understanding of what encourages and inhibits fracture healing is helpful in understanding the conditions required for healing and those interventions likely to be most effective in supporting healing. Numerous factors may mean that fractures do not heal (non-union) or heal slowly (delayed union) or do not heal in an acceptable position (malunion).

Fracture healing is encouraged by:

- adequate immobilisation of the fracture in the early stages of healing so that the gradually revascularized haematoma is not disrupted
- axial loading (weight-bearing) once the bridging callus has formed to enable new bone to be laid down along lines of stress
- good general health and diet, which provide the protein, calories, calcium and other nutrients required to physiologically support healing.

Fracture healing is inhibited by:

- excessive movement at the fracture site during the earlier stages of healing as this disrupts newly forming capillaries
- poor circulation to the fracture site reducing the availability of oxygen and the nutrients required for healing
- diseased and weakened bone in which bone cells are less active

- joint involvement: synovial fluid inhibits healing and disruption of articular (hyaline) cartilage often leads to secondary osteoarthritis is later life
- large amounts of surrounding soft-tissue damage
- infection
- some medications
- poor general health and nutrition
- smoking
- poor compliance.

These factors are taken into account when choosing methods for supporting fractures whilst they heal.

Open Fractures

Open, or compound, fractures occur when there is a break in the skin, providing a conduit between the external environment and the fracture. There are two mechanisms by which this can occur, although their clinical implications are similar:

1) *From without in*: External injury to the skin and soft tissues overlying the fracture opens a wound that connects with the fracture.
2) *From within out:* Sharp edges of the fracture lacerate overlying soft tissue and pierce the skin. This mechanism can also result in a fracture blister. Fluid-filled or blood-filled blisters lie over the fracture and, although the skin might not be broken, should be treated as an open fracture wound.

Open fractures are associated with significant soft tissue damage and as a consequence are at significant risk of infection. All open fractures must be assumed to be contaminated and the main aim of treatment is to prevent infection. Management of the open fracture depends on the site of injury, the type of fracture and the degree of soft tissue injury (with or without nerve or vascular injury). In the emergency setting, the wound should be photographed so that repeated uncovering is avoided and then covered with a sterile saline-soaked dressing. Antibiotic prophylaxis should be administered promptly and tetanus immunisation status evaluated. Irrigation of open fractures should not be performed in the emergency department for fractures of the lower limb (except for toes or forefoot injuries). Open fractures require early operation and ideally this should be performed in an operating theatre immediately for open fractures with vascular compromise or highly contaminated open fractures (e.g. agricultural, aquatic or sewage contamination), within 12 hours for other high-energy open fractures that are not highly contaminated, and within 24 hours for all other open fractures.

The aims of surgery are to:

- clean the wound
- remove contaminated or devitalised tissue (debridement)
- stabilise the fracture.

The focus is on early surgery with a combined approach and input from the orthopaedic and plastic surgery teams. This is particularly important as the externally visible skin lesion may not give a true representation of the degree of soft tissue damage beneath the surface, especially in high-energy injuries. Definitive soft tissue closure should be achieved within 72 hours and may require soft tissue transfers or flaps. Internal fixation should not be performed if soft tissue coverage has not been achieved due to the risk of infection settling on exposed metalwork. In the event that soft tissue closure cannot be achieved at the time of initially debridement, temporary stabilisation of the fracture can be achieved with external fixation, where the supporting metalwork is far from the site of skin damage. Detailed documentation of the neurovascular state should be recorded and reassessed periodically (Eccles et al. 2020).

The Gustilo–Anderson classification system (Gustilo et al. 1984) (Table 17.4) is commonly used to describe soft tissue injury associated with an open fracture and to direct treatment. The use of a classification system is important as it facilitates communication among clinicians, as well as assisting clinicians in decision-making, anticipating potential problems, predicting patient and surgical outcomes, and documenting cases. However, there are discussions regarding the inter-observer reliability of the Gustilo–Anderson classification and its ability to predict patient outcome. Other classifications systems include the mangled extremity severity score (MESS) (Johansen et al. 1990).

Table 17.4 Gustilo–Anderson classification system for compound fractures. Adapted from Gustilo et al. (1984).

Type I	An open fracture with a wound <1 cm long and clean
Type II	An open fracture with a laceration >1 cm long without excessive soft tissue damage, flaps or avulsions
Type III	Massive soft tissue damage, compromised vascularity, severe wound contamination and marked fracture instability
Type IIIA	Adequate soft tissue coverage of a fractured bone, despite extensive soft tissue laceration, flaps or high-energy trauma irrespective of the size of the wound
Type IIIB	Extensive soft tissue injury loss with periosteal stripping and bone exposure, usually associated with massive contamination
Type IIIC	Open fracture associated with arterial injury requiring repair

Management of Common Fracture Types

This section provides an overview of the common upper and lower limb fractures in adults. Spinal and hip fractures are further explored in Chapters 18–20, respectively, with Chapters 24 and 25 dedicated to fractures in the infant, child and young person.

Lower Limb Fractures

The bones of the lower limb play an important role in standing and ambulation. Fractures in this region therefore have a significant impact on patient mobility and ability to carry out activities of daily living and employment. They also commonly require admission to hospital. The femur and tibia are the major long bones that bear the most significant weight in standing and walking. They require significant force to fracture and are therefore likely to be associated with patterns of multiple injury and significant soft tissue damage, and are the most prone to complications. Fractures around the ankle and foot have different mechanisms and patterns of injury but can also have a significant impact on patient independence.

Fractures Involving the Femur

Proximal femur fractures, i.e. hip fractures, commonly occur as fragility fractures in older people. These are considered in detail in Chapters 18 and 19. Fractures of the diaphyseal shaft of the femur or distal femur fractures (including intra-articular fractures around the knee) can occur in high-energy injuries such as road traffic accidents or as fragility fractures in elderly or osteoporotic patients.

The emergency management of the patient with a fracture of the femur requires full consideration of the principles of resuscitation and advanced trauma life support (ATLS) as considered in Chapter 16. While femoral shaft fractures are associated with complications (such as blood loss) that necessitate resuscitation and ATLS principles, low-energy fragility fractures of the elderly should be considered as significant physiological strains as these patients are often frail and less able to tolerate even smaller amounts of blood loss and physiological disturbance.

Fractures of the femur are often displaced, angulated or shortened because of the action of the large muscles of the thigh. The management of femoral shaft fractures is most often by closed reduction (in an operating theatre under X-ray guidance) and fixation with an intramedullary nail. If the fixation is stable, it allows early mobilisation, reducing the risk of complications due to immobility. This is a particular priority among elderly patients, for whom being bed-bound can quickly cause chest infections, pressure sores and clots (i.e. deep venous thromboses or pulmonary emboli). The aim is therefore to allow them to weight-bear as soon as possible after surgery. Conservative management of femoral fractures is rare and generally reserved for young children and older people who are unfit for anaesthesia. Some distal femoral fractures, such as intra-articular fractures at the knee, cannot be adequately stabilised by intramedullary nailing as the nail may not be able to attach securely to a piece of bone so close to the joint surface. Internal fixation (with plates and screws) is often required but may not provide as much early stability in comparison to intramedullary nailing.

Fractures Involving the Tibia

Tibial fractures occur due to a major impact to the lower leg. The tibia is particularly vulnerable to twisting (torsion) forces and fractures are often spiral, sometimes involving the knee or ankle joint, and X-ray images should include both these joints. The anterior tibial border lies very close to the surface and is covered by only a thin layer of skin and adipose tissue. This not only increases the chance of open fractures, but the limited blood supply to the bone and the overlying soft tissue poses the risk of healing problems. As a result, open fractures, with risks of infection, delayed union and non-union, are particularly common in the tibia. Swelling and neurovascular compromise are significant problems following tibial fractures. It is essential that care includes high elevation of the lower leg, i.e. positioning the fracture site and foot above the level of the heart. The tight layers of fascia surrounding the muscle compartments of the lower leg mean that even a small amount of initial swelling or soft tissue injury can cause escalated pressure within one or more of these muscle compartments. Raised intra-compartmental pressure within these confined muscle groups can quickly prevent capillary blood flow in and out of these muscles, causing hypoxia and yet more swelling. This cycle of increasing pressure, preventing adequate perfusion to the muscles, is known as compartment syndrome and is a limb-threatening surgical emergency. It is diagnosed by clinical examination, based on pain out of keeping with the degree of injury. A high level of suspicion should be used for all lower limb injuries where pain control is difficult or analgesic requirements are greater than would normally be expected. Measurement of compartment pressures should not be used to exclude compartment syndrome, as it is technically difficult to measure the pressures of all the compartments that are at risk. Similarly, the presence of a pulse or nerve function should not be used to exclude compartment syndrome, as both these can remain after irreversible muscle ischaemia has occurred.

Tibial shaft fractures usually involve significant force among younger individuals, such as road traffic trauma and sporting injuries, and are often caused by twisting injuries. Low-energy fractures can occur as fragility fractures in the elderly or other causes of pathological weakening within the bone. Undisplaced fractures can be treated conservatively with a long leg cast. Displaced fractures often require initial closed reduction and a long leg cast. However, if an acceptable position cannot be achieved by closed reduction in the emergency department or outpatient setting, reduction under anaesthesia is generally required. Displaced and/or unstable fractures in the tibial diaphysis are most commonly treated with closed reduction and intramedullary nailing (under general or spinal anaesthesia). Tibial fractures close to the ankle or knee are more often treated with open reduction and internal fixation with specialised plates designed to minimise disturbance to the soft tissue envelope. External fixation may be used as a temporary stabilisation pending definitive management, particularly in open fractures. Circular/fine wire frames (such as Ilizarov frames) are an option for more complex fractures involving substantial intra-articular damage, substantial soft tissue injuries or bone loss.

For all leg fractures, elderly/frail patients struggle to regain mobility after a period of being unable to walk so facilitating early mobility is a priority.

Upper Limb Fractures

Fractures of the upper limb are common, particularly following a FOOSH in all age groups, especially in older people. Other common mechanisms include direct impacts and twisting injuries. Injuries often occur as a result of sport and leisure activities, workplace incidents and social violence. They can also be part of a pattern of multiple injuries following high-energy trauma associated with other significant fractures of the lower limb, pelvis, chest, spine or head.

Injury and immobility of the upper limb can cause significant problems for the patient in carrying out activities of living such as personal hygiene and eating and drinking, especially if the dominant arm is affected. Elderly frail people, in particular, need significant support in coping during the recovery period. For patients who would normally use a walking aid to mobilise (e.g. stick or walking frame), the inability to use an injured arm can result in a period of immobility that can be extremely difficult to recover from. Attention should be paid to maintaining their mobility in such situations, often with changes to their level of walking aids or assistance. Injuries of the shoulder and elbow are particularly prone to soft tissue stiffness, and early physiotherapy input is required in most elbow and shoulder injuries, regardless of non-operative or operative management. Wrist fractures are managed based on the principles of closed or open reduction as described earlier. The majority of wrist fractures (either undisplaced or achieving adequate position from closed reduction) can be managed in moulded short arm casts. As there are many bones in the hand, the methods of treatment are varied, but the principles of achieving an adequate position and maintaining it with splintage, casting or surgical stabilisation still apply to each individual bone depending on what position and degree of immobilisation is required for each bone. For example, intra-articular fractures of the first metacarpal base require accurate reduction to maintain a functioning joint, but relatively high muscle forces put it at a higher risk of displacement, often necessitating closed reduction under general anaesthesia and percutaneous wire fixation. In contrast, fifth metacarpal neck fractures can tolerate greater degrees of displacement before any effect on function occurs, meaning that less rigid support is required (e.g. a removable splint). The scaphoid has a poor blood supply so is prone to slow healing or failure of fracture healing (with resultant wrist degeneration) and can be more difficult to assess on X-ray, so should be specifically considered in cases of wrist/hand injuries. 'Neighbour' strapping is often used to immobilise finger injuries such as undisplaced and stable fractures, but splints or surgery may be needed for injuries that are more unstable. With all forms of strapping, splintage and casting, it is essential that they are not too tight as this could cause pressure to nerves, skin or blood vessels. Advice should be provided to the patients about actions to take if they have such concerns, including elevation of the limb, encouraging the patient to regularly exercise the joints that are not immobilised and seeking medical attention if they experience problems with their cast, such as loosening, tightness or damage.

As with wrist fractures, other upper limb fractures follow similar principles of achieving adequate reduction and maintaining this. Slings are adequate support for many fractures around the shoulder or elbow that are not significantly displaced, with the exception of humeral shaft fractures, which require splintage such as a humeral brace or Bohler U backslab, which can be effective in maintaining reduction in the initial stage. Closed reduction of fractures above the elbow is seldom effective due to the significant muscle forces on these and open reduction (then internal fixation) is generally required for significantly displaced fractures. Closed reduction is generally only successful for dislocations (e.g. elbow or shoulder). Midshaft fractures of the radius and/or ulna are often displaced by the significant forearm forces, and usually require open reduction and internal fixation to achieve adequate reduction as the close articulation between these two bones requires excellent reduction to maintain forearm rotation.

Complications of fractures in the upper limb and their management include neurovascular compromise, damage to tendons and compartment syndrome. Late complications include carpal tunnel syndrome, malunion, post-traumatic arthritis and residual stiffness of the elbow, wrist and fingers.

Evidence-based Practise in Fracture Care and Outcomes

Ensuring that practise is evidence-based through both conduct and use of research and audit is essential in setting standards for improving quality of care for patients and ensuring that their fracture has the best possible healing outcome. There is a large body of medical research that considers various aspects of the management of fractures. Research projects around the world are constantly comparing fracture treatment methods against others using randomised controlled trials and other robust research methods. Examples of such trials include comparing the use of percutaneous wiring versus open reduction and internal fixation of distal radius fractures, as in the UK the Distal Radius Acute Fracture Fixation Trial (DRAFFT) study by Costa et al. in 2015. There is also a good deal of research that has considered the role of physiotherapy in recovery and rehabilitation following skeletal injury. Research for nursing practise is often focused on the general aspects of fracture care considered in more detail in other chapters of this book, such as wound and pain management, the prevention of complications and rehabilitation. The care of the patient following a fragility fracture of the hip is particularly well researched (Chapter 19).

Many healthcare providers are now engaged in audit of data about fracture outcomes. Such systems aim to produce valid, accurate, consistent and timely data focusing on fracture management options and measuring performance to facilitate evidence-based practice through audit and research. Audit is a systematic way of reviewing care against explicit criteria as part of a quality improvement process that aims to improve patient care and outcomes. It is often followed by the implementation of change and practice development. The key component of clinical audit is that the performance is reviewed (or audited) to ensure that what should be done is being done and, if not, that it provides a framework to enable improvements to be made. Relevant information may be gathered regarding different types of fractures, their classifications, their treatment and the outcomes of that treatment. This provides information about the effectiveness of fracture management in a given unit, but also enables the sharing of good practice between units through benchmarking. The data necessary for audit will vary based on the service being evaluated, but these often include demographic data, accident dates and times, dates and times of presentation to health service, admission to fracture units, time to surgery, and discharge dates and times as well as discharge destinations and information about fracture management. A particularly successful example of this is provided by the National Hip Fracture Database in the UK (with many equivalents elsewhere in the world), described in more detail in Chapters 18 and 19. This has enabled the use of audit data to drive improvements in care for this specific group of patients.

Summary

In summary, this chapter informs the reader on the importance of history taking and examination in fracture patients, as well as fracture epidemiology, fracture healing and management principles that apply to various fracture types. As evidence evolves, the management of specific fractures and subgroups of fracture patterns and patients will develop, but the underlying principles of resuscitation, reduction, immobilisation and rehabilitation provide a common thread through individual management choices.

Further Reading

Note: The following texts provide the practitioner with detailed information regarding the care and management of patients with specific types of fractures.

Jester, R., Santy, J., and Rogers, J. (2021). *Oxford Handbook of Orthopaedic and Trauma Nursing*, 2e. Oxford: Oxford University Press.

McRae, R. and Esser, M. (2008). *Practical Fracture Treatment*, 5e. Edinburgh: Churchill Livingstone.

References

Black, K.J., Bevan, C.A., Murphy, N.G. et al. (2013). Nerve blocks for initial pain management of femoral fractures in children. *Cochrane Database Syst. Rev.* 17 (12): (Art. No.: CD009587). https://doi.org/10.1002/14651858.CD009587.

Costa, M.L., Achten, J., Plant, C. et al. (2015). UK DRAFFT: a randomised controlled trial of percutaneous fixation with Kirschner wires versus volar locking-plate fixation in the treatment of adult patients with a dorsally displaced fracture of the distal radius. *Health Technol. Assess.* 19 (17): 1, v–124, vi.

Dandy, D.J. and Edwards, D.J. (2009). *Essential Orthopaedics and Trauma*, 5e. Edinburgh: Churchill Livingstone/ Elsevier.

Donaldson, L.J., Reckless, I.P., Scholes, S. et al. (2008). The epidemiology of fractures in England. *J. Epidemiol. Community Health* 62 (2): 174–180.

Eccles, S., Handley, B., Khan, U. et al. (2020). *Standards for the Management of Open Fractures*. Edinburgh: Oxford University Press www.oxfordmedicine.com/view/10.1093/ med/9780198849360.001.0001/med-9780198849360.

Gustilo, R.B., Mendoza, R.M., and Williams, D.N. (1984). Problems in the management of type III (severe) open fractures: a new classification of type III open fractures. *J. Trauma* 24: 742–746.

Johansen, K., Daines, M., Howey, T. et al. (1990). Objective criteria accurately predict amputation following lower extremity trauma. *J. Trauma* 30: 568–572.

Kuntzman, A.J. and Tortora, G.J. (2010). *Anatomy and Physiology for the Manual Therapies*. New Jersey: Wiley.

Lauge-Hansen, N. (1950). Fractures of the ankle: II. Combined experimental-surgical and experimental-roentgenologic investigations. *Arch. Surg.* 60: 957–985. https://doi.org/10.1001/archsurg.1950.01250010980011.

Marquez-Lara, A., Hutchinson, I.D., Nuñez, F. Jr. et al. (2016). Nonsteroidal anti-inflammatory drugs and bone-healing: a systematic review of research quality. *JBJS Rev.* 4 (3): e4. https://doi.org/10.2106/JBJS.RVW.O.00055. PMID: 27500434.

McRae, R. and Esser, M. (2008). *Practical Fracture Treatment*, 5e. Edinburgh: Churchill Livingstone.

Stiell, I.G., McKnight, R., Greenberg, G.H. et al. (1994). Implementation of the Ottawa ankle rules. *J. Am. Med. Assoc.* 271 (11): 827–832.

Stiell, I.G., Wells, G.A., Hoag, R.H. et al. (1997). Implementation of the Ottawa knee rule for the use of radiography in acute knee injuries. *J. Am. Med. Assoc.* 278 (23): 2075–2079.

Weber, B.G. (1972). *Die verletzungen des oberen sprunggelenkes*, 2e. Bern: Huber.

Woolf, N. (2000). *Cell, Tissue and Disease. The Basis of Pathology*. Edinburgh: W.B. Saunders.

18

Fragility Fractures

Julie Santy-Tomlinson[1,2] and Karen Hertz[3]

[1] International Journal of Orthopaedic and Trauma Nursing
[2] Department of Orthopaedics, Odense University Hospitals/University of Southern Denmark, Odense, Denmark
[3] Royal Stoke University Hospital, University Hospitals of North Midlands, Stoke-on-Trent, UK

Introduction

Fragility fractures are pathological fractures that are the clinical outcome of osteoporosis (International Osteoporosis Foundation [IOF] 2021a), a major global public health problem, the cause of significant pain, distress and loss of independence for patients, and a significant challenge facing orthopaedic trauma services. Such fractures are both a sign and symptom of osteoporosis (Van Oostwaard 2018) as the condition is usually undetected until a fracture occurs. Osteoporosis is both preventable and treatable, so fragility fractures are regarded as avoidable and, because the incidence of the disease increases with age, fragility fractures are also associated with advancing age.

Fragility fractures most frequently occur at the hip, vertebrae and forearm but also occur in other bone regions commonly affected by osteoporosis, such as the proximal humerus. A fragility fracture of the hip is a significant injury that requires admission to hospital and orthopaedic surgery, which carries a high burden of complications (morbidity) and death (mortality). The older and frailer the patient who sustains a hip fracture, the more likely they are to suffer complications that can lead to death. The nursing care and management of the older person with a fragility hip fracture is considered in detail in Chapter 19.

It is widely agreed that optimal care is cheaper than suboptimal care (British Orthopaedic Association/British Geriatric Society 2007) on the basis that better care results in better outcomes as well as reduced complications and length of stay, with a greater chance of return to independent living. Focusing on high-quality, optimal care is therefore an essential aim of service/practice development. The aim of this chapter is to provide an overview of the causes, prevention, care and management of the patient with any type of fragility fracture to assist the practitioner in providing skilled, high-quality care. Prevention of fragility fractures and the management and care of a person who sustains a fragility fracture are complex processes that involve an interdisciplinary team approach and specialist age-sensitive care that is tailored to their specific needs.

Fragility Fractures

Fractures are a global public health issue, but older people are at particularly high risk (Wu et al. 2021), frequently presenting with a fragility fracture. It has been estimated that there is one fragility fracture worldwide every 3 seconds, equating to 25 000 per day (IOF 2021a), almost always resulting in attendance at an emergency department, admission to hospital or a general practitioner visit.

The main cause of fragility fractures is low bone mineral density (BMD) caused by osteoporosis. The injury may be the result of a fall or other low-energy trauma, but may also occur spontaneously because of low BMD. The incidence of fragility fractures varies by age (more common with increasing age), gender (more common in women than men by a ratio of 4 : 1), geographic location, socioeconomic status and ethnicity because of the link between these factors, osteoporosis and falls.

According to the IOF (2021a):

> Fragility fractures, which result from low energy trauma, such as a fall from standing height or less, are a sign of underlying osteoporosis. A patient who has sustained one fragility fracture is at high risk of experiencing secondary fractures, especially in the first two years following the initial fracture.

A fragility fracture is described by the National Institute for Health and Care Excellence (NICE) (2021) as a complication of osteoporosis, occurring following a fall from standing height or less, spontaneously, or because of routine activities such as bending or lifting. They are most common in those bones most likely to have reduced strength due to osteoporosis: the spine (vertebrae), hip (proximal femur), wrist (distal radius), arm (proximal humerus) and pelvis (pubic ramus). Fragility fractures often result in significant pain and severe disability, leading to reduced quality of life. Hip and vertebral fractures are also associated with decreased life expectancy. Every fragility fracture signals an increased risk of future fractures, at least doubling the risk of further fractures as well as increasing the risk of premature mortality. Figure 18.1 demonstrates how the progress of osteoporotic fractures occurs across the lifespan. A person's experience of osteoporosis is often of remorseless progression: from a Colles fracture and minor (and often minimally symptomatic) vertebral fractures to the major distress, loss of independence and disability of hip fracture. The case study presented in Boxes 18.1, 18.3 and 18.5 highlights examples of this experience.

Osteoporosis

Osteoporosis is a metabolic bone disease of later life in which there are changes in the microstructure of bone tissue leading to reduced bone mass and weakening of bone composition resulting in fragile bone that is more prone to fractures following events that would not usually be expected to result in a fracture. According to NICE (2021):

> Osteoporosis is a disease characterised by low bone mass and structural deterioration of bone tissue, with a consequent increase in bone fragility and susceptibility to fracture.

It has been estimated that 1 in 3 women and 1 in 5 men over age 50 will sustain a fracture due to osteoporosis in their lifetimes (Curtis et al. 2016). The incidence of osteoporosis in both genders is known to rise rapidly with age due to increased bone loss after the menopause in women and age-related bone loss in both women and men. This is recognised as a growing problem globally because of the ageing of the global population. Although the disease has long been understood as a problem for temperate and tundra climate countries such as in Europe and North America, in countries where the older population is growing most rapidly, such as in much of Asia and South America, incidence is rising very rapidly and expected to continue to do so (Veronese et al. 2021). As life expectancy increases globally, individuals may expect to live up to 40 years after a first fragility fracture, increasing the chances of further and more serious fractures.

The main risk factors for osteoporosis are listed in Box 18.2. Risk of osteoporosis is generated by factors that directly affect bone biology and deplete BMD (van Oostwaard 2018). Recognising such risk factors helps practitioners to identify those patients who may have osteoporosis and are consequently at risk of fragility fractures. Identifying the likelihood of osteoporosis presents opportunities for diagnosis and treatment that can ultimately prevent fractures.

Diagnosis of Osteoporosis

There are very few early signs of osteoporosis and the onset of the disease is usually asymptomatic so it is only recognised after a person sustains a fracture. Frequently, the first (index) fracture is of the wrist and other more serious fractures such as of the hip occur with increasing age, resulting in worsening pain, disability and loss of function and independence. For some people the first sign is that they have experienced a

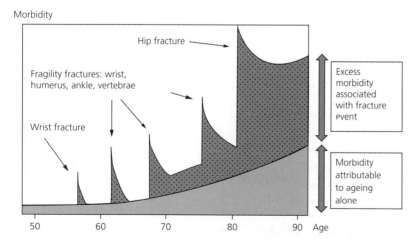

Morbidity

Figure 18.1 Fracture morbidity. *Source:* Adapted from BOA/BGS 2007.

Box 18.1   Fragility Fracture: Case Study Part 1

Background and Presentation

Ingrid is an 82-year-old woman who was admitted to the orthopaedic trauma unit at her local hospital following a fall at home. Assessment and X-ray in the emergency department indicated that she had an extracapsular (intertrochanteric) fracture of her right proximal femur (hip fracture*). She underwent surgery under spinal anaesthetic to internally fix the fracture (dynamic hip screw) the day after her admission, having been seen by the anaesthetist shortly after admission.

Social History

Ingrid lives alone in a small bungalow she moved to with her husband shortly before his death 5 years ago. She is supported by her daughter, who lives 3 miles away. She managed well for the first few years after the move, with some help with shopping, cleaning, cooking and gardening. However, since the beginning of the Covid-19 pandemic she has been largely confined to her home and has noticed that she is finding daily activities increasingly difficult to manage. She uses a rollator frame to support her in moving around her home. She confesses to having been feeling quite isolated and low lately as her social life has contracted.

Medical History

Hysterectomy age 48
Myocardial infarction at age 68, successfully treated with angioplasty, no symptoms since
Previous wrist fracture at age77, investigations for bone density/fracture risk not instigated at that time
Mild osteoarthritis in both hips
Body mass index 18

Medications

Ramipril (angiotensin-converting enzyme inhibitor to control hypertension)
Artorvastatin (statin to control cholesterol)
Timolol maleate (beta-blocker to control hypertension)
Glyceryl trinitrate spray (for angina, no angina experienced since angioplasty)
Paracetamol (for osteoarthritis pain, non-steroidal anti-inflammatory drugs are contraindicated following myocardial infarction).

Discussion

Consider these questions as you read sections 18.2 and 18.3:

Was Ingrid's hip fracture avoidable?
What should have happened after her wrist fracture?

> Further details of the case and new discussion items will be introduced later in the chapter.
> (*See Chapter 19 for further explanation of the nature and management of hip fractures.)

---

loss in height of around 4 cm/1 in. and/or a curvature of the upper back is noticed, with or without pain in the area. These are signs of osteoporotic vertebral fractures, particularly in the thoracic spine. Individuals who have sustained an injury which may be a fragility fracture and who are identified as having risk factors for osteoporosis need to be referred for diagnosis and, potentially, treatment for the condition.

The National Osteoporosis Guideline Group (NOGG) (2017) recommend that the probability of sustaining a fragility fracture should be assessed in all postmenopausal women and men aged 50 years or more who have risk factors for fracture using FRAX® (https://www.sheffield.ac.uk/FRAX/), an online tool that has been developed to evaluate fracture risk. Then individuals identified at intermediate risk should have BMD assessment and fracture probability re-estimated using FRAX®. NICE (2021) also recommend that anyone over 50 years of age with a history of fragility fracture or under 40 years of age with a

---

Box 18.2   Risk Factors for Osteoporosis (van Oostward 2018; Falaschi et al. 2021)

Fixed risk factors	Modifiable risk factors
Age >60 years	Lack of, or limited, weight-bearing exercise
Female gender	Excessive alcohol consumption
Menopause	Low body mass index (below 19)
Family history of osteoporosis	Poor nutrition/malnutrition
Previous fracture (particularly over the age of 50)	Smoking
Medications that impact on bone density, e.g. corticosteroids, chemotherapy	Vitamin D deficiency
Immobility	Low dietary calcium intake
Medical conditions, including:	Eating disorders
rheumatoid arthritis	
gastrointestinal disorders	
respirator conditions, e.g. chronic obstructive pulmonary disease, asthma	
endocrine disorders, e.g. diabetes, Cushing's syndrome, hyperparathyroidism	
chronic renal disease	
HIV/AIDS	
cancers	
haematological disorders	
mental health conditions, e.g. anorexia nervosa, dementia	

---

major risk factor for fragility fracture should have a dual-energy X-ray absorptiometry (DXA) scan to measure BMD.

Since the risk of fracture increases progressively with decreasing BMD, the clinical diagnosis of osteoporosis and associated fracture risk has, until recently, involved measurement of BMD. The most common technique for this is DXA, which involves sending two different low-radiation X-ray beams (which are absorbed differently by bones and soft tissues) through a specific bone site (usually the hip). The absorption of the beams is measured using other tissues as reference/comparison materials. The density profiles from these X-rays are used to calculate BMD. The lower the density, the greater the risk of fracture. The World Health Organization (WHO) has defined several threshold values for osteoporosis based on units of standard deviation (SD), which are usually described as *T* scores. DXA is a quick, painless, non-invasive test that has been validated by many studies as an accurate measure of fracture risk (IOF 2021b) (see Kannis et al. 2007 for more information).

Osteoporosis Prevention and Management

Non-pharmacological Prevention Measures

Osteoporosis prevention focuses on lifestyle behaviour and change related to modifiable risk factors (see Box 18.2), especially in those individuals with risk factors that cannot be modified. Osteoporosis is preventable across all global populations by achieving maximum BMD in communities by embedding two preventive behaviours across the entire lifespan: (i) adequate calcium intake and (ii) weight-bearing exercise (Nguyen 2017). Peak bone mass is reached in early adulthood. Bone health begins in utero, is consolidated during childhood and must be maintained during adulthood and into later life, hence public health interventions and education aimed at maximising calcium intake and embedding the habit of weight-bearing exercise is essential across all age groups, but especially in children and young adults. Adopting these lifestyle measures is also an important part of bone health strategies for those who are at risk of fragility fractures and/or have been diagnosed with osteoporosis.

The NOGG Guidelines (2017) recommend a daily calcium intake of 700–1200 mg that should, if possible, be achieved through dietary intake. Vitamin D deficiency should also be avoided, although this is a serious global public health concern, even in Mediterranean and tropical climate countries because of changes in lifestyle regarding spending time outdoors, especially in the young, and lack of exposure to the sunlight needed to absorb vitamin D (Horton-French et al. 2021). Postmenopausal women and older men (≥50 years) are at increased risk of fracture and benefit from the use of supplements (e.g. 800–1000 IU cholecalciferol daily) if necessary. Regular weight-bearing exercise should be advised for everyone, tailored according to the needs and abilities of the individual.

Pharmacological Management

There are a variety of pharmacological treatments available for the treatment of osteoporosis. The most common categories are bisphosphonates (e.g. alendronate, risedronate, zoledronic acid), raloxifene, denosumab and parathyroid hormone peptides; and there are others under development. All such treatments have been shown to reduce the risk of vertebral fracture alongside an adequate intake of calcium and uptake of vitamin D (needed for the absorption of calcium) (Marques 2020).

Osteoporosis treatment is, however, a long-term undertaking and the benefits of treatment are slow to take effect, so adherence has been shown to be very low. At 1 year after commencement of treatment, adherence levels have been estimated to be between 18% and 75%, resulting in increased risk of fracture, poorer outcomes after fracture and worse general health (Cornelissen et al. 2020).

Osteoporosis is a chronic disease that involves treatment over the remainder of the individual's life. Understanding and adjusting to this knowledge can be difficult for individuals and their families, especially as the problem is not visible externally until a fracture happens. A diagnosis of osteoporosis and adherence with treatment therefore needs continuous support.

Secondary Fracture Prevention Services

It is estimated that only 20% of patients with fragility fractures are assessed and treated appropriately (although this varies regionally and globally, and many patients presenting to healthcare professionals remain needlessly at risk of fractures): this is commonly called the 'treatment gap'. National and international clinical guidelines and systematic reviews recommend the use of secondary fracture prevention services to close this treatment gap by establishing an individual's risk of fracture, and determining and implementing a suitable management plan. Recognising osteoporosis as the cause of the fracture and initiating long-term management of the condition are critical in the prevention of future fractures (Fuggle et al. 2021).

There are many challenges in coordinating the key elements of fracture prevention, including (i) case-finding those at high risk of fracture, (ii) falls prevention intervention, and (iii) diagnosis and treatment of osteoporosis. Osteoporosis is often referred to as a silent disease because there are rarely any symptoms until a fracture occurs. A first fracture (known as the index fracture) is a major risk factor for a new fracture within 2 years (Kanis et al. 2018). Index fractures are often less severe injuries (e.g. wrist fractures) than those that follow (e.g. hip fracture). Previous fragility fracture at any site is associated with significant risk of further fracture, highlighting the need to identify (or case-find) those who have sustained such a fracture to initiate early clinical assessment, investigation and treatment. For patients aged over 50, proactive case-finding in acute hospitals by fracture liaison or fracture prevention services include identification by a specialist practitioner of all patients presenting with a fragility fracture at the emergency department, fracture clinics or orthopaedic wards. This can also be conducted by identification of vertebral fractures on X-rays performed for the specific purpose of identifying a fracture as well as for other purposes.

The assessment of fracture risk and availability of medication to treat osteoporosis have increased significantly over the last few decades. It is, however, evident that osteoporosis care remains suboptimal as, even in patients who have sustained a fragility fracture, it has been reported that few actually receive appropriate osteoporosis treatment in the year following the fracture (Curtis et al. 2020).

Post-fracture care (PFC) coordination programmes (also known as fracture liaison services, FLS) are secondary fracture prevention services that follow up patients who have a suspected fragility fracture. The aim of such services is to coordinate the assessment, diagnosis and treatment of osteoporosis in patients with new fragility fractures so that future fractures can be prevented. Such services are now common in some countries, such as the UK, and are made up of an interdisciplinary team of practitioners led by a dedicated coordinator (commonly a senior nurse or bone health physician). The team coordinates patient care within the orthopaedic, osteoporosis, falls prevention and primary care services. Such services ensure that all patients presenting with fragility fractures in the locality receive fracture risk assessment and treatment where appropriate. The main elements of PFC are as follows (Fuggle et al. 2021):

1) Proactively identify patients with fragility fractures (case finding).
2) Investigate fracture risk as well as bone density, should this be indicated.
3) Make personalised treatment recommendations for preventing fractures, including osteoporosis treatment and falls prevention.
4) Monitor treatment initiation and adherence.

This system has been shown to lead to fewer future fractures/refractures, fewer secondary care admissions, fewer care home admissions and healthcare benefits including reduced costs. The evidence for the benefits of FLS/PFC services is increasing and the findings of systematic reviews suggest that FLS improve rates of screening and assessment for osteoporosis, treatment for osteoporosis and reduced rates of new fractures and mortality among patients with fragility fractures, along with significant cost savings for

Box 18.3   Fragility Fracture: Case Study Part 2

Ingrid's Bone Health

Ingrid had a fracture of her wrist 5 years ago (probably an Index fracture), but she did not have any further investigation into her bone health at that time. It is likely that the wrist fracture was a fragility fracture and that this should have instigated case-finding by a fracture prevention service/FLS if one had been available in Ingrid's area at that time.

Discussion

Consider the following question:
If Ingrid had been referred into a fracture prevention/liaison service, what difference might this have made to her current situation?

health services (McLellan et al. 2011; Wu et al. 2018). The IOF (www.iof.org) has developed a global Best Practise Framework (BPF) to support healthcare providers and clinicians in developing new FLS, improve existing ones and offer recognition for excellence.

Falls

Falls are the leading cause of hospitalisation of the over 65s (Lord et al. 2021) and a third of older people fall annually (Jehu et al. 2021). Most fractures in older people are linked to a fall. Risk of falling is, in fact, more predictive of fractures than BMD, suggesting that preventing fractures should be focused on identifying risk and preventing falls as much as identifying and treating osteoporosis (Martin and Rahnhoff 2020).

Globally, an estimated 172 million falls each year result in short- or long-term disability, with significant cost to individuals, health and social care services, and societies. Fall-related deaths are most common among people aged over 60 years (WHO 2021). The consequences of falls for older people are devastating and include the physical and emotional consequences of injury, fractures, pain, impaired function, fear of falling and social isolation. There is a view within society, and even among some health professionals, that falls in older people are an inevitable part of life and particularly of the ageing process. This fatalistic view is to be avoided if the impact on quality of life and function following falls is to be avoided (WHO 2021). Evidence, however, demonstrates that falls are preventable with the right assessment, care and resources.

The NOGG guidelines (2017) recommend that falls history should be obtained in individuals at increased risk of fracture and further assessment and appropriate measures undertaken in those at risk. Fall-related risk factors add significantly to the risk of fracture and often overlap with risk factors for osteoporosis. Identifying those at risk of falls is the starting point for falls prevention. Risk is multifactorial and there are hundreds of potential individual risk factors for falls in older people. Lord et al. (2007) suggested that risk factors could be classified into seven groups:

1) balance and mobility
2) environmental
3) psychological
4) medical
5) medication
6) sensory and neuromuscular
7) sociodemographic.

Examples of risk factors for each of these groups are listed in Table 18.1.

Most inpatient units now undertake falls risk assessment for all patients admitted with fractures. Identifying the causes and risk factors for falls that have led to injury is a central principle for effective care of the injured older person. Prevention measures then must be implemented which recognise the needs of the older person who has fallen and is, therefore, at risk of further falls.

Numerous multifactorial falls risk assessment tools are now in use and many have been evaluated for their accuracy in identifying those at risk and the specific individual's risk factors that need targeted intervention. Risk assessment and

Table 18.1   Categories of risk factors and examples

Category (Lord et al. 2007)	Example specific risk factors
Balance and mobility	Previous fall/s, muscle weakness, sarcopenia, foot problems, arthritis, visual impairment, fractures, incontinence
Environmental	Home and external environment hazards increasing the risk of trips
Psychological	Delirium, dementia, depression
Medical	Hypotension, malnutrition, diabetes, respiratory and cardiovascular diseases
Medication	Polypharmacy, antihypertensive drugs, psychoactive drugs
Sensory and neuromuscular	Neuropathy, stroke, Parkinson's disease
Sociodemographic	Advanced age, female gender, poverty, dependency, poor social support, isolation

attention to individual specific risk factors must lead to multifactorial interventions that specifically address the patient's individual risk factors.

Fall Prevention Measures

Many organisations provide evidence-based guidelines for the prevention of falls in older people and a selection of these are identified in Box 18.4. The preventive measures for falls are also included in the interventions for the management of frailty that are considered in the next section. Measures for the prevention of falls have been investigated in copious research studies over several decades so there is now significant understanding of which are most likely to be successful.

NICE (2013) Guidelines recommend that:

> . . .following treatment for an injurious fall, older people should be offered a multidisciplinary assessment to identify and address future risk and individualised intervention aimed at promoting independence and improving physical and psychological function

Falls prevention measures need to take place over time to enable older people to embed them into their everyday life. In units where older people are managed following a fall that has led to a fragility fracture, it is essential that an interdisciplinary approach to assessment also leads to commencement of prevention strategies during the hospital stay so that this can be continued during rehabilitation and following discharge. Implementation of falls prevention measures should not be assumed to be the responsibility of a different service.

The NICE (2013) guidelines for falls prevention are based on strong evidence. This has consistently shown that four main strategies are most likely to be successful once an older person has been assessed for risk of falling and their individual risk factors have been identified:

- Strength and balance training: acknowledging that muscle weakness is a significant factor in falling for many older people, older people can commence the early stages of balance training while still in hospital.
- Home hazard assessment and intervention: this should take place early in the admission following fragility fracture so that issues can be resolved before discharge is likely.
- Vision assessment and referral: recognising that problems with sight are a significant factor in falling, referral for assessment should take place as soon as possible after the fracture.
- Medication review with modification/withdrawal: recognising that some types of medication and polypharmacy are significant factors in falls, medication should be reviewed during the hospital stay by a geriatrician/physician and any changes communicated to the patient's general practitioner/community team.

Fear of falling can have a significant impact on recovery following fragility fracture, especially hip fracture, which involves considerable effort for the patient in remobilisation. Fear of falling often presents as anxiety and extreme reluctance to mobilise and leads to avoidance of the activity perceived to have resulted in the fall (i.e. walking) as well as depleted motivation in the rehabilitation process, leading to a decline in function, loss of independence and reduced quality of life (Scheffers-Barnhoornet et al. 2017). Targeted interventions to reduce the impact of fear of falling lead to improved rehabilitation outcomes.

Box 18.4   Falls Prevention Guidelines

Australian Commission on Safety and Quality in Health Care (ACSQHC) (2009) Preventing falls and harm from falls in older people: Best practise guidelines for Australian hospitals. https://www.safetyandquality.gov.au/sites/default/files/migrated/Guidelines-HOSP.pdf.

British Geriatrics Society (2017) Clinical Guidelines on Falls and Fractures. https://www.bgs.org.uk/resources/clinical-guidelines-on-falls-and-fractures.

NICE (2013) Falls in older people: assessing risk and prevention. Clinical guideline [CG161]. https://www.nice.org.uk/guidance/cg161.

Public Health England (2020) Falls: Applying All our Health. https://www.gov.uk/government/publications/falls-applying-all-our-health/falls-applying-all-our-health.

Scottish Government (2019) National falls and fracture prevention strategy 2019–2024 draft: consultation. https://www.gov.scot/publications/national-falls-fracture-prevention-strategy-scotland-2019-2024/pages/6/.

Frailty and Sarcopenia

Frailty, falls and fractures are linked. Frailty increases the risk of morbidity and mortality in patients hospitalised with fragility fractures. It is a clinical syndrome characterised by increased vulnerability and diminished resistance to stressors that can cause functional impairment and increase risks (Morley et al. 2013); a minor stress or event such as a fall or acute illness can worsen a person's health condition and increase dependency and/or mortality. Frailty is both a physical and psychological phenomenon that also has significant social effects. Frailty and falls are strongly correlated (Bartosch et al. 2020): both are predictors of negative health outcomes (Chen et al. 2019) and risk factors for falls are also markers of frailty (Jeju et al. 2021). Frail individuals are at increased risk of adverse health outcomes such as falls, hospitalisation, deterioration in mobility, disability, institutionalisation, poor outcomes of treatment, complications and death (Low et al. 2021). Frailty is also negatively associated with quality of life 1 year after hip fracture (see Box 18.6). In the UK alone, approximately 64 000 adults are admitted to hospital each year with a hip fracture requiring surgery, most of whom are considered frail. Frailty is often assessed in the emergency department but is not routinely considered in most perioperative settings (BGS 2021).

Sarcopenia is a major component of frailty; it is the term used to refer to loss of muscle with ageing. Its causes and impact on mobility mean that it is linked with falls, osteoporosis and fragility fractures (Clynes et al. 2021). Because of the importance of muscle in metabolism, low muscle mass is linked with poor outcomes from acute illness, injury and surgery, so is an important consideration in the care of frail patients with significant fragility fractures (Martin and Rahnhoff 2020).

Following major fragility fractures, such as hip fracture, patients are hospitalised and almost always undergo orthopaedic surgery to manage the fracture as conservative treatment leads to an unacceptable risk of complications and surgical fixation is the most effective way to manage the pain. The outcomes and trajectory of recovery and rehabilitation are significantly affected by the degree of frailty of the patient and understanding the frailty status is a significant factor in planning care and rehabilitation, and in understanding the potential outcomes (Krishnan et al. 2014). However, nurses and other professionals involved in the peri-operative care, recovery and hospital rehabilitation of the patient do not usually routinely consider frailty as a factor, even though they often work alongside geriatricians.

Frailty status is a predictor of poor outcomes, morbidity and mortality following hip fracture surgery (Chen et al. 2019) so an understanding of this helps practitioners to identify those patients most at risk of deterioration and in need of more intensive interventions to prevent deterioration. Undertaking screening for frailty and its elements on admission to hospital following hip fracture is an important first step in designing and planning the care pathway. Timely involvement of a team with frailty expertise (such as a geriatric or orthogeriatric interdisciplinary team [see Box 18.5 for an example] who can identify and implement

---

Box 18.5   Fragility Fracture: Case Study Part 3

Post-operative Management

Ingrid receives care in an orthogeriatric unit under the collaborative care of an orthogeriatrician and her orthopaedic surgeon*. Her day-to-day care in hospital is managed by a hip fracture advanced nurse practitioner, who leads the rest of the team. Annual audits show that the evidence-based care provided in the orthogeriatric unit is some of the best in the country.

   (*See Chapter 19 for further details of post-operative care and management following hip fracture surgery.)

Functional Recovery

On admission, Ingrid was assessed by the orthogeriatric team as scoring 3 on the Clinical Frailty Scale (managing well). However, she has found the process of remobilisation after her surgery a struggle and feels weak and tired a lot of the time, lacking in energy and motivation. She can, however, walk to the ward bathroom with a walking frame and supervision within a week of her surgery. Despite every effort of the clinical team, including physiotherapy and occupational therapy, a week after her surgery she is considered to score 5 on the Clinical Frailty Scale (mildly frail). Both Ingrid and her daughter are worried about her returning home, so they have agreed that she will transfer to a residential home temporarily to give her more time to get back on her feet. Ingrid is worried about the future and she does not want to become a burden.

Discussion

Consider the following questions:

What are the clinical implications of Ingrid's current frailty status?
What needs to be in place to support her in improving her function and achieving her aim of going home in a few weeks?

interventions which aim to modify frailty can then be arranged (BGS 2021). British Geriatrics Society (BGS) guidance (2021) recommends that all patients aged over 65 years admitted for emergency surgery should have their frailty status documented on admission using the Clinical Frailty Scale (CFS) initially proposed by Rockwood (2005) and updated since. The CFS assesses several health and wellbeing domains, including comorbidity, function and cognition, to generate a frailty score ranging from 1 (very fit) to 9 (terminally ill) and has been used and evaluated in many settings, showing correlation with clinical outcomes (Church et al. 2020). Further information about the use and implementation of the CFS can be found at: https://www.dal.ca/sites/gmr/our-tools/clinical-frailty-scale.html.

The use of frailty scales in orthogeriatric units/hip fracture units has become common, but in general orthopaedic/trauma settings this is less likely to take place. Undertaking screening and assessment for frailty in older orthopaedic trauma patients helps clinical staff to recognise the part frailty plays in outcomes, as well as the benefits of expert interdisciplinary care of older people with orthopaedic injuries such as fragility fractures who are also frail.

The value of using an assessment of frailty to plan the care pathway of the patient with fragility fracture has been demonstrated in patients admitted with a hip fracture (Krishnan et al. 2014; Wilson et al. 2019). One of the challenges with assessing frailty status for patients with hip fracture is that the fall, injury and surgery will impact significantly on the patient's health and wellbeing status, and it is difficult to assess previous frailty status in this emergency situation and when the function and mobility of patients cannot be evaluated. This requires further investigation.

The normal and abnormal changes that occur with ageing negatively affect the response to trauma and subsequent surgery. Active comorbidities such as hypertension, heart disease, diabetes and dementia lead to altered immune/inflammatory responses and disordered blood clotting in older people. Polypharmacy affects the response to trauma, particularly medications such as beta-blockers and steroids, which deplete physiological responses to trauma. Medications that affect clotting (such as warfarin, direct oral anticoagulants or novel oral anticoagulants) can also lead to other problems, such as infection and chronic pain. Older people are a diverse group of individuals. Some have few health and social care needs, while many have several interconnected health, psychological and social needs.

Comprehensive geriatric assessment (CGA) is a multidimensional, interdisciplinary process designed to detect and assess frailty and to determine medical, psychological and social needs. There is evidence that CGA can improve outcomes in people with hip fractures (Eamer et al. 2018) and

that it can reduce mortality, facilitate return to home and reduce length of hospital stay (Wilson 2017).

Spirgiene and Brent (2018, p. 43) outline the principles of CGA as part of an interdisciplinary, integrated approach central to orthogeriatric care that should be embedded into the care process for all older patients hospitalised with a fragility fracture:

- The process should be person-centred.
- The older person's capacity to participate in the process voluntarily must be assessed; if capacity does not exist, there should be a system in place that considers their needs within an ethical framework.
- Links between social and healthcare need to be made so that older people who need CGA receive it efficiently in a way that considers their degree of need in a timely manner.
- Assessments should be carried out to a reliable standard within and across multidisciplinary team.

Clinical Care for those Identified as Frail

The BGS (2021) recommend three actions specific to inpatient orthopaedic trauma and orthogeriatric/hip fracture units:

1) All patients living with frailty (CFS ≥ 5) should undergo CGA and optimisation prior to surgery.
2) All hospitals should have a perioperative frailty team with expertise in CGA who provide clinical care throughout the pathway.
3) All staff working with patients at risk of frailty should receive training on frailty, delirium and dementia.

Physical, social and psychological assessment are the first steps in managing frailty and improving outcomes for those who suffer a combination of frailty and a fragility fracture. CGA is embedded in practise in geriatric units, and the same standard of care should be provided in orthopaedic units. The philosophy of CGA is a holistic approach to management and consideration of what are described as the 'geriatric giants': frailty, cognitive impairment, delirium, incontinence, malnutrition, falls and pressure injuries. The assessment should include a full and comprehensive history that identifies relevant comorbidities and medication history along with an overview of previous functional ability and personal and social history with specific focus on those domains which may be unstable, resulting in the fall or, potentially, impacting on outcomes. Many studies have shown that the incidence of fragility fractures increases as a person's age increases, that those who are frail are more likely to sustain a fragility fracture, and the older and frailer someone is the more likely they are to suffer complications and/or die in the

---

Box 18.6   Evidence Digest: Quality of Life Following Hip Fracture

van de Ree CLP, Landers MJF, Kruithof N, et al. (2019) Effect of frailty on quality of life in elderly patients after hip fracture: a longitudinal study. BMJ Open 9:e025941. doi:10.1136/bmjopen-2018-025941.

van der Ree et al. (2019) aimed to examine how health status and quality of life changed in the first year after a fragility hip fracture. They proposed that frailty (a 'clinical state of increased vulnerability') is a predictor of quality of life in this group of patients.

They conducted a prospective, observational, follow-up cohort study in secondary care settings in the Netherlands. They recruited 1091 patients with a hip fracture aged 65 years and older, of whom 696 completed the study. Data were collected regarding health status (EuroQol-5 Dimensions questionnaire) and capability/wellbeing (ICEpop CAPability measure for older people). Those who were frail pre-fracture were identified using the Groningen Frailty Indicator (GFI), with GFI ≥ 4 indicating frailty. Participants were followed up at 1, 3, 6 months and 1 year after hospital admission.

Of the patients included in the study, 371 (53.3%) were identified as frail. Frailty was negatively associated with health status (β −0.333, 95% CI −0.366 to −0.299), self-rated health (β −21.9, 95% CI −24.2 to −19.6) and capability/wellbeing (β −0.296, 95% CI −0.322 to −0.270) in patients 1 year after the hip fracture. After adjusting for confounding variables, including death, pre-fracture health status, age, pre-fracture residential status, pre-fracture mobility, American Society of Anesthesiologists grading and dementia, the associations were weakened but remained significant.

The authors concluded that frailty is negatively associated with quality of life 1 year after hip fracture, even after adjusting for confounding factors. They suggest that early identification of pre-fracture frailty in patients with a hip fracture is important for prognostic counselling, care planning and tailoring of treatment, confirming that this is an area of practise development for interdisciplinary orthopaedic trauma teams caring for patients following fragility hip fracture and other musculoskeletal injuries.

---

weeks and months following the fracture (Ravindrarajah et al. 2018). Frailty also increases the risk of falls and fractures in the first place (de Vries et al. 2013). Frailty negatively affects quality of life following fragility hip fracture (van der Ree et al. 2019, see Box 18.6) and is now being recognised as a nursing and interdisciplinary priority in all settings where older people are acutely ill, injured or receiving surgery.

Conclusion

The care of older trauma patients requires highly skilled, specialised care delivered by practitioners who have skills in orthopaedics, trauma and geriatrics (Brent et al. 2018). Although management of older people following trauma needs to follow the general considerations described in Chapter 19, there are also specific factors which must be considered when caring for an older person following significant trauma.

Orthogeriatrics is model of care involving a multidisciplinary team of health professionals with combined expertise in trauma, orthopaedics and geriatrics who co-manage and provide care for the significantly injured frail older person with a fragility fracture, especially following fragility hip fracture. This model has been shown to deliver better outcomes following significant fragility fracture (Ong and Sahota 2021). The linked speciality of orthogeriatric nursing is evolving and focuses on high-quality nursing care, focused on nurse-specific indicators, skill, education, leadership and resources that can positively influence patient outcomes in the orthogeriatric setting (Santy-Tomlinson et al. 2021). This is discussed in more detail in Chapter 19.

Further Reading

Falaschi, P. and Marsh, D. (ed.) (2021). *Orthogeriatrics. Practical Issues in Geriatrics*, 69–82. Cham: Springer https://link.springer.com/book/10.1007/978-3-319-76681-2.

Hertz, K. and Santy-Tomlinson, J. (ed.) (2018). *Fragility Fracture Nursing: Holistic Care and Management of the Orthogeriatric Patient*, 1–13. Cham: Springer https://link.springer.com/book/10.1007/978-3-319-76681-2.

Royal College of Physicians (2021). *Fracture Liaison Service Database Annual Report. Benchmarking FLS improvement and performance in 2019*. Pre-Covid https://www.rcplondon.ac.uk/projects/outputs/fls-database-annual-report-2021.

References

Bartosch, P.S., Kristensson, J., McGuigan, F.E. et al. (2020). Frailty and prediction of recurrent falls over 10 years in a community cohort of 75-year-old women. *Aging Clin. Exp. Res.* 32: 2241–2250. https://doi.org/10.1007/s40520-019-01467-1.

Brent, L., Hommel, A., Maher, A.B. et al. (2018). Nursing care of fragility fracture patients. *Injury* 49 (8): 1409–1412. https://doi.org/10.1016/j.injury.2018.06.036.

BGS (2021) Guideline for perioperative care for people living with frailty undergoing elective and emergency surgery. BGS Centre for Perioperative Care. https://www.bgs.org.uk/cpocfrailty.

British Orthopaedic Association/British Geriatric Society (2007). *Care of Patients with Fragility Fractures*. London: British Orthopaedic Association https://www.bgs.org.uk/sites/default/files/content/attachment/2018-05-02/Blue%20Book%20on%20fragility%20fracture%20care.pdf.

Chen, C.L., Chen, C.M., Wang, C.Y. et al. (2019). Frailty is associated with an increased risk of major adverse outcomes in elderly patients following surgical treatment of hip fracture. *Sci. Rep.* 9: 19135. https://doi.org/10.1038/s41598-019-55459-2.

Church, S., Rogers, E., Rockwood, K. et al. (2020). A scoping review of the clinical frailty scale. *BMC Geriatr.* 20: 393. https://doi.org/10.1186/s12877-020-01801-7.

Clynes, M.A., Gregson, C.L., Bruyère, O. et al. (2021). Osteosarcopenia: where osteoporosis and sarcopenia collide. *Rheumatology* 60 (2): 529–537. https://doi.org/10.1093/rheumatology/keaa755.

Cornelissen, D., de Kunder, S., Si, L. et al. (2020). Interventions to improve adherence to anti-osteoporosis medications: an updated systematic review. *Osteoporos. Int.* 31: 1645–1669. https://doi.org/10.1007/s00198-020-05378-0.

Curtis, E.M., van der Velde, R., Moon, R.J. et al. (2016). Epidemiology of fractures in the United Kingdom 1988–2012: Variation with age, sex, geography, ethnicity and socioeconomic status. *Bone* 87: 19–26. https://doi.org/10.1016/j.bone.2016.03.006.

Curtis, E.M., Woolford, S., Holmes, C. et al. (2020). General and specific considerations as to why osteoporosis-related care is often suboptimal. *Curr. Osteoporos. Rep.* 18 (1): 38–46. https://doi.org/10.1007/s11914-020-00566-7.

Eamer, G., Taheri, A., Chen, S.S. et al. (2018). Comprehensive geriatric assessment for older people admitted to a surgical service. *Cochrane Database Syst. Rev.* (1): (Art. No.: CD012485). https://doi.org/10.1002/14651858.CD012485.pub2.

Falaschi, P., Marques, A., and Giordano, S. (2021). Osteoporosis and fragility in elderly patients. In: *Orthogeriatrics. Practical Issues in Geriatrics* (ed. P. Falaschi and D. Marsh). Cham: Springer https://doi.org/10.1007/978-3-030-48126-1_3.

Fuggle, N.R., Javaid, K., Fujita, M. et al. (2021). Fracture risk assessment and how to implement a fracture liaison service. In: *Orthogeriatrics. Practical Issues in Geriatrics* (ed. P. Falaschi and D. Marsh). Cham: Springer https://doi.org/10.1007/978-3-030-48126-1_14.

Horton-French, K., Dunlop, E., Lucas, R.M. et al. (2021). Prevalence and predictors of vitamin D deficiency in a nationally representative sample of Australian adolescents and young adults. *Eur. J. Clin. Nutr.* 75: 1627–1636. https://doi.org/10.1038/s41430-021-00880-y.

IOF (2021a) Fragility Fractures. International Osteoporosis Foundation. https://www.osteoporosis.foundation/health-professionals/fragility-fractures (accessed 28 October 2021).

IOF (2021b) Diagnosis. International Osteoporosis Foundation. https://www.osteoporosis.foundation/health-professionals/diagnosis (accessed 2 December 2021).

Jehu, D.A., Davis, J.C., Falck, R.S. et al. (2021). Risk factors for recurrent falls in older adults: a systematic review with meta-analysis. *Maturitas* 144: 23–28. https://doi.org/10.1016/j.maturitas.2020.10.021.

Kanis, J.A., on behalf of the World Health Organization Scientific Group (2007) Assessment of osteoporosis at the primary health-care level. Technical Report. World Health Organization Collaborating Centre for Metabolic Bone Diseases, University of Sheffield, UK. https://www.sheffield.ac.uk/FRAX/pdfs/WHO_Technical_Report.pdf.

Kanis, J.A., Johansson, H., Odén, A. et al. (2018). Characteristics of recurrent fractures. *Osteoporos. Int.* 29 (8): 1747–1757. https://doi.org/10.1007/s00198-018-4502-0.

Krishnan, M., Beck, S., Havelock, W. et al. (2014). Predicting outcome after hip fracture: using a frailty index to integrate comprehensive geriatric assessment results. *Age Ageing* 43 (1): 122–126. https://doi.org/10.1093/ageing/aft084.

Lord, S., Sherrington, C., Menz, H., and Close, J. (ed.) (2007). *Falls in Older People: Risk Factors and Strategies for Prevention*, 2e. Cambridge: Cambridge University Press.

Lord, S., Sherrington, C., and Hicks, C. (2021). Epidemiology of falls and fall-related injuries. In: *Falls in Older People: Risk Factors, Strategies for Prevention and Implications for Practice*, 3e (ed. S. Lord, C. Sherrington and V. Naganathan). Cambridge: Cambridge University Press.

Low, S., Wee, E., and Dorevitch, M. (2021). Impact of place of residence, frailty and other factors on rehabilitation outcomes post hip fracture. *Age Ageing* 50 (2): 423–430. https://doi.org/10.1093/ageing/afaa131.

Marques, A.A. (2020). Osteoporosis and fractures. In: *Nursing Older People with Arthritis and Other Rheumatological Conditions* (ed. S. Ryan), 65–78. Cham: Springer.

Martin, F.C. and Ranhoff, A.H. (2020). Frailty and sarcopenia. In: *Orthogeriatrics. Practical Issues in Geriatrics* (ed. P. Falaschi and D. Marsh). Cham: Springer https://doi.org/10.1007/978-3-030-48126-1_4.

McLellan, A.R., Wolowacz, S.E., Zimovetz, E.A. et al. (2011). Fracture liaison services for the evaluation and management of patients with osteoporotic fracture: a cost-effectiveness evaluation based on data collected over 8 years of service provision. *Osteoporos. Int.* 22: 2083. https://doi.org/10.1007/s00198-011-1534-0.

Morley, J.E., Vellas, B., van Kan, G.A. et al. (2013). Frailty consensus: a call to action. *J. Am. Med. Dir. Assoc.* (6): 392–397. https://doi.org/10.1016/j.jamda.2013.03.022.

National Osteoporosis Guideline Group (2017) Clinical guideline for the prevention and treatment of osteoporosis. Updated 2019. https://www.sheffield.ac.uk/NOGG/NOGG%20Guideline%202017%20July%202019%20Final%20Update%20290719.pdf.

Nguyen, V. (2017). Osteoporosis prevention and osteoporosis exercise in community-based public health programs. *Osteoporosis and Sarcopenia* 3 (1): 18–31. https://doi.org/10.1016/j.afos.2016.11.004.

NICE (2013) *Falls in older people: assessing risk and prevention*. Clinical guideline [CG161]. https://www.nice.org.uk/guidance/cg161.

NICE (2021) *Osteoporosis – prevention of fragility fractures*. https://cks.nice.org.uk/topics/osteoporosis-prevention-of-fragility-fractures/.

Ong, T. and Sahota, O. (2021). Establishing an orthogeriatric service. In: *Orthogeriatrics. Practical Issues in Geriatrics* (ed. P. Falaschi and D. Marsh). Cham: Springer 6982. https://doi.org/10.1007/978-3-030-48126-1_5.

van Oostwaard, M. (2018). Osteoporosis and the nature of fragility fracture: and overview. In: *Fragility Fracture Nursing: Holistic Care and Management of the Orthogeriatric Patient* (ed. K. Hertz and J. Santy-Tomlinson), 1–13. Cham: Springer https://rd.springer.com/book/10.1007/978-3-319-76681-2#toc.

Ravindrarajah, R., Hazra, N.C., Charlton, J. et al. (2018). Incidence and mortality of fractures by frailty level over 80 years of age: cohort study using UK electronic health records. *BMJ Open* 8: e018836. https://doi.org/10.1136/bmjopen-2017-018836.

van de Ree, C.L.P., Landers, M.J.F., Kruithof, N. et al. (2019). Effect of frailty on quality of life in elderly patients after hip fracture: a longitudinal study. *BMJ Open* 9: e025941. https://doi.org/10.1136/bmjopen-2018-025941.

Rockwood, J., Song, X., MacKnight, C. et al. (2005). A global clinical measure of fitness and frailty in elderly people. *CMAJ* 173 (5): 489–495.

Santy-Tomlinson, J., Hertz, K., Myhre-Jensen, C., and Brent, L. (2021). Nursing in the orthogeriatric setting. In: *Orthogeriatrics. Practical Issues in Geriatrics* (ed. P. Falaschi and D. Marsh), 293–310. Cham: Springer https://doi.org/10.1007/978-3-030-48126-1_17.

Scheffers-Barnhoorn, M.N., van Haastregt, J.C.M., Schols, J.M.G.A. et al. (2017). A multi-component cognitive behavioural intervention for the treatment of fear of falling after hip fracture (FIT-HIP): protocol of a randomised controlled trial. *BMC Geriatr.* 17: 71. https://doi.org/10.1186/s12877-017-0465-9.

Spirgiene, L. and Brent, L. (2018). Comprehensive Geriatric Assessment from a Nursing Perspective. In: *Fragility Fracture Nursing: Holistic Care and Management of the Orthogeriatric Patient* (ed. K. Hertz and J. Santy-Tomlinson). Cham: Springer https://www.ncbi.nlm.nih.gov/books/NBK543827/, https://doi.org/10.1007/978-3-319-76681-2_4.

Veronese, N., Kolk, H., and Maggi, S. (2021). Epidemiology of fragility fractures and social impact. In: *Orthogeriatrics. Practical Issues in Geriatrics* (ed. P. Falaschi and D. Marsh), 19–34. Cham: Springer https://doi.org/10.1007/978-3-030-48126-1_2.

de Vries, O.J., Peeters, G.M.E.E., Lips, P. et al. (2013). Does frailty predict increased risk of falls and fractures? A prospective population-based study. *Osteoporos. Int.* 24: 2397–2403. https://doi.org/10.1007/s00198-013-2303-z.

Wilson, H. (2017). Pre-operative management. In: *Orthogeriatrics* (ed. P. Falaschi and D. Marsh), 63–79. Cham: Springer.

Wilson, J.M., Boissonneault, A.R., Schwartz, A.M. et al. (2019). Frailty and malnutrition are associated with inpatient postoperative complications and mortality in hip-fracture patients. *J. Orthop. Trauma* 33 (3): 143–148. https://doi.org/10.1097/BOT.0000000000001386. PMID: 30570618.

WHO (2021). *Step safely. Strategies for preventing and managing falls across the life-course*. Geneva: World Health Organization https://www.who.int/teams/social-determinants-of-health/safety-and-mobility/step-safely.

Wu, C.H., Kao, I.J., Hung, W.C. et al. (2018). Economic impact and cost-effectiveness of fracture liaison services: a systematic review of the literature. *Osteoporos. Int.* 29: 1227–1242. https://doi.org/10.1007/s00198-018-4411-2.

Wu, A.-M., Bisignano, C., James, S.L. et al. (2021). Global, regional, and national burden of bone fractures in 204 countries and territories, 1990–2019: a systematic analysis from the Global Burden of Disease Study 2019. *Lancet Healthy Longevity* 2 (9): e580–e592. https://doi.org/10.1016/S2666-7568(21)00172-0.

19

Fragility Hip Fracture

Karen Hertz[1] and Julie Santy-Tomlinson[2,3]

[1] *Department of Orthopaedics and Trauma, Royal Stoke University Hospital, Stoke-on-Trent, UK*
[2] *International Journal of Orthopaedic and Trauma Nursing*
[3] *Department of Orthopaedic Surgery, Odense University Hospitals/University of Southern Denmark, Denmark*

Introduction

Fragility hip fracture is a fracture of the proximal femur involving the femoral neck or intertrochanteric region caused by low-energy mechanisms of injury and low bone mass caused by osteoporosis (see Chapter 18). It is a significant injury that usually occurs in patients who are significantly older and frail. Those who have sustained this injury are admitted in ever-increasing numbers to every acute hospital across the world. Hip fracture management and care are major challenges for patients and their families, health services and care teams because of the advanced age and frailty of most patients. It can be a life-changing injury for patients, reducing their physical and psychological wellbeing, function, independence and life expectancy (see Box 19.1).

Almost all hip fractures are treated with major orthopaedic surgery and rates of complications and mortality following surgery are high. There is, however, increasing awareness of the factors which lead to improved outcomes for hip fracture patients, including collaborative, interdisciplinary care under orthogeriatric teams and the design of healthcare and hospital infrastructures and pathways which provide the best evidence-based care.

The aim of this chapter is to provide an overview of how best practice can be delivered for patients with fragility hip fracture.

Orthogeriatric Nursing

For the first time, there are 11 million people aged 65 and over in the UK and the percentage of the population in that age group is increasing globally, especially in emerging economies. Older people are remaining active for longer, but the risk of traumatic injury is also growing, whether that be major trauma or isolated injuries. There are many different mechanisms of injury in older adults that necessitate hospital attendance, including accidents in the home, slips and trips, falls downstairs or from a height, road traffic accidents and assault. However, a fall from a standing height is the most common mechanism of injury for all older people admitted with both multiple and isolated injures such as hip fracture. After the age of 70, most patients sustain their injuries indoors and the most common areas of injury for older adults following major trauma are the thorax and head (Trauma Audit and Research Network [TARN] 2017).

In many countries hip fracture is the most common reason for admission to orthopaedic trauma units. According to the National Hip Fracture Database (NHFD 2019), more than 67 000 people over the age of 60 were admitted to hospital because of a hip fracture in 2018. Orthogeriatric teams have become increasingly common in the UK and Ireland as well as in other countries, with the aims of caring for patients with fragility hip fracture collaboratively and coordinating high-quality care. This has led to sustained improvements in care processes and outcomes. Where such teams are established, the collaboration provides improved outcomes (TARN 2017; NHFD 2019).

Orthogeriatrics is an established speciality in hip fracture care that involves the collaboration of orthopaedic surgeons working in partnership with geriatricians to provide medical care that meets the best interests of the older person following hip fracture. However, as the services have evolved, the term

Box 19.1 Patient Experiences of Recovering from Fragility Hip Fracture: a Qualitative Perspective

Several qualitative studies have highlighted the impact that fragility hip fracture can have on the wellbeing and life experience of patients. Abrahamsen and Nørgaard (2021) conducted a qualitative systematic review that aimed to identify what older patients of advanced age consider important in relation to their hip fracture from qualitative research studies. The authors reviewed 16 qualitative studies that offered insight into the individual experience of recovery following a hip fracture with respect to the impact on symptoms and complications, physical health, mental health, social relationships and personal goals. They also identified several important aspects of healthcare-related experiences, including waiting times, information, participation and respect, and discharge.

They found that patients' focus was primarily on regaining physical functioning, mobility and independence. However, patients' experiences of recovery from hip fracture are often reported negatively. A common theme in qualitative research exploring these experiences is of life becoming a struggle to regain independence with a devastating impact on all aspects of life.

Reading the patient quotes in qualitative studies can help healthcare professionals to understand the patient experience, to inform healthcare that is tailored to meet patient needs effectively. For example, Bruun-Olsen et al. (2018) interviewed patients in their own homes 4 months after a hip fracture about their experience of recovery. The study revealed three overarching themes:

- feeling vulnerable
- a span between self-reliance and dependency
- disruption from normal life.

Some of the direct quotations reported in the article (see below) highlight how devastating an experience hip fracture recovery can be. The authors point out that a hip fracture 'may be seen as a minor event by health care workers, but is experienced as a disruptive event for many patients. Based on these findings, increased focus on individualized treatment and care to each patient throughout each stage in the recovery process should be emphasized' (Bruun-Olsen et al. 2018 p8). Understanding this is central to providing high-quality care that impacts positively on patient outcomes.

I felt like being in another world. Suddenly other people decided on what I should do, and I did precisely what they told me, I did not dare to do otherwise. F1 (p. 4)

After the hip fracture I have felt depressed for the first time in my life. I feel totally empty. And the gloominess persists even now (four months after the fracture). It is like having fallen into a black hole and being unable to get up again. F1 (p. 4)

My problem is that I expected this to take 14 days. I thought that after three weeks I would be able to walk without crutches. I had a friend who had a total hip arthroplasty and he walked without crutches after 14 days. I have been urgently waiting for my own functional recovery. Why is it taking such a long time? It has been very frustrating. If I had known, it would have been easier for me. M4 (p. 5)

After the fracture, my children decided that I had to sell the house and move out. Naturally, that was necessary…Everything was well before the fracture. After the fracture the consequences was a disrupted life, I have to say…suddenly I was under surveillance. F3 (p. 6)

I do not think I will return to my former life. I realise that……earlier everything was ok. M4 (p. 6)

I will never be the person I was before the fracture. I used to be in good shape, despite my age. Now I ask myself: What is there really to look forward to when you are ninety? F7 (p. 6)

'orthogeriatrics' has come to describe an interdisciplinary team, caring most often on an orthopaedic ward for older people following hip fracture. They work collaboratively across the disciplines of surgery, medicine, anaesthesia, allied health professionals and nursing, providing specialist care.

This coordinated approach, however, is not necessarily replicated with other types of injuries. Older people who are frail have multiple comorbidities, may also have dementia and are the core business of all acute hospital services. They also represent the biggest hospital costs and activity. TARN (2017) identified that older adults do not necessarily get the same treatment in trauma units as their younger counterparts. There is an increasing presence of orthogeriatric teams within major trauma centres, but this does not reflect the care older people can expect in other general hospitals and there is a need to ensure that health and social care systems are fit for older people, who have the right to equal care as established in law and ethics.

It is important to understand why we need to treat older people following falls and fractures differently, not only in terms of providing integrated orthogeriatric care but specifically in the advancement of orthogeriatric nursing. Older people rarely present with an isolated injury with no additional complexity. They are frequently frail, have multiple comorbidities and are subject to polypharmacy. Often overlooked on initial assessment is the fact that they frequently present with additional occult injuries (TARN 2017) that may relate directly to the fall and can include other fractures, head injuries and soft tissue damage. They may also have been subjected to a 'long lie' before being found, leading to pressure injuries (apparent or evolving), dehydration, acute kidney injuries and blood sugar instability.

The presence of underlying comorbidities and multiple medications also means that the older person will not react to traumatic injuries in the same way that younger patients do. Table 19.1 provides an overview of the additional considerations needed for older people when conducting a trauma primary survey as well as in the perioperative period. Further discussion of trauma management can be found in Chapter 16.

Nurses working in trauma units rarely have both the orthopaedic and geriatric knowledge/education and skills needed to provide effective orthogeriatric care. All staff working with older people following trauma should be educated to understand the effects of altered frailty, physiological reserve and comorbid diseases common in older people and the impact these have on patient outcomes. Throughout the hospital stay following hip fracture, surgery and the rehabilitation process, nurses need to consider the numerous highly complex orthogeriatric care needs and be prepared to collaborate with the team to provide skilled, compassionate nursing care that reflects the specialist nursing care needs, including those of both orthopaedic and geriatric practitioners (Brent et al. 2018).

Later in the chapter we will examine orthogeriatric nursing competencies in more detail. However, to fully understand the positive impact that nurses have within the orthogeriatric team it is important to understand the uniqueness of the nursing role while acknowledging that no healthcare professional can care for the patient in isolation and that holistic care requires interdisciplinary collaboration. Nurses spend more clinical time with patients than any other professional within the team, so they usually take on two major roles within the team: (i) the provision of safe and effective patient care, and (ii) the pivotal role of care coordinator.

Table 19.1 Additional considerations for older people in the primary survey.

	Airway
Obstruction	Dentures
	Friable tissues, especially mucosa
Neck and spine	Flexion deformities of the spine (especially cervical) due to degenerative conditions such as spondylosis and rheumatological conditions
	Breathing
Respiratory rate	>20 breaths per minute indicates the patient is struggling and <12 may indicate fatigue
Comorbidities	Older people are more likely to have pre-existing lung pathology
Rib fractures	With increased age physiological reserve decreases and a simple rib fracture that would not be significant to a younger adult may result in death due to complications
	Circulation
Hidden shock	β-blocker medication may inhibit tachycardia. Hypertension may mean that blood pressure of 120/80 mmHg is a sign of shock
Anticoagulants	Consider early reversal of anticoagulants such as dabigatran, warfarin, novel oral anticoagulant/ direct oral anticoagulant
ECG	Identify whether they fell or collapsed. There may be underlying cardiac/vascular problems leading to a collapse
	Disability
Cognition – Think delirium/ physiological cause	Is there agitation or low Glasgow Coma Score? Are any cognitive function deficits normal for them? Never assume dementia. Consider alcohol intake
	Cognitive function deficits should assume injury, not the effects of ageing
	Exposure
Hypothermia	Common in older people following trauma – recognise and manage

Source: Adapted from EMbeds (2019).

Nurses as Care Providers

Orthogeriatric nursing requires a focus on the fundamentals of nursing care such as patient comfort, improving or maintaining quality of life, ensuring safety, empowerment and satisfaction. Proficient and expert orthogeriatric nurses apply general nursing knowledge and skills (e.g. skills for pain management, delirium prevention and management, nutrition, hydration, wound and skin care) to the patient with a hip fracture. It is the synthesis and application of general nursing knowledge, values and competence to the patient with a hip fracture that demonstrate specialist orthogeriatric nursing. Having the specialist knowledge and skills to look after hip fracture patients is not sufficient in isolation, it requires nurses in an orthogeriatric team to work both autonomously and collaboratively with the interdisciplinary team to provide direct patient care, health education and promotion, providing leadership and patient and carer advocacy. Because of the vulnerability of frail older people in hospital and during the perioperative period, nurses also need to be critically aware of the prevention and management of complications to decrease mortality, improve recovery, maintain function and improve patient and carer experience.

Nurses as Care Coordinators

The sharing of care between geriatricians/physicians, orthopaedic surgeons and anaesthetists during transitions between the emergency department (ED), hospital ward, theatre, rehabilitation and home is complex and has the potential to become fragmented, directionless and overwhelming for patients and carers without the coordination role of orthogeriatric nurses. The National Institute for Health and Care Excellence (NICE 2011) describe the most effective pathway of care to be that of the hip fracture programme, a pathway of care co-ordinated from admission to the ED to discharge following rehabilitation. Coordination of care during hospital admission is usually facilitated by orthogeriatric nurses, However, few organisations have yet achieved coordination to the end of rehabilitation when transfer into rehabilitation services or community services are involved. The coordinator role is often a specialist or advanced practice nursing role and titles may include 'hip fracture nurse specialist', 'trauma coordinator' and 'nurse practitioner'. Roles vary depending on the size and culture of the hip fracture service. The key aspect of the role is to have close relationships with other members of the hip fracture team, the patient and their carers.

Fragility Hip Fracture

Fragility hip fracture is the term usually used to refer to a proximal femoral fracture (PFF) with underlying bone fragility caused by osteopenia or osteoporosis (as discussed in Chapter 18). It is a common, but serious injury that predominantly occurs in later life. Such fractures occur in the bone region between the edge of the femoral head and 5 cm below the lesser trochanter (Figure 19.1). Half of all patients admitted with a hip fracture have had a previous fragility fracture, a 'signal' fracture that gives healthcare providers the opportunity to commence treatment to reduce the likelihood of hip fracture occurring (refer to Chapter 18), aiming to reduce the number of patients sustaining a hip fracture in the future.

To contextualise the impact on orthopaedic trauma units of managing patients with a hip fracture; according to the NHFD (2017) hip fracture is the most common serious injury in older people, the most common reason for older people to need emergency anaesthesia and surgery, and the most frequent cause of death following an accident. Patients may remain in hospital for several weeks, leading to one and a half million hospital bed days being used each year. Since 2016, the overall length of stay has fallen slightly (from 20.6 to 20.0 days), but at any one time patients recovering from hip fracture still occupy over 3600 hospital beds (3159 in England, 325 in Wales and 133 in Northern Ireland), a figure equivalent to 1 in 45 of all hospital beds in England and Northern Ireland, and 1 in 33 hospital beds in Wales. The average age of a person with a hip fracture is 83 years for men and 84 years for women. In the UK about 70 000–75 000 hip fractures occur each year, and the total annual cost (including medical and social care) for all UK

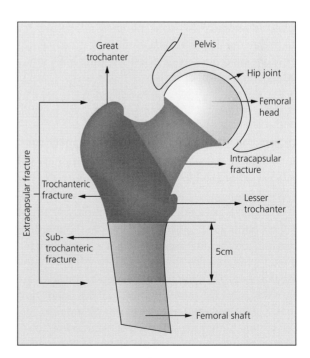

Figure 19.1 Classification of hip fracture. *Source:* From Parker and Johansen (2006) with permission.

cases is estimated to be about £2 billion (NHFD 2010). Most expenditure is accounted for by hospital bed days and by health and social aftercare costs. A similar picture is reported in many other nations, for example Australia, Canada and Sweden (Kanis et al. 2012), although statistics suggest that rates are beginning to decline in some areas (Leslie et al. 2009; Pasco et al. 2011).

For many previously fit patients, sustaining a hip fracture means loss of mobility and, for some frailer patients, the permanent loss of independence and their ability to live at home. About a quarter of patients admitted to hospital following hip fracture come from institutional care and in western nations around 10–20% of those admitted from home ultimately move to institutional care (Dyer et al. 2021).

At 1 year following hip fracture, mortality is reported to be approximately 30% (Parker and Anand 1991; Scottish Intercollegiate Guidelines Network 2009; British Orthopaedic Association/British Geriatric Society 2007) but fewer than half of deaths are attributable to the fracture itself, reflecting the frailty of individuals and associated high prevalence of comorbidities and complications. It is often the occurrence of a fall and consequent fracture that signals underlying ill-health. Hence, hip fracture is by no means an exclusively surgical concern. Its effective management requires the coordinated application of nursing, medical, surgical, anaesthetic and multidisciplinary rehabilitation skills and a comprehensive approach covering the entire journey from emergency care to discharge. Increasingly the approach of an orthogeriatric model has been adopted in caring for patients following hip fracture, demonstrating significant improvements in care and patient outcomes along with reduced mortality.

Diagnosis

Patients with a hip fracture typically present to emergency services unable to walk and may exhibit shortening and external rotation of the affected limb. Frequently, but not exclusively, they give a history of trauma and have hip pain. In some instances, patients may complain only of vague pain in their buttock, knee, thigh, groin or back, and their ability to walk may be unaffected. When it is suspected that a patient has a hip fracture, the priority is early assessment, ensuring that they are clinically stable, and then they are prioritised for an X-ray to confirm the diagnosis. Many hospitals in the UK have a fast-track protocol for patients suspected as having a hip fracture (Audit Commission 2000), and they work towards the Royal College of Emergency Medicine (2010) clinical standard that 90% of patients are X-rayed within 60 minutes of arrival in ED.

Most hip fractures are easily identified using plain X-rays, but an apparently normal X-ray does not necessarily exclude a fractured hip. Where there is doubt regarding the diagnosis (e.g. a radiologically normal hip X-ray in a patient who remains symptomatic) and where the radiographs have been reviewed by a radiologist, it is suggested that alternative imaging should be performed. The suggested diagnostic procedure is magnetic resonance imaging (MRI), but if this is not available within 24 hours, or is contraindicated, computed tomography (CT) should be undertaken (NICE 2011).

Management

Surgical intervention is the treatment of choice for almost all patients following hip fracture. Exceptions are those in whom the fracture is already healing in a satisfactory alignment and those whose expected survival is, for reasons unrelated to the hip fracture, very short. The timing of surgery has been shown to be important.

Hip fractures are divided into two main groups depending on their relationship to the capsule of the hip joint (Figures 19.1 and 19.2). Those within the joint capsule are termed *intracapsular* or *femoral neck* fractures. Those below the capsule are *extracapsular*. The extracapsular group is then further subclassified into *trochanteric* and *subtrochanteric* fractures. There is a practical basis to the division into intracapsular and extracapsular fractures relating to both the blood supply of the femoral head and the mechanics of fixation (Figure 19.3). It is therefore inaccurate to classify all hip fractures as fractures of the neck of the femur as this region is involved only in some fractures and the terminology should be used carefully to avoid confusion since the classification has a significant impact on the treatment and care required. The recommended

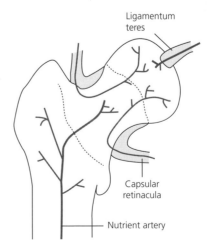

Figure 19.2 The blood supply to the head and neck of femur.

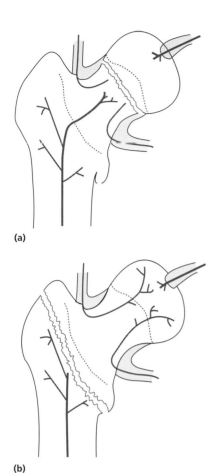

(a)

(b)

Figure 19.3 Examples of disruption of the blood supply to the head and neck of the femur following fracture. (a) Minimal disruption of the blood supply following an extracapsular fracture, e.g. intertrochanteric fracture, and (b) significant disruption of the blood supply following intracapsular fracture, e.g. subcapital fracture.

surgical procedures for the different fracture groups are described in the following sections.

Undisplaced Intracapsular Fractures

Surgical treatment is almost mandatory. Some impacted fractures may be difficult to diagnose but prognosis for impacted or undisplaced fractures is good following internal fixation conducted with a widely used method that is familiar to the surgeon such as cancellous bone screw or sliding hip screws (Mak et al. 2010).

Displaced Intracapsular Fractures

Surgical treatment is almost mandatory for displaced intracapsular fractures as they will not unite without fixation or arthroplasty. Hip replacement arthroplasty is used in patients with a displaced intracapsular fracture (hemi-arthroplasty or total hip replacement) because of the risk of avascular necrosis of the femoral head due to disruption to local blood supply resulting from displacement of the fracture. The femoral

head derives its blood supply from three sources (Figures 19.3): the nutrient artery and vessels from the joint capsule and the ligament teres. When the femoral head is displaced the blood supply from all but the foveal artery within the ligamentum teres is disrupted and this may be severe enough to cause ischaemia, resulting in avascular necrosis (bone death) and subsequent collapse of the femoral head. This leads to destruction of the joint, causing ongoing pain and deformity. Hemi-arthroplasty (Figure 19.4) is commonly performed for displaced intra-capsular fractures. Compared to uncemented arthroplasty, cemented arthroplasty is said to improve hip function and is associated with lower residual pain post-operatively. Blood loss from an intracapsular fracture at the time of injury is minimal because of the poor vascular supply at the fracture site (Association of Anaesthetists of Great Britain and Ireland [AAGBI] 2011).

There is increasing evidence to support total hip replacement (THR) (see Chapter 14) over hemi-arthroplasty in selected patients (Figures 19.4 and 19.5). This is recommended by NICE (2011), who recommend that THR is offered to patients with a displaced intracapsular fracture who prior to the fracture:

- were able to walk independently **and**
- are not cognitively impaired **and**
- are medically fit for anaesthesia and the procedure.

THR is recommended for active patients or those with preexisting joint disease (e.g. osteoarthritis) rather than hemi-arthroplasty because of potential wear of the acetabulum and inferior functional outcome achieved with a hemi-arthroplasty. THR is, however, unsuitable for patients with dementia due to their reduced ability to follow post-operative movement restrictions and a consequent

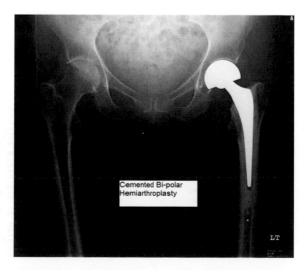

Figure 19.4 Hemiarthroplasty. *Source:* Reproduced with permission from Mr Philip John Roberts.

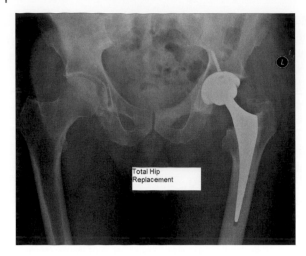

Figure 19.5 Total hip replacement. *Source:* Reproduced with permission from Mr Philip John Roberts.

higher dislocation rate. Patients need to be able to understand and follow the post-operative guidance to prevent dislocation, but if able to do so will achieve higher functional outcomes and those with underlying joint arthropathy will experience less pain.

Extracapsular Fractures

Management of extracapsular fractures should reflect the differences in presentation and symptoms. Blood loss from an extracapsular fracture is much greater than that from an intracapsular fracture; loss from the cancellous bone at this site may exceed 1 litre. The greater the degree of comminution and the larger the size of the bone fragments, the greater the blood loss. Greater periosteal disruption also causes extracapsular fractures to be considerably more painful than intracapsular fractures. They can be treated conservatively, healing after 6–8 weeks of traction and bed rest, but such management is associated with greatly increased morbidity and mortality, and a considerably reduced chance of the patient regaining independence and/or returning home (AAGBI 2011). Undisplaced extracapsular fractures are often treated with cannulated screws. Surgical intervention for other fractures is recommended as follows.

Intertrochanteric Fractures

Extra medullary implants such as a sliding hip screw are used in the fixation for patients with trochanteric fractures above and including the lesser trochanter (Figure 19.6) (NICE 2011). This stabilises the fracture, reduces pain and allows early mobility. The movement allowed by the implant in only one plane and axial loading of the fracture encourages bone healing.

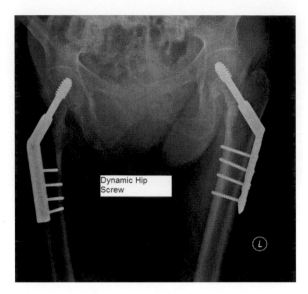

Figure 19.6 Dynamic hip screw. *Source:* Reproduced with permission from Mr Philip John Roberts.

Subtrochanteric Fractures

These fractures are less common, accounting for about 5–10% of all hip fractures. They present a considerable challenge to the surgeon as the high mechanical forces in this region lead to an increased risk of fixation failure. NICE (2011) recommend the use of an intramedullary nail to treat patients with a subtrochanteric fracture such as the proximal femoral nail (Figure 19.7), which requires shorter duration of surgery and

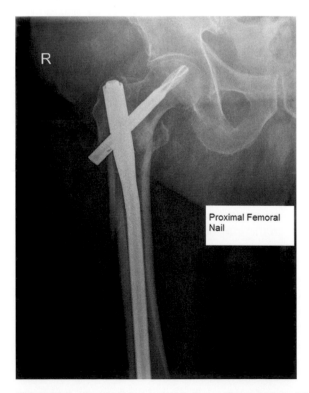

Figure 19.7 Proximal femoral nail. *Source:* Reproduced with permission from Mr Philip John Roberts.

shorter hospital stay. It also results in fewer orthopaedic complications and there is less need for major re-operations than with other types of fixation (Mak et al. 2010).

Atypical Femur Fractures

Atypical femoral fractures are unusual fragility fractures in the subtrochanteric region of the femur and along the femoral diaphysis with unusual radiological appearance. They tend to occur in patients who are being treated with antiresorptive medications (e.g. bisphosphonates) for osteoporosis although the link with these is uncertain (Black et al. 2020). Although rare, these fractures are being reported more often and require a different approach to management. There is also considerable debate about whether to continue antiresorptive treatment for osteoporosis (Shane et al. 2014).

Orthogeriatric Nursing Competencies

Patients with hip fractures represent a significant challenge for the healthcare team because of the complexity of patient needs, especially as nursing teams are struggling to provide adequate fundamental and expert nursing care due to a global shortage of nurses. Nurses spend the most clinical time directly with patients and represent the largest group of healthcare professionals, so are in a central position to have a significant impact on patient care and outcomes. Surgery for hip fracture is now so well-crafted that its direct complications are unusual. Patients who struggle to recover do so due to pre-existing problems such as frailty and, cognitive and nutritional problems that worsen following surgery and can be significantly impacted by effective nursing care.

Despite improving standards, however, there remains significant mortality and morbidity for patients following hip fracture. The factors that increase the risk of complications have been studied in great detail and many care pathways take these into account. Every attempt is made in services where there are audit and quality improvement measures in place to optimise patient care in the peri-operative period, particularly concerning surgical techniques, skill and timing of surgical procedures, anaesthetic practice and co-managed orthogeriatric care. What has not been studied is the impact of the nursing care that is not delivered due to operational issues such as inadequate staffing resources, skill mix and competing care priorities. High patient acuity can contribute to the prioritisation of medical tasks over basic nursing tasks that can lead to difficulties for nurses in maintaining the wellbeing of frail elderly patients and complying with evidence-based care guidelines (Fitzgerald et al. 2020).

This patient group are at increased risk of the more familiar peri-operative complications such as venous thromboembolism, pneumonia and urinary tract infections (see Chapter 9). Normal age-related changes, the physiological and psychological stress of the injury event and fracture, hospitalisation and chronic medical conditions also predispose them to other serious problems, including inappropriately managed pain, malnutrition, dehydration, constipation, pressure ulcers, delirium, functional decline and death (Koval and Zuckerman 1994; Mak et al. 2010).

Nurses should be mindful of the complications that can occur in older patients and must monitor them closely at the same time as liaising with family and carers to promptly detect changes in patient condition. The most significant care issues relate to pain, malnutrition, dehydration, constipation, delirium, pressure ulcers and mobility/function. The quality of care is reflected in these aspects of care, and they are issues that respond to nursing management strategies, so can be referred to as *nurse sensitive quality indicators*. The following evidence-based principles of care following hip fracture have been identified in a set of international guidelines (Meehan et al. 2019).

Pain

Hip fracture is painful and early surgical fracture fixation provides the most effective pain relief. Accurate pain assessment is the foundation for successful pain management, but assessment of pain in older adults needs a multidimensional stepwise approach and although standardised tools can be used, the information they provide needs to be individualised for specific patient needs (Fischer et al. 2018). Good pain management in the early stages of care will promote comfort and confidence in movement for the patient as well as reduce the incidence of complications. Later, if pain is poorly controlled, mobilisation will be delayed, bringing with it the complications of prolonged immobility, leading to increased dependency and an associated rise in the risk of post-operative delirium.

A local evidence-based analgesia protocol should be followed. Simple analgesics such as paracetamol should be prescribed and administered regularly (unless contraindicated), and additional opioids or nerve blocks used in conjunction with the paracetamol to provide pain relief as required. NICE (2011) suggest that pain assessment should be conducted immediately on presentation at hospital and analgesia should be given routinely at that time. Within 30 minutes of administering initial analgesia, a further assessment should be made, followed with additional analgesia if required. Assessment and PRN administration of analgesia should occur hourly until the patient is settled and then regularly as part of routine care. The aim of analgesia should be to give sufficient pain relief to allow the movement necessary for nursing care, investigations and rehabilitation.

Many studies support the administration of regional nerve blocks (femoral nerve block or fascia iliac nerve block) on admission to hospital and in the early post-operative period. Nerve blocks are known to be effective in reducing pain and muscle spasm, meaning that less opioid analgesia is needed and that the potential effects of opioid administration are reduced, including delirium, respiratory depression and constipation (Griffiths et al. 2021).

Pain in older people is often under-reported, undetected and even ignored by practitioners, with cognitive impairment increasing this risk of this. Pain assessment scales alone do not provide all the essential information needed to guide management; understanding pain type, onset, duration, location, predisposing factors and influences is essential. The acute pain of the fracture is often combined with chronic pain related to other comorbid conditions such as osteoarthritis or malignancy. It is essential that pain is assessed both at rest and on movement. Visual analogue pain scores (VAPSs) should be recorded before and after the administration of analgesia (RCP/British Geriatric Society/Pain Society 2007). This form of self-reporting is the single most reliable measurement of pain. Verbal reports of pain are also valid and reliable in patients with mild to moderate dementia or delirium. The diagnosis of pain in a patient with cognitive impairment due to dementia or delirium may be particularly difficult and requires familiarity with the patient and information from relatives or carers.

Many studies have shown that patients with cognitive impairment are given less analgesia than their unimpaired counterparts. Nursing and medical staff rely on self-reporting of pain and often fail to consider other indicators of pain such as moaning, sighing or holding a guarded posture, tachycardia and high blood pressure (British Orthopaedic Association 2007). The use of a tool to tell staff about the individual needs of a person with dementia, such as the 'This is Me' tool available from the Alzheimer's Society (2021), encourages relatives and carers to document individual patient information and personal behaviours. Working with families of patients with dementia or delirium to complete this document will support pain assessment. See Chapter 11 for further consideration of general issues related to pain management.

Malnutrition

Malnutrition (MN) is observed in a third of hospital inpatients and is directly associated with adverse outcomes and mortality (Holst et al. 2021). It has many causes and is defined as:

> . . . deficiencies, excesses or imbalances in a person's intake of energy and/or nutrients. Undernutrition includes energy or macronutrient deficiencies (protein-energy malnutrition) and micronutrient deficiencies or insufficiencies, while overnutrition is routinely associated with overweight, obesity and diet-related noncommunicable diseases. (Geirsdóttir et al. 2021 p4)

Malnutrition is a common clinical problem in patients with a hip fracture, placing them at increased risk of complications (Han et al. 2021). It is often associated with ageing and is also linked with falls, osteoporosis and frailty, and characterised by diminished hunger and thirst, along with chronic illness patterns.

The Determinants of Malnutrition in Aged Persons (DoMAP) model (Volkert et al. 2019a; see Figure 19.8) highlights the factors that lead to malnutrition in older people, including those with hip fracture. Understanding these factors is a critical aspect of nutritional assessment. All the factors represented in the model are possible causes of malnutrition, individually and collectively. The levels within the model denote different requirements for intervention, described by Volkert et al. (2019a, p. 4) as follows:

- *Level 1 (dark green)*: Central etiologic mechanisms.
- *Level 2 (light green)*: Factors in this level directly lead to one of the three mechanisms in Level 1 (e.g. swallowing problems may directly cause low intake).
- *Level 3 (yellow)*: Factors in this level may indirectly lead to one (or more) of the three central mechanisms through one (or more) of the direct factors in the light green triangle (e.g. stroke may cause low intake via dysphagia or difficulties with eating).
- *Surrounding factors in red* are age-related changes and general aspects which also contribute to the development of malnutrition, but act even more indirectly or subtle.

Many older people do not eat and drink adequate amounts while in hospital, putting their health and recovery at risk; hospitalised hip fracture inpatients do even less well. During hospitalisation, hip fracture patients have been shown to only receive half their recommended daily energy, protein and other nutritional requirements (Roigk 2018). Bonjour et al. (1996) identified that there is a high prevalence of malnutrition in hip fracture patients at the time of fracture and admission. There is then a rapid deterioration in nutritional status whilst in hospital that is

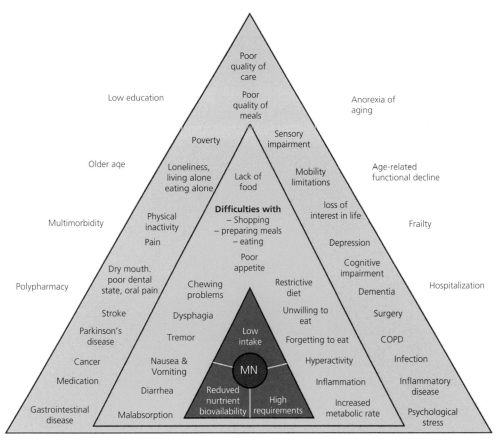

Figure 19.8 DoMAP model: Determinants of malnutrition in aged persons. *Source:* Volkert et al. (2019a) / Springer Nature / CC BY 4.0.

associated with increased metabolic requirements due to the injury, fracture and surgery (Enroth et al. 2006).

Routine nursing care must include an assessment of nutritional intake: a best practice standard required in all hip fracture audits. Identification of malnourished patients (or those at risk) needs to then initiate a plan and action for enhanced nutrition and, where appropriate, referral for dietetic advice. General issues related to nutrition and the orthopaedic patient are considered in more detail in Chapter 10.

Malnutrition is an interdisciplinary concern that requires effective collaboration, liaison and communication between all members of the team (Santy-Tomlinson et al. 2021a). It is crucial that all staff understand the importance of adequate nutritional intake for patients recovering from hip fracture and that specific attention is given to helping people to eat. Simple practical measures such as engaging additional carers or volunteers to assist in nutrition can be effective, as well as other strategies such as mealtimes protected from disturbance and systems that highlight patients at risk of malnutrition, such as coloured meal trays.

Collaborating with older adults themselves, as well as within the team providing their care, is pivotal to providing effective nutritional care for those with, or at risk of, malnutrition. Nurses, in collaboration with interdisciplinary team members, are vital for this process as they spend the most clinical time with patients and are often the supervisors of eating and drinking (Geirsdóttir et al. 2021).

In the absence of adequate oral nutrition, several approaches to nutritional support have been studied (Avenell et al. 2016) and the strongest evidence for the effectiveness of nutritional supplementation exists for oral protein and energy and multinutrient feeds (providing energy, protein, vitamins and minerals), which may reduce the risk of complication and possibly the length of stay within the first year following hip fracture (Holst et al. 2021).

Dehydration and Acute Kidney Injury

Dehydration is depletion in total body water content due to pathological fluid loss, diminished water intake or a combination of both (Meehan et al. 2019). It is common among hip fracture patients (Ekman et al. 2020), carrying with it significant risk of adverse consequences. Dehydration decreases the circulating blood volume, reducing perfusion of organs and tissues, potentially leading to delirium, acute kidney injury (AKI), pressure ulcers, falls, venous thromboembolism and urinary tract infections. Older adults admitted to hospital from home or other care facilities can present with dehydration for several reasons, categorised as:

1) low intake dehydration
2) volume depletion dehydration.

Dehydration and its associated terms are defined by The European Society for Clinical Nutrition and Metabolism (Volkert et al. 2019b, p. 35) as:

Dehydration: A shortage of water (fluid) in the body caused by insufficient intake of water (*low-intake dehydration*) or excessive loss of water (*volume depletion*) or a combination of both.

Low-intake dehydration: A shortage of water caused by low intake. Leads to loss of both intracellular and extracellular fluid, raises osmolality.

Volume depletion: An excessive loss of water and salts caused by bleeding, fever, vomiting, diarrhoea or other causes. Leads to loss of extracellular fluid but not intracellular fluid, keeps osmolality normal or low.

Low-intake dehydration includes pre-existing (prior to hospitalisation) restricted fluid intake, which may relate to normal age-related changes such as diminished thirst reflex and subsequent diminished fluid intake. Many patients who suffer from incontinence or frequency self-regulate fluid intake to reduce the risk of incontinence and because of difficulty accessing toilet facilities. A long post-fall lie on the floor can also result in significantly reduced fluid intake. Diuretic administration and peri-operative or post-trauma fluid loss from bleeding, fever and/or gastrointestinal disturbances can also result in volume depletion dehydration. Box 19.2 provides an overview of a study that explored the signs of dehydration.

Immediately following admission, optimised peri-operative fluid management helps to reduce the incidence of dehydration and therefore reduces morbidity and hospital stay (Lewis et al. 2016; Kusen et al. 2021). Intravenous fluid replacement must be prescribed on admission and administered accurately. Strict fluid balance monitoring of both intake and output along with shortest possible periods of pre-operative fasting also reduce the chances of dehydration and its associated pre- and post-operative complications. Pre-existing comorbid conditions, age and complex polypharmacy (e.g. diuretics and nephrotoxic medication such as angiotensin-converting enzyme [ACE] inhibitors used in the management of hypertension and heart failure and non-steroidal anti-inflammatory drugs [NSAIDs] used for pain relief) affect renal function.

Box 19.2 Recognising Dehydration

Ekman L, Johnson P, Hahn RG (2020) Signs of dehydration after hip fracture surgery: An observational descriptive study. Medicina (Kaunas) 56(7):361. 10.3390/medicina56070361.

Ekman et al. (2020) acknowledge that dehydration is an issue following hip fracture surgery but argue that the optimal tools to identify dehydration have not been published.

The aim of their study was to compare the characteristics of older people who had undergone surgery for hip fracture and were classified as dehydrated according to data collected during patient assessment. Thirty-eight patients aged between 65 and 97 (mean 82) years were studied after being admitted to a geriatric department for rehabilitation after hip fracture surgery. Each participant underwent blood analyses, urine sampling and clinical examination. Three indices were used to identify dehydration:

hyperosmolality: defined as ≥ 300 mosmol/kg ($n = 7$)
low fluid intake: patients who drank ≤ 800 ml of liquid on the day of admission
concentrated urine: urine-specific gravity ≥ 1.025

The results demonstrated that patients drank a mean of 1008 ml (standard deviation 309 ml) of fluid during their first day. Serum osmolality increased significantly with plasma concentrations of sodium, creatinine and urea. Seven patients had high serum osmolality (≥ 300 mosmol/kg) that correlated with the presence of tongue furrows ($P<0.04$), poor skin turgor ($P<0.03$) and pronounced albuminuria ($P<0.03$). Eight patients had concentrated urine (urine-specific gravity ≥ 1.025) that correlated with a low intake of liquid and a decrease in body weight during the past month of -3.0 kg (25–75th percentiles, -5.1 to -0.9) versus $+0.2$ kg (-1.9 to $+2.7, P<0.04$).

The authors concluded that renal fluid conservation of water, in the form of either hyperosmolality or concentrated urine, was found in 40% of the patients in the study. Hyperosmolality might not indicate a more severe fluid deficit than is indicated by concentrated urine but suggests an impaired ability to concentrate the urine.

The findings of the study help us to understand the parameters that might be useful in making a clinical assessment of dehydration. It is helpful that the study focused on patients who have undergone hip fracture surgery as dehydration is particularly common in this population and much needs to be done in developing care bundles that prevent and treat dehydration, particularly following admission and in the peri-operative period.

AKI is seen in 13–18% of all people admitted to hospital, with older people being particularly at risk, often in specialties such as orthopaedics and trauma where practitioners may not be familiar with the optimum care, leading to care deficiencies in prevention and management (NICE 2019). AKI is a significant cause of death following hip fracture (Rantalaiho et al. 2019), particularly in the frail patient, and is largely attributable to dehydration. Baseline renal function assessment alongside a medication review is an important part of recognising those patients who need intensive intervention to prevent deterioration. Establishing renal function may be difficult following hip fracture as patients may be acutely dehydrated on admission with or without the presence of previously existing chronic renal dysfunction. Close monitoring of fluid balance and blood biochemistry is essential to prevent and/or identify renal injury.

NICE (2019) (see Box 19.3) provide guidelines for the prevention, detection and management of AKI on which practice following hip fracture and surgery should be based.

Constipation

Constipation is a significant risk for patients following hip fracture and can lead to other complications, including fatal bowel obstruction. Constipation prevention and recognition are often overlooked aspects of practice. Assessment and prevention should be fundamental aspects of care from early in the pathway. The effect of ageing, frailty, use of opioid analgesics including codeine (even in low doses), dehydration, altered diet (particularly decreased fibre in the diet) and lack of mobility all increase this risk (Trads and Pedersen 2015). Constipation is considered in more detail in Chapter 9.

Box 19.3   NICE (2019) Acute Kidney Injury: Prevention, Detection, and Management

NICE (2019) Acute kidney injury: prevention, detection, and management. ng148 National Institute for Health and Care Excellence, www.nice.org.uk/guidance/ng148

The guideline emphasises early intervention along with risk assessment, prevention measures, early recognition and treatment of AKI. It is aimed particularly at the non-specialist setting, where care deficiencies are most common.

Altered Cognitive Function

The cognitive syndromes of dementia, delirium and depression are common in patients following hip fracture. Refer to the further reading and resources at the end of this chapter for more information on these cognitive syndromes. Such is the frequency and effect of delirium on hip fracture patients that it warrants additional consideration here. Delirium is terrifying for the patient, with approximately 50% remembering the episode later.

Delirium (sometimes called acute confusional state) is a common clinical syndrome characterised by disturbed consciousness, cognitive function and/or perception that has an acute onset and fluctuating course (Young and Inouye 2007) that usually develops over 1–2 days. It is a serious condition that is associated with poor outcomes, but it can be prevented and treated if staff are vigilant for the warning signs and prompt action is taken.

Delirium may be present on arrival to hospital or it may develop during the hospital stay. It can be hypoactive or hyperactive, but some people show signs of both (mixed delirium). People with hyperactive delirium have heightened arousal and can be restless, agitated and aggressive. People with hypoactive delirium become withdrawn, quiet and sleepy. Hypoactive and mixed delirium can be more difficult to recognise. It can be difficult to distinguish between delirium and dementia, and some people may have both conditions. If clinical uncertainty exists over the diagnosis, the person should be managed initially for delirium (Cross 2018).

Older people and people with dementia, severe illness or a hip fracture are more at risk of delirium. The prevalence of delirium in people is approximately 10–50% of people having surgery. It is suggested that it may be as high as 60% in patients admitted with a hip fracture (NICE 2010).

There is a significant burden associated with this condition. Compared with people who do not develop delirium, people who develop delirium may (Cross 2018):

- need to stay longer in hospital or in critical care
- have an increased incidence of dementia
- have more hospital-acquired complications, such as falls and pressure ulcers
- be more likely to need to be admitted to long-term care if they are in hospital
- be more likely to die.

Assessment

Assessment and establishment of baseline cognition is an important, but often challenging, first step in delirium detection. Close communication between the nursing team and family or carers is essential. Assessment of patients following hip fracture who will be proceeding swiftly to surgery requires

Table 19.2 Predisposing and precipitating factors for delirium (Meehan et al. 2019).

Predisposing factors	Precipitating factors
• Age	• Change in environment
• Dementia or cognitive impairment	• Sleep deprivation
• Depression	• Loss of sensory aids/clues
• History of delirium	• Physical restraints
• Severe illness or hip fracture	• Constipation
• Polypharmacy	• Urinary retention
• Malnutrition/dehydration	• Sepsis
• Functional dependency	• Acute illness (e.g. myocardial infarction)
• Sensory impairment	• Untreated pain or excess use of analgesics

tools that allow rapid identification of those at risk. Best practice guidance (NICE 2011) expects that all patients have an abbreviated Mental Test Score pre-operatively. Although this is not an assessment tool for delirium, it will provide baseline information relating to cognitive function. Post-operatively assessment continues, along with documentation of a 4AT (rapid clinical test for delirium), an easy-to-use validated tool used to assess for the presence of delirium. Table 19.2 provides a list of predisposing (currently existing) and precipitating (potential causes) for delirium. The prompt recognition of predisposing factors is essential because (i) many of these factors are modifiable or can be improved and (ii) the non-modifiable risk factors raise awareness of the risk of delirium, providing the impetus for interventions.

Prevention and Management of Delirium

It has been suggested that prevention of delirium is possible in up to 30% of cases (Inouye et al. 1999; Marcantonio et al. 2001). Attention to risk factors, particularly in patients with underlying dementia, should be addressed early and good communication with patients, family and carers can help practitioners to recognise subtle changes. Alongside comprehensive geriatric assessment, interventions targeting risk factors such as promoting the use of glasses and hearing aids, maintaining normal night and day routines, and using prompts such as clocks or calendars to orientate to time and place help reduce delirium risk.

Nursing interventions are important in reducing the incidence and intensity of delirium. If delirium is suspected, it is important to identify and manage any potential individual or combination of underlying causes (British Geriatric Society 2005) by:

- seeking early comprehensive orthogeriatric review
- withdrawing or reducing culprit drugs such as opioids, where appropriate

- effective management of pain
- monitoring and screening for infection
- avoiding the use of devices that increase the risk of infection, such as urinary catheters
- identifying and managing alcohol withdrawal as this increases the likelihood of patients developing delirium
- communicating in an effective and reassuring manner which is reorientating (e.g. explaining where the person is, who you are and what your role is)
- inviting and encouraging family, friends and carers to participate in care
- considering medication and other methods to maintain safety, such as low beds and higher levels of supervision, if a person with delirium is distressed or considered a risk to themselves or others and verbal and non-verbal de-escalation techniques are ineffective or inappropriate.

Pressure Injuries

Development of pressure injuries is a frequent complication of hip fracture and surgery, ageing skin, multiple comorbidities, impact skin injury and wound healing, Pressure injuries are significant breaches in patient safety but remain common following hip fracture, resulting in short- and long-term pain and distress for patients (Hommel and Santy-Tomlinson 2018).

Patients with pressure ulcers following hip fractures require significantly more nursing care, longer hospital stay, increased hospital costs and use more healthcare resources following discharge compared to patients without pressure ulcers (Chaves et al. 2010). Given the very high risk, prevention and management of pressure ulcers in this group of patients is central to effective, high-quality care. Chapter 12 provides detailed evidence-based advice for both prevention and management of pressure ulcers applicable to a patient with a hip fracture.

Rehabilitation of the Older Person Following Hip Fracture

Although Chapter 6 considered rehabilitation for patients with orthopaedic conditions and following orthopaedic surgery or injury, specific aspects of rehabilitation must be considered specifically for patients following hip fracture. Patients of advanced age are more likely to have comorbid medical conditions that will adversely affect rehabilitation abilities and outcomes if the rehabilitation process is not managed appropriately. After hip fracture surgery, an older person's recovery is enhanced if they are provided with an optimistic, well-coordinated rehabilitation programme.

The rehabilitation approach should be part of the care process from as early as possible to help prevent functional decline and complications. Rehabilitation should be managed by a multidisciplinary team (physiotherapy, occupational therapy, dietician, social work, psychology and medicine) with the integration of orthogeriatric and rehabilitation services (Dyer et al. 2021).

Rehabilitation needs to be a collaborative process that involves professionals, patients and their carers. Effective rehabilitation programmes begin pre-operatively, when realistic expectations and timings should be discussed with patients and their carers. The main facilitator of rehabilitation in orthogeriatrics is comprehensive geriatric assessment (CGA). The central concept of CGA is a holistic, patient-centred care approach that focuses on assessment of older people with complex problems, emphasises functional status and utilises the interdisciplinary skills of the whole orthogeriatric team. The information gained from CGA is used by the team to set realistic rehabilitation goals in collaboration with patients and their carers.

Such is the importance of early mobilisation as a first step in rehabilitation that the National Hip Fracture Database (2019) has included as a standard the assessment by a physiotherapist on the first post-operative day and the necessity to record if the patient was able to get out from their bed on the first post-operative day in the database and this forms part of the best practice guidance.

In the NHFD report for 2018 (NHFD 2019), in approximately 20% of recorded cases this standard was not achieved.

In the hospital setting rehabilitation is mainly a role for the nursing team working alongside their allied healthcare colleagues; the presence of nurses over the entire 24 hours means that rehabilitation actions can be continued and repeated throughout the day as an integral part of care. Rehabilitation is not, however, only focused on remobilisation, but includes motivation, regaining confidence, overcoming the fear of falls and achieving functional ability on all levels.

Orthopaedic rehabilitation models are often fragmented and have not been well evaluated in relation to functional outcomes when compared to length of hospital stay. There are, however, three main pathways for patients following hip fracture described by NICE (2011):

1) The traditional pathway of care is that a patient with hip fracture is admitted to a trauma ward where the orthopaedic surgical team lead both surgical care and subsequent rehabilitation. Geriatrician input to such wards is limited, with referrals and medical queries being dealt with on a consultative basis by the on-call medical registrar or on occasional geriatrician visits. This results in the absence of a proactive geriatrician lead within the multidisciplinary team.

2) A more collaborative model of care through formal orthogeriatric care, with older trauma patients admitted to a trauma ward or specialised unit under the joint care of both geriatricians and orthopaedic surgeons.

3) Hip fracture programmes, with the orthogeriatric medical team contributing to joint pre-operative patient assessment and increasingly taking the lead for post-operative medical care, multidisciplinary rehabilitation and discharge planning, with ongoing governance for rehabilitation in hospital or as part of a community rehabilitation scheme as described below.

After initial surgical care and mobilisation in the first two models of care, early post-operative transfer to an orthogeriatric rehabilitation unit or mixed rehabilitation unit for ongoing treatment is another option. This may be additionally supported by community rehabilitation as early supported discharge or intermediate care at home. Patients are discharged home from the acute trauma ward or, in some cases, a rehabilitation ward within the hospital supported with a 4–6-week rehabilitation package. This service may include patients living in care homes but may be limited to patients returning to live independently in their own homes.

Cohort studies suggest that following hip fracture only 40–60% of people who survive are likely to recover their pre-fracture level of mobility. Up to 70% may recover their level of independence for basic activities of daily living, but this is variable and less than half of all people experiencing a hip fracture may regain their ability to perform instrumental activities of daily living (ADLs). The extent to which these outcomes can be improved with greater access to rehabilitation is not clear (Dyer et al. 2021).

Palliative and End-of-life Care for Patients Following Hip Fracture

Although palliative care originally focused on patients with cancer, it is now acknowledged that consideration for a palliative care approach should be made for people at the end of their lives for non-malignant as well as malignant disease. Palliative care is defined by the World Health Organization (2011) as:

> . . .an approach that improves the quality of life of patients and their families facing the problems associated with life threatening illness, through the

prevention and relief of suffering by means of early identification and impeccable assessment and treatment of pain and other problems, physical, psychosocial and spiritual. Palliative care affirms life and regards dying as a normal process and intends neither to hasten nor to prolong death. Using a team approach palliative care addresses the needs of patients and their families, including bereavement counselling if necessary.

This philosophy of care allows for physical, psychological, social and emotional care for patients, their families and carers when the patient with a hip fracture is frail and does not have the physical resilience to survive the trauma of the fracture and ensuing surgery. For some people the hip fracture may be an event that will hasten the end of life. The Covid-19 pandemic has demonstrated the vulnerability of older people following hip fracture: in 2019 (before the pandemic) the 30-day mortality for patients following hip fracture in the UK was 6.5% compared to 2020 when, for the first time since NHFD had been recording such data, an increase in recorded deaths to 8.3% was seen, meaning that over 1000 more people died following hip fracture during this first year of the COVID-19 pandemic (30-day mortality was three times higher for patients with COVID-19 than seen in those without the infection) (NHFD 2020).

Effective models of care for patients with hip fracture lend themselves to the inclusion of patient-centred palliative care when appropriate. Typically, palliative care is provided by an interdisciplinary team who focus on the assessment and treatment of pain and other symptoms while ensuring that care is enhanced by patient-centred communication and decision-making across the continuum of care settings, from hospital to home.

Identifying patients for whom a palliative care approach is most appropriate is difficult. Many patients presenting with hip fracture also have multiple comorbidities. In the 2011/12 NHFD report 67% of patients were graded at American Society of Anaesthesiologists Grade III or above, those who have severe systematic disease that limits activity or is life threatening. These may be the people for whom palliative care should be considered, but many such patients recover well post-operatively, leave hospital and have a good functional outcome and ongoing quality of life. Appropriate models of end-of-life care are currently a matter of considerable discussion.

End-of-life care is a key aspect of the support orthopaedic and orthogeriatric teams provide to patients and their families. In the NHFD Facilities Audit of 2018 (NHFD 2018), two-thirds of units reported that a treatment escalation plan, commonly known as 'ceilings of care', was routinely discussed with the patient or those important to them as a part of the admission assessment process. Since 2017, the NHFD has asked hip fracture teams to review the care offered to people who died as an inpatient following hip fracture; a request is designed to stimulate investigation by local teams, so that the root cause of each death is identified and can inform clinical governance and quality improvement processes. The audit also identifies which patients died following a resuscitation attempt as opposed to those in whom the end of life had been anticipated and managed following appropriate discussion of care priorities with the patient, their family and their carers. During 2017, 4541 people (6.9%) died as an inpatient. In 74.3% of patients death had been anticipated and appropriate end-of-life care was already in place.

It is the responsibility of the orthogeriatric or hip fracture team, through good communication with patients' families and carers, to identify those people who have been noticed to have a period of decline pre-fracture and for whom the physical insult of fall, fracture, surgery and hospitalisation may lead to the hastening of end of life. It then becomes the responsibility of the team to prepare the patient and family both physically and emotionally, but also to ensure that ongoing care and treatment is appropriate for the patient's needs. This may or may not include surgical intervention. If a hip fracture complicates or precipitates a terminal illness, surgery should be considered as part of a palliative care approach to minimise pain and other symptoms, not necessarily to regain functional ability (NICE 2011). Surgery provides significant pain relief that not only allows nursing interventions to be undertaken more comfortably but will facilitate transfer from an acute orthopaedic unit to either home or another care setting in keeping with the patient's and/or carers' end-of-life wishes.

Ethical Considerations in Treatment of Patients with Hip Fracture

Because of potential physical and mental vulnerability, a significant consideration in the care of patients with a hip fracture is their decision-making capacity. Many decisions need to be made along the pathway of care, including consent for surgery, discussion regarding escalation plans, ceilings of care and resuscitation status, and ongoing discharge planning, which may result in transition to long-term care facilities. It is suggested that there are high levels of delirium and dementia among patients with hip fractures. Among elderly hip fracture patients, the incidence of delirium is estimated to be 5–56% (Mitchell et al. 2017; Mosk et al. 2017). Dementia and delirium often coexist in patients with a hip fracture, with a detrimental effect on outcomes (Mitchell et al. 2017). Both conditions increase vulnerability and affect decision-making capacity.

In healthcare settings, capacity is assessed in the UK using the Mental Capacity Act (Department of Health 2005), using the following principles:

- Always presume the patient has capacity.
- Capacity changes over time in both directions.
- Support people to have capacity through education and timing (e.g. pain must be managed, the effect of opioids should be considered).
- People can make bad decisions, despite having decision-making capacity.
- Treatment decisions must be in the patient's best interest.
- Where a decision is to be made without involvement of the patient, the least restrictive option should be made.

Assessment of capacity is specific to the decision being made at any given time, for example if a patient is assessed in the ED to lack capacity for surgery consent, this does not mean that they can be presumed as lacking capacity to refuse participation in a rehabilitation programme. The mental capacity assessment is a two-stage process:

Stage 1
- Is there a disturbance of the consciousness? (This could include delirium, dementia, intoxication etc.)

Stage 2
- Can the patient understand the information given relevant to the decision (such as potential complications of surgery or anaesthesia)?
- Can they retain the information?
- Can they weigh up the risks and benefits?
- Can they communicate their decision to others?

For the patient to consent to, or refuse, hip fracture surgery, they must be able to give consent voluntarily, based on a decision made following presentation and understanding of information about the procedure. The patient must be judged as having capacity to make that decision: they must be able to understand the information, remember it and use it to reach a decision. In older age groups the ability to assimilate information and communicate decisions may additionally be impaired by poor vision, hearing or speech, and steps should be taken to overcome these problems (AAGBI 2011). In some circumstances the operating team may be unable to satisfy themselves that the patient can give consent. If the patient does not have an advocate with a legal responsibility for decision-making on their behalf, an alternative approach needs to be found. Depending on national law and guidance, and following close liaison with family or carers, surgery may progress if two surgeons agree that it is in the patient's best interests.

The Mental Capacity Act also influences care in terms of identifying safeguarding and deprivation of liberty standards. It is an amendment to the Mental Capacity Act 2005, and applies to people in care homes and hospitals in England and Wales to whom proportionate restrictions and restraints may need to be applied in their best interests. In circumstances where a person's liberty might be deprived (e.g. using frequent physical or chemical restraint to help a person with hip fracture through a period of post-operative delirium), a hospital can apply for a standard authorisation from a local authority to have a third party appointed with legal powers to represent that person. This is commonly used where a patient may have a hyperactive delirium and is being denied leaving the room/ward or care is being provided under close observation.

Guidance on anticipatory decisions relating to whether or not cardiopulmonary resuscitation (CPR) should be attempted was updated in 2016 jointly by the British Medical Association, the Resuscitation Council (UK) and the Royal College of Nursing (UK) (BMA 2016), and it provides clarity on decision-making where the patient does not have capacity. Such decisions should be made using the ReSPECT Process (Recommended Summary Plan for Emergency Care and Treatment). While the patient retains capacity, the process aims to establish a summary of personalised recommendations for the person's clinical care in a future emergency in which they do not have capacity to make or express choices. Such emergencies may include death or cardiac arrest but are not limited to those events and may involve specific actions such as not wanting to be admitted to hospital, artificial feeding or any further active treatment. The process is intended to respect patient preferences as well as providing room for clinical judgement. The agreed realistic clinical recommendations that are recorded include a recommendation on whether or not CPR should be attempted if there is a cardiopulmonary arrest. Equally, the patient can decide (in collaboration with the clinician) an ethos of care along a continuum, for example strongly focusing on active treatment or strongly focusing on comfort or symptomatic management, or something in between.

Involvement of patients who have capacity is empowering and clinical teams are encouraged to use this approach. Where the patient is assessed as not having capacity, the Mental Capacity Act (Department of Health 2005) recommends the appointment of an advocate, a court-appointed individual with lasting power of attorney for care and welfare who has been identified as the patient's decision-maker if they lack capacity, or an advocate, normally a family member or friend, who can provide opinion and information that the clinical team can use in their decision-making in the patient's best interests

Hip Fracture Audit

Older people who sustain a hip fracture deserve to receive the best healthcare possible every time they present to a hospital, but there are variations in the quality of care that patients receive locally, nationally and globally. There have been increasing numbers of hip fracture audits taking place globally, but the process has been well-established in the UK and Ireland and several other countries for some years.

Where it has taken place and its results used to improve practice, hip fracture audit has had a significant impact on the quality of medical and surgical care, but with only a limited focus on nursing so far. It is essential that measures/indicators of the quality and value of nursing care are developed so that the impact of nursing care be measured, improved and monitored (MacDonald et al. 2018). The overall contribution of healthcare delivery is often measured in terms of the patient's resulting health status, outcomes, readmissions rates, length of stay, complication rates and mortality, but these do not always help to capture the specific contribution of nursing care (Santy-Tomlinson et al. 2021b). Assessment of baseline nutrition and development of pressure ulcer graded stage 2 or above are the only nurse-sensitive indicators within the NHFD, representing the impact of nursing in only a limited way. There is a need to develop a critical set of nurse-sensitive indicators for hip fracture care which specifically identify the role that nursing plays in patient outcomes.

Conclusion

Fragility hip fracture is a serious injury with potentially devastating and lasting effects on patients, especially those who are frail. Such fractures are caused by a combination of a fall and bone fragility due to osteoporosis. They carry a high burden of complications and patient outcomes can be poor, often resulting in poorer health, depleted physical and social function, depression, loss of independence and admission to residential care or death. The experience for the patient and their family is often described in terms of a devastating impact on daily life and wellbeing.

Standard management of fragility hip fracture, in all but a few cases, is surgical repair. This places the patient at risk of complications and health deterioration, especially if they are already frail. Nursing priorities following fragility hip fracture focus on fundamental assessment and care of the older adult as part of an orthogeriatric, collaborative and interdisciplinary approach in addition to meeting the needs of the frail older person with a major fracture and undergoing orthopaedic surgery.

Further Reading

Falaschi, P. and Marsh, D. (ed.) *Orthogeriatrics. Practical Issues in Geriatrics.* Cham: Springer https://link.springer.com/book/10.1007/978-3-030-48126-1.

Geirsdóttir, Ó.G. and Bell, J.J. (ed.) *Interdisciplinary Nutritional Management and Care for Older Adults. Perspectives in Nursing Management and Care for Older Adults.* Cham: Springer https://doi.org/10.1007/978-3-030-63892-4_1.

Hertz, K. and Santy-Tomlinson, J. (ed.) *Fragility Fracture Nursing. Perspectives in Nursing Management and Care for Older Adults.* Cham: Springer https://link.springer.com/book/10.1007/978-3-319-76681-2.

Resources

Dementia. A dementia game from Dementia NI that aims to raise awareness of the public regarding people living with dementia. www.dementiagame.com.

Delirium. Information from the Royal College of Psychiatrists for anyone who has experienced delirium, knows someone with delirium or is looking after people with delirium. www.rcpsych.ac.uk/mental-health/problems-disorders/delirium.

Depression in older adults. Information fromk the Royal College of Psychiatrists for people over 65 who have depression and their relatives, friends and carers. www.rcpsych.ac.uk/mental-health/problems-disorders/depression-in-older-adults.

References

AAGBI (2011) Management of Proximal Femoral Fractures. Association of Anaesthetists of Great Britain and Ireland. http://www.aagbi.org/sites/default/files/femoral%20fractures%202012_0.pdf.

Abrahamsen, C. and Nørgaard, B. (2021). Elderly patients' perspectives on treatment, care and rehabilitation after hip fracture: a qualitative systematic review. *Int. J. Orthopaedic Trauma Nurs.* 41: 100811. https://doi.org/10.1016/j.ijotn.2020.100811.

Audit Commission (2000). *United they Stand: Co-ordinating Care for Elderly Patients with Hip Fractures.* London: HMSO.

Avenell, A., Smith, T.O., Curtain, J. et al. (2016). Nutritional supplementation for hip fracture aftercare in older people. *Cochrane Database Syst. Rev.* (11): https://doi.org/10.1002/14651858.CD001880.pub6.

Black, D.M., Geiger, E.J., Eastell, R. et al. (2020). Atypical femur fracture risk versus fragility fracture prevention with bisphosphonates. *N. Engl. J. Med.* 383: 743–753. https://doi.org/10.1056/NEJMoa1916525.

BMA (2016) Decisions relating to cardiopulmonary resuscitation. BMA London. www.bma.org.uk/media/1816/bma-decisions-relating-to-cpr-2016.pdf.

Bonjour, J.P., Schurch, M.A., and Rizzoli, R. (1996). Nutritional aspects of hip fractures. *Bone* 18 (3): 139S–S144.

Brent, L., Hommel, A., Maher, A.B. et al. (2018). Nursing care of fragility fracture patients. *Injury* 49 (8): 1409–1412. https://doi.org/10.1016/j.injury.2018.06.036.

British Geriatric Society (2005) Guidelines for the Prevention, Diagnosis and Management of Delirium in Older People in Hospital. www.bgs.org.uk/index.php

British Orthopaedic Association (2007). *Standards for Trauma (BOAST). BOAST 1: Hip Fracture in the Older Person.* London: British Orthopaedic Association www.boa.ac.uk/LIB/LIBPUB/Documents/BOAST%201%20%20Hip%20Fracture%20in%20the%20Older%20Person%20Version%201%20-%202008.pdf (accessed 19 November 2013).

British Orthopaedic Association/British Geriatric Society (2007). *Care of Patients with Fragility Fractures.* London: British Orthopaedic Association www.bgs.org.uk/sites/default/files/content/attachment/2018-05-02/Blue%20Book%20on%20fragility%20fracture%20care.pdf.

Bruun-Olsen, V., Bergland, A., and Heiberg, K.E. (2018). "I struggle to count my blessings": recovery after hip fracture from the patients' perspective. *BMC Geriatrics* 18 (18): https://doi.org/10.1186/s12877-018-0716-4.

Chaves, L.M., Grypdonck, M., and DeFloor, T. (2010). Protocols for pressure ulcer prevention: are they evidence-based? *J. Adv. Nurs.* 66 (3): 562–572.

Cross, J. (2018). Nursing the patient with altered cognitive function. In: *Fragility Fracture Nursing. Perspectives in Nursing Management and Care for Older Adults* (ed. K. Hertz and J. Santy-Tomlinson). Cham: Springer https://doi.org/10.1007/978-3-319-76681-2_9.

Department of Health (2005). *Mental Capacity Act.* London: HMSO.

Dyer, S.M., Perracini, M.R., Smith, T. et al. (2021). Rehabilitation following hip fracture. In: *Orthogeriatrics. Practical Issues in Geriatrics* (ed. P. Falaschi and D. Marsh). Cham: Springer https://doi.org/10.1007/978-3-030-48126-1_12.

Ekman, L., Johnson, P., and Hahn, R.G. (2020). Signs of dehydration after hip fracture surgery: an observational descriptive study. *Medicina (Kaunas, Lithuania)* 56 (7): 361. https://doi.org/10.3390/medicina56070361.

EMbeds (2019) Silver Trauma Embeds. www.embeds.co.uk/2019/10/21/silver-trauma.

Enroth, M., Olsson, U.B., and Thorngren, K.G. (2006). Nutritional supplementation decreases hip fracture-related complications. *Clin. Orthopaedics Relat. Res.* 451: 212–217.

Fischer, T., Sirsch, E., Gnass, I., and Zwakhalen, S. (2018). The assessment of pain in older people. In: *Pain Management in Older Adults. Perspectives in Nursing Management and Care for Older Adults* (ed. G. Pickering, S. Zwakhalen and S. Kaasalainen). Cham: Springer https://doi.org/10.1007/978-3-319-71694-7_3.

Fitzgerald, A., Verrall, C., Henderson, J., and Willis, E. (2020). Factors influencing missed nursing care for older people following fragility hip fracture. *Collegian* 27 (4): 450–458. https://doi.org/10.1016/j.colegn.2019.12.003.

Geirsdóttir, Ó.G., Hertz, K., Santy-Tomlinson, J. et al. (2021). Overview of nutrition care in geriatrics and orthogeriatrics. In: *Interdisciplinary Nutritional Management and Care for Older Adults. Perspectives in Nursing Management and Care for Older Adults* (ed. Ó.G. Geirsdóttir and J.J. Bell). Cham: Springer https://doi.org/10.1007/978-3-030-63892-4_1.

Griffiths, R., Babu, S., Dixon, P., et al. (2021) *AAGBI Guideline for the management of hip fractures.* Association of Anaesthetists. https://anaesthetists.org/Home/Resources-publications/Guidelines/Management-of-hip-fractures-2020.

Han, T.S., Yeong, K., Lisk, R. et al. (2021). Prevalence and consequences of malnutrition and malnourishment in older individuals admitted to hospital with a hip fracture. *Eur. J. Clin. Nutr.* 75: 645–652. https://doi.org/10.1038/s41430-020-00774-5.

Holst, M., Geirsdóttir, Ó.G., and Bell, J.J. (2021). Nutrition support in older adults. In: *Interdisciplinary Nutritional Management and Care for Older Adults. Perspectives in Nursing Management and Care for Older Adults* (ed. Ó.G. Geirsdóttir and J.J. Bell). Cham: Springer https://doi.org/10.1007/978-3-030-63892-4_5.

Hommel, A. and Santy-Tomlinson, J. (2018). Pressure injury prevention and wound management. In: *Fragility Fracture Nursing. Perspectives in Nursing Management and Care for Older Adults* (ed. K. Hertz and J. Santy-Tomlinson).

Cham: Springer https://doi. org/10.1007/978-3-319-76681-2_7.

Inouye, S.K., Bogardus, S.T., Charpentier, P.A. et al. (1999). A multicomponent intervention to prevent delirium in hospitalized older people. *N. Engl. J. Med.* 340 (9): 669–676.

Kanis, J.A., Oden, A., McCloskey, E.V. et al. (2012). A systematic review of hip fracture incidence and probability of fracture worldwide. *Osteoporosis Int.* 23 (9): 2239–2256.

Koval, K.J. and Zuckerman, J.D. (1994). Hip fractures: overview and evaluation and treatment of femoral neck fractures. *J. Am. Acad. Orthopaedic Surgeons* 2 (3): 141–149.

Kusen, J.Q., van der Vet, P.C.R., Wijdicks, F.J.G. et al. (2021). Does preoperative hemodynamic preconditioning improve morbidity and mortality after traumatic hip fracture in geriatric patients? A retrospective cohort study. *Arch. Orthop. Trauma Surg.* 141: 1491–1497. https://doi. org/10.1007/s00402-020-03601-5.

Leslie, W.D., O'Donnell, S., Jean, S. et al. (2009). Trends in hip fractures in Canada. *J. Am. Med. Assoc.* 302 (8): 883–889.

Lewis, S.R., Butler, A.R., Brammar, A. et al. (2016). Perioperative fluid volume optimization following proximal femoral fracture. *Cochrane Database Syst. Rev* 3 (3): CD003004. https://doi.org/10.1002/14651858. CD003004.pub4. PMID: 26976366; PMCID: PMC7138038.

MacDonald, V., Maher, A.B., Mainz, H. et al. (2018). Developing and testing an international audit of nursing quality indicators for older adults with fragility hip fracture. *Orthopaedic Nurs.* 37 (2): 115–121. https://doi. org/10.1097/NOR.0000000000000431.

Mak, J., Cameron, I., and March, L. (2010). Evidence-based guidelines for the management of hip fractures in older persons: an update. *Med. J. Aust.* 192 (1): 37–41.

Marcantonio, E., Flacker, J., Wright, J., and Resnick, N. (2001). Reducing delirium after hip fracture: a randomized trial. *J. Am. Geriatrics Soc.* 49: 516–522.

Meehan, A.J., Maher, A.B., Brent, L. et al. (2019). The international collaboration of orthopaedic nursing (ICON): best practice nursing care standards for older adults with fragility hip fracture. *Int. J. Orthopaedic Trauma Nurs.* 32: 3–26. https://doi.org/10.1016/j.ijotn.2018.11.001.

Mitchell, R., Harvey, L., Brodaty, H. et al. (2017). One-year mortality after hip fracture in older individuals: the effects of delirium and dementia. *Arch. Gerontol. Geriatrics* 72: 135–141. https://doi.org/10.1016/j.archger.2017.06.006.

Mosk, C.A., Mus, M., Vroemen, J.P. et al. (2017). Dementia and delirium, the outcomes in elderly hip fracture patients. *Clin. Interv. Aging* 12: 421–430.

NHFD (2010) *The National Hip Fracture Database National Report 2010*. www.nhfd.co.uk/20/hipfracturer.nsf/c9a99d 2f189bd1be8025875b0059f78d/7de8dac5ec3b468980257d4 f005188f2/$FILE/NHFD2010Report.pdf.

NHFD (2017) *NHFD Annual Report 2017*. www.nhfd.co.uk/ files/2017ReportFiles/NHFD-AnnualReport2017.pdf.

NHFD (2018) *NHFD 2018 Annual Report*. www.nhfd. co.uk/2018report.

NHFD (2019) *NHFD 2019 Annual Report*. www.nhfd. co.uk/20/hipfracturer.nsf/docs/2019Report.

NHFD (2020) *NHFD Annual Report – A review of 2019 NHFD data*. www.nhfd.co.uk/20/hipfractureR.nsf/docs/ reports2020.

NICE (2010) Delirium: prevention, diagnosis and management. Clinical guideline [CG103] www.nice.org.uk/guidance/cg103.

NICE (2011). *Hip Fracture: The Management of hip Fracture in Adults. NICE Clinical Guideline 124*. London: NICE www.nice.org.uk/guidance/cg124.

NICE (2019) *Acute kidney injury: prevention, detection, and management*. NG148 National Institute for Health and Care Excellence. www.nice.org.uk/guidance/ng148.

Parker, M. and Anand, J.K. (1991). What is the true mortality of hip fractures? *Public Health* 105 (6): 443–446.

Parker, M. and Johansen, A. (2006). Hip fracture. *BMJ* 333 (7557): 27–30. https://doi.org/10.1136/bmj.333.7557.27.

Pasco, J.A., Brennan, S.L., Henry, M.J. et al. (2011). Changes in hip fracture rates in South-Eastern Australia spanning the period 1994–2007. *J. Bone Miner. Res.* 26 (7): 1648–1654.

Rantalaiho, I., Gunn, J., Kukkonen, J., and Kaipia, A. (2019). Acute kidney injury following hip fracture. *Injury* 50 (12): 2268–2271. https://doi.org/10.1016/j.injury.2019.10.008. Epub 2019 Oct 4. PMID: 31623901.

Roigk, P. (2018). Nutrition and hydration. In: *Fragility Fracture Nursing: Holistic Care and Management of the Orthogeriatric Patient* (ed. K. Hertz and J. Santy-Tomlinson). Cham: Springer Chapter 8. https://www.ncbi. nlm.nih.gov/books/NBK543833. http://dx.doi. org/10.1007/978-3-319-76681-2_8.

Royal College Emergency Medicine (2010) Clinical Standards for Emergency Departments. https://heeoe.hee.nhs.uk/ sites/default/files/cem_clinical_standards_august_2010.pdf.

Royal College of Physicians, British Geriatrics Society and the British Pain Society (2007). *The Assessment of Pain in Older People*. London: RCP/BGS/BPS.

Santy-Tomlinson, J., Laur, C.V., and Ray, S. (2021a). Delivering interprofessional education to embed interdisciplinary collaboration in effective nutritional care. In: *Interdisciplinary Nutritional Management and Care for Older Adults. Perspectives in Nursing Management and Care for Older Adults* (ed. Ó.G. Geirsdóttir and J.J. Bell). Cham: Springer https://doi.org/10.1007/978-3-030-63892-4_12.

Santy-Tomlinson, J., Hertz, K., Myhre-Jensen, C., and Brent, L. (2021b). Nursing in the orthogeriatric setting.

In: *Orthogeriatrics. Practical Issues in Geriatrics* (ed. P. Falaschi and D. Marsh). Cham: Springer https://doi.org/10.1007/978-3-030-48126-1_17.

Scottish Intercollegiate Guidelines Network (2009) Management of Hip Fracture in Older People. National Clinical Guideline 111.

Shane, E., Burr, D., Abrahamsen, B. et al. (2014). Atypical subtrochanteric and diaphyseal femoral fractures: second report of a task force of the American Society for Bone and Mineral Research. *J. Bone Miner. Res.* 29: 1–23. https://doi.org/10.1002/jbmr.1998144S.

TARN (2017) Major trauma in older people in England and Wales. www.tarn.ac.uk/content/downloads/3793/Major%20Trauma%20in%20Older%20People%202017.pdf.

Trads, M. and Pedersen, P.U. (2015). Constipation and defecation pattern the first 30 days after hip fracture. *Int. J. Nurs. Pract.* 21 (5): 598–604. https://doi.org/10.1111/ijn.12312.

Volkert, D., Kiesswetter, E., Cederholm, T. et al. (2019a). Development of a model on determinants of malnutrition in aged persons: a MaNuEL project. *GGM* 5: 1–8. https://doi.org/10.1177/2333721419858438.

Volkert, D., Beck, A.M., Cederholm, T. et al. (2019b). ESPEN guideline on clinical nutrition and hydration in geriatrics. *Clin. Nutr.* 38 (1): 10–47.

World Health Organization (2011). *Palliative Care for Older People: Better Practice*. Geneva: WHO http://www.euro.who.int/__data/assets/pdf_file/0017/143153/e95052.pdf.

Young, J. and Inouye, S.K. (2007). Delirium in older people. *BMJ* 334: 842. https://doi.org/10.1136/bmj.39169.706574.AD.

20

Spinal Cord Injury

Sian Rodger

Royal National Orthopaedic Hospital, Stanmore, Middlesex, UK

Introduction

Spinal cord injury (SCI) is a life-changing event often resulting in permanent neurological loss below the level of cord damage as the spinal cord is the main channel through which motor and sensory information travels between the brain and body. The care of the individual following SCI is complex and often provided by specialist practitioners. Sometimes, however, it is provided in general hospitals by practitioners who care for people with SCI rarely or intermittently. This chapter aims to provide an overview of the care a patient with SCI requires, focusing on the essential role of the nurse in this process as part of the wider multi-disciplinary team (MDT) and will provide practitioners working in orthopaedic and musculoskeletal trauma settings with the evidence, guidance and knowledge required to underpin effective practise for the person with SCI.

SCI is a chronic condition that is complex in nature (Singh et al. 2019). Disruption to the spinal cord caused by trauma or dysfunction can result in permanent neurological loss below the point of damage. SCI can affect people of all genders at any time of life and at present there is no cure (Chen et al. 2016).

There are approximately 16 new cases per million of traumatic SCI (TSCI) and two to three new cases per million of spinal cord dysfunction (SCD) (non-traumatic in mode of injury) per year. This equates to in excess of 1200 new cases every year (McDaid et al. 2019), making the economic and individual cost (physical and psychological) huge. A recent study by McDaid et al. (2019) conservatively estimated lifetime costs for an expected 1270 new cases of SCI per annum to be £1.43 billion (2016 prices).

The global trend across developed nations is to care for patients with SCI at specialist spinal centres due to its complexity and the specialist services needed (Maharaj et al. 2016). Although the rates of mortality caused by SCI have been decreasing since the 1950s, patients are at significant risk of injury-related complications. In a systematic review by Maharaj et al. (2016), a German study showed that 50% of participants ($n = 45\,000$) had post discharge hospital readmissions to treat complications. Common post-injury complications include bowel dysfunction, pressure ulcers, urinary tract infections (UTIs), respiratory issues, sexual dysfunction, pain and psychological issues (Sezer et al. 2015).

Patterns of Injury

Typically SCI affects young males, with a male to female ratio of 2 : 1 (Alizadeh et al. 2019), involved in trauma (e.g. road traffic collision, falls or violence) resulting in complete loss of neurological function below the level of injury to the spinal cord (World Health Organization 2013). This is now starting to change due to an ageing population, more effective emergency treatment and in recent years a large increase in the number of patients who have sustained damage to their spinal cord due to SCD (New et al. 2016). SCD can be caused by metastatic cord compression, degenerative disorders or infection (Rodger 2019).

The average age of people affected by SCD is generally older compared to TSCI and there also seems to be a more even split between genders. SCD is more likely to cause an incomplete SCI, which occurs when some messages are able to get to and from the brain past the spinal cord damage (New et al. 2016). Women are at higher risk of sustaining in SCI during adolescence and in their 70s with men mostly affected in early adulthood (30s) or late adulthood (80s) (Alizadeh et al. 2019).

Orthopaedic and Trauma Nursing: An Evidence-based Approach to Musculoskeletal Care, Second Edition. Edited by Sonya Clarke and Mary Drozd.
© 2023 John Wiley & Sons Ltd. Published 2023 by John Wiley & Sons Ltd.

Clinical outcomes are very much dependant on severity and location of damage to the spinal cord. It should be noted, however, that adults over 60 years of age have worse outcomes than younger patients, with falls and age-related bone changes.

During April 2018 to December 2021, the London SCI centre had approximately 397 new SCI admissions for intensive rehabilitation: 183 caused by trauma, 214 caused by SCD.

The primary injury to the spinal cord is the initial mechanical forces delivered to the cord at the time of injury. Alizadeh et al. (2019) report that there are four main characteristic mechanisms of primary injury: impact and persistent compression, impact and transient compression, distraction and laceration/transaction (although most injuries do not completely sever the spinal cord), and the most common cause is impact with persistent compression.

The forces from the primary injury damage the ascending and descending pathways in the spinal cord and disrupt blood vessels and cell membranes regardless of how the SCI occurred.

Early surgical decompression (within 24 hours) is to date the most effective clinical treatment to limit further tissue damage (Alizadeh et al. 2019).

Anatomical Considerations

As discussed in Chapter 4, the spinal column comprises the bony elements from cervical vertebra (C1–7), thoracic vertebra (T1–12), lumbar vertebra (L1–5), sacral vertebra (S1–5, fused in adults) and the coccyx (four fused). This surrounds the vertebral canal, which, in turn, surrounds the spinal cord. Ligaments surround all the bony surfaces, the key ones being the anterior longitudinal ligament, the posterior longitudinal ligament and the ligamentum flavum. This creates a corset-like effect that stabilises the whole spinal structure.

The spinal cord is surrounded by cerebrospinal fluid (CSF) and enclosed by meninges, providing a flexible, protective system within a semi-rigid frame that allows movement of the spine while protecting the cord and spinal nerves. Most movement occurs at the craniocervical, cervico-thoracic or thoraco-lumbar junction where the most rigid part of the structure (e.g. the thoracic region) meets a movable region (e.g. the cervical or lumbar). In the cervical region, the cord is enlarged and passes through a relatively narrow vertebral canal. Numerous neurones that supply the upper limbs arise from this section of the cord. This contributes to cervical injuries being the most common, accounting for approximately 59% of injuries in the USA since 2015 (National Spinal Cord Injury Statistical Center 2021) and 51% in the United Kingdom in 2017/18 (NHS England 2019), with the remainder being spread between the thoracic, thoracolumbar and lumbosacral regions.

Two-thirds of the blood supply to the cord is provided by the anterior artery. The posterior arteries and radicular arteries provide the final third, with input provided at different levels in the cervical and thoracic regions. Injury to the anterior artery can result in ischaemia of the cord and has a far greater impact on a larger area of tissue (two-thirds of the anterior aspect of the cord). Traumatic or non-traumatic injury that results in a space-occupying lesion such as a haematoma or foreign body can cause compression to the cord and ischaemia that results in neurological damage.

In children, the vertebral facets have a shallow angulation and the vertebral bodies, particularly cervical, are more wedge-shaped. The structure is also more cartilaginous, providing much more ligamentous laxity. This can lead to false-negative X-ray results. This is known as spinal cord injury without radiologic abnormality (SCIWORA) and is considered in more detail in Chapter 25. Children may be inadvertently sent home with little or no intervention. Younger children are less able to participate in neurological examinations and may present several days or even weeks later with evidence of delayed onset neurological changes. It is recommended to always maintain a high index of suspicion in cases where there may be relatively minor trauma.

Older people may have concurrent conditions such as osteoporosis, ankylosing spondylitis and spinal stenosis, making them more vulnerable to spinal cord compression from minor trauma such as falls from standing or a low height. Forced hyperextension is a classic example that results in stretching of the cord and compression from subsequent oedema and haematoma, often presenting as spinal cord injury without radiographic evidence of trauma (SCIWORET).

Pathophysiology of the Injury

There are several stages of injury within the cord itself: primary, secondary and chronic (Quadri et al. 2020). Immediately following the primary injury (within minutes), there is disruption to cell bodies and axonal activity, leading to haemorrhage and oedema in and around the site of injury, releasing inflammatory mediators. This results in a neurochemical cascade, leading to further injury and damage to the cord secondary to the primary injury (within hours). This can eventually result in a CSF-filled cyst in the centre of the cord (weeks to years), with the potential for elongating the damage caused from the initial injury that can result in neurological loss higher than that initially sustained. The resulting scar tissue in the cord prevents any growing nerve fibres from crossing and with inhibitory substances and lack of nerve growth factors in the surrounding tissues the adult spinal cord does not regenerate spontaneously after injury. Neuro-protection and neuro-regeneration are currently being researched but, at this time, SCI remains 'incurable'.

Emergency Care and Management

The British Orthopaedic Association (2021) specify that all patients (above the age of 16 years) involved in trauma must be assumed to have an unstable injury to their spine with or without damage to spinal cord, although as previously stated this could lead to spinal cord damage if not managed effectively. Approximately 2% of conscious patients increasing to 34% of unconscious patients have unstable spinal injuries, 50% affecting the thoracic or lumbar region.

Care at the trauma site should start with the use of a prioritising sequence, for example airway, breathing, circulation, disability, exposure (ABCDE), whilst maintaining spinal alignment to minimise secondary damage to the cord. Life-threatening injuries take priority (NICE 2016a).

Full details on the assessment and initial management of spinal injury can be assessed in the NICE guideline (2016b) Spinal Injury: assessment and initial management, NICE guideline on major trauma (2016a) and the British Orthopaedic Association Standards for Trauma and Orthopaedics (BOAST 2021).

Subsequent Care and Rehabilitation

On diagnosis of an SCI, referral to a specialist spinal cord injury rehabilitation centre (SCIC) should be completed. Whilst waiting for a bed at the SCIC, information and support can be accessed through the SCIC acute outreach team. The aim of the acute outreach team is to provide clinical assessment, education, advice and support to the SCI patient, their family and non-specialist healthcare professionals. Due to the demand for beds, the wait for admission to the SCIC can be lengthy, therefore it is imperative that SCI patients receive the care that will minimise post-injury complications such as pressure ulcers and allow them to begin their rehabilitation. The acute outreach team is able to visit the referring hospital to speak to the patient and care team face to face or liaise over the telephone.

Assessing and documenting neurological loss is essential. The International Standard for Neurological Classification of SCI (ISNCSCI), more commonly known as the American Spinal Injuries Association (ASIA) Impairment Scale (AIS), is carried out to assess where the spinal cord is damaged and the severity of neurological loss, including the lowest sacral segments (deep anal pressure and deep anal contraction). This should be completed on admission, at 72 hours following admission, prior to and post any surgical intervention, prior to transfer to SCIC and on admission to the SCIC. This assessment is much more accurate than using magnetic resonance imaging scans to diagnose the severity of neurological loss. The assessment can only be completed by specially trained healthcare professionals for accuracy of diagnosis. The ASIA assesses where the last 'normal' neurological motor and sensory levels are on both sides of the body and the last sacral segments, enabling diagnosis of 'complete' and 'incomplete' SCI as shown (Figure 20.1).

As the cord is an extension of the brain from the medulla oblongata, it has many characteristics that the brain has. Not only does it relay messages up the cord to the brain (sensory/ascending pathways) and relay messages back down the cord (motor/descending pathways), it also sends messages within the cord via interneurons. Following SCI this creates a reflex and allows electrical messages to move quickly within the cord without the brain controlling it. With injuries in the region of the conus medullaris (the base of the cord) there can be a mixed picture of some reflex activity and some flaccidity. This is often referred to as a conal injury. Injury above this level is referred to as a supraconal injury. If injury is sustained in the cauda equina region, there is no ability to create this connectivity between neurones, as the cord (as a single entity) no longer exists. There are only peripheral spinal nerves exiting the cord from approximately L1 bony level and thus no reflex activity can be seen in injuries that affect this level and below (generally below L1).

Understanding if the patient's cord injury is complete or incomplete and from which level provides predictive information for nursing care and will enable nurses to effectively plan and carry out the care and management regimes required for the SCI patient.

When nursing a patient with a SCI there are many factors that need to be considered:

- neurogenic/spinal shock
- respiration
- swallowing
- orthostatic hypotension
- autonomic dysreflexia
- bladder

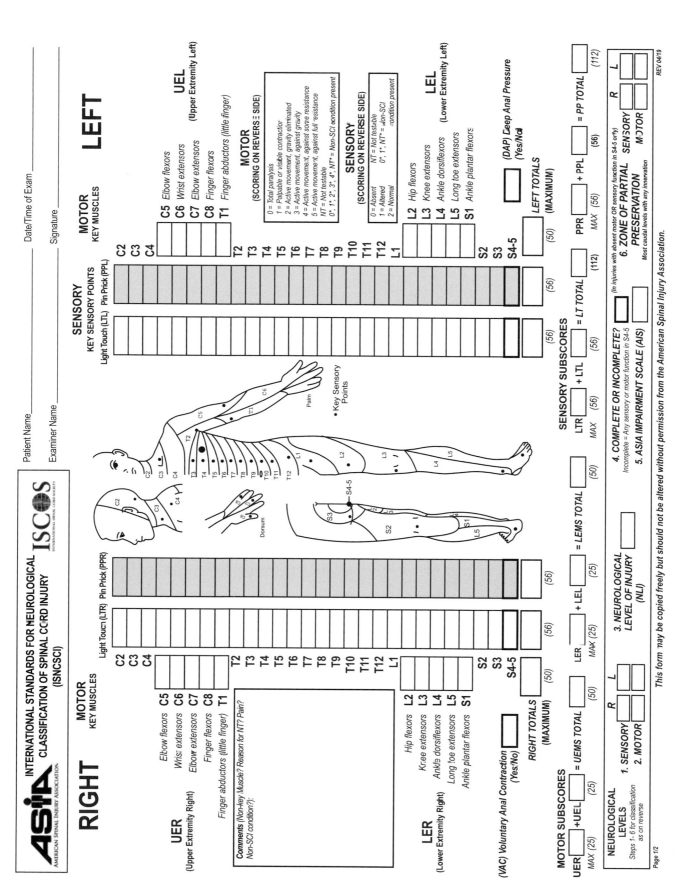

Figure 20.1 American Spinal Injuries Association Impairment Scale (2019). *Source:* Reproduced with permission from American Spinal Injury Association

Muscle Function Grading

0 = Total paralysis

1 = Palpable or visible contraction

2 = Active movement, full range of motion (ROM) with gravity eliminated

3 = Active movement, full ROM against gravity

4 = Active movement, full ROM against gravity and moderate resistance in a muscle specific position

5 = (Normal) active movement, full ROM against gravity and full resistance in a functional muscle position expected from an otherwise unimpaired person

NT = Not testable (i.e. due to immobilization, severe pain such that the patient cannot be graded, amputation of limb, or contracture of > 50% of the normal ROM)

0*, 1*, 2*, 3*, 4*, NT* = Non-SCI condition present [a]

Sensory Grading

0 = Absent   1 = Altered, either decreased/impaired sensation or hypersensitivity

2 = Normal   NT = Not testable

0*, 1*, NT* = Non-SCI condition present [a]

[a] Note: Abnormal motor and sensory scores should be tagged with a '*' to indicate an impairment due to a non-SCI condition. The non-SCI condition should be explained in the comments box together with information about how the score is rated for classification purposes (at least normal / not normal for classification).

When to Test Non-Key Muscles:

In a patient with an apparent AIS B classification, non-key muscle functions more than 3 levels below the motor level on each side should be tested to most accurately classify the injury (differentiate between AIS B and C).

Movement	Root level
Shoulder: Flexion, extension, abduction, adduction, internal and external rotation **Elbow:** Supination	C5
Elbow: Pronation **Wrist:** Flexion	C6
Finger: Flexion at proximal joint, extension **Thumb:** Flexion, extension and abduction in plane of thumb	C7
Finger: Flexion at MCP joint **Thumb:** Opposition, adduction and abduction perpendicular to palm	C8
Finger: Abduction of the index finger	T1
Hip: Adduction	L2
Hip: External rotation	L3
Hip: Extension, abduction, internal rotation **Knee:** Flexion **Ankle:** Inversion and eversion **Toe:** MP and IP extension	L4
Hallux and Toe: DIP and PIP flexion and abduction	L5
Hallux: Adduction	S1

ASIA Impairment Scale (AIS)

A = Complete. No sensory or motor function is preserved in the sacral segments S4-5.

B = Sensory Incomplete. Sensory but not motor function is preserved below the neurological level and includes the sacral segments S4-5 (light touch or pin prick at S4-5 or deep anal pressure) AND no motor function is preserved more than three levels below the motor level on either side of the body.

C = Motor Incomplete. Motor function is preserved at the most caudal sacral segments for voluntary anal contraction (VAC) OR the patient meets the criteria for sensory incomplete status (sensory function preserved at the most caudal sacral segments S4-5 by LT, PP or DAP), and has some sparing of motor function more than three levels below the ipsilateral motor level on either side of the body.
(This includes key or non-key muscle functions to determine motor incomplete status.) For AIS C – less than half of key muscle functions below the single NLI have a muscle grade ≥ 3.

D = Motor Incomplete. Motor incomplete status as defined above, with at least half (half or more) of key muscle functions below the single NLI having a muscle grade ≥ 3.

E = Normal. If sensation and motor function is graded as normal in all segments, and the patient had prior deficits, then the AIS grade is E. Someone without an initial SCI does not receive an AIS grade.

Using ND: To document the sensory, motor and NLI levels, the ASIA Impairment Scale grade, and/or the zone of partial preservation (ZPP) when they are unable to be determined based on the examination results.

Steps in Classification

The following order is recommended for determining the classification of individuals with SCI.

1. Determine sensory levels for right and left sides.
The sensory level is the most caudal, intact dermatome for both pin prick and light touch sensation.

2. Determine motor levels for right and left sides.
Defined by the lowest key muscle function that has a grade of at least 3 (on supine testing), providing the key muscle functions represented by segments above that level are judged to be intact (graded as a 5).
Note: in regions where there is no myotome to test, the motor level is presumed to be the same as the sensory level, if testable motor function above that level is also normal.

3. Determine the neurological level of injury (NLI).
This refers to the most caudal segment of the cord with intact sensation and antigravity (3 or more) muscle function strength, provided that there is normal (intact) sensory and motor function rostrally respectively.
The NLI is the most cephalad of the sensory and motor levels determined in steps 1 and 2.

4. Determine whether the injury is Complete or Incomplete.
(i.e. absence or presence of sacral sparing)
If voluntary anal contraction = No AND all S4-5 sensory scores = 0 AND deep anal pressure = No, then injury is Complete.
Otherwise, injury is Incomplete.

5. Determine ASIA Impairment Scale (AIS) Grade.

Is injury Complete?   If YES, AIS=A

NO ↓

Is injury Motor Complete? If YES, AIS=B

NO ↓   (No=voluntary anal contraction OR motor function more than three levels below the motor level on a given side, if the patient has sensory incomplete classification)

Are at least half (half or more) of the key muscles below the neurological level of injury graded 3 or better?

NO ↓   YES ↓

AIS=C   AIS=D

If sensation and motor function is normal in all segments, AIS=E
Note: AIS E is used in follow-up testing when an individual with a documented SCI has recovered normal function. If at initial testing no deficits are found, the individual is neurologically intact and the ASIA Impairment Scale does not apply.

6. Determine the zone of partial preservation (ZPP).
The ZPP is used only in injuries with absent motor (no VAC) OR sensory function (no DAP, no LT and no PP sensation) in the lowest sacral segments S4-5, and refers to those dermatomes and myotomes caudal to the sensory and motor levels that remain partially innervated. With sacral sparing of sensory function, the sensory ZPP is not applicable and therefore "NA" is recorded in the block of the worksheet. Accordingly, if VAC is present, the motor ZPP is not applicable and is noted as "NA".

AMERICAN SPINAL INJURY ASSOCIATION

INTERNATIONAL STANDARDS FOR NEUROLOGICAL CLASSIFICATION OF SPINAL CORD INJURY

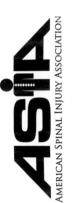
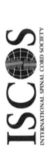

INTERNATIONAL SPINAL CORD SOCIETY

Figure 20.1 (Continued)

- bowels
- skin
- spasms/spasticity
- pain
- psychological wellbeing
- patient education.

Neurogenic and Spinal Shock

These two terms are often used interchangeably, but they present quite differently. After trauma to the spinal cord there is often a period of spinal 'shock', which is a transient physiological disruption in function and reflexes resulting from the primary injury. This can result in a shutdown of functions controlled by that area of the cord, resulting in an absence of reflexes, i.e. flaccid paralysis of all skeletal muscle and loss of all spinal reflexes below the level of injury. This is a temporary state and will resolve in hours or weeks from the injury. Spinal shock does not indicate the severity of paralysis in the long term and neurological recovery will vary as cord oedema subsides and spinal neurons regain excitability.

Neurogenic shock should be suspected if there is a cervical or high thoracic injury with hypotension and bradycardia with no signs of systemic fluid loss. With the initial flaccid paralysis and neurogenic shock, it is common for there to be a low resting blood pressure (BP) recording (e.g. 80/50 or 90/60). This is due to passive vasodilation of the blood vessels, lack of sympathetic tone and reflex activity below the level of injury. It may also lead to blood pooling in the extremities, resulting in oedema in the hands and feet (Ruiz et al. 2018).

Neurogenic shock may require inotropic therapy to keep the cardiovascular system supported whilst it is in crisis. The autonomic reflexes that normally control BP can be unreliable in maintaining the body's equilibrium while in shock and increasing fluid input may simply result in overloading a system that already has full circulating volume (providing no hypovolaemia has been diagnosed). Conservative use of crystalloids, principally normal saline, is often adequate and fluids should be given based on urine output (approximately 0.5 mg/kg/h). Incomplete injuries may have less significant changes if any.

As well as close monitoring of the BP and pulse, frequent monitoring of body temperature is also advisable. Passive vasodilation of the blood vessels and inability to moderate temperature below the level of injury through the usual mechanisms, such as shivering, may lead to poikilothermia (assuming the ambient temperature of the environment), resulting in hypo- or hyperthermia.

In higher level SCI, usual signs and symptoms of venous thromboembolism (VTE), such as leg pain and chest pain, may be absent due to loss of sensory pathways. VTE may present as persistent tachycardia with recurrent fevers in the absence of sepsis. Prophylaxis with low molecular weight heparin (LMWH) and use of usual VTE prevention regimes is mandatory along with other prophylactic measures such as passive and or active limb movements and deep breathing. Regular measurements of calf and thigh width to identify unilateral increase can give early indication of VTE (see Chapter 9 for further information).

During this time of flaccidity, it is essential to use the correct handling of vulnerable limbs. It is most important for practitioners to understand that poor handling/mishandling may have detrimental future outcomes for hand and arm function and lower limb function. For example, a poorly placed hand on a pillow can lead to the patient losing the ability to grip that will be required later during rehabilitation for feeding and holding utensils. Unsupported feet can lead to foot drop.

In cervical SCI, while in neurogenic shock, the unopposed activity of the parasympathetic vagus (10th cranial) nerve results in bradycardia and there is a risk of asystole secondary to stimulation such as with pharyngeal suction, attempted intubation, endotracheal suction, passing of nasogastric tubes or turning the patient during or following surgery. Exaggerated vagal responses, however, tend to be temporary and reduce over time (Kripa and Khanal 2021).

Respiratory

The degree of respiratory dysfunction following an SCI is dependent on where the cord has been damaged. Flaccid paralysis of the respiratory muscles and cord oedema are the causes of this directly following SCI (Respiratory Information for Spinal Cord Injury [RISCI] 2017). The level and completeness of SCI determine the patient's ability to breathe deeply and cough forcefully following SCI, with greater dysfunction seen at higher injury levels (Table 20.1).

Ventilatory failure is rapid in high cervical SCI when diaphragmatic and scalene activity is lost; couple this with excessive bronchial secretions and a likelihood of bronchoconstriction due to autonomic disruption, and respiratory failure is likely, resulting in the patient needing to be intubated and mechanically ventilated for a period of time or, in a small number of cases, for life. If a patient is intubated, a tracheostomy is recommended due to the complexities of extubating these patients (RISCI 2017). A tracheostomy also allows effective clearance of secretions and provides the patient with the ability to communicate.

The RISCI recommend a slow and cautious respiratory weaning programme focusing on vital capacity to guide the process. This process can take time due to setbacks like fatigue and pneumonia.

Table 20.1 Summary of respiratory function dependant on level of SCI.

Level of injury	Muscles affected	Likely effect
C1 and 2	Accessory muscles, intercostal muscles, diaphragm and abdominals	Will require a ventilator for breathing and manual treatments[a] to clear secretions as unable to cough and clear secretions independently.
C3, C4 and C5	Accessory muscles (partially affected), intercostal muscles, diaphragm (partially affected) and abdominals	May require a ventilator for breathing some or all of the time. Will require manual treatments[a] to clear secretions as unable to cough and clear secretions independently.
C6, C7 and C8	Accessory muscles (partially affected), intercostal muscles and abdominals	Unlikely to require ventilator assistance to breathe. Likely to require manual treatments[a] to clear secretions as unable to cough and clear secretions independently.
T1–T5	Intercostal muscles (partially affected) and abdominals	Independent breathing. May require manual treatments[a] to clear secretions as unable to cough and clear secretions independently.
T6–T12	Intercostal muscles (partially affected) and abdominals (partially affected)	Independent breathing. Less likely to require manual treatments[a] to clear secretions but may occasionally need an assisted cough due to weak abdominals.
L1–S4	No respiratory muscles are affected	No effect on breathing.

[a] Manual treatments include endotracheal suctioning, manual assisted coughs, manual chest oscillation and intermittent positive pressure breathing devices, which should be carried out by trained healthcare practitioners.

Communication requires special attention to enable patients to interact with healthcare professionals whether verbally or non-verbally (if the tracheostomy cuff is inflated). Other considerations are any associated injuries at the time of SCI, for example acquired brain injury, age or pre-existing respiratory conditions.

Swallowing

The link between cervical SCI and the development of dysphagia is well documented (Lee et al. 2016), with a 17–41%

occurrence of swallowing dysfunction in this patient group. Dysphagia (swallowing dysfunction) is characterised by the abnormal movement of food or liquid from the oral cavity to the oesophagus and increases the patient's risk of aspiration pneumonia and airway obstruction. This can have a huge detrimental effect on an already comprised respiratory system due to the cord injury (McRae et al. 2019).

As well as the vital role swallowing has in the body's nutrition, it also aids the clearing of the naso- and oral pharynx (Chaw et al. 2012) and closure of the nasopharynx and larynx to prevent aspiration.

Anterior cervical spinal surgery, respiratory interventions such as tracheostomy and ventilator use increase the likelihood of dysphagia as anterior spinal muscles involved in swallowing may be disrupted, becoming stretched or oedematous (Chew et al. 2012) and making swallowing difficult. It is therefore imperative that any dysphasia is diagnosed early and appropriate referrals are made to the wider MDT (speech and language therapist [SALT], respiratory team). Early interventions from the SALT may include insertion of a nasogastric tube or percutaneous endoscopic gastrostomy feeding tube. Oral hygiene care should be executed to the highest standard to avoid any aspiration.

Stress gastric ulceration is common in victims of major trauma. In patients with SCI, multiple causes could be responsible, with one being unopposed sympathetic activity resulting in increased gastric acid. Haemorrhage and ulceration are therefore possible. Stress ulcer prophylaxis should be considered, as should any predisposing risks to gastrointestinal bleed such as anticoagulants, non-steroidal anti-inflammatory drugs and excessive smoking.

Orthostatic Hypotension

Orthostatic hypotension (OH) is defined as a drop in systolic BP of least 20 mmHg and/or a drop in diastolic BP of at least 10 mmHg when a person changes position from lying to upright (BMJ 2020).

For patients with a higher level thoracic or cervical SCI, OH can be a common complication due to the inability of the nervous system to automatically constrict the blood vessels to balance the BP after a change of position. Decreased lower limb movement hinders blood flow back to the heart and the rest of the body, increasing the likelihood of OH.

Common signs and symptoms of OH:

- lightheadedness
- blurred vision
- dizziness
- fainting.

OH is usually managed with a combination of pharmacological and non-pharmacological treatments (Wecht 2022). Prior to mobilising, patients should be gradually sat up in bed until in an upright position for 15–20 minutes to enable the BP to adapt to the change of position. The use of an abdominal binder, compression stockings (knee or thigh), and increased fluid and salt intake (as advised by the medical team) can also help to reduce symptoms.

Autonomic Dysreflexia

This is a medical emergency. Autonomic dysreflexia (AD) is an exaggerated response of the sympathetic nervous system to any noxious or painful stimuli. This is most likely when the SCI is above T6 and is unlikely to develop if the injury is below T10. Noxious stimuli include bladder outflow obstruction, constipation, pressure ulceration or even restrictive clothing, anything that would cause pain or uncomfortable sensations in those who are without SCI. The most common cause is bladder issues: UTI, blocked catheter and distended bladder. The stimuli are picked up by the sympathetic nervous system and trigger reflex responses that cause vasoconstriction of the large blood vessels in the gut. This rapidly elevates the BP, which then continues to rise. In a patient with SCI the normal compensatory parasympathetic response cannot travel below the level of the cord damage so vasoconstriction continues below the level of injury, leading to systemic hypertension. The compensatory parasympathetic response has an impact above the level of the SCI, causing bradycardia and vasodilation in an attempt to lower the BP by sweating and dilating the vessels of the skin of the face, head and shoulders (which appear flushed), and the nose. Associated bradycardia is due to stimulation of the parasympathetic nervous system (via the vagus nerve). If the stimulus that triggered the AD is not removed, the patient may have a myocardial infarction or stroke, leading to death.

Once spinal shock has resolved and reflexes have returned, AD can present at any time and must be considered whenever the BP is elevated. In a tetraplegic (neurological deficit in upper and lower limbs) patient, the resting BP may be as low as 80/50 mmHg due to passive vasodilation of peripheral blood vessels below the level of injury. The higher the level of injury the more likely that there will be autonomic changes and altered observations. AD should be suspected with a rise of 15–20 mmHg in BP above the usual for that patient. Initial management is to find the stimulus and remove it. Sitting the patient up (if the spine is stable) may help to reduce the BP while the cause is sought, such as urinary outflow, obstruction, constipation or pressure ulcer. Further stimulus to the bowel or bladder in performing evacuations to resolve the AD can actually trigger further stimulus and reflexes, potentially exacerbating the problem. Using local anaesthetic gel to perform the examination can help to reduce local stimuli in the rectum. If the stimulus cannot be found, removed or resolved, a quick-acting antihypertensive agent such as nifedipine can be given sublingually (up to twice) to reduce the BP. It is important to be aware the BP will drop rapidly once the cause has been resolved. If the problem cannot be resolved, such as ingrowing toenails or pressure ulcer, advice and action from senior medical staff or the resuscitation team should be sought. Regular administration of antihypertensive agents may be required to keep the BP under control until the stimulus is treated or resolved (Wecht 2022).

Recap

Signs of AD
- A severe pounding headache that gets worse.
- High BP: usually there is a 20–40 mmHg rise in BP above the patient's normal level but it may be much higher.
- Red blotches above the level of injury (face, neck, arms).
- Sweating above the level of injury.
- Goosebumps above the level of injury.
- Stuffy nose.

(Lakra et al. 2021)

Treatment
- Call for assistance.
- Sit patient up.
- Identify cause by checking for distended bladder or bowel and any other stimuli that could cause AD.
- Eliminate the cause if possible (once eliminated, BP will drop).
- If cause unknown, administer nifedipine sublingually and seek medical assistance.
- BP should be monitored throughout and when AD has resolved for 24 hours.

(Wecht 2022; Lakra et al. 2021)

Bladder

Bladder dysfunction is a common associated condition in SCI (Kuris et al. 2021). During spinal shock, the bladder becomes atonic (without tone). When this happens the bladder should be managed with an indwelling urethral catheter (IDUC) to allow free drainage and avoid overdistention of the bladder, urinary incontinence and UTI caused by stagnation of urine. If priapism (prolonged erection of the penis) is present and has not resolved, urethral catheterisation should not be attempted and a suprapubic catheter inserted instead. Once spinal shock has resolved, an appropriate bladder management regime can be commenced.

The purpose of effective bladder management is to:

- ensure the bladder is emptied
- maintain renal function and protect the kidneys (high detrusor pressure and reflux are responsible for renal damage and renal failure) (Roth et al. 2019)
- reduce risk of UTI
- reduce risk of AD (in patients with SCI T6 and above)
- reduce episodes of incontinence
- maintain an independent lifestyle.

Genitourinary function is both autonomic (involuntary) and somatic (voluntary). The level of SCI and diagnosis (complete or incomplete and upper motor neurone [UMN] or lower motor neurone [LMN]) as well as hand function and patient choice will define the treatment programme put in place. In a person without an SCI the bladder fills, the stretch receptors in the detrusor (bladder) muscle stretch and a conscious urge to void is triggered, which is usually received and controlled by the brain until the person finds a socially acceptable time and place to void. Following SCI these processes are interrupted, voluntary control is impaired and autonomic control remains with either a reflex or flaccid presentation (UMN above T 12 or LMN usually below T12/L1).

Understanding the AIS will help to predict what type of input the healthcare professional will need to plan. For example, if the patient is an AIS B then the patient may have some degree of sensation but will not have voluntary control of the sacral nerves that control the urinary sphincter. They may report that they feel the urge to void but will have no ability to relax the muscle in order to void. A reflexic (UMN) cord injury will usually lead to the detrusor muscle contracting involuntarily and not being able to coordinate with the external sphincter (detrusor sphincter dyssynergia) and this will lead to a high-pressure system where damage can be caused to the kidneys by refluxed urine under pressure. Involuntary escape of urine (firing off) under pressure in this type of bladder should not be perceived as complete voiding as it would in a person without an SCI. It usually leads to incomplete emptying.

Types of Bladder Management

- IDUC: Although advocated for use during spinal shock an IDUC is not advocated for long-term use due to the risk of urethral damage and increased risk of UTIs.
- Superpubic catheter (SPC): Commonly used as long-term bladder management for patients with a high-level SCI resulting in reduced hand function. An SPC will not damage the urethra or interfere with sexual activity.

- Intermittent self-catheterisation (ISC): This is the preferred method of bladder management post-SCI. The patient needs to have some degree of hand function to be able to undertake this. This management mimics the bladder's natural function of filling and emptying. Patients perform four or five ISCs per day at set times using a clean technique. UTIs can cause patients to leak urine in between catheters so men can apply convene drainage to prevent incontinence and women may have an IDCU inserted for a short time.

(Taweel and Seyam 2015)

When a patient's bladder is managed with a long-term catheter, whether it be an SCP or an IDUC, the catheter should be clamped daily (when infection-free) for short periods to stretch the bladder and maintain capacity.

SCI patients should be under the care of a urology team to monitor bladder/kidney function and advise best management.

Bowel Management

Neurogenic bowel dysfunction is a common and distressing associated condition of SCI and requires an established individualised management programme to minimise the risk of complications such as faecal incontinence, constipation, impaction and perforated bowel to name a few (Multidisciplinary Association for Spinal Cord Injury Professionals [MASCIP] 2018).

During the first 48 hours post-injury paralytic ileus is possible as a result of neurogenic shock and the gut wall being unresponsive to stimuli (Johns et al. 2021). During this period the patient should be nil by mouth. On return of bowel sounds, diet can be reintroduced. If the patient is unable to take an oral diet, other forms of nutritional support should be commenced as metabolic changes following severe injury can impact on the nutritional status for several weeks after injury.

It is important to check bowel sounds daily, perform a daily rectal check and perform digital removal of faeces (DRF) to ensure that the rectum is clear of faeces as well as observing for abdominal distension. A free-draining nasogastric tube is recommended, with observation for bradycardia and vagal stimulation when it is being passed.

As the patient's condition improves and bowel sounds return, a bowel management regime should be established in light of the AIS to ensure that faeces are of the right consistency to enable DRF. There should be continued observation for signs of paralytic ileus, which can return at any time. As reflexes return, autonomic dysreflexia can occur in response to rectal stimulation for those persons with SCI above T6.

The process of defecation and micturition is a complex and coordinated process in a person without SCI. Voluntary control is mostly via sacral nerves S2–S4. Any SCI is, therefore, likely to cause disconnection between the brain and the anorectal structures. The rectum is normally empty and when faeces arrive in the rectum a conscious urge to defecate is triggered, which is usually controlled by the brain until a socially acceptable time for elimination. The internal anal sphincter is composed of smooth involuntary muscle and the external anal sphincter is composed of skeletal voluntary muscle (refer to the MASCIP Bowel Management Guidelines 2012 for further information; MASCIP 2012). As reflex activity returns and the patient commences mobilisation, a bowel management regime can be commenced based on the AIS with the aim of ensuring the person is able to empty their bowel fully within an acceptable timeframe on a regular basis. Consideration of past bowel patterns and medical/surgical history is crucial. Assistance will be required to ensure appropriate stool consistency and passage of stool through the gut as well as emptying of the rectum.

Depending on the level of neurological damage some enteric reflexes may exist and digestion, absorption and peristalsis will be slower, leading to an increased transit time of faeces. Stools can become hard due to reabsorption of fluid from the bowel and the risk of constipation is high. Appropriate fluids and diet are essential elements in counteracting this and use of the gastrocolic reflex (reflex contraction of the colon in response to ingestion of warm food or fluid 15–20 minutes earlier) is also useful. Aperients may be commenced to ensure stools are the right consistency for evacuation and that the patient does not become constipated or impacted. DRF is an appropriate and required procedure for the emptying of the neurologically damaged bowel (MASCIP 2012). Refer to Box 20.1 for additional bowel management evidence.

Care should include a daily assisted bowel movement using DRF until such time as sphincter reflexes appear in an UMN reflex lesion (usually above T12). If the person has a complete SCI and has a reflexic sphincter (the sphincter contracts involuntarily when a per rectum check is done, and they have a strong positive bulbospongiosis reflex test) it can be assumed it is likely to be an UMN or reflex lesion. For this type of lesion the bowel will have reflex overstimulation of the external anal sphincter, pelvic floor and colon, meaning that there is less compliance or stretch and the sphincter is tightly contracted. Intervention is required to ensure the rectum is fully emptied on a regular basis as sphincter dyssynergia (lack of coordination between the contraction and relaxation of the sphincters) may result in stool being retained in the rectum. The person may appear to be evacuating their bowel by themselves, but this may not mean it is emptying fully as it is being evacuated through a reflex contraction and not a coordinated contraction and expulsion. The bowel regime will consist of regular aperients or laxatives for stimulation and softening of faeces, massage of the abdomen, use of the gastrocolic reflex and suppositories. Anal stimulation for the UMN neurogenic bowel involves insertion of a lubricated, gloved finger into the rectum and gently circling the finger for 15–20 seconds or until the external anal sphincter can be felt to relax (through overstimulation of skeletal muscle) and the internal anal sphincter contracts. The finger is then removed as the faeces are expelled. The external anal sphincter will contract again by reflex and this process may be repeated several times until the rectum is empty or the reflexes tire and DRF can be used to ensure the rectum is empty. Failure to completely empty the rectum may result in an unplanned bowel evacuation later which is emotionally and physically distressing.

For those persons with a SCI that results in a flaccid presentation (LMN, generally below T12/L1), the external anal sphincter will appear soft and does not contract by reflex when a gloved lubricated finger is inserted and no bulbospongiosis reflex will be seen. The colon has increased compliance and there is little intrinsic peristalsis. The pelvic floor is relaxed as is the internal anal sphincter. This means there is a high risk of faecal incontinence as the external gateway mechanisms are impaired and any abdominal pressure can result in loss of faeces if the rectum is not emptied regularly. The bowel regime will consist of regular aperients or laxatives for stimulation and softening of faeces and massage of the abdomen. Use of the gastrocolic reflex may be of some

---

Box 20.1 Evidence Digest: Neurologic Bowel Management

In an evidence-based systematic review of the literature on digital rectal stimulation as an intervention in persons with SCI and upper motor neurone neurogenic bowel (UMN-NB) by Nelson and Orr (2021), 11 articles met the inclusion criteria and were included. The Johns Hopkins Nursing evidence-based practise model was used to critically examine the articles. This review suggests that management has not significantly changed in the last 20 years, with digital rectal stimulation remaining as an effective management alongside other techniques. This review therefore continues to support recommendations for the use of multiple techniques for successful evacuation of the bowels at set times of the day tailored to patients as the optimal management.

help for enteric reflexes but suppositories will be of little help as no reflex emptying or stimulation of the rectum will be gained. DRF will be required to ensure emptying of the bowel.

The aim in all instances is to ensure that the faeces are in the rectum at the established time and of the right consistency to ensure complete emptying, so timing of the bowel evacuation and the ingestion of laxatives (8–12 hours prior) is important. A single digital check 5–10 minutes after the last faeces have been expelled is important in ensuring faeces are not left in the rectum. Bowel management is mostly performed on the bed due to the risks involved for the carer in moving, handling and positioning for DRF. Use of gravity by using toilets or commodes, if appropriate, is also useful. Phosphate enemas should be used with caution as there is a risk of autonomic dysreflexia with an SCI above T6.

Quality of life for the SCI person is positively affected by having an effective bowel and bladder regime. It is crucial this is established as soon as possible, and education and involvement of the person in this process is key. They may not wish or be able to provide their own care, but the options should be discussed and education be provided so that problem solving and decisions regarding their future choice of bowel management are in their control. Persons with SCI at C4 and above will have no or very limited ability to self-care for bowel evacuation, but they can direct carers to provide this assistance if educated to do so. Other options for bowel evacuation are available, such as transanal irrigation, retrograde colonic irrigation, nerve stimulator or stoma, but these are not usually offered as the initial choice. Being aware of all options offers awareness, choice and discussion. The medical practitioner or specialist nurse can help with decision making as people living with SCI can change their bowel evacuation methods and bladder evacuation methods over time depending on need and lifestyle (Table 20.2).

Myth Busters

- It is illegal to perform digital rectal examination and DRFs: FALSE
  The Royal College of Nursing (2019) guidelines for bowel care including digital rectal examination and DRFs state that for some patients, such as those with SCI, these procedures are an integral part of their routine and should not be interrupted, regardless of the setting in which care is provided.
- It is abuse to perform digital rectal examination and digital removal of faeces: FALSE
  If a patient has freely given informed consent and has the mental capacity to make informed decisions it is not abuse (RCN 2019).

Table 20.2 Example of a daily bowel management routine.

Gain patient consent	NMC code 4.2 (2018) states 'Make sure you get properly informed consent and document it before carrying out any action'
Glycerine suppositories	To stimulate the bowel, assist colonic transit and produce a spontaneous result – only for patients with reflexic/upper motor neurone bowel
Warm drink	To promote gastrocolic reflex and encourage stools to move through the bowel into the rectum
Digital rectal stimulation	To stimulate the bowel and assist colonic transit – only for patients with reflexic/upper motor neurone bowel
Digital removal of faeces	To empty bowel to reduce occurrence of accidents later in the day

Source: Adapted from MASCIP (2012).

- Only nurses with special training can perform DRE and DRFs: TRUE
  These procedures can only be undertaken by a health professional who demonstrates professional competence in them (RCN 2019). Training should be provided and experienced healthcare staff should be available at all times to teach the procedure in order for nursing staff to facilitate bowel care for people with SCI.
- Bowels can be managed with medication only: FALSE
  This can lead to ineffective bowel emptying and bowel accidents, while continuous passive soiling or diarrhoea increases the risk of skin breakdown (MASCIP 2018).
- If a patient is having bowels open onto a pad, a DRFs is not required: FALSE
  This will lead to ineffective and irregular bowel emptying, which could in turn lead to an episode of AD (RCN 2019).

Skin

Pressure ulcer prevention is a very significant aspect of care for patients with SCI. Significant weight loss due to metabolic and nutritional status, and the loss of superficial tissues, subcutaneous fat and muscle to cushion the bony prominences, together with a lack of sensation, makes the SCI patient one of the most vulnerable groups. From the beginning of the SCI, immunity, skin integrity, vasomotor control and sensation will all be different to the pre-injury state and will make the SCI person more vulnerable to acquiring pressure ulcers. Risk assessment on admission along with an associated plan of care is essential. Both of these must be reviewed regularly and as the patient's condition changes, especially if there is any sign of sepsis or extreme weight loss or after spinal surgery. The principles of pressure ulcer prevention discussed in more detail in Chapter 12 also apply to the person with SCI.

Skin observation or signs of damage should begin immediately on admission. A baseline observation should be recorded as soon as the skin can be visualised with the patient's clothing removed. There may be tissue damage from lacerations, bruising etc. and this should also be noted. As soon the skin state has been assessed, a pressure ulcer prevention plan should be instigated. It is safe to position the patient in a side-lying position as long as spinal alignment is maintained and pillows are used to support the position firmly. Maintaining spinal alignment makes the use of the 30° tilt discussed in Chapter 12 inappropriate in patients with SCI. A regular turning plan should be instigated along with use of pressure redistributing mattresses and cushions. Alternating pressure mattresses should not, however, be used if the spinal fracture is unstable (reference needed). Many SCICs use specialist 'turning' beds when prolonged immobilisation of the unstable spine is likely. Such equipment can facilitate care in the general hospital, but should only be used if staff are trained to use it in a safe and effective manner. Regular care should consist of good nutrition, adequate hydration, skin inspection, keeping the skin clean and dry, and action planning. When a patient is able to mobilise in a wheelchair, a gradual mobilisation programme should be commenced and adhered to, starting with 15 minutes and increasing daily by 15 minutes if there is no adverse effect to skin. This allows the skin to build up its tolerance to pressure. Once the patient is up for an hour, a plan for pressure relief in the wheelchair should be instigated, such as tilting laterally to each side for 2 minutes or bending forwards for 2 minutes in each hour. If the skin is reddened at all after sitting, especially over the bony prominences, a further check should be made within 30 minutes of return to bed. If the mark remains non-blanching the time in the wheelchair should not be increased but reduced to a time that does not produce a non-blanching skin reaction. This can then gradually progress to sitting up all day with pressure-relieving position changes every hour for 2 minutes as long as there is no skin deterioration. Increasing skin tolerance to pressure needs to continue gradually to ensure that eventually the person can sleep overnight without requiring position changes. Education to ensure the SCI person develops the ability to manage or perform their own skin checks with a mirror or carer assistance is crucial. Once a pressure ulcer has been sustained there is a higher likelihood of sustaining more damage, particularly in same area. Living with the risk of pressure ulcers significantly impacts on home and work life, affecting the feasibility of holding down a job and maintaining life satisfaction.

Spasm

Spasm can occur once spinal and neurogenic shock have subsided. It is a velocity-dependent increase in the muscle stretch reflex usually stimulated by touching the SCI person's skin or movement during daily patient care. It can present in complete and incomplete injuries but is most prevalent in sensory incomplete lesions. If the patient is still considered as unstable or is being managed conservatively, then maintaining spinal alignment and staff safety during care provision can be an additional challenge. Spasticity should be expected and discussed with the patient and their family, and information about the cause and physiology should be provided. It is not a sign of return of normal movement but is a reflex-initiated response to a stimulus. Spasm can be useful in providing clues as to injury, pain or infection below the level of the lesion (e.g. full bladder or bowel) and can be used for standing and transferring. Too much reflex activity and spasm can also be detrimental and needs to be monitored and treated as appropriate. Correct positioning in bed, physiotherapy for stretching and exercising limbs and use of antispasmodic medication such as baclofen can be used initially until the rehabilitation team explore the benefits and use of spasm for the patient.

Consequences of Spasticity

- Spasticity itself is not harmful, but some of the things it causes can be.
- For some, the movement caused by spasticity is often seen as helpful and spasticity can help maintain the size of muscles.
- Pain can result either from the spasms or the position the body is put in as a result.
- Breathing can feel difficult during spasms in the trunk as they can push into the chest.
- Spasticity can be inconvenient and sometimes dangerous when it moves the patient and affects their balance.
- Moving can feel harder work when the patient is trying to move against the resistance of their muscles. This can also be difficult for nurses when assisting patients with activities of daily living.
- Spasticity can push the body into a set of characteristic positions. Untreated this can lead to contractures. This then makes the spasticity worse and can cause deformity.

For some patients the appearance of the deformity is distressing and it can make function more difficult or impossible over time.

- Skin can be damaged by spasticity due to friction and shearing. Contractures can cause skin damage when it becomes hard to keep skin creases clean and dry. When sitting or lying for long periods in an awkward position caused by spasticity and contractures, pressure can increase on the skin and eventually result in pressure ulcers.

Pain

Pain after SCI is often misunderstood. Some people think that because the person is paralysed that they will not feel any pain. The reality is quite the opposite.

Ongoing pain is common following SCI, with Widerström-Noga et al. (2016) reporting approximately 80% experiencing some form (neuropathic/musculoskeletal) within 1 year post-injury, furthermore for some neurogenic pain can persist over a lifetime. Neuropathic pain can occur from damage to the neural tissues and nociceptive pain can result from damage to non-neural tissues following SCI and lead to comorbidities such as insomnia, depression and anxiety, which can have a negative effect on life post-injury, e.g. social reintegration and returning to work. Pain management and assessment are considered in more detail in Chapter 11.

Psychological Wellbeing

As many patients become dependant on others to perform simple tasks following SCI, psychological effects such as loss of self-esteem and self-worth are common issues. Furthermore, the physical changes caused by SCI can also contribute to an extensive array of psychological effects.

Smyth et al. (2016) report that following SCI, prevalence rates for post-traumatic stress are 20–25% for clinically significant anxiety and 30–40% for depression.

Receptiveness to rehabilitation can be affected by patients' emotional responses to their SCI, such as sadness, confusion, anxiety, fear and anger.

During early rehabilitation, the patient will receive information about their SCI and what they will require, with a view to moving towards being as independent as possible whether that be physically or verbally. For example, it is hoped patients can be independent and in charge of their SCI, so for those who have high-level injuries and rely on carers for all care they are able to verbally direct what they need, thus making them verbally independent.

These conversations can be difficult and distressing for patients and need to be handled by experienced staff with appropriate sensitivity and honesty.

Patient Education

A vital element of rehabilitation is the provision of information and education to decrease the gap in the patient's knowledge on the impact of their SCI (Bailey et al. 2012). Patient education optimises the patient's participation in their own decision-making and care process, and promotes concordance with agreed plans, reducing the risk of post-injury complications, promoting independence and improving quality of life (Harvey and Davidson 2011).

During rehabilitation patients not only need to learn self-care management techniques but also develop skills in critical thinking and coping mechanisms to deal with health challenges after discharge (Bailey et al. 2012). Essentially, education gives patients the knowledge needed to successfully reintegrate into the community and live as independently as possible (Wyk et al. 2015).

Educating the patient on how their SCI affects their body will (along with intensive therapies) help prepare them for reintegration into the community. Preparing for the transition to community and home using open and clear communication between the patient, family, MDT and rehabilitation team is key. Goal planning and case conferences are the usual means to keep this communication and the ensuing rehabilitation process moving forwards.

Expert Patients

The aim of specialist rehabilitation is to enable the patient to understand the impact of their SCI on their body, what they need to do to remain healthy and how to be as independent as possible (physically and/or verbally). People with SCI spend a great deal of time refining their care routines to avoid complications and successfully reintegrate into their community and lives. Because of this, people with SCI can become very directorial about their care routines, which can appear inflexible to non-SCI specialist healthcare professionals. The expertise of SCI patients in managing their SCI should be recognised and acknowledged in line with the Nursing and Midwifery Council Code (Nursing and Midwifery Council 2018), which requires nurses to listen to patients, respond to their preferences and concerns, and work in partnership with them, and acknowledges the contribution they can make to their own healthcare.

Post-injury Complications

Complications such as pressure ulcers, bowel-related issues such as constipation, and recurrent urinary tract and chest infections have a devastating impact on the SCI individual, affecting their quality of life. These complications can also lead to life-threatening infections, which are not only costly to the SCI individual but also to the NHS. Prevention of costly complications is therefore paramount, as prevention has been reported to cost approximately one-tenth of the cost of treatment. Patients who are under the care of an SCIC have lifelong follow-up to ensure that they continue to receive expert advice and support throughout their life following SCI.

Children and Young People SCI

Although children and young people (CYP) SCI is rare, it can have a devastating effect on the growing skeleton. In a literature review, New et al. (2019) estimated that the incidence of CYP SCI for Western Europe was 3.3/million population/year for TSCI, with falls, road traffic collisions and sports injuries being the most common, and 6.2/million population/year for non-traumatic aetiologies, with tumours and inflammatory/autoimmune conditions being the most common causes.

The child and young person's spine is less ossified, with lax ligaments, which results in different patterns of injury. Cervical SCI are common due to the weight of the head in relation to less muscular development and greater elasticity of the soft tissue (Saul and Dresing 2018).

CYP SCI patients experience the same secondary health conditions as adult patients and should be managed similarly to avoid post injury complications. CYP with an SCI have to adjust to their SCI whilst progressing through the various stages of physical and psychological development.

Throughout the rehabilitation period, support and education also need to be given to the patient's family for them to adjust to the impact of the SCI.

CYP SCI patients should have a specialised MDT to facilitate and support their rehabilitation. SCICs are always willing to advise and educate non-specialist healthcare professionals if the patient is not an inpatient at a specialist centre.

Complications specific to CYP SCI patients include scoliosis, especially if the SCI happened prior to the adolescent growth spurt and hip deformity. Scoliosis occurs as a result of the lack of muscular support due to the reduced invertation of the trunk caused by the SCI. Careful monitoring is required throughout child/adolescent development to reduce the risk of muscular skeletal complications. Specialist interventions/equipment may be required, for example a thoracal lumbar spinal orthosis may be advised for prevention/treatment of scoliosis. It is imperative that child/adolescent SCI patients are under the care of a specialist MDT and have regular reviews.

Specialist Support Following SCI

Because of the complexities of SCIs, specialist SCICs offer their patients lifelong follow-up. As part of this, SCICs are able to offer advice and support to staff in non-specialist healthcare settings. Collaboration between the two healthcare settings and the patient in planning care can reassure the patient their SCI needs will be addressed. If care routines cannot be adhered to due to a patient's condition, for example acute illness, an explanation should be given to the patient and an alternative plan agreed. For example, if intermittent catheterisation cannot be managed during an acute illness, the patient may require a urethral indwelling catheter and a clamping regime to maintain bladder capacity.

Conclusion

Care and management of the patient following SCI is complex. However, a fundamental understanding of the pathophysiology of injury to the spinal cord can help the practitioner to make sense of the fundamentals of that care. Ideally, such care should be provided in a specialist SCI centre, but where this is not possible the practitioner working in the general hospital setting can seek advice and support from their nearest centre and from various organisations that specialise in this aspect of care.

Further Reading

As the scope of this chapter has been limited, the recommended further reading should be accessed. The following are examples that may be supplemented by other, locality-specific sources in the reader's own country.

American Spinal Injury Association Learning Center. https://asia-spinalinjury.org/learning/ (accessed 26 January 2022).

British Association for Spinal Cord Injury Specialists (2022) http://www.bascis.org.uk (accessed 26 January 2022). Includes good practice guides.

British Orthopaedic Association Standards for Trauma and Orthopaedics (2014) The management of traumatic spinal cord injuries. https://www.boa.ac.uk/resources/boast-8-pdf.html. A website for medical and paramedical professionals working in the field of spinal cord injury. Contains elearning modules.

Harrison, P. (ed.) (2007). *Managing Spinal Cord Injury: The First 48 Hours*. Milton Keynes: Spinal Injuries Association.

Multidisciplinary Association of Spinal Cord Injury Professionals. http://www.MASCIP.co.uk or https://www.

mascip.co.uk/sci-charities/sci-resources/ (accessed 27 January 2022).

Royal College of Nursing (2019) Bowel Care: Management of Lower Bowel Dysfunction, including Digital Rectal Examination and Digital Removal of Faeces. https://www.rcn.org.uk/professional-development/publications/pub-007522 (accessed 23 January 2022).

Spinal Cord Injury Charities have a wealth of educational material and resources, e.g.

Spinal Cord Injury Association (UK), http://www.spinal.co.uk/

Back Up, https://www.backuptrust.org.uk

Aspire, https://www.aspire.org.uk

References

Alizadeh, A., Dyck, S.M., and Karimi-Abdolrezaee, S. (2019). Traumatic spinal cord injury: an overview of pathophysiology, models and acute injury mechanisms. *Front Neurol. Mar* 22 (10): 282. https://doi.org/10.3389/fneur.2019.00282. PMID: 30967837; PMCID: PMC6439316.

Bailey, J., Dijkers, M.P., Gassaway, J. et al. (2012). Relationship of nursing education and care management inpatient rehabilitation interventions and patient characteristics to outcomes following spinal cord injury: The SCIRehab project. *J. Spinal Cord Med.* 35 (6): 593–610.

BMJ (2020) *Orthostatic Hypotension. BMJ Best Practice.* https://bestpractice.bmj.com/topics/en-gb/972 ().

British Orthopaedic Association (2021). BOA Standards for Trauma and Othopaedic (BOASTs). https://www.boa.ac.uk/standards-guidance/boasts.html.

Chaw, E., Shem, K., Wong, S.L. et al. (2012). Dysphagia and associated respiratory considerations in cervical spinal cord injury. *Top Spinal Cord Inj. Rehabil.* 18 (4): 291–299. https://doi.org/10.1310/sci1804-291.

Chen, Y., He, Y., and DeVivo, M.J. (2016). Changing demographics and injury profile of new traumatic spinal cord injuries in the United States, 1972–2014. *Arch. Phys. Med. Rehabil.* 97 (10): 1610–1619.

Harvey, M. and Davidson, J. (2011). Long term consequences of critical illness: a new opportunity for high impact critical care nurses. *Crit. Care Nurse* 31 (5): 12–15.

Johns, J., Krogh, K., Rodriguez, G.M. et al. (2021). Management of neurogenic bowel dysfunction in adults after spinal cord injury: clinical practice guideline for health care providers. *Top Spinal Cord Inj. Rehabil.* 27 (2): 75–151.

Kripa, K.C. and Khanal, S. (2021). Use of midodrine and fludrocortisone in neurogenic shock: A case report. *Ann. Med. Surg* 70: https://doi.org/10.1016/j.amsu.2021.102811. https://www.sciencedirect.com/science/article/pii/S2049080121007615.

Kuris, E.O., Alsoof, D., Osorio, C., and Daniels, A.H. (2021). Bowel and bladder care in patients with spinal cord injury. *J. Am. Acad. Orthop. Surg.* 30 (6): 263–272.

Lakra, C., Swayne, O., Christofi, G., and Desai, M. (2021). Autonomic dysreflexia in spinal cord injury. *Pract. Neurol.* 21 (6): 532–538. https://doi.org/10.1136/practneurol-2021-002956.

Lee, J.C., Gross, B.W., Rittenhouse, K.J. et al. (2016). A bitter pill to swallow: dysphagia in cervical spine injury. *J. Surg. Res.* 201 (2): 388–393. https://doi.org/10.1016/j.jss.2015.11.031.

Maharaj, M.M., Hogan, J.A., Phan, K., and Mobbs, R.J. (2016). The role of specialist units to provide focused care and complication avoidance following traumatic spinal cord injury: a systematic review. *Eur. Spine J.* 25 (6): 1813–1820.

MASCIP (2012). *Guidelines for Management of Neurogenic Bowel Dysfunction in Individuals with Central Neurological Conditions*. Peterborough: Coloplast Ltd.

MASCIP (2018) Statement on Spinal Cord Injury Bowel Management. https://www.mascip.co.uk/wp-content/uploads/2019/11/SCI-Bowel-Management-01-Nov-2018.pdf (accessed 15 January 2022).

McDaid, D., Park, A., Gall, A. et al. (2019). Understanding and modelling the economic impact of spinal cord injuries in the United Kingdom. *Spinal Cord* 57: 9.

McRae, J., Smith, C., Beeke, S. et al. (2019). Oropharyngeal dysphagia management in cervical spinal cord injury patients: an exploratory survey of variations to care across specialised and non-specialised units. *Spinal Cord Ser. Cases* 5: 31. https://doi.org/10.1038/s41394-019-0175-y.

National Spinal Cord Injury Statistics Center (2021) *Spinal cord injury facts and figures at a glance.* https://www.nscisc.uab.edu/Public/Facts%20and%20Figures%20-%202021.pdf.

Nelson, M. and Orr, M. (2021). Digital rectal stimulation as an intervention in persons with spinal cord injury and upper motor neuron neurogenic bowel. An evidenced-based systematic review of the literature. *J. Spinal Cord Med.* 44 (4): 525–532. https://doi.org/10.1080/10790268.2019.1696077.

New, P., Reeves, R., Smith, E. et al. (2016). International retrospective comparison of inpatient rehabilitation for patients with spinal cord dysfunction: differences according to etiology archives of physical medicine and rehabilitation. *Arch. Phy. Med. Rehab.* 97 (3): 380–385.

New, P.W., Lee, B.B., Cripps, R. et al. (2019). Global mapping for the epidemiology of paediatric spinal cord damage: towards a living data repository. *Spinal Cord* 57: 183–197. https://doi.org/10.1038/s41393-018-0209-5.

NHS England (2019) Spinal Cord Injury Services (Adults and Children). https://www.england.nhs.uk/wp-content/uploads/2019/04/service-spec-spinal-cord-injury-services-all-ages.pdf.

NICE (2016a) Spinal Injury: assessment and initial management. https://www.nice.org.uk/guidance/ng41 (accessed 5 January 2022).

NICE (2016b) Major Trauma: Assessment and Initial Management. https://www.nice.org.uk/guidance/ng39 (accessed 5 January 2022).

Nursing and Midwifery Council (2018). *The Code: Professional Standards of Practice and Behaviour for Nurses, Midwives and Nursing Associates.* London: Nursing & Midwifery Council.

Quadri, S.A., Farooqui, M., Ikram, A. et al. (2020). Recent update on basic mechanisms of spinal cord injury. *Neurosurg. Rev.* 43 (2): 425–441.

RISCI (2017) Weaning Guidelines for spinal cord injured patients. http://risci.org.uk/weaning-guidelines-for-spinal-cord-injured-patients-in-critical-care-units/ (accessed 10 January 2022).

Rodger, S. (2019). Management of patients with non-traumatic spinal cord injury. *Nurs. Times [online].* 115 (3): 34–37.

Roth, J.D., Pariser, J.J., Stoffel, J.T. et al. (2019). Patient subjective assessment of urinary tract infection frequency and severity is associated with bladder management method in spinal cord injury. *Spinal Cord* 57 (8): 700–707.

Royal College of Nursing (2019) Bowel Care: Management of Lower Bowel Dysfunction, including Digital Rectal Examination and Digital Removal of Faeces. https://www.rcn.org.uk/professional-development/publications/pub-007522 (accessed 23 January 2022).

Ruiz, I.A., Squair, J.W., Phillips, A.A. et al. (2018). Incidence and natural progression of neurogenic shock after traumatic spinal cord injury. *J. Neurotrauma* 35 (3): 461–466. http://doi.org/10.1089/neu.2016.4947.

Saul, D. and Dresing, K. (2018). Epidemiology of vertebral fractures in pediatric and adolescent patients. *Pedia. Rep.* 10 (1): 17–23. https://doi.org/10.4081/pr.2018.7232.

Sezer, N., Akkus, S., and Gulcinugirlu, F. (2015). Complications of spinal cord injury. *J. World Orthop.* 6 (1): 24–33.

Singh, G., MacGillivray, M., Mills, P. et al. (2019). Patients' perspectives on the usability of a mobile app for self-management following spinal cord injury. *J. Med. Systems* 44 (1): 26.

Smyth, C., Spada, M.M., Coultry-Keane, K., and Ikkos, G. (2016). The stanmore nursing assessment of psychological status: understanding the emotions of patients with spinal cord injury. *J. Spinal Cord Med.* 39 (5): 519–526. https://doi.org/10.1080/10790268.2016.1163809.

Taweel, W.A. and Seyam, R. (2015). Neurogenic bladder in spinal cord injury patients. *Res. Rep. Urol.* 7: 85–99. https://doi.org/10.2147/RRU.S29644. PMID: 26090342; PMCID: PMC4467746.

Van Wyk, K., Backwell, A., Townson, A.A. et al. (2015). Narrative literature review to direct spinal cord injury education programming. *Top. Spinal Cord Inj. Rehabil.* 21 (1): 49–60.

Wecht, J.M. (2022). Management of blood pressure disorders in individuals with spinal cord injury. *Curr. Opin. Pharmacol.* 62: 60–63. https://doi.org/10.1016/j.coph.2021.10.003.

Widerström-Noga, E., Anderson, K.D., Perez, S. et al. (2016). Living with chronic pain after spinal cord injury: a mixed-methods study. *Arch. Phys. Med. Rehab.* 98 (5): 856–865.

World Health Organization (2013) Spinal Cord Injury Factsheet. https://www.who.int/news-room/fact-sheets/detail/spinal-cord-injury.

21

Soft Tissue, Peripheral Nerve and Brachial Plexus Injury

Julie Craig[1], Beverley Gray Linnecor[2], and Martyn Neil[1]

[1] *Trauma and Orthopaedic Department, Belfast Health and Social Care Trust, Belfast, UK*
[2] *International Journal of Orthopaedic and Trauma Nursing*

Introduction

The aim of this chapter is to provide evidence-based guidance for the assessment, investigation, surgical and conservative care, management and rehabilitation for patients who have sustained a soft tissue injury, peripheral nerve injury or injury to the brachial plexus. Each section will also provide a brief overview of the associated anatomy.

Soft Tissue Injuries

Soft tissue injuries have several mechanisms of injury but are often caused by either overuse of musculoskeletal soft tissue or a single specific injuring event. With the exception of degenerative tears, most injuries present with a clear history of direct trauma or a change from usual activities. The impact on the patient of such injuries can be underestimated and it is important to make a full assessment and follow this with an effective plan of care.

Ligaments and Tendons

Ligaments and tendons are collagenous tissues that have an important role in the musculoskeletal system, providing strength and mechanical stability to joints.

Ligaments form attachments between bones, and tendons are the strong collagenous end-portions in continuity with muscles. Tendons usually attach muscles to bones, but can attach to other tendons in the case of lumbricals. Muscles therefore exert their action on bones through their tendon attachments. The patellar tendon, between the patella and the tibial tuberosity on the proximal tibia, is still considered to be a tendon as the patella is a sesamoidal bone (a bone encased within a tendon), so the patellar tendon is a continuation of the quadriceps muscles and quadriceps tendon.

Tendons are strong and have little elasticity, allowing them to transmit the forces from muscles efficiently. They have few blood vessels, making them difficult to heal if inflamed, and unlikely to heal without surgery if completely ruptured/severed. As tendons often act as 'pulley ropes', they often have cushioning pads around bony prominences to reduce friction from abrasion.

Sprains and Strains

Soft tissue injuries are often treated in primary and secondary care settings. Strains and sprains are both soft tissue injures, but the tissue affected is different.

A *sprain* is an injury to a ligament supporting a joint. A twisting mechanism usually causes damage to fibres of the affected ligament and/or the joint capsule itself, resulting in decreased joint stability. Three grades of ligament injury/sprain are recognised (Altizer 2003):

- *Grade I, Mild*: Stability is maintained, but can be decreased. The injury is often caused by a wrenching or twisting mechanism and commonly seen at the ankle. The site may be tender, with bruising and mild oedema. In the case of sprains around the foot or ankle, the patient can usually walk, but with some discomfort.
- *Grade II, Moderate*: Partial rupture or tear. Some fibres are torn, but some remain intact although with some loss of stability. More than one ligament may be torn, increasing the severity of the injury and affecting the treatment regime that follows. The joint is tender, painful and difficult to move, usually with some swelling and bruising.
- *Grade III, Severe*: Complete rupture with loss of continuity of one or several ligaments. This causes loss of stability and a weakened, painful joint with significantly decreased

range of movement. The patient is unable to actively move the joint or to weight bear, and the injury has a significant impact on mobility and activities of living.

A *strain* is an injury caused by overstretching of the muscle and may be severe enough to cause a partial or complete tear. These may also be mild, moderate or severe:

- *Mild*: Pain and stiffness lasting a few days.
- *Moderate*: Partial tears causing more pain and swelling, with bruising with symptoms lasting for 1 to 3 weeks.
- *Severe*: Complete tears resulting in significant swelling, bruising and pain.

Complete tears of tendons often require surgical repair, but muscle tears are usually not suitable for surgical repair due to their more fragile consistency.

Management and Care

There are some general principles of management for all soft tissue injuries.

Pain Management

The most obvious symptom of soft tissue injury is pain, caused by the traumatic damage to tissue, cell hypoxia and release of chemicals such as histamine, bradykinin and prostaglandin as well as pressure on local nerve endings from swelling. Pain relief is usually provided with simple analgesia and/or non-steroidal anti-inflammatory drugs (Chapter 11). However, anti-inflammatories should generally be avoided if a fracture is suspected due to the risk of impaired bone healing. Cryotherapy (the application of cold) has also been shown to have a positive effect on pain relief (Airaksinen et al. 2003) as the cold reduces nerve conductivity.

Control of Swelling

Swelling is due to the release of chemicals, including prostaglandin, histamine and serotonin, which increases the permeability of the cell membrane resulting in protein escaping into the interstitial space. This increases the osmotic pressure and causes increased oedema and associated pain and discomfort. The control of swelling is facilitated by rest, ice, compression and elevation.

Rest, Ice, Compression and Elevation (mnemonic: RICE)

- *Rest*: It is important to maintain the normal correct anatomical alignment of the injured structures while immobilising the area until a full clinical examination and diagnosis is made. This will dictate the recovery time that can be expected and the subsequent plan of care. This may include a period of non-weight-bearing or supported weight-bearing with mobility aids, the application of a cast, brace, splint or supporting bandage and advice on when to return to physical activities.
- *Ice*: In an acute phase of injury, ice can help reduce pain and inflammation and muscle spasm. It decreases the inflammatory responses and cold-mediated vasoconstriction can help to decrease oedema. Ice should not be applied directly to the skin due to the risk of ice burns. The ice is best applied frequently for moderate periods of time and for a minimum of 3 days (Airaksinen et al. 2003).

- *Compression*: This can be applied using an elastic tubular bandage or equivalent with the aim of controlling the oedema at the injury site and to aid venous return. The evidence for this practise is, however, limited. Care is advised with the amount of compression applied to avoid other complications such as the tourniquet effect and compartment syndrome. The aim is to assist with venous and lymphatic drainage and the dispersal of inflammatory fluid whilst preventing an accumulation of oedema.
- *Elevation*: This assists in lymphatic and venous drainage and reduces pain by reducing pressure on the capillaries and tissues. The injured part should be elevated above the level of the heart, but caution is advocated with any suspected compartment syndrome.

The goal of treatment, management and rehabilitation is to improve the condition of the injured area to allow a return of functional ability so that the patient can return to full daily activities. Depending on the level of mobility of the patient, significant nursing support may be needed along with assisted personal care.

Nerve Injuries

Principles of Nerve Injuries

All nerves in the body can be traced back to either the brain or the spinal column. For all the nerves of the limbs, they begin where spinal nerve roots exit the spinal column between the vertebrae though the vertebral foramina, with one spinal nerve root leaving from the left side and one from the right at the level of each junction between vertebrae. These spinal nerves are named based on the level at which they leave the spinal column. Nerves leaving from the cervical spine are named based on the bone they exit above (i.e. the C3 nerve root exits above vertebra C3 and below vertebra C2), with the exception of nerve root C8, which exits below the C7 vertebra as there is no eighth cervical vertebra. Nerves exiting from the thoracic spine or lumbar spine are named based on the bone they exit below (i.e. the L4 nerve root exits below vertebra L4 and above vertebra L5). Embryologically, the sacrum develops as a fusion of several bones, so the nerves exiting from the sacrum (the sacral nerves) are named S1–S5, with the top of the sacrum generally referred to as level S1 in spinal surgery (hence the nerve root L5 exits at the junction of L5 and S1).

Many nerves in the upper and lower limbs are formed from the merging and dividing of spinal nerve roots that emerge from the spinal column. A network of nerves (or vessels) joining and dividing can be described as a plexus. The nerves of the arm derive from the brachial plexus and the nerves of the leg derive from the sacral plexus. In each case, spinal nerve roots merge and separate, ultimately giving rise to peripheral nerves. The anatomical structure of the brachial plexus and individual peripheral nerves is discussed below.

Nerve injuries can occur anywhere along the long route from their starting point at the spinal nerve roots to the ends of the peripheral nerves. However, the principles of how nerves can be damaged and their treatment follow some common themes regardless of the point of injury.

The spinal cord ends at the level of L1, so the spinal nerve roots which have not exited by that level continue down within the spinal column as the cauda equina (literally meaning horse's tail), with each nerve root exiting at the relevant level. For this reason, compression of the spinal columns above the level of L1 causes spinal cord compression, but below this level causes compression of nerve roots before they exit. This can be seen in the case of large vertebral disc prolapses or spinal tumours.

The Anatomy of the Brachial Plexus

A *plexus* is a network of nerves or blood vessels and *brachial* is an adjective relating to or affecting the arm. The *brachial plexus* is a network of nerves that provide muscle control

(motor function) and feeling (sensory function) to all of the shoulder and arm. The brachial plexus is formed from five spinal nerve roots: spinal nerve roots from the four lowest cervical roots (C5, C6, C7 and C8) and the first thoracic root (T1) (Figure 21.1). The spinal nerves leave the spinal column through the vertebral foramina between the vertebrae, and then undergo a complex process of joining and division of nerve fibres to form the brachial plexus. As the nerve fibres merge and divide, the various sections are referred to as roots, trunks, divisions, cords and branches (the latter being peripheral nerves). This network of nerves weaves around one of the large arteries between the back of the neck and the axilla. (This artery is called the subclavian artery above the lateral edge of the first rib and called the axillary artery beyond this.) As a result, brachial plexus injuries should be assessed for possible damage of the adjacent artery. Each section is also named in terms of its position in relation to the artery.

After leaving the spinal column, the spinal nerve roots (C5–C8 and T1) form three trunks:

- C5 and C6 spinal nerve roots merge to form the upper trunk
- C7 spinal nerve root forms the middle trunk
- C8 and T1 spinal nerve roots merge to form the lower trunk.

These trunks are relevant as some injuries (particularly traction injuries) only involve the upper or lower trunk.

Each of these three trunks then divides into two branches called divisions: anterior and posterior. The three posterior divisions merge to form the posterior cord, which gives rise to the axillary and radial nerves. These control the abduction of the shoulder (axillary nerve), elbow extension (radial nerve) and wrist extension (radial nerve), which is easily remembered by the posterior location of the latter muscle groups.

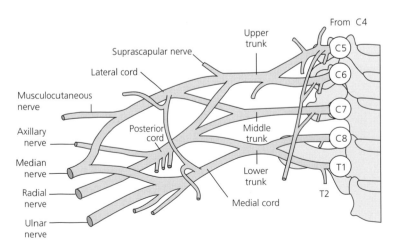

Figure 21.1 The brachial plexus. *Source:* Scottish National Brachial Plexus Injury Service, Information for patients, Dec 2012. Medical Illustration Services, NHS Greater Glasgow and Clyde.

The three anterior divisions form two cords: medial (from the anterior division of the lower trunk) and lateral (from the merging of the two other divisions).

The lateral cord divides to form the musculocutaneous nerve and a component of the median nerve. The musculocutaneous nerve supplies the flexor muscles of the elbow.

The medial cord divides to form the ulnar nerve and the main component of the median nerve. The median nerve therefore has components of the medial and lateral cords, so is contributed to by spinal roots C6, C7, C8 and T1.

The median nerve controls most of the flexor muscles of the wrist and some of the muscles in the hand and thumb base.

The ulnar nerve controls most of the small muscles within the hand and a small portion of the forearm muscles that flex the wrist.

The nerves derived from the medial cord are therefore responsible for most muscles causing flexion of the wrist and digits.

The five main peripheral nerves in the upper arm are:

the axillary nerve
the radial nerve
the musculocutaneous nerve
the median nerve
the ulnar nerve.

All these nerves have roles in motor function (muscle movement) and sensory function (feeling, particularly to the skin), although many divide into separate motor and sensory branches near the end of their course. The area of sensation supplied by a nerve often matches fairly closely with the location of the muscles supplied by the nerve. Table 21.1 provides a summary of the origins of the main peripheral nerves of the arm. Peripheral nerve injuries are usually associated with another musculoskeletal injury such as a fracture and can have far-reaching effects for the patient. The practitioner needs an understanding of the peripheral nerve supply to understand the impact of nerve injury on the patient.

Table 21.1 The origins of the main peripheral nerves of the arm.

Spinal nerve root	Cord	Peripheral nerve
C5, C6	Posterior	Axillary
C5, C6, C7, C8	Posterior	Radial
C5, C6, C7	Lateral	Musculocutaneous
C6, C7, C8, T1	Lateral and medial	Median
C8, T1	Medial	Ulnar

Radial Nerve Injury

The radial nerve is the most commonly injured nerve of the upper limb, often alongside fractures of the humerus. The radial nerve curls along the back of the humerus from medial to lateral beneath the triceps. It then continues round the lateral side of the distal humerus to the front of the elbow, anterior to the radial head, where it divides into a motor branch and a sensory branch. This position makes it prone to injury when the arm suffers trauma at either the level of the humerus or the elbow.

The radial nerve supplies motor function to the triceps (which extends the elbow) on the posterior aspect of the humerus and the main forearm muscles that cause extension of the wrist, as well as sensation to the posterior aspect of the arm and forearm, back of the hand and dorsal aspect of the thumb base.

The causes of radial nerve injury are closely associated with its anatomical position and include:

- injury associated with fracture of the midshaft or distal humerus, or radial head dislocation
- pressure damage from poor application technique or prolonged use of a tourniquet or blood pressure cuff, or casting/bracing that is too tight around the humerus. Such pressure can also occur when the arm is left hanging over the side or back of a chair, bed or trolley (often associated with alcohol intoxication and poor sleep posturing).

Patients usually present with weakness in their wrist extension and finger extension (called 'wrist drop') and may also have reduced or absent sensation over the dorsum of the thumb base and first web space. Conservative management of the wrist drop is provided with a wrist support/splint and specific physiotherapy exercises to prevent contractures.

Ulnar Nerve Injury

The ulnar nerve is derived from spinal nerve roots C8 and T1. The ulnar nerve travels along the posteromedial aspect of the humerus but does not provide any muscle control or sensation above the elbow. It curls around the back of the medial epicondyle of the elbow. It then enters the flexor compartment of the forearm, supplying movement to flexor carpi ulnaris (FCU, a wrist flexor), running close to the ulnar bone. The ulnar nerve also supplies the long flexors to the little and ring finger (flexor digitorum profundus), most of the muscles within the hand, and sensation to the ulnar side of the hand, the little finger and medial half of the ring finger.

The causes of ulnar nerve injury are closely associated with its anatomical position and include:

- compression by tight soft tissue bands at the elbow, such as when it passes through the cubital tunnel
- stretching around the medial epicondyle of the humerus
- injury during elbow/distal humerus fractures or elbow dislocation.

Patients usually experience paraesthesia or numbness in the ring and little fingers. They may also be unable to spread the fingers apart, flex the metacarpophalangeal joints or extend the interphalangeal joints. Severe entrapment or complete severing of the ulnar nerve can present with wasting of the muscles that provide these movements and development of a 'claw hand'. Conservative management of ulnar clawing of the fingers is provided with splinting to maintain functional position and specific exercises to prevent further joint stiffness. Ulnar nerve symptoms resulting from areas of localised soft tissue pressure on the nerve (e.g. cubital tunnel syndrome) may be suitable for surgical release.

Median Nerve Injury

The median nerve is derived from spinal nerve roots C5–T1. The median nerve travels down the medial side of the upper arm, alongside the brachial artery, between the biceps brachii and brachialis muscles. It then crosses the artery near the elbow, crossing the anterior aspect of the elbow just medial to the tendon of biceps brachii, to the flexor group of muscles on the anteromedial aspect of the forearm. It continues along the forearm and enters the hand on the palmar side of the wrist through the narrow space of the carpal tunnel (between the carpal bones and the transverse carpal ligament of the wrist). The median nerve supplies most of the flexor muscles in the forearm that are responsible for most of the wrist and finger flexion, as necessary for strong grip. Within the hand, it supplies motor innervation to the lateral two lumbricals (i.e. to the index and middle fingers) and three muscles in the thenar eminence at the base of the thumb (opponens policies, abductor pollicis brevis and flexor pollicis brevis). These latter three muscles are responsible for thumb opposition (moving the thumb across the palm towards the base of the little finger), thumb abduction (moving the thumb at 90° from the palm) and flexion at the interphalangeal joint in the thumb. The median nerve provides sensation to the palmar surfaces of the thumb, the index and middle fingers, and the lateral half of the ring finger.

The causes of median nerve injury are closely associated with its anatomical position and include:

- above the elbow, an injury may result in loss of pronation and a reduction in flexion of the wrist, as well as pincer grip where the interphalangeal joints within the thumb

and finger bend. The 'Okay' sign, of making a circle with the index finger and thumb, is therefore used to assess for damage to the anterior interosseous branch of the median nerve injury in supracondylar elbow fractures.
- at the wrist, compression at the carpal tunnel causes carpal tunnel syndrome.

Carpel tunnel syndrome involves paraesthesia (tingling and 'pins and needles') in the thumb, index and middle fingers, and the adjacent half of the ring finger, and often a dull aching and discomfort in the hand. Thumb movements, specifically thumb abduction and opposition, can become weak and the muscles of the thenar eminence may eventually become wasted.

Mild cases of carpal tunnel syndrome may be treated nonoperatively with wrist splints or steroid injection, or treatment of underlying reversible underlying causes. Surgical management involves decompression of the median nerve by releasing the tight soft tissues of the transverse carpal ligament, which forms the roof the carpel tunnel.

Tinel's test is commonly used to assess for impaired nerve function. It involves tapping over the affected nerve to elicit a reaction such as paraesthesia. This can be used to help identify the level of nerve irritation, such as by tapping over the region of the carpal tunnel to see if neurological symptoms are likely to be related to pressure at that site. Alternatively, in nerves which had not displayed any function due to substantial injury, eliciting a response from tapping over the nerve may be a sign of early nerve recovery.

Sciatic Nerve Injury

As the brachial plexus involves the joining and separating of nerves to form the nerves of the arm, so the lumbar and sacral nerve roots form the lumbar plexus to form the nerves of the legs. The sciatic nerve arises from the sacral plexus from the roots of spinal nerves L4 and L5 and S1–S3. It crosses behind the hip joint, descends along the back of the femur and divides just above the knee to form the tibial nerve and common fibular nerve. Due to its proximity to the hip joint, it is at risk of injury in hip fractures (i.e. proximal femoral fractures), acetabular fractures and hip surgery (particularly joint replacement surgery, either electively or for fracture). Dislocation of a hip replacement prosthesis or, more rarely, a patient's native hip can also injure the sciatic nerve.

The symptoms of sciatic nerve damage include paraesthesia and/or loss of sensation over the medial side of the leg below the knee (except in the medial border of the foot supplied by the saphenous nerve). The patient may also have severe weakness or paralysis of the hamstring muscles, causing an inability to flex the knee and weakness of ankle dorsiflexion resulting in 'foot drop'. As few sciatic nerve injuries involve the nerve being completely severed, most are managed non-operatively with the use of orthotics or splints such as ankle-foot orthosis (AFO) splints, walking aids and lifestyle adaptation advice. As the lumbar nerve roots that contribute to the sciatic nerve (L4 and L5) can be compressed at the level of the spine, most commonly due to vertebral disc prolapses, care should be taken in history-taking, examination and investigation to differentiate between sciatic nerve and lumbar nerve root irritation as some symptoms may be similar.

All peripheral nerve injuries require a complete patient history and thorough clinical examination (see also Chapter 7) to establish the level of the injury. A tool used to grade muscle power and sensory function is the Medical Research Council (MRC) scale (Table 21.2).

The British Orthopaedic Association (https://www.boa.ac.uk/) recently released the British Orthopaedic Association Standards for Trauma (BOAST) on Peripheral Nerve Injuries (2021), a one-page guidance document focused on the practicalities, which is a valuable resource for readers of this chapter. The recent Standard for Practice provides background and justification, inclusion and exclusion followed by the key sections:

- Identification of peripheral nerve injury
- Response to identification of peripheral nerve injury
- Audit.

Table 21.2 MRC scale for assessment of muscle power.

Motor function	
M 0	No muscle contraction is visible
M 1	Return of perceptible contraction in proximal muscles
M 2	Return of perceptible contraction in proximal and distal muscles
M 3	Return of proximal and distal muscle power to act against resistance
M 4	Return of function as stage 3 + independent movement possible
M 5	Complete recovery
Sensory function within the autonomous area	
S 0	Absence of sensibility
S 1	Return of deep cutaneous pain
S 2	Return of some degree of superficial cutaneous pain and touch
S 3	Return of some degree of superficial cutaneous pain and touch with disappearance of previous overreaction
S 3/4	As stage 3 with some recovery of two-point discrimination
S 4/5	Complete recovery

Source: Adapted from Medical Research Council (1981).

The BOAST 2021 guidance is available at https://www.boa.ac.uk/resources/boast-peripheral-nerve-injury.html.

Brachial Plexus Injuries

Mechanisms of Injury

Nerve injuries can be classified in different ways and are often referred to as being open or closed injuries, the latter being either high-energy or low-energy injuries:

- *Open injuries* occur as a result of a penetrating wound that can lacerate the nerves, e.g. stabbing or falling through a glass door.
- *Closed injuries* occur as a result of either high-energy or low-energy injuries, and occur without breaching the skin.
- *High-energy injuries* are often associated with motor vehicle collisions or falls from a height, and can be caused by violent stretching or pulling, typically around the neck or shoulder in the case of nerve root or brachial plexus injuries. Traction injuries can affect mainly upper nerve roots (Erb's palsy, causing paralysis of shoulder abduction and elbow flexion) or mainly lower nerve roots (Klumpke's palsy, causing paralysis to the muscles within the hand). These can also occur as obstetric injuries to the newborn during vaginal delivery. Nerve injuries can occur with or without concurrent injuries such as fractures.
- *Low-energy injuries* are usually the result of blunt trauma to the neck or upper limb causing crushing of the nerves, such as nerve damage caused by a prolonged period of pressure, particularly in patients who are not mobile and alert. This can occur in anaesthetised patients (e.g. ventilated patients in intensive care) who have prolonged periods of prone positioning with their arms positioned above their head.

If the injury was sustained due to a high-velocity accident, e.g. a motorcycle collision, the likelihood of a more serious pathology is much greater than when the injury is sustained from a comparably low-velocity fall. Patients involved in high-velocity accidents are also more likely to sustain other injuries such as fractures to the spine, pelvis and/or limbs, head injuries (with or without skull fracture) and vascular injuries (see Chapters 16 and 19 for further information). These other injuries have to be considered when prioritising care for the newly injured patient, as neurological injuries seldom cause immediate threat to life, but injuries causing loss of consciousness (including conscious control of airway patency), breathing difficulties and blood loss can be immediately life-threatening.

In the absence of obvious trauma, other neurological conditions should be considered. For example, brachial plexus neuritis (also called idiopathic brachial plexus neuropathy, brachial neuritis or Parsonage Turner syndrome) is an inflammatory condition which can occur without any trauma or obvious cause. Similarly, upper motor neurone causes such as stroke should be considered.

Grades of Injury

While injuries at different points along the course of a nerve will have specific consequences, some general principles are common to most nerve injuries. Three broad categories of severity of nerve injury can be explained by the structure of nerves.

1) Neuropraxia involves damage to the myelin sheath, which aids conduction of impulses through the nerve. The axons remain intact, so recovery is possible over time, depending on the degree of demyelination.
2) Axonotmesis results from damage to the axons, although the surrounding layers such as the endoneurium remain intact. Recovery is therefore possible, but much more slowly than in neuropraxia.
3) Neurotmesis is the complete rupture/severing of a nerve and its surrounding layers, and spontaneous recovery would not be expected.

It can be difficult to tell the difference between these options in the early stages on the basis of examination only, although nerves which retain some function (e.g. motor function but with reduced sensation) are generally not completely cut (i.e. not neurotmesis).

Nerve Root Injuries

Injuries at the level of the nerve root may involve avulsion from the attachment to the spinal cord, rupture due to stretching or dysfunction of the nerves due to stretching or bruising without complete rupture. Injuries at the level of the nerve root are rare and generally managed by specialist centres. Surgical management options are limited. Horner's syndrome, classically involving ptosis (eyelid drooping), miosis (reduced pupil size), anhydrosis (reduced sweating to the face) and enophthalmos (sinking of the eyeball into the eye socket), can occur with nerve root avulsions to C8 and T1 due to disruption of the sympathetic nerve supply in this area.

Plexus Injuries

Patients who have sustained an injury or damage to the brachial plexus will present with motor and sensory loss in all or part of the upper limb depending on the extent of the injury.

Brachial plexus injuries can be caused by a traction injury to the brachial plexus (e.g. in a motorcycle accident where the shoulder or neck is forcibly stretched or longer periods of stretching as during prone positioning during anaesthesia), adjacent bony injuries (e.g. proximal humerus fracture or shoulder dislocation) or direct injury (e.g. stabbing or gunshot wound). Common patterns of supraclavicular injury can be subdivided into three groups:

1) *Upper plexus*: mainly affecting nerves derived from the roots of C5 and C6
2) *Lower plexus*: mainly affecting nerves derived from the roots of C8 to TI
3) *Total plexus*: there is damage to the whole plexus and all peripheral nerves derived from it.

Upper plexus injuries can result in Erb's palsy, typified by weakness in shoulder abduction (C5), elbow flexion (C5) and wrist extension (C6), resulting in a straight downward hanging arm.

Lower plexus injuries can result in Klumpke's palsy, typified by weakness in the small muscles within the hand responsible for flexion of the fingers at the metacarpophalangeal joints (C8) and abduction of the fingers (T1) resulting in clawing of the fingers.

Peripheral Nerve Injuries

Neuropraxia is the most common type of peripheral nerve injury caused by blunt trauma or stretching. Complete tears of peripheral nerves are less common and can be directly repaired, but without any guarantee of recovery. If there is a gap between the ends of a cut nerve, reconstruction with a graft from another nerve may be considered in specialist centres, although this is rare and also without guarantee of restoration of function.

Diagnosis and Investigations

A thorough clinical examination is essential, recording the motor and sensory function of each nerve. In the context of potential spinal injuries or plexus injuries (rather than likely peripheral nerve injuries), it is especially important to fully document the function of individual spinal nerve roots motor functions (myotomes) and sensory function (dermatomes). An established tool used to grade muscle power and sensory function is the MRC Scale (refer to Table 21.2), which should be documented in detail according to muscle group. However, the American Spinal Injuries Association (ASIA) Impairment Scale is now more commonly used (Kirshblum et al. 2020). The two-page updated resource (ASIA 2019) presented in Figure 21.2

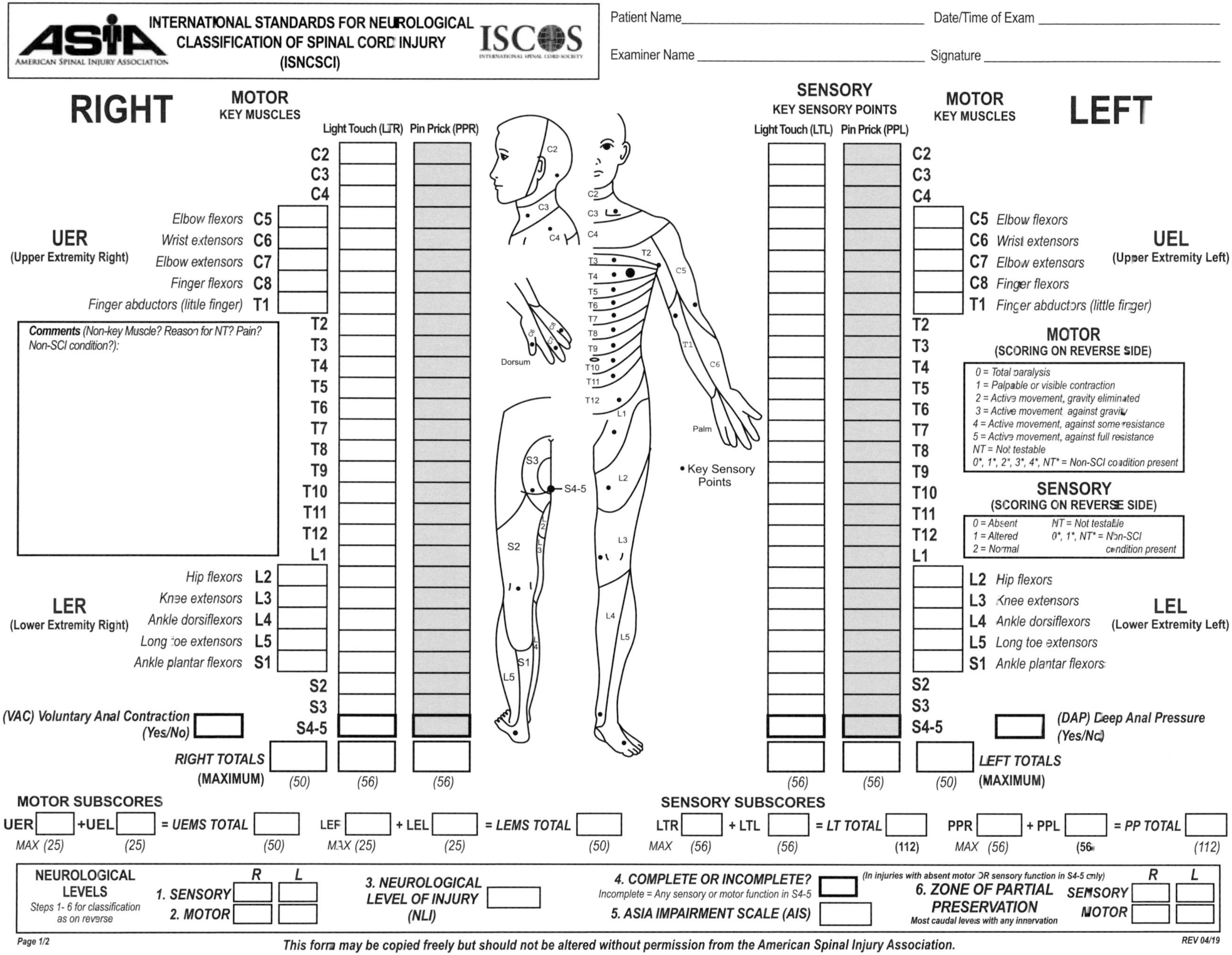

INTERNATIONAL STANDARDS FOR NEUROLOGICAL CLASSIFICATION OF SPINAL CORD INJURY (ISNCSCI)

ASIA — American Spinal Injury Association | ISCOS — International Spinal Cord Society

Patient Name ______ Date/Time of Exam ______

Examiner Name ______ Signature ______

RIGHT

MOTOR KEY MUSCLES

	Motor	Light Touch (LTR)	Pin Prick (PPR)
C2			
C3			
C4			
UER (Upper Extremity Right): Elbow flexors C5			
Wrist extensors C6			
Elbow extensors C7			
Finger flexors C8			
Finger abductors (little finger) T1			
T2			
T3			
T4			
T5			
T6			
T7			
T8			
T9			
T10			
T11			
T12			
L1			
LER (Lower Extremity Right): Hip flexors L2			
Knee extensors L3			
Ankle dorsiflexors L4			
Long toe extensors L5			
Ankle plantar flexors S1			
S2			
S3			
S4-5			
RIGHT TOTALS (MAXIMUM)	(50)	(56)	(56)

Comments (Non-key Muscle? Reason for NT? Pain? Non-SCI condition?):

(VAC) Voluntary Anal Contraction (Yes/No)

SENSORY KEY SENSORY POINTS

LEFT

MOTOR KEY MUSCLES

	Light Touch (LTL)	Pin Prick (PPL)	Motor
C2			
C3			
C4			
C5 Elbow flexors — UEL (Upper Extremity Left)			
C6 Wrist extensors			
C7 Elbow extensors			
C8 Finger flexors			
T1 Finger abductors (little finger)			
T2			
T3			
T4			
T5			
T6			
T7			
T8			
T9			
T10			
T11			
T12			
L1			
L2 Hip flexors — LEL (Lower Extremity Left)			
L3 Knee extensors			
L4 Ankle dorsiflexors			
L5 Long toe extensors			
S1 Ankle plantar flexors			
S2			
S3			
S4-5			
LEFT TOTALS (MAXIMUM)	(56)	(56)	(50)

MOTOR (SCORING ON REVERSE SIDE)

0 = Total paralysis
1 = Palpable or visible contraction
2 = Active movement, gravity eliminated
3 = Active movement, against gravity
4 = Active movement, against some resistance
5 = Active movement, against full resistance
NT = Not testable
0*, 1*, 2*, 3*, 4*, NT* = Non-SCI condition present

SENSORY (SCORING ON REVERSE SIDE)

0 = Absent
1 = Altered
2 = Normal
NT = Not testable
0*, 1*, NT* = Non-SCI condition present

(DAP) Deep Anal Pressure (Yes/No)

MOTOR SUBSCORES

UER ___ + UEL ___ = UEMS TOTAL ___ MAX (25) (25) (50)

LER ___ + LEL ___ = LEMS TOTAL ___ MAX (25) (25) (50)

SENSORY SUBSCORES

LTR ___ + LTL ___ = LT TOTAL ___ MAX (56) (56) (112)

PPR ___ + PPL ___ = PP TOTAL ___ MAX (56) (56) (112)

NEUROLOGICAL LEVELS
Steps 1- 6 for classification as on reverse

	R	L
1. SENSORY		
2. MOTOR		

3. NEUROLOGICAL LEVEL OF INJURY (NLI)

4. COMPLETE OR INCOMPLETE?
Incomplete = Any sensory or motor function in S4-5

5. ASIA IMPAIRMENT SCALE (AIS)

6. ZONE OF PARTIAL PRESERVATION
(In injuries with absent motor OR sensory function in S4-5 only)
Most caudal levels with any innervation

	R	L
SENSORY		
MOTOR		

Page 1/2

REV 04/19

Figure 21.2 ASIA scale.

Muscle Function Grading

0 = Total paralysis

1 = Palpable or visible contraction

2 = Active movement, full range of motion (ROM) with gravity eliminated

3 = Active movement, full ROM against gravity

4 = Active movement, full ROM against gravity and moderate resistance in a muscle specific position

5 = (Normal) active movement, full ROM against gravity and full resistance in a functional muscle position expected from an otherwise unimpaired person

NT = Not testable (i.e. due to immobilization, severe pain such that the patient cannot be graded, amputation of limb, or contracture of > 50% of the normal ROM)

0*, 1*, 2*, 3*, 4*, NT* = Non-SCI condition present [a]

Sensory Grading

0 = Absent   1 = Altered, either decreased/impaired sensation or hypersensitivity

2 = Normal   NT = Not testable

0*, 1*, NT* = Non-SCI condition present [a]

[a] Note: Abnormal motor and sensory scores should be tagged with a '*' to indicate an impairment due to a non-SCI condition. The non-SCI condition should be explained in the comments box together with information about how the score is rated for classification purposes (at least normal / not normal for classification).

When to Test Non-Key Muscles:

In a patient with an apparent AIS B classification, non-key muscle functions more than 3 levels below the motor level on each side should be tested to most accurately classify the injury (differentiate between AIS B and C).

Movement	Root level
Shoulder: Flexion, extension, abduction, adduction, internal and external rotation **Elbow:** Supination	C5
Elbow: Pronation **Wrist:** Flexion	C6
Finger: Flexion at proximal joint, extension **Thumb:** Flexion, extension and abduction in plane of thumb	C7
Finger: Flexion at MCP joint **Thumb:** Opposition, adduction and abduction perpendicular to palm	C8
Finger: Abduction of the index finger	T1
Hip: Adduction	L2
Hip: External rotation	L3
Hip: Extension, abduction, internal rotation **Knee:** Flexion **Ankle:** Inversion and eversion **Toe:** MP and IP extension	L4
Hallux and Toe: DIP and PIP flexion and abduction	L5
Hallux: Adduction	S1

Figure 21.2 (Continued)

ASIA Impairment Scale (AIS)

A = Complete. No sensory or motor function is preserved in the sacral segments S4-5.

B = Sensory Incomplete. Sensory but not motor function is preserved below the neurological level and includes the sacral segments S4-5 (light touch or pin prick at S4-5 or deep anal pressure) AND no motor function is preserved more than three levels below the motor level on either side of the body.

C = Motor Incomplete. Motor function is preserved at the most caudal sacral segments for voluntary anal contraction (VAC) OR the patient meets the criteria for sensory incomplete status (sensory function preserved at the most caudal sacral segments S4-5 by LT, PP or DAP), and has some sparing of motor function more than three levels below the ipsilateral motor level on either side of the body. (This includes key or non-key muscle functions to determine motor incomplete status.) For AIS C – less than half of key muscle functions below the single NLI have a muscle grade ≥ 3.

D = Motor Incomplete. Motor incomplete status as defined above, with at least half (half or more) of key muscle functions below the single NLI having a muscle grade ≥ 3.

E = Normal. If sensation and motor function as tested with the ISNCSCI are graded as normal in all segments, and the patient had prior deficits, then the AIS grade is E. Someone without an initial SCI does not receive an AIS grade.

Using ND: To document the sensory, motor and NLI levels, the ASIA Impairment Scale grade, and/or the zone of partial preservation (ZPP) when they are unable to be determined based on the examination results.

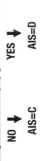

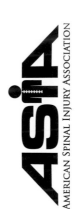

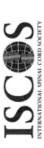

AMERICAN SPINAL INJURY ASSOCIATION

INTERNATIONAL STANDARDS FOR NEUROLOGICAL CLASSIFICATION OF SPINAL CORD INJURY

INTERNATIONAL SPINAL CORD SOCIETY

Page 2/2

Steps in Classification

The following order is recommended for determining the classification of individuals with SCI.

1. Determine sensory levels for right and left sides.
The sensory level is the most caudal, intact dermatome for both pin prick and light touch sensation.

2. Determine motor levels for right and left sides.
Defined by the lowest key muscle function that has a grade of at least 3 (on supine testing), providing the key muscle functions represented by segments above that level are judged to be intact (graded as a 5).
Note: in regions where there is no myotome to test, the motor level is presumed to be the same as the sensory level, if testable motor function above that level is also normal.

3. Determine the neurological level of injury (NLI).
This refers to the most caudal segment of the cord with intact sensation and antigravity (3 or more) muscle function strength, provided that there is normal (intact) sensory and motor function rostrally respectively.
The NLI is the most cephalad of the sensory and motor levels determined in steps 1 and 2.

4. Determine whether the injury is Complete or Incomplete.
(i.e. absence or presence of sacral sparing)
If voluntary anal contraction = **No** AND all S4-5 sensory scores = 0 AND deep anal pressure = **No**, then injury is **Complete**.
Otherwise, injury is **Incomplete**.

5. Determine ASIA Impairment Scale (AIS) Grade.

Is injury Complete?   If YES, AIS=A

NO ↓

Is injury <u>Motor</u> Complete?   If YES, AIS=B

NO ↓   (No=voluntary anal contraction OR motor function more than three levels below the <u>motor level</u> on a given side, if the patient has sensory incomplete classification)

Are at least half (half or more) of the key muscles below the <u>neurological level of injury</u> graded 3 or better?

NO ↓   YES ↓

AIS=C   AIS=D

If sensation and motor function is normal in all segments, AIS=E
Note: AIS E is used in follow-up testing when an individual with a documented SCI has recovered normal function. If at initial testing no deficits are found, the individual is neurologically intact and the ASIA Impairment Scale does not apply.

6. Determine the zone of partial preservation (ZPP).
The ZPP is used only in injuries with absent motor (no VAC) OR sensory function (no DAP, no LT and no PP sensation) in the lowest sacral segments S4-5, and refers to those dermatomes and myotomes caudal to the sensory and motor levels that remain partially innervated. With sacral sparing of sensory function, the sensory ZPP is not applicable and therefore "NA" is recorded in the block of the worksheet. Accordingly, if VAC is present, the motor ZPP is not applicable and is noted as "NA".

may be copied freely but should not be altered without permission from the American Spinal Injury Association.

X-rays of the cervical spine, shoulder and clavicle may be taken to exclude any skeletal/bony injury. An MRI may be considered, but often shows no structural damage in the case of neuropraxia. Nerve root avulsions may cause leakage of cerebrospinal fluid (CSF), which may be seen on MRI scanning of the cervical spine. An MR angiogram can show vascular injuries in the axillary artery, signifying local injury and the potential for injury to the adjacent brachial plexus. Neurophysiology or electrical nerve conduction tests are more accurate in demonstrating the passage of electrical signals along nerves in the limbs using small electrical pulses on the skin. This may include a recording of the electrical activity of muscles using fine needles. These tests can be used to diagnose a variety of nerve or muscle problems.

Non-surgical Management

Most non-penetrating injuries involve neuropraxia or axonotmesis, but this can be difficult to assess on a clinical basis at the early stages. Patients should be counselled regarding the potential for a prolonged period of recovery or the potential for persistent dysfunction.

It is essential that the patient understands the importance of maintaining the range of joint movement while waiting for recovery. Early signs of recovery are sometimes difficult to detect and this highlights the importance of accurate record keeping. Once a flicker of muscle contraction can be detected the patient should then commence prescribed exercises to maximise this improvement. This can include passive and gravity-assisted exercises and/or electrical muscle stimulation (via pads applied to the overlying skin to electrically stimulate muscle contraction, although this does not replace an exercise programme).

It may be necessary to provide some form of splinting to maintain joint position and avoid contractures and/or aid function. There may be a need for an orthosis to be fitted to aid in supporting a paralysed arm that is not functional. Some splints can be used to reduce pain, as in reducing the risk of subluxation in a paralysed shoulder, or for cosmetic purposes, allowing a limb to rest in a more natural position when long-term recovery is not expected.

Surgical Management

While most nerve injuries will not benefit from surgery, even those with a potential benefit from surgery offer a limited prospect for recovery. There are a number of factors that are collectively considered prior to surgery, including the level or grade of injury, the age and fitness of the patient and any other comorbidities.

Primary surgical options include:

- *Direct repair*: This is suitable if there is minor damage to the nerve and the ends are in approximation and can be directly sutured.
- *Nerve graft*: This may be considered where there is a gap between the ends of a severed nerve. A sensory nerve from elsewhere may be used to breech the gap to provide a route for any potential nerve regeneration to follow. The nerve graft acts as a guide through which new nerve fibres can grow and cross the gap caused by the injury. Growth is very slow, recovery time is lengthy and complete recovery may be impossible due to the way that each individual microscopic nerve fibre grows. Common nerve donor sites are the cutaneous nerves in the forearm or the sural nerve in the lower leg. These are sensory nerves and will leave a feeling of paraesthesia or numbness over the harvested nerve's distribution area, but have little effect on function.
- *Nerve transfer*: Undamaged nerves in the area that are performing less valuable functions can be transferred to other parts (e.g. within the brachial plexus) to try and regain some function within the limb. As the nerves used in this transfer start to recover, the patient needs to work very hard at retraining these nerves to move the arm and initially they may have to engage different movements to make the arm function. However, results are often poor.

These primary surgical options are undertaken as soon as is reasonably possible after full investigations and preparation of the patient. Recovery following primary surgery varies according to the individual, the level of injury and the type of surgery performed, but can be prolonged. Therefore, secondary surgery is generally not considered until around 2 years after injury or primary surgery as it is unlikely to achieve much further symptomatic recovery beyond 2 years.

Secondary surgical procedures fall into three categories:

- bony/joint fusion (arthrodesis), e.g. wrist
- tendon transfer
- muscle transfer.

Arthrodesis

Arthrodesis is fusion of the bones in a joint to provide stability, resulting in no movement at that joint. It is rarely used in the context of nerve injuries unless there is better function more distally in the affected limb, whereby a firm 'foundation' would permit better function, such as where radial nerve injury has caused weakness in the wrist but finger flexion beyond that is maintained by other functioning nerves.

Tendon Transfer

Tendon transfer surgery is necessary when the function of a specific muscle is lost due to damage to the nerve controlling that muscle. Tendon transfer surgery can be used to attempt to replace that function by moving the distal attachment (insertion) of another functioning tendon to a new insertion site, either to the tendon of the paralysed muscle or close to the insertion site of the paralysed muscle. The repositioned tendon will then produce a different action to previously, depending on where it has been inserted. Rehabilitation involves the re-education of function, occasionally with trick movements or with the coordination of other movements, e.g. wrist extension with finger flexion.

Muscle Transfer

A variety of muscles may be used as free transfers or transplantations and this surgery is often performed by a plastic surgeon. The aim is often to restore elbow flexion or wrist extension. The muscles used include latissimus dorsi and gracilis. Some degree of function may be restored, but return to pre-injury function would not be expected.

Rehabilitation and Ongoing Care and Support

Many patients will experience neuropathic pain, which can be difficult to treat and requires specific neuro-analgesics. Some of these drugs have another mode of use as antidepressants or antiepileptics. The use of a TENS device may also be useful where skin sensation is intact. This is a small portable electrical device that is designed to help relieve pain. It works by sending a harmless electrical current through pads that are placed on the skin. This is felt as pins and needles, and these sensations can help to block pain messages. General pain management issues are considered in more detail in Chapter 11. The use of other techniques in addition to drug therapy can be useful to help the patient 'live with' the pain. These may include psychological exercises such as relaxation, visualisation of pain and guided imagery, cognitive behavioural therapy and specific directed counselling. Acceptance of the effects of the injury and changes to body image should be addressed with counselling support. The purpose of therapy is to address the effects of pain on behaviour, mood, function and activity, and consider ways to set and achieve goals such as being more active, returning to previous activities and improving the individual's ability to function and regain quality of life (QoL). There are many ways of adapting activities to allow a return to leisure activities and work which can benefit well-being and self-esteem, although it may be necessary to consider different types of hobbies and work from those engaged in pre-injury. QoL issues for patients with brachial plexus injury are considered in Box 21.1.

Even though brachial plexus injury is uncommon, practitioners working in the trauma setting are likely to care for

---

Box 21.1   Evidence Digest

Quality of life following traumatic brachial plexus injury: A questionnaire study (Gray 2016)

Reproduced with permission from Elsevier

This paper builds on the previous work by Wellington (2009, 2010) which explored the QoL for patients following a traumatic brachial plexus injury and published the findings in a series of two papers. This study by Gray used the World Health Organization (WHO 2022) QoL-BREF questionnaire to assess the QoL experiences of patients with traumatic brachial plexus injuries. The WHO QoL-BREF questionnaire is a self-reported questionnaire of 26 questions with Likert scale responses relating to QoL in four domains: physical health, psychological, social relationships and environmental. You can download the WHO Qol-BREF tool free at https://www.who.int/toolkits/whoqol

Patients were identified from the database for the Scottish National Brachial Plexus Injury Service, a national tertiary referral service, between 2011 and 2013. Of 47 questionnaires distributed, 22 were returned.

Questionnaire responses displayed a broad range of results. The majority of patients reported that pain had some effect on restricting daily activities and more than half-required medications in order to function in their daily lives. The majority of respondents ($n = 19$) reported being mostly to completely able to accept the change to their body appearance and 17 were neutral or very satisfied with themselves in general. However, 12 respondents reported some degree of negative experiences in thought processes. Seven respondents reported issues regarding having enough money to live on, but the study recognised that the questionnaire did not collect information on other factors that may influence income such as employment status or geographic distribution of participants.

In summary, the findings reinforce that this group of patients continue to have similar issues of concern that have been highlighted and documented from previous research. The distribution of responses also highlights the need for an awareness of the needs of individual patients of brachial plexus injuries and a holistic approach in their care. For additional information visit www.brachialplexus.scot.nhs.uk.

patients in the early stages of their recovery. The complexity of brachial plexus injuries can provide a challenge to the healthcare professional. A holistic approach to the assessment, treatment, care and support of the patient and their family is best provided by an interdisciplinary team with specialist knowledge and expertise. Team members will include consultant medical staff, nurse specialists and therapy practitioners as well as other professionals such as psychologists, pain specialists and orthotists.

Further Reading

Anscomb, S.J. (2007). Managing sprains and strains. *Pract. Nurs.* 33 (5): 44, 46, 48–49.

Bailey, R., Kaskutas, V., Fox, I. et al. (2009). Effect of upper extremity nerve damage on activity participation, pain, depression and quality of life. *J. Hand Surg.* 34 (a): 1682–1688.

Elton, S.G. and Rizzo, M. (2008). Management of radial nerve injury associated with humeral shaft fractures: an evidence-based approach. *J. Reconstr. Microsurg.* 24 (8): 569–573.

Hems, T. (2015). Brachial plexus injuries. In: *Nerves and Nerve Injuries*, 681–706. Academic Press.

Hems, T. (2016). Nerve injury: classification, clinical assessment, investigation, and management. In: *Living Textbook of Hand Surgery* (ed. E.V. Handchirurgie

Weltweit and R. Böttcher). Cologne: German Medical Science GMS.

Norris, B.L. and Kellam, J.F. (1997). Soft tissue injuries associated with high-energy extremity trauma: principles of management. *J. Am. Acad. Orthop. Surg.* 5 (1): 37–46.

Tortora, G.J. and Derrickson, B. (2020). *Principles of Anatomy and Physiology*. New York: Wiley.

Wardrope, J., Barron, D., Draycott, S., and Sloan, J. (2008). Soft tissue injuries: principles of biomechanics, physiotherapy and imaging. *Emerg. Med. J.* 25: 158–162.

Wellington, B. and McGeehan, C. (2015). A case study from a nursing and occupational therapy perspective – Providing care for a patient with a traumatic brachial plexus injury. *Int. J. Orthop. Trauma Nurs.* 19 (1): 15–23.

References

Airaksinen, O.V., Kyrklund, N., Latvala, K. et al. (2003). Efficacy of cold gel for soft tissue injuries. *Am. J. Sports Med.* 31 (5): 680–684.

Altizer, L. (2003). Strains and sprains. *Orthop. Nurs.* 22 (6): 404–409.

ASIA (2019). *International Standards for Neurolgical Classification of Spinal Cord Injury Worksheet*. American Spinal Injury Association. ASIA-ISCOS-Worksheet_10.2019_PRINT-Page-1-2.pdf (asia-spinalinjury.org).

British Orthopaedic Association (2021). *Peripheral Nerve Injury*. BOA Standard, London. https://www.boa.ac.uk/resources/boast-peripheral-nerve-injury.html (accessed 4 January 2022).

Gray, B. (2016). Quality of life following traumatic brachial plexus injury: a questionnaire study. *Int. J. Orthop. Trauma Nurs.* 22: 29–35. https://doi.org/10.1016/j.ijotn.2015.11.001. Epub 2015 Nov 27. PMID: 27091305.

Kirshblum, S., Snider, B., Rupp, R., and Read, M.S. (2020). International Standards Committee of ASIA and ISCoS. Updates of the international standards for neurologic classification of spinal cord injury: 2015 and 2019. *Phys. Med. Rehabil. Clin. N. Am.* 31 (3): 319–330. https://doi.org/10.1016/j.pmr.2020.03.005. Epub 2020 Jun 3. PMID: 32624097.

Medical Research Council (1981). *Aids to the Examination of the Peripheral Nervous System*. Memorandum 45. London: Her Majesty's Stationery Office.

Wellington, B. (2009). Quality of life issues for patients following traumatic brachial plexus injury – Part 1. *J. Orthop. Nurs.* 13 (4): 194–200.

Wellington, B. (2010). Quality of life issues for patients following traumatic brachial plexus injury – Part 2. *Int. J. Orthop. Trauma Nurs.* 14 (1): 5–11.

World Health Organization (WHO) (2022). WHOQOL-BREF Files. https://www.who.int/toolkits/whoqol (accessed 7 February 2022).

Part V

Children and Young People

22

Key Issues in Caring for the Child or Young Person with an Orthopaedic or Musculoskeletal Trauma Condition

Sonya Clarke

Queen's University Belfast, Belfast, UK

Introduction

Even though the final part of this book sits within the early stages of a person's life span, it is pivotal and designed to inform all nurses. This chapter, although dedicated to children, continues to build on the transferable knowledge and skills discussed in the earlier chapters of this book. The terms 'child', 'children' and 'CYP' will be used collectively to refer to the neonate, infant, child and young person. The common concepts of informed consent, pain assessment/management and safeguarding are explored. This is in addition to the assessment and planning of care alongside educational and psychological issues pertinent to this client group. Additional team members who help to create a positive child and family experience are also introduced. In summary, the chapter introduces the reader to the fundamental aspects of care pertinent to orthopaedics and trauma from a child perspective, e.g. caring for the child in spica cast (Figure 22.1). Subsequent chapters will then build on caring for the CYP presenting with a common orthopaedic condition or injury. Juvenile idiopathic arthritis is explored in Chapter 13.

The United Nations Convention on the Rights of the Child (1989) recognises that children are a vulnerable group who need special consideration in all respects, including healthcare. Children's nurses are therefore committed to safeguarding vulnerable children and improving standards of care. A significant review of the UK National Health Service (NHS) (Kennedy 2010) in respect of meeting the needs of children and young people in light of widespread concerns expressed about a particular case

(Laming 2009) found many services needing improvement, with only a minority deemed excellent. The report also found that general practitioners had little or no experience of paediatrics as part of their professional training. Safeguarding was also considered an ongoing challenge alongside the transition into adult services, with parents who were frustrated due to poor sharing of information by health professionals. The report stated that children were a low priority in healthcare and that they needed a 'champion' within such complex care organisations. The Kennedy report (2010) was positive about the value of benchmarking to develop a range of standards. A benchmark is a process of comparison between the performance characteristics of separate, often competing, organisations intended to enable each participant to improve its own performance. An example in Box 22.1 specifically relating to children's musculoskeletal wellbeing, although dated, remains pertinent to practice. That said, it should be used in conjunction with the more recent Competence Framework for Orthopaedic and Trauma Practitioners, developed and published by the Royal College of Nursing (RCN) in 2019. The recent document is intended to provide a framework for orthopaedic and trauma practitioners in clinical practice across the lifespan. It remains recognised that orthopaedic and trauma practitioners require specific, specialist knowledge and skills reflecting different levels of practice and job roles (Clarke and Santy-Tomlinson 2014), and that appropriate education and training are essential to support practitioners' development and competence. Barnard et al. (2020) also published a supporting document around the process of developing the competency RCN framework.

Orthopaedic and Trauma Nursing: An Evidence-based Approach to Musculoskeletal Care, Second Edition. Edited by Sonya Clarke and Mary Drozd.
© 2023 John Wiley & Sons Ltd. Published 2023 by John Wiley & Sons Ltd.

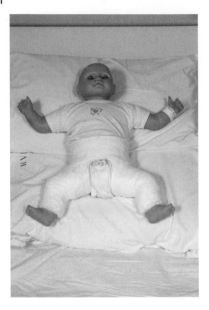

Figure 22.1   Spica cast/hip spica in human position.

Box 22.1   Evidence Digest: Benchmarks for Children's Orthopaedic Care, RCN Guidance (2007a)

Reproduced with permission from RCN

This inspiring publication offers a portfolio of succinct evidence on the key elements required to effectively care for the infant, child and young person requiring orthopaedic and fracture trauma-related nursing care. The indicators of best practice are identified as factors (F) for each of the nine benchmarks. The RCN guidance document was developed by an expert group of children's nurses experienced in orthopaedic-related nursing care.

1) *Pre-op assessment*: F1 screening and assessment; F2 practitioner competence; F3 informing child/young person and carers; F4 implementation of an individualised plan.
2) *Cast care*: F1 education and training; F2 patient care; F3 upper body cast; F4 lower body cast; F5 discharge planning.
3) *Neurovascular assessment*: F1 education and competence; F2 recording and documentation; F3 communication and information; F4 clinical action; F5 discharge planning.
4) *Traction*: F1 education and application of traction; F2 education, management of traction and nursing care; F3 communication and information
5) *Pin site care*: F1 screening and assessment; F2 education; F3 evidence, knowledge and competence; F4 clinical care; F5 discharge planning.

6) *Kirchner wire removal*: F1 competence and knowledge; F2 preparation of chid/young person and carers.
7) *Bone or joint infection*: F1 admission; F2 assessment and screening; F3 treatment; F4 discharge planning.
8) *Spinal injury*: F1 assessment of injury; F2 stabilisation; F3 acute care and rehabilitation programme; F4 psychological impact of a spinal cord injury; F5 discharge planning.
9) *Spinal surgery*: F1 pre-operative assessment; F2 nursing care plan; F3 pain management; F4 post-surgical mobility.

The nine benchmarks reflect pertinent areas relating to this client group and the speciality of orthopaedics and fracture trauma.

Age Definitions

Variations exist, but a consensus suggests that key phases in respect of age are:

- *neonate*: a newborn infant less than 4 weeks old
- *infant*: less than 1 year but more than 4 weeks old
- *child*: over 1 year old but before puberty
- *young person/adolescent*: between puberty and adulthood (up to 18 years old).

Psychosocial and educational issues that relate to the infant, child and young person are central to their wellbeing and the outcomes of the care they receive. The term 'psychosocial' refers to the child's ability to consciously or unconsciously adjust and relate themselves to their social environment. The term 'educational' refers to the provision of knowledge or instruction required as part of the child's development that must be incorporated into the care process.

The overarching family dynamics, culture, language and age of a child affect their physical and cognitive development and the achievement of expected milestones. Age is central, as the needs of an infant are very different from those of a young person. For example, a young person may experience anxiety and fear related to insults to dignity and altered body image and need acceptance within their peer group. They have a right to have a voice, to be heard and to have their vulnerability acknowledged regardless of their presenting condition and treatment. At the opposite end of the age continuum, the infant has increased vulnerability and dependence, and their growth and development must be central to ensure individualised and holistic nursing care. The CYP's experience of health professionals, hospital admission and pain, is an important consideration for the nurse when caring for them in all health care settings.

Box 22.2 The Importance of Telling the Truth to Children

An example of a challenging admission to hospital taken from practice involved a 6-year-old child carrying a suitcase, who appeared somewhat confused on arrival to the ward. The assessment process exposed parents who thought their child unable to cope with the truth, leading to them to tell the child they were going on holiday. The lack of parental truth telling had the potential to negatively impact on the child's hospital experience of minor orthopaedic surgery. Using a child-centred approach, with the child a rights holder and service user, the children's nurse requested involvement from the play specialist and 'clown doctors'. The child was enabled to deal with their experience, resulting in a positive outcome.

Key fact: One of the most helpful things a parent and health professional can do is to be honest with the child and provide developmentally appropriate information ahead of time regarding what is happening and why.

Assessment of the child on admission to hospital must include involvement of the parent and child when possible. History taking can be confounded by the child and parents failing to remember old or previous conditions and incidents, which remain pertinent to anaesthetic, surgery and planning of care. Honesty should be maintained whenever possible as children do not often forgive or forget if an untruth is revealed, affecting the nurse/child relationship and leading to an anxious or non-compliant child and an angry parent (Box 22.2). Resources, culture, language, social services, school, peer group, age, body image and discharge planning can present barriers to parent and child education and communication. Benchmarks (RCN 2007a) identify a number of areas that relate to this (Box 22.1).

Assessment of Children and Young People

The needs of the infant, child and young person have been charted across the decades by a variety of government reports (Platt Report 1959; Laming 2003; HMSO 2004). Even with the differences and similarities of children and adult patients acknowledged and continually debated, there is a widely accepted recognition that a children's nurse is best placed to care for this client group (Clarke 2007, 2017). It must be noted, nonetheless, that not all children will have a children's nurse caring for them in all healthcare settings. Pre-registration children's nursing programmes have evolved with increasing degrees of

academic demand, e.g. undergraduate and postgraduate. Registered nurses can be dual qualified, i.e. having a professional and academic award in both children's alongside either adult/general nursing, learning disability nursing or mental health nursing. Depending on individual need, children requiring continued care in the community are ideally placed under the care of a children's community nurse (CCN) or public health nurse. Many adult registered nurses and other fields of nursing may be able to care for this client group effectively but often not in a child-friendly environment. Clarke (2007) has established the children's nurse should have equal opportunity to complete recognised continuing education in caring for the child with orthopaedic conditions and fracture trauma, but adult orthopaedic and trauma nurses currently have better access to such continuing professional development.

Hydration and nutrition are key components of child health and wellbeing. The child's immature and developing skeletal system can result in an extreme metabolic response to injury, surgery and fasting, resulting in a high risk of poor outcomes if diet and hydration are not carefully considered. The practitioner needs to be aware of the importance of a balanced diet in maintaining normal childhood development and expected milestones. Dietary assessment history is essential in identifying the child's likes and dislikes for food texture and presentation. While body mass index charts are used in adult patients, standard practice with children is to plot the child's weight and height on centile charts, which provide better indicators of child growth and development. STAMP, the Screening Tool for the Assessment of Malnutrition in Paediatrics, provides a simple way of determining whether a child is at risk of malnutrition (https://www.stampscreeningtool.org/downloads/index.html). Hydration is equally as important as diet but assessing fluid balance can be problematic in the child. For example, assessing urinary output can be difficult due to the use of nappies and obtaining a midstream specimen of urine can be problematic due to lack of understanding and anxiety associated with using a bedpan for the younger child. Diet and hydration are explored in greater detail in Chapter 10.

Children receiving orthopaedic or trauma care come from a variety of diverse patient groups, ages and cultures. Challenges often exist in communicating with the child and family in respect to cultural and language barriers and difficulties, for example the use of touch in some cultures. Family dynamics, especially where there is obvious dysfunction, can also have an impact on the care process. Equality, diversity and inclusion (EDI) also applies to all CYP in healthcare. For example, a child may state they are non-binary (someone whose gender is not male or female).

Unfortunately, the infant, child and young person can struggle to have a say in their care and the practitioner caring for children is best placed to advocate for the patient (Nursing and Midwifery Council 2018). The management of disclosure of sensitive information needs to be carefully handled. The child who presents with a fracture and has a learning disability may present specific challenges to the assessment and delivery of care, particularly in the acute environment, which may not be well organised to address their specific needs. The complex or special needs child reinforces the need for a multidisciplinary team approach with the children's nurse as the key worker within the team. This group of children requires additional knowledge and skill in providing safe and effective care.

Assessment of risk is fundamental to wellbeing and positive outcomes in all parts of the journey of care and in all settings (Corkin et al. 2012). All children undergoing surgery, for example, require care that gives a high priority to their ASA level (the American Society of Anaesthesiologists grade given to each patient using a scale in relation to their fitness for undergoing an anaesthetic) as this predicts the need for 24-hour paediatric intensive care unit support (see Chapter 14 for further details).

The Care Environment

Children are cared for in a wide range of settings with an emphasis on home care with the intention of reducing hospital acquired infections and keeping the child within the family home and normal routine. Even so, children are often cared for within acute hospital settings, day procedure units, outpatient clinics, hospices and residential units. Because of concerns about child safety, children should be cared for in units that have specific security measures in place, including closed-circuit television surveillance and locked doors to promote safety. The ideal environment should meet the specific needs of children: it should be light, spacious and colourful with appropriate decoration, pictures and toys for young children and a dedicated area for young people. Bathroom and toilet facilities need to meet the needs of the child and specifically the child with mobility problems. Sensory rooms can provide a relaxing atmosphere for those with special needs.

A recent empirical study published by Clarke in 2021 explores children's experiences of hospital from the perspective of the child and children's nurses using child-centred methodology. The paper reaffirms 'globally the needs of children differ to those of adults', consequently, the 'voice' of children in healthcare delivery is paramount to its effectiveness as a service. The qualitative study presents a contemporary slice of life in four children's wards in a typical UK children's hospital in the twenty-first century from the perspective of the service user (child) and significant service giver (registered children's nurse). Phase one of the study involved the development of a child research advisory group (CRAG) with five local primary school children (aged 10–11 years) to assist in the co-production of research questions and data collection tool for child participants: two talking cartoon characters (Sprinkle Cupcake and Ronaldo Football) via an app/iPad. In phase two (main study), hospitalised children ($n = 18$) and registered children's nurses ($n = 8$) were interviewed on one occasion within their ward setting using a semi-structured approach in July 2017.

The emerging broad themes (using thematic analysis) were (1) children, the child's needs, relationships, fears and concerns, alongside (2) nurses, children's nursing, job pressures, safe and effective care. The themes were then presented as tensions in that they represent the relationship between variables where the different elements in the relationship are held in tension, such that a change in one impacts on the other. Similarities between the children and nurse participants included issues with the environment, lack of time to care (nurse), effects of nurse-led interventions and valued role of play. Differences are largely around the role of the parent. The development and work of the CRAG and use of tensions to more effectively present the complexity of the findings are unique to this study. In conclusion, this study contributes to the development of a generalised knowledge base for policy, nursing education and clinical practice by shedding light on how the complex hospital environment can be challenging for the child and children's nurse (see Box 22.3 for examples of evidence relating to the child's experience of hospital). Clarke's 2019 open-access narrative review and 2020 paper focus on how technology can be used to seek the vulnerable and marginalised child's voice in hospital(Clarke 2019, 2020).

The Team

A wealth of health professionals and lay persons participate in the care of the child, from the specialist/advanced nurse to the allied health professional working within a multidisciplinary team, CCN, parent and beyond. Chapter 5 provides an overview of the team approach and nursing roles within orthopaedics and fracture trauma with some principles that can be transferred to the care of the child. Additional roles have been developed to promote effective care of children. The fundamental role of play in child wellbeing and development must be considered in providing the right care environment for children, again with a specific focus on the child who has difficulty

---

Box 22.3 Evidence Digest

The study by Clarke (2021) adds to a growing body of knowledge. This evidence digest presents the demographics of seven of the 18 child participants who were admitted to hospital with either a 'musculoskeletal' condition or injury. It attempts to give those children a voice in matters that affect them by publishing their views on being hospitalised and of the nurses who care for them. Their views are insightful.

Demographics: Seven child participants

Reason for admission: Juvenile idiopathic arthritis, fracture, spinal or crush injury

Gender: Four girls and three boys

Ages: 8–12 years

Narrative views of being in hospital (mixed)
'Bored'
'Happy'
'Staff is helpful'
'Safe, feel in good care, the nurses are very nice'
'Bad, because I got an operation and it hurts'
'This place is comfortable'

The children's views on parental presence (positive…)
'I do not really mind if they are here or not [now] but it was really important [when admitted]'
'Alright', [mum can go home, child would like] 'some peace'
'I feel a lot safer when mum around'
'Sad when not there'
'Good as I have someone to talk to'
'Really good, safer, fun, I love them [if not there] sad and lonely'
'Good because I feel more confident'
'Safe, really safe [if not there] sad and upset'

Views on children's nurses (positive)
'Funny, really nice, I love them all'
'Pleasant'
'Kind and really safe, fun to play with'
'Sometimes kind'

'Kind, helpful, always there if you need them'
'Friendly, I like them, make me laugh a bit'

Do the children's nurses listen to you? (positive)
'Yeah, they are always there to talk about stuff'
'They always there to listen'
[Laughs] 'I asked for beans and toast and it took them 2 days'
'Yes, I asked to get my thing out [cannula[, they only took one'
'Yes, they do this project "what matters to you"'

Do the children's nurses ask your opinion? (mixed)
'Yeah, they ask you, what you want us to do?'
'Never really [they ask mummy and it annoys me]'
'Sometimes and sometimes not. Plain nurses great fun, they get you toys like the play nurses [students]'

Worst things about being in hospital!
'You are always badly injured or sick and you cannot go outside and play with your friends as you usually would'
'Not being able to go out to play'
'Definitely not being able to go outside'
'Being away from home, miss brother and sister'
'Heat, noise smell and pain'
'TV too small, yucky food, cannot sleep at night, too warm, do not like the side room',
'Trying to get asleep, baby crying over there, not their fault'
'Nothing, not a thing…'

If you had one wish in hospital, what would it be?
'Not to break my arm…'
'Get me better quick'
'Being in a room of my own'
'More toys'
'Quicker service [waiting 2 days to go home – bed to be delivered]'
'I would love to see my wee baby niece'
'A play place for children, bring my cat, my cousin, my auntie, my granny'

---

mobilising. Play is a familiar activity for most children and central to relieving stress and boredom. Stonehouse et al. (2018) reinforce play in children to be important in all healthcare settings, with nurses having a key role in facilitating play. Dissimilar to adult care but highly valued within children's nursing, the parent, play specialist/therapist and arts-based 'clown doctors' are engaged to generate a more positive hospital experience for the child – children want to feel safe.

- *Play specialists*: Holland (2020) reports on hospital play specialists working with children in an inclusive and family-centred way through providing a secure space for meaningful play. They plan and supervise activities that help the child to express their feelings through play and encourage the development of creative skills to provide an outlet for the child's thoughts and worries, offering ways to adapt to the new environment. This involves managing preadmission clubs, using play to welcome children to hospital and preparing them to cope with surgery or other procedures. This enables the child to express and manage their fears about separation from parents and encourages the child to maintain their usual interests whilst using specific play techniques to minimise stressful events by acting them out in advance. Clarke's (2021) study reported that the role of play and play specialists positively impacts on the child's experience of hospitalisation.

- *Clown doctors* are professional performers who are specially trained to work in hospitals with the aim of creating fun, laughter, play, communication and creativity in clinical environments. They visit children who are chronically and acutely ill and who are hospitalised, children who are in hospice care, children and young people with severe or profound disabilities and those with life-limiting conditions. Further information can be found at www.tinarts.co.uk/current-projects/the-clown-doctors. It is important to note, however, that not all children like clowns.
- *The parent or guardian* has parental responsibility for a child. Clarke (2021) reports that while most children want their parent present during their time in hospital, it can be challenging for the nurse. Unfortunately a minority of parents and guardians do not act in the best interest of their child. The RCN have provided key information on safeguarding the CYP, available at www.rcn.org.uk/clinical-topics/children-and-young-people/safeguarding-children-and-young-people. Like Simons et al. (2001), Clarke's (2021) recent study also recognised that a child's siblings and other family members such as grandparents can play an important part in the child's wellbeing and in maintaining social links in hospital.

Planning Care

Effective care planning through all care phases and healthcare settings is pivotal in achieving positive outcomes for the child and family. The complexity of modern families, however, makes this challenging, especially when the child's long-term care transfers to adult services as they become older. Transition is often not seamless and can be problematic for the service provider, young person and family, as developed relationships within the child's service are family-centred, and built on trust and respect. A variety of frameworks, models and approaches to care planning are available (Corkin et al. 2012) and a joint approach is commonly adopted when planning care for children, for example Casey's partnership model (Casey 1988) and the Roper et al. (2000) model of care. Whilst Casey's model

endorses a partnership with the parent/carer, the Roper Logan Tierney model encompasses the 12 activities of living with an overarching aim to move the person's level of care from dependence to independence.

An essential aspect of care planning is assessment. Chapter 23 discusses the commonly applied look, feel and move approach with ears that listen to the child and parent, underpinned by a holistic and family-centred approach. Family-centred care (FCC) recognises that the parent is a valued part of the child's care team but should not be taken for granted. Some parents adopt an 'expert' role when their child has complex needs. Examples of FCC include the following:

- Parental facilities: kitchen, shower and overnight facilities or purpose-built parent accommodation.
- One parent is routinely expected and welcomed in the anaesthetic and recovery room. This parent needs to be educated and supported by the nurse as an anaesthetised or recovering child can be upsetting for the parent.
- One parent should be present during routine, painful and stressful procedures, e.g. wound dressings, cast removal and venepuncture. The child is given a choice, but the rights of the child and consent are complex and challenging issues within all healthcare settings.

Consent and Capacity

Adults

At 18 years of age, mentally competent adults are considered able to make all decisions in relation to their medical care providing they have the capacity to do so. This right does not diminish with age and all mentally competent adults have the right to refuse treatment even when it will clearly benefit them. The Mental Health Capacity Act (2005) introduced in England and Wales in 2007 permits courts to appoint a proxy decision maker who has the power to grant consent to medical treatment if the patient becomes incapacitated.

For consent to be valid, the person must have *capacity*, the consent must be *voluntary* and it must not be given under *duress*. Furthermore, the person must have received *sufficient information* on which to base their decision. The person must also be able to communicate their decision. No adult is able to give consent for another adult. Here, 'surgical, medical or dental treatment' includes any procedure undertaken for the purposes of diagnosis and applies to any procedure (including, in particular, the administration of an anaesthetic) that is ancillary to any treatment as it applies to that treatment.

Young Person: 16–17 Years of Age

In many localities, 16–17 year olds are legally entitled to consent to their own medical treatment (without parental involvement). However, in certain circumstances they may not be permitted to refuse therapeutic care where they are at risk of suffering harm as a result of their decision.

Young Person: Under 16 Years of Age

A high-profile test case of child consent (*Gillick v West Norfolk and Wisbech Area Health Authority* 1985) saw Victoria Gillick attempting to set a legal precedent in England and Wales that would have meant that medical practitioners could not give young people under the age of 16 treatment or contraceptive services without parental permission. After initial success, the House of Lords ruled that under-16s who are fully able to understand what is proposed, and its implications, are competent to consent to medical treatment regardless of age. This test case led to 'Gillick competence', which states:

> As a matter of law, the parental right to determine whether or not their minor child below the age of 16 will have medical treatment terminates if and when the child achieves sufficient understanding and intelligence to enable him to understand fully what is proposed.

This also establishes that a child who is competent to consent to a course of treatment is entitled to the same obligation of confidentiality. Disclosures, however, need be considered against:

- the young person's right to privacy
- the degree of current harm or likely harm
- what any such disclosure is likely to achieve
- what the potential benefits are to the young person's wellbeing and, of course, the criminal law in this regard.

Those under 16 years may be able to consent if they are Gillick competent, meaning they have sufficient understanding and intelligence to make relevant decisions. In under 16s, parental involvement is desirable but not always essential (e.g. contraception) except where it is in the child's best interests (e.g. sexual abuse). If a person with parental responsibility consents, they are subject to the same tests for capacity, duress and information as all adults. It is routine practice to gain consent from only one person with parental responsibility, i.e. parent or guardian.

Pain

Childhood may require hospital admission and surgical intervention as a result of developmental disorders, disease or injury. The 'total pain' concept which considers the physical, psychological, spiritual and social aspects should be valued, with the last three being met only after pain and related symptoms (e.g. anxiety) are controlled. Anxiety and fear are often overlooked or cause confusion for those caring for the child in pain. Chapter 11 concentrates on the fundamentals and exploration of orthopaedic and musculoskeletal trauma conditions. There is a need, however, to consider specific issues for the child in pain.

Twycross (2017:17) reports 'Unrelieved pain in children has undesirable physical and psychological consequences that can affect them in both the short and longer term'. With the perception of pain in children, undergoing orthopaedic surgery can be determined by the individual child's threshold for pain (Pedwesen et al. 2020). It is well established within the literature that pain is an individual and subjective phenomenon, with three approaches commonly used in isolation or in combination to assess child pain, i.e. self-report (what the child says), behavioural (how the child behaves) and physiological (how the child's body reacts) indicators. Self-report of pain intensity is a valuable source of information although there are many sources of bias and error (von Baeyer 2006). Twycross et al. (2009) reported that children younger than 5 years of age can point to where they hurt but may be unable to accurately offer a reliable description of pain intensity due to age-related development. Consequently, behavioural and physiological approaches are also commonly used. A one-dimensional approach is limited whereas multidimensional approaches promote optimal pain management. The child's ability to describe pain increases with age, experience and changes throughout their development.

Commonly adopted child-specific assessment tools in the UK include the following:

- FLACC: face, legs, activity, crying and consolability, an observer-rated pain scale for the non-verbal child developed by Merkel et al. (1997). McKay and Clarke (2012) reported it was suitable for children with a learning disability within the orthopaedic and trauma setting.
- Wong and Baker (1988) devised a six-point cartoon face rating scale, with each face equating to a numerical value, i.e. 0, 2, 4, 6, 8 and 10, and representing the level of hurt. The tool is designed for younger children.
- A numerical 11-point scale from 0–10, where 0 means no pain and 10 is the worst possible pain. Used by older children and young people (plus adults).

Pain management for children following orthopaedic trauma and surgery is further complicated by it commonly being difficult to obtain self-report of the pain experience of the younger child (Clarke 2003). Such complexity has historically led to nurse-reporting of pain. Parents commonly adopt a central or supportive role when their child is too young to self-report their pain. However, parents' and nurses' judgements of facial expression or 'how the patient looks' mean that children's pain is frequently underestimated (Goubet et al. 2009). Twycross et al. (2009) demonstrate that practices can be suboptimal when children are asked to report on how well their pain is managed. This problem may relate to nurses' continuing belief in misconceptions about children's pain, for example that a sleeping child cannot be in pain. There is evidence to suggest, however, that a sleeping child may, in fact, be exhausted because of persistent pain. If pain management is dependent solely on nurse assessment then the outcome may be suboptimum. The role of the parent within the domain of family-centred care is deemed paramount (Corkin et al. 2012), with seminal and contemporary literature openly debating the value of the parent to score pain equal to the child post-surgery. That said, the child and young person are service users with an increasing expectation they should participate in health and social care decisions that affect them (Franklin and Sloper 2009). The subjective nature of reporting pain severity and a reliance on the use of nurse and parent report when communication and cognition is absent questions how effectively and consistently the documenting nurse and parent assess a child's pain. Caution is advised due to the impact of fear and anxiety and not actual pain, alongside a need to identify pain location as the child could be reporting pain associated with, for example, their cannula. Children communicate their pain in many different ways, for example a child may hide under their duvet, stop talking or become vocal, aggressive or lash out.

Misconceptions around children's pain continue to impact on practice, pain outcomes and wellbeing, for example:

- neonates do not feel pain
- children experience pain differently to/less than adults
- children cannot express their pain
- children do not remember pain
- it is not safe to give children opiates due to the risk of respiratory depression.

In the first edition of this book, Harrop (2007) reported there to be widespread inadequate prevention and relief of pain, supporting findings documented by the National Service Framework for Children in 2004. Conversely, at that time Clarke and Richardson (2007) reported on evolving practice that included the recognition and deeper understanding of the child's individual pain experience and the benefits of using an age-appropriate pain assessment tool that demonstrates validity and reliability and is taught preoperatively to the child (if possible) with parental involvement. Other evolving practices include recent pharmacological advances such as intravenous (IV) paracetamol, continuous epidural infusions, caudal and nerve blocks, and recognising the benefits of non-pharmacological interventions. Non-pharmacological options include behavioural and supportive methods such as information, empathy, belief and choices. Psychological treatment should be an integral part of orthopaedic and fracture trauma pain management with cognitive methods such as imagery and hypnosis potential options. Deep breathing and progressive relaxation should not be used in isolation for intense pain. Parents sometimes need to be given permission to touch and stroke their child. Sadly, a narrative review by Twycross et al. in 2015 found nurses' assessment and management of children's pain post surgery to be not consistent with published guidelines.

Fear and anxiety management play key roles in children's pain management and the nurse needs to take into account the stage of child development, cognitive abilities, gaining child and family trust, and ensuring pain intensity is being measured and not the anxiety or fear. Influences on the pain experience for any child include past experiences, socialisation (how they see pain managed at home), personal values, cultural patterns and differences in assessment and intervention of pain (e.g. phobia of needles due to previous analgesic injections). Developments and innovative practice should be managed by a dedicated integrated multidisciplinary pain team (Clarke 2003) with the contribution of a children's nurse educated in orthopaedics and fracture trauma. Pain management continues to challenge practitioners caring for children but particularly within orthopaedics and trauma as surgical intervention often produces pain of medium to severe intensity.

Safeguarding Children: Everybody's Business

Working together to safeguard children (2018) defines safeguarding as protecting children from maltreatment, preventing impairment of health or development, ensuring that children grow up in circumstances consistent with the provision of safe and effective care, and taking action to enable all children to have the best outcomes. Child protection is therefore part of safeguarding and refers to action taken to protect children who are suffering or likely to suffer significant harm. Article 19 in the United Nations Convention of the Rights of the Child (UNICEF 1989), ratified by the UK in 1991, states that all children have a right to be protected from 'all forms of physical or mental violence, injury or abuse, neglect or negligent treatment, maltreatment or exploitation including sexual abuse, while in the care of parent(s), legal guardian(s) or any other person who has the care of the child'. Martin et al. (2020, p. 379) recently defined safeguarding as, 'the action taken to protect children from harm is an important aspect of paediatric care'.

This section of the chapter aims to provide an overview of safeguarding plus the signs of child abuse and neglect. It will also identify the key government policies and guidelines that have been produced for all health professionals. The focus will be on physical abuse as it is aligned to the field of orthopaedics and trauma, with an emphasis on fractures in young children who present to emergency departments and surgical wards.

The case of Victoria Climbie has had a significant impact on children's services in the UK over the last decade. Victoria suffered maltreatment at the hands of her great aunt and partner (Laming 2003). A wide range of agencies was involved, and they missed opportunities to protect Victoria. Laming (2003) made multiple recommendations regarding assessment and observation, documentation and communication between all agencies and clearly stated that this was a lesson to be learned and never to happen again. However, it did happen again; in August 2007, a 17-month-old boy, Baby P, died having suffered fatal injuries at the hands of his mother and her boyfriend (Laming 2009). Baby P was visited 60 times by health and social care professionals and had been on the child protection register for 9 months. There was a public outcry and a national review of child protection. The message was clear, it must not happen again.

During the period 2007–2012 a further 100 children have died in similar circumstances in the UK alone (www.nspcc.org.uk). In 2020, it was reported that within the last 5 years there had been an average of 62 child deaths a year by assault or undetermined intent in the UK (https://learning.nspcc.org.uk).

These statistics show that the publishing of further guidelines to help health professionals to recognise, assess and protect children who may be at risk of significant harm appears, so far, to have had little effect.

Recognition of Child Abuse

The categories of child abuse fall into the following areas:

- physical abuse
- sexual abuse
- emotional abuse
- neglect.

All staff involved need to be alert to signs of child abuse and act accordingly following the guidelines set out by government and professional bodies.

Physical Abuse

This type of abuse may involve hitting, slapping, throwing, burning or scalding, poisoning or suffocating the child, resulting in the injury or death of the infant or child. Signs and symptoms include:

- bruising
- broken bones
- bites, scratches
- burns, scalds
- black eyes.

Additional mediating factors include (Corkin et al. 2012):

- where there is delay in seeking medical attention
- where there is conflicting history as to what has happened
- where a pattern appears linked to recurrent injuries
- where there is poor parental anxiety shown.

National Institute for Health and Care Excellence guidance (NICE 2009) suggests a focus on the concepts of 'alerting features', 'consider' or 'suspect':

- *Alerting features* are symptoms, signs and patterns of injury or behaviour that may indicate child abuse.
- *Consider* means that abuse is one possible explanation for an alerting feature (but there are other possible diagnoses).
- *Suspect* means there is a serious level of concern about abuse, but not proof. It may trigger a child protection investigation. This may lead to child protection procedures being put in place, offering the family more support, or to alternative explanations being found.

More recent NICE (2017) guidance states:

'Suspect child maltreatment if a child has one or more fractures in the absence of a medical condition that predisposes to fragile bones (for example, osteogenesis imperfecta, osteopenia of prematurity) or if the explanation is absent or unsuitable. Presentations include:

- fractures of different ages
- X-ray evidence of occult fractures (fractures identified on X-rays that were not clinically evident). For example, rib fractures in infants.'

Fractures are a common manifestation of child abuse that may be found incidentally on X-rays ordered for another reason. A majority of non-accidental fractures occur in children under 18 months old. There are few genuine accidental fractures in this age group as fracture requires significant force in a child with normal bone development and does not occur during normal childcare. Nurses are often one of the first to assess a child with an injury or fracture, so they require a good level of knowledge of bone and child development.

When a child has a fracture, concerns are raised by the following issues:

- age/developmental level: fractures in non-ambulatory children are unusual
- location: metaphyseal, post-ribs, scapula, vertebrae and sternum fractures are highly suggestive of nonaccidental injury
- pattern: e.g. multiple fractures or complex skull fractures may suggest non-accidental injury
- age of injury: delay in seeking medical attention, fractures of different ages.

Eighty-five percent of fractures from non-accidental injury occur in children under the age of 3 years and 69% under the age of 1 year. Fractures under the age of 1 year are highly associated with non-accidental trauma, as the infant would not have the ability to exert the force required to cause a fracture (Shrader et al. 2011). Long bone fractures can be suggestive of non-accidental injury. Long bone fracture may present initially with a cry/scream, and then the child may be irritable with decreased movement/use of limb and crying on movement of the affected area (i.e. changing, bathing) along with swelling. Fractures usually occur as a result of a twisting fall with foot planted, i.e. less force than expected. Fractures that occur due to traction/torsional forces can sometimes be attributed to forceful yanking or tugging with twisting, which rarely occur accidentally and can suggest non-accidental injury.

Spiral humeral fractures and metaphyseal fractures of the distal femur and tibia are thought to be more likely to be caused by non-accidental injury. If an infant is pulled sharply, the corner of the metaphyseal region of the bone can be torn; this is referred to as 'bucket handle' fracture. Finding spiral fractures in a bone shaft is indicative of a twisting injury. Violent squeezing of the rib cage can result in anterior and posterior rib fractures, which are difficult to acquire, as children's ribs are quite flexible. Additionally, skull fractures such as linear fractures in the parietal bone are uncommon in a child under 18 months and result from a direct force to the skull (refer to Chapter 25 for an Evidence Digest that highlights the incidence of non-accidental fractures in infants).

Assessment for Non-accidental Injury

The assessments of children following local and national guidance are a fundamental part of recognising non-accidental injury. Assessment frameworks set out to improve the quality of assessment and to assist in communicating the needs of children across all agencies involved. They also aim to avoid the escalation of a 'child in need' in relation to child protection through early identification and effective intervention. Guidance provides information to practitioners on how and when to refer a child to the dedicated child protection agency/team. A detailed documented assessment can lead to action that ensures child protection is maintained. Throughout the process, the child is the main focus and the child's views must be listened to throughout. The family's circumstances must also be considered, including their strengths, needs and potential risks, to make robust plans that can lead to improving the outcomes for the child. All practitioners must be aware of the assessment tool in use and be responsible for ensuring that the assessment process and subsequent action are carried out effectively and in a timely manner to ensure the safety of the child.

Role and Responsibilities of Practitioners

The guidance *Safeguarding Children and Young People: Roles and Competencies for Healthcare Staff* (RCN 2019) is an intercollegiate document that provides a clear framework and identifies the competencies required for all healthcare staff. Levels 1–3 relate to different occupational groups, while levels 4 and 5 are related to specific roles. All practitioners must be aware they have a role to play in recognising abuse or neglect in infants and children. They must work closely with other disciplines and act accordingly. They must place the interests of the child at the centre of their work and act on the child's behalf if they have concerns (Department for Education and Skills 2006). UK nurses, for example, must adhere to the Nursing and Midwifery Council Code, which states that:

> Nurses, midwives and nursing associates must act in line with the Code, whether they are providing direct care to individuals, groups or communities or bringing their professional knowledge to bear on nursing and midwifery practice in other roles, such as leadership, education, or research. The values and principles set out in the Code can be applied in a range of different practice settings, but they are not negotiable or discretionary. *(Nursing and Midwifery Council 2018)*

As well as having the skills of recognition and communication, all staff must have good record-keeping and report-writing skills. Records must be clear, comprehensive, accurate, accessible, dated and signed in a chronological order (RCN 2007b). The nurse's responsibility around safe-guarding children is summarised in Box 22.4.

Summary

The first chapter in this section highlights the rights and needs of the CYP (and their family) presenting with either an orthopaedic condition or fracture to be, ideally, cared for by a children's nurse who has received post-qualifying education in orthopaedics and trauma. Key issues within this client group include challenges around assessment and planning care, informed consent, safe-guarding, separation from parents, change of environment, anxiety and fear, and the effective assessment and management of pain. The wider team of healthcare and non-healthcare professionals should adopt a person-centred approach (supported by the parent or guardian) when delivering safe and effective care to the CYP. To fully appreciate the wider context of caring for children and young people within orthopaedic and fracture

Box 22.4   Nurse Responsibility: Safeguarding
• Refer to hospital policies and procedures
• Inform line manager
– Consultant
– Hospital social worker
– Child protection nurse specialist
– Follow up with a written referral, including names of child and carer, date of birth, address, general practitioner, health visitor, school, language spoken
• State concerns/issues/reason for referral
• All referrals must be followed up in writing within 24 hours
• Observe and document anything that may be of significance
• Never confront a suspected abuser
• Do let parents know you are concerned
• Document
• Note outcome

trauma the reader should review Chapters 23, 24 and 25 while taking into account the principles covered in this chapter.

Further Reading

Glasper, A., Richardson, J., and Randall, D. (2021). *A Textbook of Children and Young People's Nursing, 3*. London: Elsevier Press.

NSPCC www.nspcc.org.uk (accessed September 2012).

References

von Baeyer, C.L. (2006). Children's self-reports of pain intensity: scale selection, limitations, and interpretation. *Pain Res. Manag.* 11 (3): 157–162.

Barnard, K., Judd, J., Clarke, S. et al. (2020). Updating the UK competence framework for orthopaedic and trauma nurses 2019. *Int. J. Orthop. Trauma Nurs.* https://doi.org/10.1016/j.ijotn.2020.100780.

Casey, A. (1988). A partnership with child and family. *Senior Nurse* 8 (4): 8–9.

Clarke, S.E. (2003). Postoperative pain in children: a retrospective audit of continuous epidural analgesia in a paediatric orthopaedic ward. *J. Orthop. Nurs.* 7 (1): 4–9.

Clarke, S. (2007). Changing paediatric orthopaedic education and certification for the RN in Northern Ireland? *Orthop. Nurs.* 26 (2): 126–129.

Clarke, S. (2017). The history of children's nursing and its direction within the United Kingdom. *Compr. Child Adolesc. Nurs.* 40 (3): 200–214. https://doi.org/10.1080/24694193.2017.1316790.

Clarke, S. (2019). Children's experiences of staying in hospital from the perspectives of children and children's nurses: a narrative review. *Nurs. Health Care* 4: 62–70. https://doi.org/10.33805/2573.3877.141.

Clarke, S. (2020). Using technology to seek the vulnerable and marginalized child's voice in hospital: co-working with a Child Research Advisory Group (CRAG). *Compr. Child Adolesc. Nurs.* https://doi.org/10.1080/24694193.2020.1832626.

Clarke, S. (2021). An exploration of the child's experience of staying in hospital from the perspectives of children and children's nurses using child-centered methodology. *Compr. Child Adolesc. Nurs.* https://doi.org/10.1080/24694193.2021.1876786.

Clarke, S.E. and Richardson, O. (2007). Using intravenous paracetamol in children following surgery: a literature review. *J. Child. Young People's Nurs.* 1 (6): 273–280.

Clarke, S. and Santy-Tomlinson, J. (2014). *Orthopaedic and Trauma Nursing: An Evidence Based Approach to Musculoskeletal Care.* Oxford: Wiley-Blackwell.

Corkin, D., Clarke, S., and Liggett, L. (ed.) (2012). *Care Planning in Children and Young People's Nursing.* Oxford: Wiley Blackwell.

Department for Education and Skills (2006). *What to Do if You Are Worried a Child Is Being Abused.* London: Department for Education and Skills.

Franklin, A. and Sloper, P. (2009). Supporting the participation of disabled children and young people in decision-making. *Children and Society* 23 (1): 3–15. https://doi.org/10.1111/j.1099-0860.2007.00131.x.

Gillick v West Norfolk and Wisbech Area Health Authority (1985) UKHL 7 British and Irish Legal Information Institute. www.nspcc.org.uk/Inform/research/briefings/gillick_wda101615.html#How_is_Gillick_competency_assessed? (accessed 7 April 2014).

Goubet, L., Vervoort, T., Cano, A., and Crombez, G. (2009). Catastrophizing about their children's pain is related to higher parent-child congruency in pain ratings: an experimental investigation. *Euro. J. Pain* 13 (2): 196–201.

Harrop, J.E. (2007). Management of pain in childhood. *Arch. Dis. Childh.* 92: 101–108.

HMSO (2004). *The Children Act*, Chapter 31. London: HMSO.

Holland, C. (2020). Play specialist practice and the value of play. *Dissector* 48 (1): 16–17.

Kennedy, I. (2010). *Getting it Right for Children and Young People: Overcoming Cultural Barriers in the NHS So as to Meet Their Needs.* London: Department of Health.

Laming, R. (2003). *The Victoria Climbie Inquiry: Report of an Inquiry by Lord Laming.* Norwich: The Stationery Office.

Laming, R. (2009). *The Protection of Children in England. A Progress Report.* London: The Stationary Office.

Martin, E., Kraft, J., Wilder, R., Bryant, H. (2020). Safeguarding children in trauma and orthopaedics. *Ortho. Trauma* 34 (6): 379–389.

McKay, M. and Clarke, S. (2012). Pain assessment tools for the child with severe learning disability: a review and application to orthopaedic practice. *Nurs. Child. Young People* 24 (2): 14–19.

Mental Health Capacity Act (2005) The Stationary Office, London.

Merkel, S.I., Voepel-Lewis, T., Shayevitz, J.R., and Malviya, S. (1997). The FLACC: A behavioral scale for scoring post-operative pain in young children. *Pediatr. Nurs.* 23 (3): 293–297.

NICE (2009). *When to Suspect Maltreatment: Clinical Guideline CG89.* London: National Institute for Health and Care Excellence.

NICE (2017). *Child Maltreatment: When to Suspect Maltreatment in under 18s. Clinical Guideline CG89.* London: National Institute for Health and Care Excellence.

Nursing and Midwifery Council (2018). *The Code: Professional Standards of Practice and Behaviour for Nurses, Midwives and Nursing Associates.* London: Nursing and Midwifery Council.

Pedwesen, L., Matinkevich, P., Rahek, O. et al. (2020). Pressure pain thresholds in children before and after surgery: a prospective study. *Scand. J. of Pain* 20 (2): 339–344. TTPS://DOI-ORG.QUEENS.EZP1.QUB.AC.UK/10.1515/SJPAIN-2019-0130.

Platt Report (1959). *The Report of the Committee on the Welfare of Children in Hospital.* London: Ministry of Health.

Roper, N., Logan, W., and Tierney, A.J. (2000). *The Roper-Logan-Tierney Model of Nursing: Based on Activities of Living.* Edinburgh: Elsevier Health Sciences.

Royal College of Nursing (2019) *Safeguarding children and young people: roles and competencies for healthcare staff.* www.rcn.org.uk/professional-development/publications/007-366 (accessed April 2019).

RCN (2007a) *Benchmarks for Children's Orthopaedic Nursing Care – RCN guidance.* Royal College of Nursing. www.rcn.org.uk/__data/assets/pdf_file/0007/115486/003209.pdf (accessed 15 April 2013).

RCN (2007b). *Safeguarding Children and Young People – Every Nurse's Responsibility.* London: Royal College of Nursing.

Shrader, W.M., Nicholas, M.D., Bernat, B.A. et al. (2011). Suspected non accidental trauma and femoral shaft fractures in children. *Orthopaedics* 34: 5.

Simons, J., Frank, L., and Robertson, E. (2001). Parent involvement in children's pain care: views of parents and nurses. *Journal of Advanced Nursing* 36 (4): 591–599.

Stonehouse, D., Piper, C., Briggs, M., and Brown, F. (2018). Play within the pre-registration children's nursing curriculum within the United Kingdom: a content analysis of programme specifications. *J. Pediatr. Nurs.* 41: e33–e38. https://doi.org/10.1016/j.pedn.2018.01.013.

Twycross, A. (2017). Guidelines, strategies and tools for pain assessment in children. *Nurs. Times* [online] 113 (5): 18–21.

Twycross, A., Dowden, S.J., and Bruce, E. (2009). *Managing Pain in Children: A Clinical Guide.* London: Wiley Blackwell.

Twycross, A., Forgeron, P., and Williams, A. (2015). Paediatric nurses' postoperative pain management practices in hospital based non-critical care settings: a narrative review. *Int. J. Nurs. Stud.* 52 (4): 836–863. https://doi.org/10.1016/j.ijnurstu.2015.01.009. Epub 2015 Jan 24. PMID: 25661526.

UNICEF (1989). *A New Charter for Children 3/88.* UNICEF/UK Information Sheet No. 8. UNICEF, London.

Wong, D. and Baker, C. (1988). Pain in children: comparison of pain assessment scales. *Paediatr. Nurs.* 14 (1): 9–17.

HM Government *Working Together to Safeguard Children* (2018) A guide to interagency working to safeguard and promote the welfare of children. http://www.gov.uk/government/publications/working-togetherto-safeguard-children.

23

Common Childhood Orthopaedic Conditions, Their Care and Management
Julia Judd

University Hospital Southampton, Child Health. Tremona Rd Southampton, SO16 6YD, UK

Introduction

The purpose of this chapter is to review current knowledge and management of neonate, infant, child and young people's orthopaedic conditions and discuss some of the health issues that affect bone development in this part of the lifespan. This will serve as a source of information for nurses caring for children with a musculoskeletal condition in hospital, in the outpatient setting and in primary care. The selected topics, description of the subject matter and the child's pathway of care are of value to the practitioner in the advancement of their knowledge. The evidence base for this is represented through current literature in the subspecialty of paediatric orthopaedics, although in some areas the evidence may be old or lacking.

Musculoskeletal Assessment

In the assessment of children, it is important to use your ears, eyes and hands along with listening to the history given by the family and the child. It is vital to obtain a clear history about the presenting problem. The term 'OLD CART' is a useful tool for clinical examination (Dawson et al. 2012). Each letter aims to prompt the recall of a series of statements that encourage the practitioner to ask the child and family about the **O**nset of the problem, **L**ocation of problems, **D**uration and **C**haracteristics of symptoms, **A**ssociated factors that contribute to the problem, **R**elieving factors that make the problem better and **T**reatment so far.

Throughout the assessment the practitioner must take into account the family dynamics and involve the child, however young they are, listening to their description of the problem, using language that is age appropriate and using toys or favourite items to help the child to understand what is being asked. Information needs to be accessible in a variety of forms, including written, visual and through play (Dawson et al. 2012). The environment should be friendly and welcoming to alleviate any fear that the child may have in coming into the hospital.

Try to build a rapport with the child before examining them. If they are very young, it may be more appropriate to examine them on the parent's lap. One format for examination is to use the *look, feel, move* approach to assess the presenting problem. This involves looking at the problem area, feeling and moving where the problem is and assessing associated joints whilst observing the child's facial expressions and noticing pain or discomfort.

The orthopaedic practitioner should have sound domain-specific knowledge to be able to clinically assess the child and reach conclusions (Judd 2005). This means knowing what the normal musculoskeletal development for different age groups is and being able to interpret X-rays dependent on the child's age and the bone or joint that is being assessed. Collectively the history and clinical examination should lead the practitioner to a plan for investigations and diagnosis.

A systematic approach is helpful when assessing a child. Look at the overall appearance, taking note of the child's colour (pale or healthy), their stature and posture. How does the child stand? Look at the leg alignment. Is there evidence of asymmetry, such as genu varum/valgum (Figure 23.1), an abnormal rotational profile or leg length difference? Is there evidence of dysfunction, for example tripping up, a limp, reduced range of motion in a joint or disability.

Orthopaedic and Trauma Nursing: An Evidence-based Approach to Musculoskeletal Care, Second Edition. Edited by Sonya Clarke and Mary Drozd.
© 2023 John Wiley & Sons Ltd. Published 2023 by John Wiley & Sons Ltd.

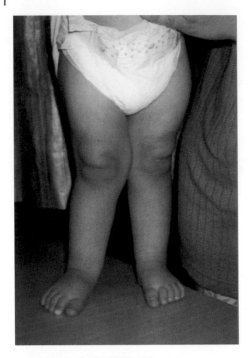

Figure 23.1 Genu valgum.

Normal Variants

Many referrals from general practitioners to orthopaedic services relate to concerns regarding deviation from what parents believe to be the norm. Moloney et al. (2006) determined that half of child referrals (53%) to the hospital present with normal variants, predominated by in-toeing gait and flexible flat feet. In-toeing may be caused by femoral anteversion, tibial torsion or metatarsus adductus (forefoot adduction). An out-toeing gait may be due to femoral retroversion, external tibial torsion or flat feet. All of these are normal variants and are expected to resolve naturally with growth (Yeo et al. 2015).

Developmental dysplasia of the hip, a neuromuscular problem, club foot or a slipped capital femoral epiphysis, however, contribute to in-toeing or out-toeing torsional abnormalities and will require orthopaedic intervention. Flat feet are commonly referred as a result of concern raised by a shoe shop. If the foot is flexible with the arch restored on tip toe standing, then parents can be reassured. The normal age for arch development is by age 6 years, although if the child has ligamentous laxity, they may always have normal flexible flat feet. Orthotics are not required to restore an arch in a normal foot and are used only for the symptomatic foot.

Genu varum (bow legs) and genu valgum (knock knees) deformities can be physiological or pathological and diagnosis is made based on the age of the child, X-ray appearances and progression versus resolution. At birth, a baby's legs are naturally bowed and this can look progressively worse, especially if the child walks at a young age. By the age of 2 years, the legs will straighten, followed by valgus deformity between the ages of 3 and 4 years, and gradual correction to normal by age 6. It is important to exclude pathology such as rickets, Blounts disease or a metaphyseal dysplasia and to be aware that a unilateral deformity is probably pathological in origin.

Common Conditions Presenting in the Neonate, Infant, Child and Young Person

Congenital Muscular Torticollis

Congenital muscular torticollis is a benign condition that is usually detected in early infancy. The baby tilts their head towards the affected side and turns their face in the opposite direction. This is caused by a fibrous tissue mass within the sternocleidomastoid muscle (SCM). The reason for this is unclear but may be due to in utero crowding or a decrease in the blood supply to the muscle. On palpation a firm tumour can be felt in the neck and there may be accompanying plagiocephaly (Luther 2002). Hollier et al. (2000) report a high incidence of 1 per 250 live births, associating difficult births as a causative factor. Resolution is usually within 4–6 months with stretching exercises if the condition is without other association. The incidence of developmental dysplasia of the hip in an infant with torticollis varies between 2% and 29% and should be excluded with a hip scan at 6 weeks of age (von Heideken et al. 2006). Physiotherapy is the mainstay of treatment and parents are taught stretching exercises to continue at home. For those who do not respond favourably by 12 months, a surgical release of the SCM is performed.

Developmental Dysplasia of the Hip

Developmental dysplasia of the hip (DDH) is the term used to describe a spectrum of disorders affecting the infant hip. Previously known as congenital dislocation of the hip (CDH), the term was changed to DDH to reflect that the condition is dynamic, can change and is not always detectable at birth. The hip joint may be dysplastic with a shallow acetabulum (acetabular dysplasia) that is unstable and subluxing or completely dislocated. Early recognition and appropriate treatment by skilled practitioners predetermines a good outcome. Clinical guidelines (NIPE 2021) promote a uniform approach to infant screening and detecting abnormality promptly. Treatment decisions are determined by abnormal clinical and sonographic examination (Clarke and Castaneda 2012) and are reliant on the competence of the practitioner (Royal College of Nursing 2012). The primary aim of DDH treatment is to achieve a concentric and stable hip joint, and ultimately normal development of the acetabulum and proximal femur with minimal possibility for subsequent reconstructive surgical intervention (Bolland et al. 2010). Early osteoarthritis, chronic pain and a reduction in activity levels are all possible sequelae of DDH and the earlier the intervention the more likely a successful outcome.

Aetiology and Epidemiology

DDH is the most common congenital newborn defect (75%). The cause is unknown, although there are multifactorial traits and gender, hormonal influence, race, hyperlaxity, uterine malposition, geographic and environmental influences. Box 23.1 outlines some of the associated risk factors. The incidence of true DDH is difficult to determine accurately as the definition lends itself to a broad spectrum of the condition, giving variance to the accurate incidence. Over the years, authors have strived to clarify the terminology and there have been improved methods of detection and diagnosis. The introduction of screening of neonates at risk and sonography has improved diagnostic techniques (Kokavec and Bialik 2007). Ultimately clinical examination of the infant with a risk factor is unreliable and hip ultrasound should be employed in these cases (Harper et al. 2020). Reported incidence of hip instability is as high as 20 per 1000 live births and varies depending on geographic location. Many of these are due to ligamentous laxity and stabilise within the first couple of weeks. The incidence of true hip dislocation in the UK is reported as one to two per 1000 live births (Clarke and Taylor 2012).

DDH is more common in females, with increased prevalence in firstborn infants. The latter is believed to be due to the tight structure of the uterus and subsequent reduced capacity for foetal movement. The risk of late DDH was found to be 29% in breech presentation at 4–6 months follow-up (Imrie et al. 2010), despite normal ultrasound at

6 weeks. Research studies to assess prophylactic hip abduction splints for this category of patient are ongoing (Clarke and Judd 2013).

The infant hip is at risk of DDH if the baby is subject to the recognised risk factors. Early appropriate intervention will result in normal hip development in the majority of babies.

Diagnosis

A routine part of the neonate's postpartum check is hip examination. The practitioner assesses for equal leg length and looks for asymmetry of the gluteal and thigh folds. More importantly, reduced hip abduction and instability are indicative of DDH (Vaquero-Picado et al. 2019). In the UK, the NHS Newborn and Physical Examination Programme (NIPE) recommend examiners be trained and are competent in the Ortolani and Barlow tests (NIPE 2021). The Barlow test demonstrates hip instability as the hip displaces posteriorly out of the actebulum and the Ortolani test produces an audible clunk as the dislocated hip is relocated back into the acetabulum. Babies with a positive clinical examination and those that meet the screening criteria are referred to a specialist clinic for hip ultrasound (see Box 23.2 and Figure 23.2).

As an adjunct to clinical assessment, ultrasound clarifies clinical findings. It is not feasible, however, to scan all babies' hips due to the inordinate expense and requirement for resources (American Academy of Pediatrics 2000). Guidelines ensure practitioners make appropriate referrals at the correct time (Box 23.2).

It is important to obtain a good family and birth history (Judd 2012a) prior to a clinical and sonographic examination. The ossific nucleus (secondary ossification centre) is normally present in the infant's hip at the approximate age of 4 months but later in an infant with DDH. An X-ray

---

Box 23.1 Associated Risk Factors for DDH

- Breech presentation
- Firstborn child
- Large baby for gestational age
- Packaging disorders, e.g. torticollis, positional/structural club foot
- Caesarean section delivery
- Cerebral palsy
- Oligohydramnios

Box 23.2 Infant Hip Screening Criteria (NIPE 2021)

Babies with a Positive Clinical Examination

Abnormal/unstable hips
↓
Refer for expert paediatric orthopaedic consultation and hip ultrasound by 3 weeks of age

Positive Risk Factors

Family history of DDH
Breech presentation
In utero postural deformities (torticollis, club foot)
Multiple births
↓
Refer for ultrasound by 4–6 weeks of age

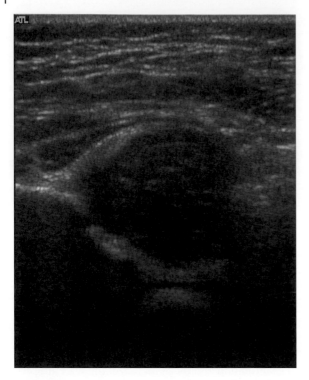

Figure 23.2   Hip ultrasound showing a dysplastic hip.

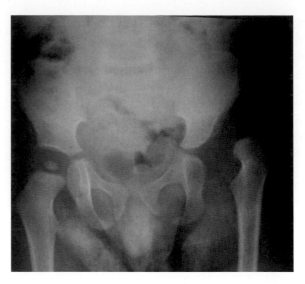

Figure 23.3   X-ray showing a dislocated left hip: the ossific nucleus is absent.

therefore is not helpful in determining the hip structure and ultrasound is the gold standard to show true hip dislocation or dysplasia. A static coronal view can be measured using the Graf method to assess for dyplasia (Eastwood and de Gheldere 2010). A further dynamic stress test in the transverse plane will assess for instability. Combined, the two images detect the degree of abnormal hip morphology.

Late diagnosis of DDH is commonly detected by the parent, who notices their child has a short leg or a limp when there is a unilateral presentation. A child with bilateral dislocated hips will present with a waddling gait. Confirmation is made by X-ray (see Figure 23.3) and clinical examination. Hip abduction is markedly reduced and if unilateral, the affected side shows a shortened limb. The later the diagnosis, the more interventional the treatment and potential for the development of degenerative joint disease. Because DDH is often neglected or treated in appropriately it has become the most common cause of secondary osteoarthritis of the hip.

Guidelines (NIPE 2021) advise the practitioner when to refer to a specialist paediatric orthopaedic doctor and tested algorithms of treatment are available in the literature (Clarke and Taylor 2012). Multicentred research studies aim to amalgamate findings to improve knowledge of DDH management and to test new theories. The Institute of Infant Hip Dysplasia (IHDI) strives to create a gold standard for referral and treatment, looking at timing of intervention, method of treatment, failure and complication rates.

Treatment

Treatment of DDH is dependent on the age of the child at presentation (Clarke and Taylor 2012; Clarke et al. 2016).

Newborn to 4 Months

The Pavlik harness is the most common hip abduction orthosis for the treatment of DDH. Reported as having a 95% success rate, it is effective for dysplastic and unstable hips. It should be abandoned early if a fixed irreducible hip fails to respond to treatment in the first week as there is an increased risk of subsequent avascular necrosis (AVN). It is also contraindicated in neurological hip dislocation (Taylor and Clarke 1997; Clarke and Taylor 2012). The harness consists of shoulder and leg straps secured to a chest band (Figure 23.4).

The optimum position for treatment and prevention of complications, such as femoral nerve palsy and AVN, is 90° of hip flexion and 60° of hip abduction. Weekly ultrasound scans confirm successful treatment and allows the practitioner to check and adjust the harness position and ensure

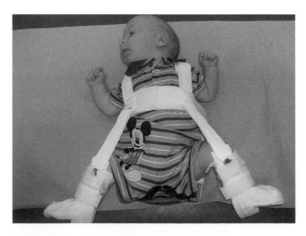

Figure 23.4   Pavlik harness. *Source:* Reproduced with permission from John Wiley & Sons.

compliance. The infant wears the harness for 6 weeks full time, following which they are gradually weaned out of it. Follow-up is recommended with serial X-rays until the age of 5 years to exclude residual dysplasia and late onset complications.

Parents are often upset by the diagnosis and the visual appearance of their baby in the harness. Close observation of the infant and reassurance and support of the parents are required to ensure successful treatment (Atalar et al. 2007; Jennings et al. 2016). The consequence of not treating the infant's hip is extremely detrimental and will condemn the child to significant surgical intervention later. It is important to give parents written information on how to care for their baby (Box 23.3 shows an abbreviated sample information leaflet) and advice on appropriate and useful websites (for further information of the care of a baby in a harness, see www.stepsworldwide.org).

Early Years Treatment

Between the ages of 4 and 12 months, surgical correction is necessary to reduce the hip. For these infants either the Pavlik harness failed and was abandoned early, or the diagnosis was not detected on initial clinical examination. Surgical correction is usually deferred until the ossific nucleus is evident on scan to prevent the potential for subsequent AVN (Luedtke et al. 2000).

There is some consensus that a week of pre-operative gallows traction to stretch the vascular supply to the femoral head reduces the risk of post-operative AVN although this is not proven (Luedtke et al. 2000). Gallows traction is not a pre-requisite and does not affect whether the hip reduces by closed manipulation or by open surgery. An arthrogram and adductor tenotomy is performed as part of the surgical procedure and if the hip does not reduce concentrically with a closed manipulation, the hip joint is opened to remove obstructing soft tissue such as the labrum. The hip position may be confirmed post-operatively by CT scan to confirm concentric reduction. A hip spica in the human position maintains the femoral head in the acetabulum for 6 weeks if an open reduction or 12 weeks for a closed reduction (Chapter 22). Sequential broomstick casts (6 weeks) and night splint casting (6 weeks) may be used to complete the surgical programme (Table 23.1) or as an alternative ring splints or a hip abduction orthosis. For the older child who presents late (aged >18 months) a femoral shortening is required in addition to the open hip reduction to reduce the tension on the hip and protect from AVN. The 18-month-old child is too heavy for gallows traction as they would be heavier than the upper weight limit of 16 kg (Davis and Barr 1999).

Further Surgical Procedures

Children who have undergone a closed or open hip reduction for either late presentation or failed Pavlik harness may subsequently need further surgery to improve acetabular

---

Box 23.3 Parent's Information: Care of your Baby in a Pavlik Harness (NIPE 2021)

The harness does not hurt your baby. It is designed to gently position your baby's hips normally.

Cuddle and feed them as you would normally do.

Do not remove the harness or adjust it.

The harness will be checked and adjusted weekly when you come to clinic.

Your baby will have an ultrasound scan to check the hip position each week.

Clothing

- It is recommended that a vest be worn underneath to prevent skin chafing.
- To change the vest: first loosen the chest band. Undo one shoulder strap. Take the vest up the body and off one arm. Do up this shoulder strap.
- Undo the second shoulder strap and remove the vest.
- Check your baby's skin and wash with a cloth or cotton wool and water.
- The new vest can be put on in the same way as when taking it off.
- Replace the chest band to its marked position.
- Each day remove the legs one at a time from its straps to wash and replace socks.

General Care

- The best position for your baby's health and hips is to place them on their back.
- If the harness is soiled, clean with detergent and a nailbrush. Dry with hairdryer on a cool setting, taking care not to harm your baby's skin.
- All clothes on top of the harness need to be loose around the legs to maintain the correct position.
- Do not swaddle your baby's legs tightly as this prevents normal hip development.
- Contact the team at the hospital if you have any questions or concerns.

Table 23.1 An example surgical programme.

Gallows traction		
Closed reduction	**Open reduction**	
6 weeks hip spica	6 weeks hip spica	
6 weeks hip spica		Changed under general anaesthetic
6 weeks broomstick plasters	6 weeks broomstick plasters	Changed under general anaesthetic
6 weeks night splints	6 weeks night splints	Changed under general anaesthetic

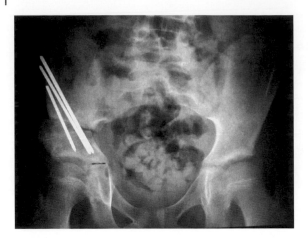

Figure 23.5 X-ray showing a pelvic osteotomy – the graft is secured with pins.

cover. Residual hip dysplasia following treatment for DDH has a reported incidence of 2–17% (Cashman et al. 2002). Of those children requiring pelvic osteotomy 60% previously underwent a closed reduction of the hip and 20% open reduction. This is usually by the age of 3–4 years to prevent progressive dysplasia, instability and eventual early osteoarthritis. The most important predictive factor for further surgery was found to be the initial achievement of a stable concentric reduction at closed or open reduction (Bolland et al. 2010).

A pelvic osteotomy aims to realign the bony structure of the hip joint and therefore the weight-bearing forces. A triangular shaped bone graft taken from the iliac crest is inserted into the osteotomy site above the acetabulum. This is fixed with two pins, which are removed at 6 weeks under general anaesthetic (Figure 23.5). Post-operatively the child is nursed in a one and half hip spica cast to immobilise the hip joint until the bone graft has fused. The optimum timing is before school age, giving the femoral head and acetabulum opportunity to remodel with growth.

Specific Nursing Considerations

The child in a hip spica requires considerable care. It is a stressful time for the parents, who require support emotionally and practically as well as needing written information on caring for their child (Clarke and McKay 2006).

An epidural is effective pain management for the first 48 hours if the child has had an open hip reduction after which paracetamol is usually sufficient. This modality can provide excellent pain relief but can also be problematic. The line can migrate (comes out of epidural space), and the child requires close observation and monitoring as the epidural site cannot be visualised due to being covered by the spica.

The spica needs to dry naturally and the child is nursed on pillows alternating from front to back for the first

24 hours. A fibreglass covering is applied on day 1 post-operatively and waterproof tape is secured around the edges of the spica cast for protection (Sparks et al. 2004). The parents are taught nappy care and instructed on the frequency of checking the nappy for dampness and changing promptly to prevent the spica from becoming soiled. The parents should check their child's skin daily for signs of friction or rash. They can use a cloth to wash their child, taking care not to get the cast wet. Hair washing is possible with the child resting on the legs of an adult who sits beside the bath. Holding the child's head over the edge of the bath, another adult can use the shower attachment to wash the hair.

The child in a spica cast is both heavy and awkward to lift; refer to Chapter 22 to view a picture of a hip spica in the human position. The occupational therapist can teach the parents handling techniques and how to turn their child safely. An assessment of the home will highlight issues early. A hoist may be required in the home. If the child cannot be securely and safely transported in the car, it may be necessary to arrange ambulance transfer home.

There are a number of ways to clothe a child in a spica. Trousers can be split and Velcro added to secure seams. Dresses are the easiest clothing for girls. Online companies advertise specific clothing made especially for children in spica casts.

Intervention for the Young Person

As the child gets older, a hip with residual dysplasia will give intrusive pain. A total hip arthroplasty for young and active patients, however, is not the best option. There is a risk of loosening and the revision rates are high. Alternative non-arthroplasty choices for the young patient include proximal femoral and periacetabular osteotomies to realign the femoral head or reposition the acetabulum to delay the onset of arthritis. Surgical management of the problematic hip in adolescent and young adult patients can be challenging and technically difficult to do. As well as hip pain, the patients may also have associated chronic instability. The optimum time for operative intervention is before there is too much wear on the cartilage and before arthritis sets in.

Legg Calvé Perthes Disease

Legg Calvé Perthes disease (LCPD) (also known as Perthes disease) is a condition of the child's hip of unknown aetiology which results in a deformed femoral head due to avascular necrosis. The condition is believed to be due to ischemia of the femoral head due to an interruption of its blood supply. Studies suggest that the articular cartilage, the bony femoral epiphysis, the growing physis and the metaphysis are all affected (Catterall et al. 1982). The aim of treatment, whether conservative or surgical, is to manage the child's symptoms and preserve hip joint congruency throughout the approximate 2-year disease process (Herring 1998). Outcomes of Perthes disease are largely dependent on age at diagnosis as well as on treatment modalities (Daly et al. 1999). Studies suggest that >50% of patients will develop osteoarthritis in their 60s (Perry et al. 2012a) and require early total hip replacements. Recent research has investigated the effect of bisphosphonates on animals with induced Perthes. Early results of ongoing research have shown effectiveness on increasing bone density, bone mineral content and strength (Little and Kim 2011).

Aetiology and Epidemiology

The cause of Perthes is unknown, although theories exist regarding relationship with possible comorbidities, congenital genito-urinary ad inguinal region abnormalities, behavioural disorders and asthma (Perry et al. 2012b). A study by Glueck et al. (1996) found 75% of participants had abnormal coagulation properties. Thrombophilia as a cause, however, has not been proven and debate regarding the reason for the temporary deficient blood supply of the femoral head continues (Kim 2010). Studies of epidemiology indicate a varied incidence of between 6 and 15.6 per 100 000. A higher incidence is reported in lower socioeconomic and urban areas and a lower incidence in rural areas. Ethnicity may be a factor as Caucasians are affected more than other races with fewer numbers affected in the African and Chinese populations. It is also more common in the Japanese and in some parts of central Europe (Nochimson 2011). The condition predominantly affects boys from 4 to 8 years and children who are small for their age and have a low BMI (body mass index) (Judd and Wright 2005). The condition is bilateral in 10% of cases.

Diagnosis

The child usually presents to the general practitioner with a history of limp and complaints of pain in either their hip or knee. Clinical examination frequently reveals reduced hip abduction with pain at the extreme of movement on the affected side. An initial radiograph may show evidence of the disease, but often it is the subsequent X-rays or an MRI which demonstrates changes in the appearance of the femoral head and confirms the diagnosis (Dillman and Hernandez 2009) (see Figure 23.6). There a number of classification systems are used to grade the stage of the disease

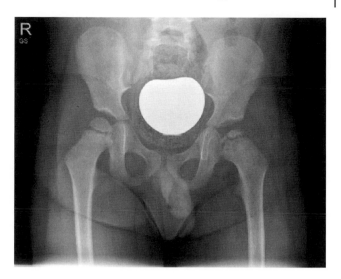

Figure 23.6 X-ray showing Perthes disease of the left hip – note the collapsing femoral head.

and in the further monitoring of the disease status (Box 23.4). A bone age (left hand X-ray) is also useful in determining the child's actual skeletal and chronological ages which assists with treatment planning strategies. MRI can also be used.

The disease process covers an approximate 2-year period from when the femoral head starts to collapse to the remodelling phase; eventually with the blood supply re-innervated (see Figure 23.6 and Box 23.5). The duration of the disease and its course is variable and treatment outcomes are therefore difficult to predict (Maxwell et al. 2004). During

---

Box 23.4 Herring Classification for Grading Stage of Perthes Disease (Herring et al. 2004)

Group A: Lateral pillar of femoral head not involved. No loss in femoral head height. No changes in bone density.
Group B: Lateral pillar of femoral head shows lucency and a loss of height of up to 50%.
Group C: Lateral pillar of femoral head has increased lucency and collapse of over 50%.

Box 23.5 Four Stages of Perthes Disease

Stage 1: Necrosis: increased radiodensity of the femoral head. The joint space is wider.
Stage 2: Fragmentation: subchondral fracture of the femoral head. Metaphyseal cysts. Bone resorption
Stage 3: Reossification: healing phase
Stage 4: Remodelling: residual deformity with new femoral head shape dependent on hip joint congruency

the early stages, when the femoral head is collapsing and softening, there is a risk of extrusion beyond the outer rim of the acetabulum. Left untreated the enlarged femoral head can impinge and become deformed. The best treatment for Perthes disease is debated. The aim of treatment is to prevent femoral head deformity, containing it within the acetabulum to allow for optimal remodelling and resulting in a better long-term outcome (Bowen et al. 2011). However, the expected result is worse if the child is over the age of 8 years at diagnosis.

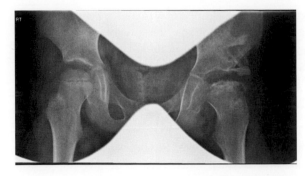

Figure 23.7 X-ray showing shelf acetabuloplasty of the left hip.

Treatment

The treatment of Perthes disease is dependent on the age of the child, the stage of the disease, the X-ray appearance, and the child's symptoms and clinical evaluation. The aim is to maintain femoral head containment through the disease process either non-operatively or operatively. Conservative management includes non-steroidal therapy such as ibuprofen to minimise inflammation of the hip joint synovium, 'slings and springs' traction to maintain hip joint movement, non-adhesive traction and physiotherapy with hydrotherapy. Hip abduction orthoses are used in some centres to protect the femoral head.

Under 5 years: Treatment is usually non-operative with 3–6-monthly X-rays monitoring the hip's progression. Symptoms are managed with simple analgesics and a change in lifestyle. The child needs to refrain from impact sports and activities that are likely to cause pain, such as jumping from a height. Swimming is recommended to prevent stiffness in the hip and maintain the joint's range of movement. If symptoms become severe and unmanageable at home, the child may be admitted to hospital. A period of bed rest and hydrotherapy (with or without simple skin traction) is normally sufficient to settle pain and muscle spasm (Judd and Wright 2005). The child may need to use crutches or a Zimmer frame to assist mobility and offload the affected hip when symptomatic. Occasionally, if symptoms are relentless, the hip can be protected by applying broomstick plasters (Petrie cast) for 4–6 weeks. This is a temporary measure that in many units has been replaced with a surgical shelf acetabuloplasty.

Over 5 years: There are a variety of surgical options to treat Perthes, ranging from femoral or pelvic procedures to improve both hip containment and articular congruence.

Shelf acetabuloplasty: The aim is to provide additional cover for the extruding femoral head (Figure 23.7) and facilitate maintenance of a free range of hip movement. In turn, the femoral head will remodel in the revascularisation phase of the disease to the shape of the new hip socket. A hip arthrogram is performed to show the cartilaginous component of the femoral head and the degree of subluxation. The shelf is a corticocancellous graft taken from the ilium. It is inserted into a previously made notch on the outer edge of the acetabulum and secured in position by reattaching the reflected head of the rectus femoris muscle (van der Geest et al. 2001). Post-operatively the child may be nursed on simple skin traction for 48 hours to allow muscle spasm to settle prior to application of a single hip spica to immobilise the hip joint and reduce post-operative pain.

Varus derotation femoral osteotomy: Reserved for the older child with residual deformity at the end of treatment. The proximal femur is realigned, tilting the femoral head into the acetabulum to achieve improved containment and facilitate femoral remodelling ability. This prevents subluxation and redirects the force through the hip when weight bearing.

Arthrodiastasis: Designed to protect the femoral head and preserve its height during the early fragmentation stage of the disease. The hip joint is distracted using an external monolateral fixator for 2–6 months. The distraction causes the hip joint to open, thereby increasing the space, reducing the weight-bearing forces and encouraging restoration of the synovial circulation. Although good results have been achieved, this significant interventional procedure is not without complications, including pin site infection and residual stiffness in the hip and knee joint (Chapter 8). Studies are of small numbers and long-term follow up to skeletal maturity is required to assess whether arthrodiastasis results is a better outcome (Maxwell et al. 2004). From the child's point of view the fixator is unsightly and cumbersome and psychological support from the outset is recommended.

Slipped Capital Femoral Epiphysis

A slipped capital femoral epiphysis (SCFE) is a condition where the head of the femur appears to slip off the physis. The neck or the metaphysis of the femur is the section that actually moves, normally migrating anteriorly and superiorly (Sun et al. 2011), while the femoral head maintains its normal position in the acetabulum. The slip occurs through the widened hypertrophic zone of the growth plate and may be acute (sustained after a traumatic episode) or chronic (occurring slowly over a period of time), 25% of cases are bilateral, half of which present sequentially.

Aetiology and Epidemiology

The incidence of SCFE is two to three per 100000 and it is more common in male adolescents. Although the cause is unknown, risk factors and associated traits include obesity, delayed skeletal maturity, hypothyroidism, endocrine abnormalities, puberty and vitamin D deficiency (Clarke and Page 2012; Perry et al. 2018). It is suggested that the growth plate plays a part in the cause. The perichondral fibrocartilaginous ring which surrounds the physis contributes to its strength. It is at its strongest during infancy, diminishing as the child gets older. In addition, the physis is widened and therefore potentially weakened during the adolescent growth spurt, which is the most common time for a slip to occur. The condition is more common in boys, with a ratio of 2.4 per female, and more prevalent in the 10–16-year-old age group in boys (average 13.4 years) and 10–14-year-old age group in girls (average 11.5 years). Children presenting outside these age perimeters should be investigated for causative factors such as endocrine or systemic disorders.

Diagnosis

A child who presents with pain and a limp over the age of 8 years should be investigated for SCFE with an anteroposterior (AP) and frog lateral X-ray views. The AP view is not always helpful and will be normal in 14% of cases (Benson et al. 2002). For a suspected SCFE that is not evident on X-ray, an MRI is useful in detecting a pre-slip (Lalaji et al. 2002) in a child who presents with symptoms.

SCFE can be classified as (Southwick, 1967):

- acute: symptoms <2 weeks
- chronic: symptoms >2 weeks
- acute-on-chronic: long-term pain with a sudden episode of acute pain.

The X-ray findings are described according to the degree of displacement:

- mild: grade 1, 0–30° of displacement
- moderate: grade 2, 30–60°
- severe: grade 3, 60–90°+.

On presentation with an acute slip the child will complain of pain of less than 3 weeks' duration in their

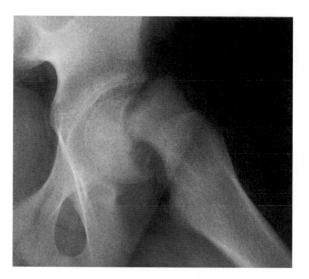

Figure 23.8 X-ray showing slipped left femoral capital epiphysis where Kleins line does not intersect the epiphysis.

groin, thigh or knee. They will limp and have an out-toeing gait. With a chronic slip their symptoms will have been more insidious in nature (Uglow and Clarke 2004). They may be able to weight bear, indicating that the slip is stable. If there is an unstable slip the child is unable to bear weight due to pain. In a severe unstable slip, the examination will show a shortened leg lying in external rotation with markedly restricted range of movement. X-ray findings may be subtle or obvious. The AP view will show widening of the physis and a loss of epiphyseal height. There is increased density in the femoral neck (Blanch sign) and Klein's line drawn up the superior aspect of the femoral neck does not cross the femoral head (see Figure 23.8).

Treatment

The prognosis of SCFE is linked to the prompt recognition of the condition and the severity of the slip. The aim of treatment is to reduce the complication rate of AVN and chondrolysis (Uglow and Clarke 2004). Early intervention within 24 hours of diagnosis reduces the rate of AVN to 7% with surgery; after this time the rate of AVN increases to 87.5% (Walter et al. 2011). It is important to determine whether the slip is stable or unstable. The latter has a poorer prognosis with increased probability of avascular necrosis whilst a stable slip may deteriorate and become unstable if not treated. Attempting to realign the femoral head will damage the blood supply and risk AVN. Stabilisation of the slip with single screw fixation (see Figure 23.9) is advocated for mild to moderate slips to prevent further slipping and maintain position until physeal fusion (Judd and Wright 2005).

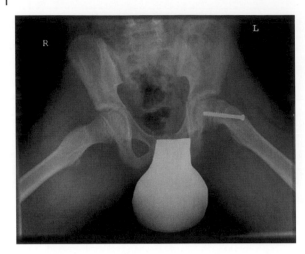

Figure 23.9 X-ray showing slipped left femoral capital epiphysis, fixed with a left screw.

Moderate and severe slips are difficult to manage. Gentle intra–operative reduction of the hip, taking care not to damage the blood supply, is advocated by some surgeons prior to screw fixation. Osteotomies of the femoral neck can be performed to realign the femoral neck in a severe slip but subsequent AVN, chondrolysis and reduced range of hip movement are all significant complications (Lawane et al. 2009). There is some debate whether the contralateral hip of a child with a unilateral slip should be fixed at initial presentation. A study by Riad et al. (2007) demonstrated that the younger the patient, the greater the probability of increased development of a contralateral slip.

Post-operatively the child mobilises non-weight bearing with crutches for the first 6 weeks, progressing to partial weight bearing for another 6 weeks. X-rays are taken at each stage to assess the position of screw fixation and possible AVN. Patients are followed up radiographically until the physis has fused, negating the possibility of further slippage. The average time for this is approximately 9 months but has been demonstrated to be as much as 25 months in patients with deficient or insufficient vitamin D levels (Judd et al. 2016).

Vitamin D Deficiency

Vitamin D deficiency is associated with rickets, fractures and musculoskeletal symptoms (Judd 2011). Previously thought of as a condition of the past, it is no longer a rarity and is linked to a number of health issues. Studies suggest a concerning association with deformity and generalised bone and muscle pain. In the UK the increase in vitamin D deficiency is attributed to the varied ethnic population, poor diet and lifestyle choices made by families.

Accepted sufficient blood serum levels of vitamin D have been agreed as >75 nmols/l (Pearce and Cheetham 2010), with some variance according to population and environmental factors. Below 20 nmols/l is considered deficient. Approximately, 80–90% of vitamin D is made through synthesis in the skin and the remaining 10–20% is acquired through diet. In efforts to protect children from sun exposure parents use high-factor sun protection creams and cover children's skin with clothing. A reduction in time spent outdoors due to a preference for indoor activities also contributes to lack of sunlight exposure, as do cultural dress codes (Judd and Wright 2011). The best source of vitamin D is exposure to sunlight, with 20–30 minutes a day recommended without application of sunscreen (Judd and Wright 2011). Dark-skinned children do not synthesise vitamin D well due to increased melanin and are therefore prone to deficiency. In addition to reduced synthesis in the skin, hypovitaminosis D is the primary cause of rickets as it results in poor absorption of calcium and phosphorus minerals from foods. Circulating blood levels of vitamin D are low, resulting in bone softening, non-specific musculoskeletal symptoms and deformity.

Vitamin D deficiency is a global problem and is not restricted to culture, race or demographics. Low vitamin D levels have been associated with musculoskeletal problems such as SCFE, cerebral palsy, fractures and poor bone healing (Clarke and Page 2012). Guidance (Department of Health 2012) advises practitioners to be aware of at-risk groups within the population and recommends that older people, pregnant women, infants and young children receive vitamin D supplementation.

An X-ray of a child with rickets will show evidence of widened growth plates which have a cupped and splayed appearance (see Figure 23.10). Due to loading on the leg's long bones, genu varum and valgum is noticeable, with

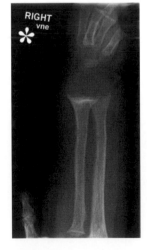
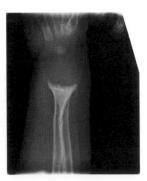

Figure 23.10 Wrist X-ray showing widened and cupped physis.

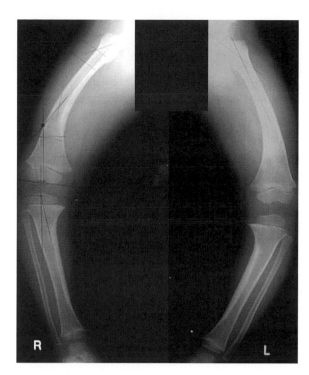

Figure 23.11 X-ray showing rickets.

abnormality depicted on leg alignment radiographs (see Figure 23.11). Clinical findings are of bowed legs (tibia vara) or knock knees (genu valgum). Skeletal deformity may be symmetric or asymmetric. The wrists and ankles are swollen and enlarged due to reduced mineralisation of the physis. The incidence of fracture and re-fracture rates are increased. There may be permanent skeletal deformities such as rachitic rosary (ends of the ribs are enlarged) and scoliosis. Children may present due to a delay in walking, have poor muscle development and tone, and complain of muscle pain.

Management

Vitamin D deficiency is an ever-increasing problem, with new evidence linking it to a number of health issues. Shared care of the child and family is important, with both orthopaedic and endocrinology teams contributing to the overall management. Where levels are simply insufficient (20–75 nmols/l) supplementation of 400 international units (IU) per day is recommended. At-risk population groups (pregnant women, infants, young children and older people) should receive supplements routinely (Gillie 2006). Deficient levels of vitamin D require a treatment dose of 6000 IU of cholecalciferol daily for 3 months with calcium supplements for 2 weeks. Dosages are adjusted according to the results of repeated blood tests at the end of 3 months (Judd 2012b). Supplementation should be supported by maintaining a dietary intake of vitamin D-rich foods (Chapter 10) and adequate exposure to the sun.

Poor diet, whether an excess of the 'wrong' foods or a reduced intake of the 'right' foods, can contribute to both vitamin D deficiency and future osteoporosis. Obese children tend to have low vitamin D as it is a fat-soluble vitamin and obesity may prevent the storage of the vitamin (Elizondo-Montemayor et al. 2010). An excess consumption of carbonated drinks affects the body's ability to absorb calcium due to the presence of phosphoric acid (Wyshak 2000). This results in poor bone density and an increased risk of fracture as well as poor fracture healing (Tucker et al. 2006). Eating disorders can result in a reduced intake of calcium and vitamin D; if there is concern, review by a dietician, who can advise parents and monitor the child, should be requested.

Vitamin D deficiency is a recognised health concern in the UK. Parents lack awareness of the role vitamin D plays in supporting good bone and muscle health, and on how to improve their child's vitamin D intake. Education and information on dietary supplements, vitamin D-fortified foods and safe sun exposure are an important role of the health professional (Day et al. 2019).

Uncorrected deformity following treatment with 25-hydroxyvitamin D may need surgical intervention. A classical picture of rickets is deformed leg alignment. Genu varum or valgum can be simply corrected through a minimally invasive procedure using guided growth plates. These slow down the physeal growth on one side whilst the other continues to grow. They are removed when the limbs are clinically straight (Ballal et al. 2010). More invasive procedures are reserved for residual tibia vara requiring proximal tibial and/or femoral osteotomies (Zaki and Rae 2009). An alternative is to correct the deformity using an external fixator following the osteotomy. The literature reports nonunion of the osteotomy, the possibility of fracture through the regenerate and the recurrence of the deformity (Petje et al. 2008; Fucentese et al. 2008; Choi et al. 2002).

Congenital Talipes Equino Varus

Congenital talipes equino varus (CTEV), or club foot, is the most common structural deformity of the lower limb present at birth (see Figure 23.12).

The name comes from:

- congenital – at birth
- talipes (talus = ankle bone)
- pes (pes = foot)
- equino – characteristic of a horse; the term describes the position of the heel
- varus – inward turning.

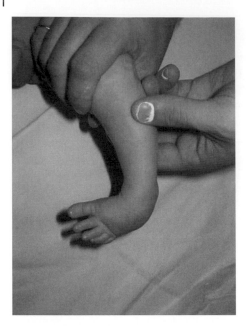

Figure 23.12 Club foot (congenital talipes equino varus).

The condition involves abnormal alignment of the foot bones and contractures of the joint capsules, ligaments and tendons:

- The deformity is seen at the hindfoot and forefoot.
- The heel is in equinus (high) and in varus (turned inward).
- The forefoot is supinated (rotated) and adducted (turned inwards).

The core problem of the foot deformity is the abnormal positioning of the talus and subsequent malaligned relationship with the calcaneus and navicular bones. Muscle, tissue and vascular structure are all abnormal (Cummings et al. 2002). The deformity may be detected antenatally on the mother's 20-week ultrasound scan or noted at birth. Pre-natal counselling has proven to be valuable for the expectant parents, giving an explanation of the proposed treatment and reassurance of the excellent functional outcomes (Bar-on et al. 2005). They should be made aware that as the child grows, they will notice the affected foot to be shorter by 1–2 sizes and the calf muscle to be thinner.

Aetiology

The CTEV is unknown. It occurs in one per 1000 births in Caucasians but varies in different races, with an incidence in Polynesians of 6.8 per 1000, for example. It is bilateral in 50% of cases and more common in males. Strong genetic links are reported in the literature: a sibling has a 30% chance of having club-foot deformity and a reported 24% of children with CTEV will have a positive family medical history.

Treatment

Treatment for idiopathic club foot is primarily non-operative, although this may be dependent on place of birth and treatment availability (Judd and Wright, 2005). The overall aim of treatment is to give the child a pain-free, functional foot-shaped foot, so they are able to wear normal shoes and perform normal daily activities (Ponseti 1992). At birth the foot will have varying degrees of stiffness in the hind-foot and forefoot. For the best results, early intervention before the age of 1 month is advocated since much of the skeleton is cartilaginous, allowing the ligaments, tendons and muscles to be readily stretched (Hart et al. 2005; Ponseti and Smoley 2009).

Prior to initial orthopaedic assessment parents can be taught simple stretching exercises and massage to maintain suppleness in the foot. They are usually extremely keen for their baby to be reviewed by a paediatric orthopaedic specialist and to commence treatment. Information available via the Internet has meant parents have enhanced knowledge and choice regarding their baby's treatment (Judd 2004).

The management of the foot begins with an assessment of its severity using a grading system. Different assessment tools exist to classify the foot deformity and are useful in the evaluation of patient outcomes (Judd 2004). The *Pirani scoring system* is a recognised and universally accepted simple tool to use (Dyer and Davis 2006). Divided into sections to give a score for the hindfoot and for the forefoot, it gives an assessment of the flexibility in the foot as a whole (Figure 23.13). An audit of outcomes using the Pirani score as an assessment tool demonstrated that higher total scores and a high hindfoot score predicted a potential relapse of deformity (Goriainov et al. 2010).

The *Ponseti method* is a conservative technique for the treatment of club foot which is well established and evidenced based. Commenced ideally before 1 month of age, weekly gentle manipulation and application of above-knee

		Right					Left			
		0	0.5	1		0	0.5	1		
					Posterior crease					
Total					Empty Heel					Total
					Ankle DF					
					Medial crease					
					Lateral Head Talus					
					Lateral Border					

Figure 23.13 Pirani score.

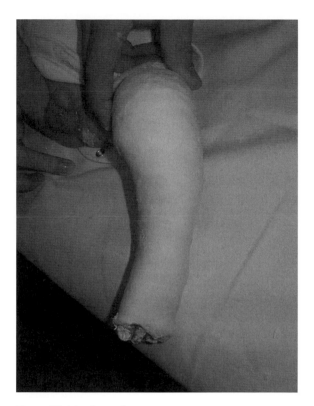

Figure 23.14 Ponseti cast.

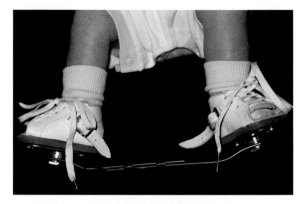

Figure 23.15 Boot on a bar. NHS, https://www.nhs.uk/conditions/club-foot/.

moulded serial casts, will gradually correct each component of the foot deformity (Figure 23.14). The average number of casts is five, with more or fewer required depending on the severity of the foot deformity. Parents can remove the casts in the bath on the morning of the clinic, but if removed earlier the foot may relapse from its new position. Parents should be reassured that the treatment is not painful, but their baby will dislike having their leg held still. Feeding at the same time as the procedure is calming (Faulks and Luther 2005).

Approximately 70% of babies will require a percutaneous Achilles tenotomy to correct the heel equinus (Ponseti 1992; Goriainov et al. 2010). This is commonly performed in the clinic using a topical anaesthetic cream, following which a final cast is applied for 3 weeks, holding the ankle in a dorsi-flexed position while the tendon heals in its new position. The final stage of the correction is maintained by the infant wearing 'boots on a bar' in the overcorrected position of 70° of abduction (Figure 23.15). These are worn for 3 months for 23 hours per day and then at night-time only until the age of 4 years.

The child is reviewed in the clinic at 3–4-monthly intervals to review the progress of the foot as it grows. Compliance with the boots and bar can sometimes be problematic and it is vital to ensure they fit correctly, with the heel positioned snuggly down in the boot. Poor outcomes

of club-foot correction using the Ponseti method have been attributed to lack of compliance with the boot and bar for the 4-year duration (Ponseti 1992).

Approximately 20–40% of children will require a tibialis anterior tendon transfer to correct dynamic forefoot supination. Considered to be part of the Ponseti technique, the problem is usually detected in the early years when the child is up and running around. The tendon is transferred into the lateral cuneiform, adjusting the muscle pull to bring the forefoot around. Post-operatively a cast is required for 6–8 weeks.

Assessment of the Atypical Club Foot

The atypical club foot commonly coexists with other diagnoses, such as arthrogryposis. It is important to examine the baby by fully assessing the upper and lower limbs, spine and hips, looking for associated anomalies. Assessment of the foot demonstrates a deep posterior heel crease and a deep plantar crease that extends across the entire sole of the foot, creating tightness in the plantar aspect. Treatment requires identification of the difference between the idiopathic and the atypical club foot, with modification of the Ponseti method to address the components of the deformity (Gupta et al. 2015). This type of foot may require minimal surgical intervention (Faulks and Luther 2005).

Surgical Correction

Surgical correction is reserved for the recalcitrant club foot when there is little or no progression in correction with manipulation. The procedure may be minimal, with a soft tissue release, or more interventional addressing all the components of the deformity and requiring a posteromedial plantar lateral release (Cummings et al. 2002). Surgery may be performed in either one or two stages, the latter proven to reduce the incidence of wound infection (Uglow and Clarke 2000). The corrected position is held with casts for 3 months (Judd and Wright 2005).

Relapsed Club Foot

Bradish and Noor (2000) report a 20% recurrence rate of club-foot deformity. Severely stiff feet have a greater tendency to relapse. The child needs regular follow-up throughout growth to detect deformity recurrence, which commonly occurs in the hind foot with reduced ankle dorsiflexion and heel varus. With walking on the lateral border of the foot, forefoot supination may also feature (Ponseti 2002). Surgery may involve capsular releases, tendon transfers or osteotomies. Plaster casts hold the corrected foot for 6–12 weeks depending on the surgery. Routine plaster care and neurovascular observations should be carried out. Pain is controlled with a nerve block and oramorph initially, with subsequent simple analgesics. If the child has had bony surgery an epidural for 48 hours is optimal (Judd and Wright 2005).

Amplified Musculoskeletal Pain Syndrome

Amplified musculoskeletal pain syndrome (AMPS) is also known as:

- chronic regional pain syndrome
- reflex sympathetic dystrophy
- fibromyalgia.

Everyone interprets pain differently. The International Association for the Study of Pain states that pain is, 'An unpleasant sensory and emotional experience normally associated with, or resembling that associated with, actual or potential tissue damage' (IASP). There is no assumed cause and the pain is increased to a point that the child can no longer manage. Commonly AMPS in children is initiated by minor insignificant trauma, psychological stress or an illness. The trauma maybe a simple fracture or a soft tissue injury and, although the injury itself heals, the pain does not resolve within the expected time frame. The pain pathway is dysfunctional. There is an abnormal short circuit within the spinal cord so that the transmission of pain to the brain is also transmitted to the neurovascular nerves. The signal causes the blood vessels to constrict, resulting in a reduced blood flow and deprivation of oxygen to the bones, muscles and skin. The result is a build-up of acid waste products such as lactic acid, with the subsequent production of pain. The new pain signal transmits across the abnormal circuit, further reducing the blood flow and

consequently produces more pain (Sherry 2008). How pain is perceived and how individuals cope with pain is influenced by a number of external factors (Chapter 11). The child with AMPS is noted to experience higher levels of stress. The pain, however, not only affects the individual but also has a psychological and social impact on the immediate family.

Signs and symptoms of AMPS may include some or all of the following (Miller 2003):

- allodynia: pain that comes from a stimulus that is not normally painful, e.g. wearing a sock or gentle light touch
- hyperalgesia (increased sensitivity to a pain): pain that is disproportionate to the injury
- burning sensation
- muscle cramps
- X-rays may reveal some osteoporosis as a result of disuse
- intermittent colour changes of the skin
- shiny appearance or mottling of the skin
- clammy skin or increased sweating
- diffuse swelling
- coolness or warmth of the affected limb
- reduced mobility.

Epidemiology

The majority of children who present with AMPS are female and are from higher socioeconomic backgrounds. It is more common in the adolescent population, with a mean age of onset at 12–13 years. In a study by Perquin et al. (2000) of 6636 Dutch children, 25% reported recurrent or continuous pain for >3 months. Similarly, Roth-Isiqkeit et al.'s (2005) study of 749 children in Germany gave a result of 30.8% reporting symptoms for >6 months. The prevalence is significantly higher in females and is increased with age. The site of symptoms is frequently the lower limb and overall AMPS is the most common reason for school non-attendance. Predisposing factors to AMPS have been reported as:

- hypermobility
- significant previous pain experiences
- family members response to pain and their coping strategies
- emotional personality: high achievers, pleasers, high anxiety levels.

Management

The patient pathway begins immediately on diagnosis. Early recognition of the problem and prompt action are the key to success in treatment (Taylor 2002; Littlejohn 2004). Once all investigations such as bloods, radiographs and scans have proven that there is no organic cause for the pain, medical intervention should be stopped, with emphasis placed on rehabilitation (Clinch and Ecclestone 2009). Management of children with AMPS involves the whole family. A clear discussion with the child and family supported with written information regarding the diagnosis and requirement for involvement with the rehabilitation programme is vital to a successful outcome. It is important to get the child and family onboard (Clinch and Ecclestone 2009) and help them to understand the necessity of physiotherapy and continued compliance. Early intervention for mild symptoms that are suggestive of impending AMPS will abate further deterioration with a reassuring prognosis.

Background history may reveal a role model within the family who has chronic pain (Littlejohn 2004), a major life event as a trigger to symptoms, such as parental marital problems or a house or school move, sporting stressors and high parental expectations. All of these can affect the child's response to their pain and their involvement and progression with rehabilitation. Family interactions can be intense, with enmeshment between the child and mother or sometimes the father.

A major part of the rehabilitation programme is the emphasis on ownership. The child needs to acknowledge that to get better they have to participate at all levels and work with practitioners and therapists to improve. The perception from the child and family may be an expectation that the health professionals will solve the problem. A usual course of action would be to identify the problem, to review what the child can or cannot do and discuss treatment that has failed. This problem-focused approach is negative whereas the aim is for positivity.

Solution-focused Approach

The solution-focused approach encourages ownership of the problem, involving the child in their rehabilitation. The focus is to get to the problem via the solution, utilising positive discussion, which always focuses on strengths and achievements (Iveson 2002; Sherry et al. 1999). The child is encouraged to think forward to the future and where they would like to be in terms of wellness and activity. 'Scaling' is used where the child allocates a score to where they are currently and where they are aiming to get to in their rehabilitation. The aim of the practitioner is to empower the child and encourage them to aim high. A successful tool is to use a scenario where the child endeavours to climb a mountain on which they have placed goals to reach at each stage of improvement. It is crucial that the team have a unified approach, with the nurses and therapists working with the child and family to build a rapport, aiming to help them to reach their goals. Early psychological support may also be useful, especially if progress is slow. Guided imagery, externalising the pain, distraction techniques and teaching the child relaxation methods can all be employed with the assistance of the play specialist. It is important for the team to stress their understanding of the symptoms and not to ignore the fact that the pain exists. However, the pain that the child feels is not harmful or protective of the body. Pain medication is gauged and is dependent on symptoms and progress. It varies from simple analgesics to antidepressants (amitriptyline) and anticonvulsants (gabapentin). The latter two are used for neuropathic pain (nerve damage) (Sherry 2008).

Further Reading

Glasper, E.A., McEwing, G., and Richardson, J. (ed.) (2007). *Oxford Handbook of Childrens and Young Peoples Nursing*. Oxford: Oxford University Press.

Kelsey, J. and McEwing, G. (ed.) (2008). *Clinical Skills in Child Health Practice*. Edinburgh: Churchill Livingstone Elsevier.

Peck, D.M., Voss, L.M., and Voss, T. (2017). Slipped capital femoral epiphysis: diagnosis and management. *Am. Fam. Physician* 95 (12): 779–784. www.aafp.org (accessed 7 June 2021).

Sherry, D.D., Sonagra, M., and Gmuca, S. (2020). The spectrum of pediatric amplified musculoskeletal pain syndrome. *Pediatr. Rheumatol. Online J.* 18 (1): 77. https://doi.org/10.1186/s12969-020-00473-2. PMID: 33046102; PMCID: PMC7552512.

References

American Academy of Pediatrics, Committee on Quality Improvement, Subcommittee on Developmental Dysplasia of the Hip (2000). Clinical practice guideline: early detection of developmental dysplasia of the hip. *Pediatrics* 105 (4): 896–905.

Atalar, H., Sayli, U., Yavuz, O.Y. et al. (2007). Indicators of successful use of the Pavlik harness in infants with developmental dysplasia of the hip. *Int. Orthop.* 31 (2): 145–150.

Ballal, M.S., Bruce, C.E., and Nayagam, S. (2010). Correcting genu varum and genu valgum in children by guided growth: temporary hemiepiphysiodesis using tension band plates. *J. Bone Joint Surg., Br.* 92 (2): 273–276.

Bar-On, E., Mashiach, R., Inbar, O. et al. (2005). Prenatal ultrasound diagnosis of club foot. Outcome and recommendations for counselling and follow up. *J. Bone Joint Surg.* 87-B (7): 990–993.

Benson, M.K.D., Fixsen, J.A., Macnicol, M.F., and Parsch, K. (2002). *Children's Orthopaedics and Fractures*, 2e. London: Churchill Livingstone.

Bolland, B.J., Wahed, A., Al-Hallao, S. et al. (2010). Late reduction in congenital dislocation of the hip and the need for secondary surgery: radiologic predictors and confounding variables. *J. Pediatr. Orthop.* 30 (7): 676–682.

Bowen, J.R., Guille, J.T., Jeong, C. et al. (2011). Labral support shelf arthroplasty for containment in early stages of Legg-Calve-Perthes disease. *J. Pediatr. Orthop.* 31 (2 Suppl): S206–S211.

Bradish, C.F. and Noor, S. (2000). The Ilizarov method in the management of relapsed clubfeet. *J. Bone Joint. Surg., Br.* 82B: 387–391.

Cashman, J.P., Round, J., Taylor, G., and Clarke, N.M. (2002). The natural history of developmental dysplasia of the hip after early supervised treatment in the Pavlik harness: a prospective, longitudinal follow-up. *J. Bone Joint. Surg., Br.* 4-B: 418–412.

Catterall, A., Pringle, J., Byers, P.D. et al. (1982). A review of the morphology of Perthes' disease. *J. Bone Joint. Surg., Br.* 64 (3): 269–275.

Choi, I.H., Kim, J.K., Chung, C.Y. et al. (2002). Deformity correction of the knee and leg lengthening by Ilizarov method in hypophosphataemic rickets: outcomes and significance of serum phosphate level. *J. Orthop. Nurs.* 22: 626–631.

Clarke, N.M.P. and Castaneda, P. (2012). Strategies to improve non-operative childhood management. *Orthop. Clin. North Am.* 43: 481–489.

Clarke, N.M.P. and Judd, J. (2013). *La cadera neonatal limítrofe: observación versus Pavlik. Rev. Mexicana de Ortop. Pediátrica* 15 (1): 14–18. www.medigraphic.org.mx.

Clarke, S. and McKay, M. (2006). An audit of spica cast guidelines for parents and professionals caring for children with developmental dysplasia of the hip. *J. Orthop. Nurs.* 10 (3): 128–137.

Clarke, N.M.P. and Page, J.E. (2012). Vitamin D deficiency: a paediatric orthopedic perspective. *Curr. Opin. Pediatr.* 24 (1): 46–49.

Clarke, N.M.P. and Taylor, C.C. (2012). Diagnosis and management of developmental hip dysplasia. *Paediatr. Child Health* 22 (6): 235–238.

Clarke, N.M.P., Taylor, C., and Judd, J. (2016). Diagnosis and management of developmental hip dysplasia. *Paediatr.*

Child Health. Symposium: Surgery and Orthopaedics 26 (6): 252–256.

Clinch, J. and Ecclestone, C. (2009). Chronic musculoskeletal pain in children: assessment and management. *Rheumatology* 48 (5): 466–474.

Cummings, R.J., Davidson, R.S., Armstrong, P.F., and Lehman, W.B. (2002). Congenital clubfoot. An instructional course lecture, American Academy of Orthopaedic Surgeons. *J. Bone Joint Surg.* 84A (2): 290–308.

Daly, K., Bruce, C., and Catterall, A. (1999). Lateral shelf acetabuloplasty in Perthes'disease. A review at the end of growth. *J. Bone Joint Surg. Br.* 81: 380–384.

Davis, P. and Barr, L. (1999). Principles of traction. *J. Orthop. Nurs.* 3 (4): 222–227.

Dawson, P., Cook, L., Holliday, L.J., and Reddy, H. (2012). *Oxford Handbook of Clinical Skills for Children's and Young People's Nursing*. Oxford: Oxford University Press.

Day, R.E., Krishnarao, R., Sahota, P., and Christian, M.S. (2019). We still don't know that our children need vitamin D daily: a study of parents' understanding of vitamin D requirements in children aged 0–2 years. *BMC Public Health* 19: 1119. https://doi.org/10.1186/s12889-019-7340-x.

Department of Health (2012). *Vitamin D: Advice On Supplements For At Risk Groups*. www.dh.gov.uk/en/Publicationsandstatistics/Lettersandcirculars/Dearcolleagueletters/DH_132509 (accessed 03 March 2012).

Dillman, J.R. and Hernandez, R.J. (2009). MRI of Legg-Calvé-Perthes disease. *Am. J. Roentgenol.* 193 (5): 1394–1407.

Dyer, P.J. and Davis, N. (2006). The role of the Pirani scoring system in the management of club foot by the Ponseti method. *J. Bone Joint Surg. Br.* 88-B(8): 1082–1084.

Eastwood, D.M. and de Gheldere, A. (2010). Clinical examination for developmental dysplasia of the hip in neonates: how to stay out of trouble. *Br. Med. J.* 340: c1965.

Elizondo-Montemayor, L., Ugalde-Casas, P.A., Serrano-González, M. et al. (2010). Serum 25-hydroxyvitamin D concentration, life factors and obesity in Mexican children. *Obesity (Silver Spring)* 18 (9): 1805–1811.

Faulks, S. and Luther, B. (2005). Changing paradigm for the treatment of clubfeet. *Orthop. Nurs.* 24 (1): 25–30.

Fucentese, S.F., Neuhaus, T.J., Ramseier, L.E., and Ulrich Exner, G. (2008). Metabolic and orthopedic management of X-linked vitamin D-resistant hypophosphatemic rickets. *J. Child. Pediatr.Orthop.* 2 (4): 285–291.

van der Geest, I.C.M., Kooijman, MA.P., Spruit, M., Anderson, P.G., De Smet, P.M.A. (2001). Shelf acetabuloplasty for Perthes disease: 12 year follow up. *Acta Orthop. Belg.* 67 (2): 126–131.

Gillie, O. (2006). A new health policy for sunlight and vitamin D. In *Health Research Forum Occasional Reports: No 2*. www.healthresearchforum.org.uk/reports/sunbook.pdf (accessed 13 April 2013).

Glueck, C.J., Crawford, A., Roy, D. et al. (1996). Association of antithrombotic deficiencies and hypofibrinolysis with Legg-Calve Perthes' disease. *J. Bone Joint Surg. Br.* 78A: 3–13.

Goriainov, V., Judd, J., and Uglow, M. (2010). Does the Pirani score predict relapse in clubfoot? *J. Child. Pediatr.Orthop.* 4 (5): 439–444.

Gupta, A., Hakak, A., Singh, R. et al. (2015). Atypical clubfoot: early identification and treatment by modification of standard Ponseti technique. *Int. J. Adv. Res.* 3 (7): 1229–1234.

Harper, P., Brijil, M., Clarke, N. et al. (2020). Even experts can be fooled: reliability of clinical examination for diagnosisng hip dislocations in newborns. *J. Pediatr. Orthop.* 40 (8): 408–412.

Hart, E.S., Grottkau, B.E., Rebello, G.N., and Allbright, M.B. (2005). The newborn foot. Diagnosis and management of common conditions. *Orthop. Nurs.* 24 (5): 313–321.

von Heideken, J., Green, D.W., Burke, S.W. et al. (2006). The relationship between developmental dysplasia of the hip and congenital muscular torticollis. *J. Pediatr. Orthop.* 26: 805–808.

Herring, J.A. (1998). Legg-Calve Perthes disease. In: *Pediatric Orthopaedic Secrets* (ed. L.T. Staheli). Philadelphia: Hanley and Belfus.

Herring, J.A., Kim, H.T., and Browne, R. (2004). Legg-Calve-Perthes disease. Part I: classification of radiographs with use of the modified lateral pillar and Stulberg classifications. *J. Bone Joint Surg. Am.* 86-A(10): 2103–2120.

Hollier, L., Jeong, K., Grayson, B., and McCarthy, J. (2000). Congenital muscular torticollis and associated craniofacial changes. *Plast. Reconstr. Surg.* 105 (3): 827–834.

International Association for the Study of Pain. http://www.iasp-pain.org/Content/NavigationMenu/GeneralResourceLinks/PainDefinitions/default.htm.

Imrie, M., Scott, V., Stearns, P. et al. (2010). Is ultrasound screening for DDH in babies born breech sufficient? *J. Child. Orthop.* 4 (1): 3–8. Institute of Infant Hip Dysplasia (IHDI). www.hipdysplasia.org.

Iveson, C. (2002). Solution-focused brief therapy. *Adv. Psychiatr. Treat.* 8: 149–156. http://apt.rcpsych.org/content/8/2/149.full (accessed 3 March 2012).

Jennings, H.J., Gooney, M., O'Beirne, J., and Sheahan, L. (2016). Exploring the experiences of parents caring for infants with developmental dysplasia of the hip attending dedicated clinic. *Int. J. Orthop. Trauma Nurs.* 25: 48–53.

Judd, J. (2004). Congenital talipes equino varus – evidence for using the Ponseti method of treatment. *J. Orthop. Nurs.* 8 (3): 160–163.

Judd, J. (2005). Strategies used by nurses for decision-making in the paediatric orthopaedic setting. *J. Orthop. Nurs.* 9 (3): 166–171.

Judd, J. (2011) Rickets: a 21st-century disease? *Nursing in Practice* (March/April). www.nursinginpractice.com (accessed 3 March 2012).

Judd, J. (2012a). History taking. In: *Oxford Handbook of Clinical Skills for Children's and Young People's Nursing* (ed. P. Dawson, L. Cook, L. Holliday and H. Reddy), 485. Oxford: Oxford University Press.

Judd, J. (2012b). Rickets in the 21st century: A review of the consequences of low vitamin D and its management. *Int. J. Orthop. Trauma Nurs.* 17: 199–208.

Judd, J. and Wright, E. (2005). Joint and limb problems in children. In: *Orthopaedic and Trauma Nursing*, 2e (ed. J. Kneale and P. Davis). Edinburgh: Churchill Livingston.

Judd, J. and Wright, E. (2011). Vitamin D deficiency in the paediatric orthopaedic patient: the epidemiology and evidence of sunlight exposure – a follow-up audit on the sun habits of families. Poster presentation, Pediatric Orthopedic Society of North America Conference (11–14 May 2011) Montreal, Quebec, Canada.

Judd, J., Welch, R., Clarke, A. et al. (2016). Vitamin D deficiency in slipped upper femoral epiphysis: time to physeal fusion. *J. Pediatr. Orthop.* 36 (3): 247–252.

Kim, H. (2010). Legg-Calvé-Perthes disease. A review article. *J. Am. Acad. Orthop. Surg.* 18: 676–686.

Kokavec, M. and Bialik, V. (2007). Developmental dysplasia of the hip. Prevention and real incidence. *Bratisl. Lek. Listy* 108 (6): 251–254. http://www.bmj.sk/2007/10806-03.pdf (accessed 16 September 2012).

Lalaji, A., Umans, H., and Schneider, R. (2002). MRI features of confirmed 'pre-slip' capital femoral epiphysis: a report of two cases. *Skeletal Radiol.* 31: 362–365.

Lawane, M., Belouadah, M., and Lefort, G. (2009). Severe slipped capital femoral epiphysis: the Dunn's operation. *Orthop. Traumatol. Surg. Res.* 95 (8): 588–591.

Little, D.G. and Kim, H.K. (2011). Potential for bisphosphonate treatment in Legg-Calve-Perthes disease. *J. Pediatr. Orthop.* 31 (2): S182–S188.

Littlejohn, G.O. (2004). Reflex sympathetic dystrophy in adolescents: lessons for adults. *Arthritis Care and Res.* 51 (2): 151–153.

Luedtke, L.M., Flynn, J.M., and Pill, S.G. (2000). Review of avascular necrosis in developmental dysplasia of the hip and contemporary efforts at prevention. *Univ. Pa. Orthop. J.* 13: 22–28.

Luther, B.L. (2002). Congenital muscular torticollis. *Orthop. Nurs.* 21 (3): 21–28.

Maxwell, S.L., Lappin, K.J., Kealey, W.D. et al. (2004). Arthrodiastasis in Perthes' disease. Preliminary results. *J. Bone Joint Surg. Am.* 86 (2): 244–250.

Miller, R.L.S. (2003). Reflex sympathetic dystrophy. *Orthop. Nurs.* 22 (2): 91–99.

Moloney, D., Heffernan, G., Dodds, M., and McCormack, D. (2006). Normal variants in the paediatric orthopaedic population. *Ir. Med. J.* 99 (1): 13–14.

NIPE (2021). *Newborn and Infant Physical Examination (NIPE) screening programme handbook.* http://www.gov.uk/government/publications/newborn-and-infant-physical-exmination-programme-handbook (accessed 0 June 2021).

Nochimson, G. (2011). *Legg-Calve-Perthes Disease in Emergency Medicine.* http://emedicine.medscape.com/article/826935 (accessed 16 September 2012).

Pearce, S.H.S. and Cheetham, T.D. (2010). Diagnosis and management of vitamin D deficiency. *Br. Med. J.* 340: b5664.

Perquin, C.W., Hazebroek-Kampschreur, A.A.J.M., Hunfeld, J.A.M. et al. (2000). Pain in children and adolescents: a common experience. *Pain* 87 (1): 51–58.

Perry, D.C., Green, D.J., Bruce, C.E. et al. (2012a). Abnormalities of vascular structure and function in children with Perthes disease. *Pediatrics* 130 (1): 126–131.

Perry, D.C., Bruce, C.E., Pope, D. et al. (2012b). Comorbidities in Perthes' disease: a case control study using the general practice research database. *J. Bone Joint Surg. Am. Br.* 94 (12): 1684–1689.

Perry, D.C., Metcalfe, D., Lane, S., and Turner, S. (2018). Childhood obesity and slipped capital femoral epiphysis. *Pediatrics* 142 (5): http://www.Aapublications.org/news (accessed 7 June 2021).

Petje, G., Meizer, R., Radler, C. et al. (2008). Deformity correction in children with hereditary hypophosphatemic rickets. *Clin. Orthop. Relat. Res.* 466 (12): 3078–3085.

Ponseti, I.V. (1992). Treatment of congenital clubfoot. *J. Bone Joint Surg. Am.* 74A (3): 448–454.

Ponseti, I.V. (2002). Relapsing clubfoot: causes, prevention, and treatment. *Iowa Orthop. J.* 22: 55–56.

Ponseti, I.V. and Smoley, E.N. (2009). The classic congenital club foot: the results of treatment. *Clin. Orthop. Relat. Res.* 467 (5): 1133–1145.

Riad, J., Bajelidze, G., and Gabos, P.G. (2007). Bilateral slipped capital femoral epiphysis: predictive factors for contralateral slip. *J. Pediatr. Orthop.* 27 (4): 411–414.

Roth-Isigkeit, A., Thyen, U., Stöven, H. et al. (2005). Pain among children and adolescents: restrictions in daily living and triggering factors. *Pediatrics* 115 (2): e152–e162.

Royal College of Nursing (2012). *A Competence Framework for Orthopaedic and Trauma Practitioners.* London: Royal College of Nursing.

Sherry, D. (2008). Amplified musculoskeletal pain: treatment approach and outcomes. *J. Pediatr. Gastroenterol. Nutr.* 47 (5): 693–694.

Sherry, D., Wallace, C., Kelley, C. et al. (1999). Short and long-term outcomes of children with complex regional pain syndrome type I treated with exercise therapy. *Clin. J. Pain* 15: 218–223.

Southwick, W.O. (1967). Osteotomy through the lesser trochanter for slipped capital femoral epiphysis. *J. Bone Joint Surg.* 49-A: 807–835.

Sparks, L., Rush Ortman, M., and Aubuchon, P. (2004). Care of the child in a body cast. *J. Orthop. Nurs.* 8 (4): 231–235.

Sun, W., Li, Z., Shi, Z. et al. (2011). Early and middle term results after surgical treatment for slipped capital femoral epiphysis. *Orthop. Surg.* 3 (1): 22–27.

Taylor, L.M. (2002). Complex regional pain syndrome: comparing adults and adolescents. *Top. Adv. Pract. Nurs.* 2 (2): http://www.medscape.com/viewarticle/430537_1 (accessed 3 March 2012).

Taylor, G.R. and Clarke, N.M.P. (1997). Monitoring the treatment of developmental dysplasia of the hip with the Pavlik harness. *J. Bone Joint Surg. Br.* 79-B: 719–723.

Tucker, K.L., Morita, K., Qiao, N. et al. (2006). Colas, but not other carbonated beverages, are associated with low bone mineral density in older women: the Framingham osteoporosis study. *Am. J. Clin. Nutr.* 84 (4): 936–942.

Uglow, M.G. and Clarke, N.M.P. (2000). Relapse in staged surgery for congenital talipes equinovarus. *J. Bone Joint Surg. Br.* 82B (5): 739–743.

Uglow, M.G. and Clarke, N.M.P. (2004). The management of slipped capital femoral epiphysis. *J. Bone Joint Surg. Br.* 86-B (5): 631–635.

Vaquero-Picado, A., Gonzalez-Moran, G., Garay, E.G., and Moraleda, L. (2019). Developmental dysplasia of the hip: update on management. *Effort Open Rev* 4 (9): online. boneandjoint.org.uk/doi/full/10.1302/2058-5241.4.180019 (accessed 6 June 2021).

Walter, K.D., Lin, D.Y. and Schwartz, E. (2011). *Slipped Capital Femoral Epiphysis.* http://emedicine.medscape.com/article/91596-overview (accessed 16 September 2011).

Wyshak, G. (2000). Teenaged girls' carbonated beverage consumption and bone fractures. *Arch. Pediatr. Adolesc. Med.* 154 (6): 610–613.

Yeo, A., James, K., and Ramachandran, M. (2015). Normal lower limb variants in children. *BMJ* bmj.com/content/351/bmj.h3394.full (accessed 6 June 2021).

Zaki, S.H. and Rae, P.J. (2009). High tibial valgus osteotomy using the Tomofix plate – medium-term results in young patients. *Acta Orthop. Belg.* 75: 360–367.

24

Fracture Management in the Infant, Child and Young Person

Elizabeth Wright

University Hospital Southampton, Southampton, UK

Introduction

Children are not small adults but 'different' due to their state of development and growth, resulting in physiological differences between the child and adult skeleton. The growing skeleton has an enormous capacity for more rapid healing and remodelling. Injuries that involve skeletal growth plates can potentially cause permanent growth irregularities. Children sustain more fractures than healthy adults (Jones et al. 2002) and Schalamon et al. (2011) estimated that 10–25% of all children's injuries worldwide will be fractures. In a study of 3421 children's fractures 34.7% were sport related, 17.6% occurred at home and 16.7% happened outdoors. The incidence of childhood fractures varies across the age spectrum. This is influenced by a child's physical mobility, language development, their comprehension of danger, ability to identify risk in their immediate environment and more adventurous behaviour with age. Obesity, which is now more prevalent, has been found to increase the likelihood and severity of fractures (Kosuge and Barry 2015) and vitamin D insufficiency and deficiency is also known to effect fracture occurrence and healing (Mullis et al. 2021). Throughout the life span, beginning in childhood, a healthy lifestyle involving regular physical exercise with prudent dietary consumption is proven to increase bone mass density and reduce fracture occurrence (Sheng et al. 2021). The principles of fracture management are considered in Chapter 17 while this chapter, along with Chapter 25, focuses specifically on fractures in the infant, child and young person.

The Pre-ambulant Child

The pre-ambulant child, newborn to around 13 months of age, is dependent and vulnerable, with crying the only means of communication. This can sometimes seem relentless and frustrating for carers. This age group has minimal capacity to place themselves in danger, therefore for any child from this age group presenting with a fracture, there should be a high index of suspicion for non-accidental injury (Clarke et al. 2012). Skellern et al. (2000) report 24% of fractures in children under 1 year of age to be due to non-accidental injury. It is essential that practitioners working with this age group always obtain a full medical history and seek continuity between the mechanism of injury and the actual injury (Clarke et al. 2012) (see Chapter 23 for further discussion). Notably Blatz et al. (2019) reviewed the management of children under 3 years of age with a femoral fracture and found that assessment for non-accidental injury only occurred in 41% of 281 patients, suggesting that there is scope for improvement by healthcare professionals assessing for non-accidental injury. Accidents that do happen are often attributed to unexpected mobility by the child, for example the first time a baby independently rolls over and falls from a surface or unexpectedly crawls and falls downstairs. Other accidents are inadvertently caused by the child's carer, for example dropping the child while carrying them or placing a child seat on a high surface from which it can fall. It is known that pre-school age children are most likely to sustain fractures in the home environment (Majori et al. 2009) and there is a role here for parental/carer education in accident prevention.

The Pre-school Child

Pre-school children, aged 13 months to 5 years of age, are gradually becoming independently mobile. They are inquisitive about their environment and need to interact with things to learn. It is in their nature to be impetuous, excitable, trusting, naïve and quick. However, they have little knowledge of what can potentially harm them. Language skills are developing but they may not fully comprehend instructions. For those 3–5 years of age the most likely reason for emergency department attendance for 1- to 2-year-olds is accidental poisoning followed by musculoskeletal injury (Orton et al. 2012). Valerio et al. (2010) researched paediatric fracture patterns in 382 subjects and found that 19.9% of pre-school children sustained a fracture, 83% of these injuries were to the upper limb, there was no gender difference and 68% of the fractures occurred in the home environment.

The School-age Child

School-age children, aged 5 to 12 years, continue to interact with the environment and gradually form some independence. It is at this age they start to play outside away from direct supervision. Their understanding of risk is developing but is still limited. They form friendships and may start to engage in risk-taking behaviours to impress their friends. Language comprehension has developed and instructions can be followed unless the child chooses to be disobedient. This is reflected in the injury patterns for this age group. Most injuries still occur in the home (46%) but 28% of fractures are sustained at playgrounds and 18% at sports facilities (Valerio et al. 2010). Children are seen with injuries that relate to trends in their play activities, such as skating (Ruth et al. 2009), trampolining and skateboards (Lustenberger et al. 2010). It is important to look at these trends and consider health and safety initiatives to help reduce the number of fractures that children sustain, such as the type of surfaces in playgrounds (Howard et al. 2009). Such initiatives have health benefits but are also important because school attendance is reduced when a child has a limb immobilised in a cast (Hyman et al. 2011) and this may impact on their education. Young children often do not pay attention and are at particular risk of injury from road traffic accidents (Doong and Lai 2012; Dunbar 2012). Children at the younger end of this age group are short in stature and have small body mass, rendering them more vulnerable to significant injury if involved in a road traffic accident. Often the child is a pedestrian, possibly playing in the street or on a bike, and because of their smaller size they are harder to see, the main trunk of their body comes into contact with the vehicle and they can be thrown further. Even at slow speeds, the child involved in a road traffic accident is likely to sustain injuries that are more significant.

The Young Person/Adolescent

Adolescents are known for being adventurous and engaging in risk-taking behaviours. Many are thrill seeking, attention seeking, respond to peer pressure and confidently believe that they are indestructible. Most adolescents have adult appearance, but it is important to remember that they have not fully reached skeletal maturity. Wang et al. (2010) suggest the higher fracture incidence in this age group is related to the very rapid pubertal growth spurt that weakens the bone cortex. Mathison and Agrawal (2010) attribute the recent increase in the number of paediatric fractures to the emergence of more adventurous sporting activities that appeal to this age group. Most adolescent fractures are sustained when participating in contact sports such as rugby and football or more adventurous activities like skiing and mountain biking (Aleman and Meyers 2010). More recently adolescents are sustaining orthopaedic injuries whilst being distracted using a mobile phone (Wagner et al. 2019) and there is an increased association between alcohol consumption and injury in this age group (Milczarek et al. 2021).

Key Stages of Musculoskeletal Development of Bone and Fracture Healing

Childhood Skeletal Growth

Skeletal formation commences in the embryo and continues until skeletal growth is complete at around 21 years of age. Before 8 weeks' gestation the foetal skeleton is formed entirely of fibrous membranes and hyaline cartilage. Two types of bone tissue development occur: intramembranous ossification, when bone develops from a fibrous membrane and is called membranous bone, and endochondral ossification, when bone develops from hyaline cartilage and is called cartilage or endochondral bone. Interstitial growth at the epiphyseal plates or physis lengthens bone and appositional growth widens bones. During bone lengthening the epiphyseal plate cartilage that abuts the diaphysis produces new cartilaginous cells that transit towards the diaphysis and then form new bone. Appositional growth occurs along the periosteum. Osteoblasts form new bone on the inner side of the periosteum whilst osteoclasts erase bone along the outer edge of the endosteum. Osteoblast formation is more prolific than osteoclast activity. The end result is a thicker and stronger bone shaft and a widening medullary canal in proportion to the bone diameter. Bone growth is said to be complete when the epiphyseal plates fuse. Growth of the young child's femoral head demonstrates this. Figure 24.1 shows a series of radiographic images of the hip illustrating development from birth to skeletal maturity.

At birth, the femoral head is a cartilaginous template that is not evident on X-ray. By 8 months of age the ossific nuclei of the femoral head (secondary centre of ossification) is evident. At around 8 years of age the femoral heads are fully formed, with the epiphyseal plate (physis) clearly evident. At skeletal maturity, the physis of the proximal femur is fused.

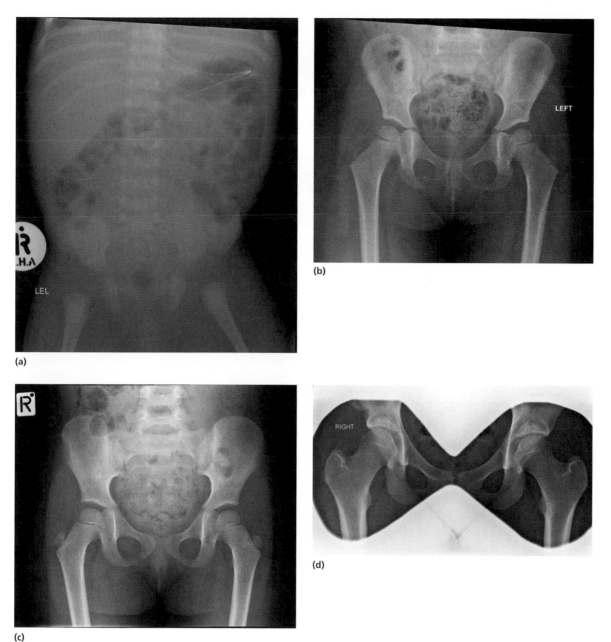

Figure 24.1 Series of child hip X-rays from birth to skeletal maturity: (a) Child hip x-ray at 2 months of age, (b) Child hip xray at 3 years of age, (c) Child hip x-ray at 6 years of age, (d) Child hip x-ray at 14 years of age.

Bone Repair and Remodelling

Bone repair and remodelling occurs throughout life. Remodelling is controlled in two ways:

1) A hormonal negative feedback mechanism in which parathyroid hormone and calcitonin control the blood calcium concentration. When blood calcium concentration falls, parathyroid hormone stimulates osteoblasts to release calcium from the skeleton. When blood calcium levels rise the thyroid gland releases calcitonin, which stimulates the calcium to be deposited into bone. Calcium is essential for many physiological processes and this mechanism exists to maintain the blood calcium level rather than assist with skeletal wellbeing.

2) A response to mechanical stress. A bone grows or remodels according to the forces or demands made of it (Wolff's law). Bones are thicker and stronger at the points of maximum weight bearing and muscle attachment/pull. Long bones are thickest mid shaft, curved bones are thickest at the bend point and form bony projections for muscle attachment (i.e. neck of femur),

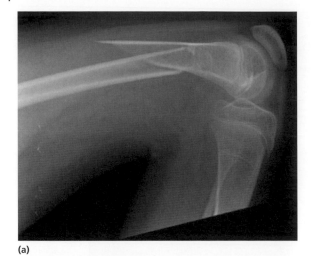

(a)

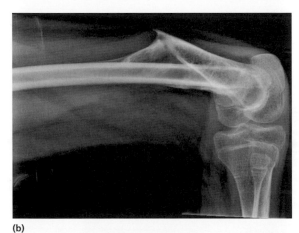

(b)

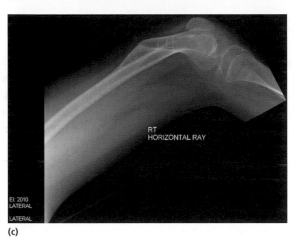

(c)

Figure 24.2 Series of X-rays to show fracture remodelling in a femur: (a) new injury, (b) 2 months post-injury and (c) 8 months post-injury.

spongy bone forms struts (bony bridges) along areas of compression. Thus, the negative feedback mechanism controls when remodelling occurs and mechanical stresses control where remodelling occurs (see Chapter 4 for musculoskeletal structure and development).

Fracture healing in the child fundamentally follows the same process as in adults (Chapter 17) with some differences. Younger children have a greater capacity for fracture remodelling and so angulated and/or displaced fractures can be treated conservatively. After initial callus formation more bone is laid down in the plane with the greatest mechanical stress. As a general rule fractures within the sagittal plane remodel well whereas fractures with axial rotation are unlikely to remodel. In adults, similar injuries would require surgical correction. Figure 24.2 provides a pictorial overview of the healing process.

Children have a growing skeleton, consequently fracture healing is faster in children than adults. It is estimated that a 2-year old will heal a long bone fracture in 3 weeks whereas a 10-year-old will take 3 months and children have a greater capacity for fracture remodelling. When managing children's fractures, it is acceptable for the fracture fragments not to be in true alignment and/or have some degree of angulation. It is important to know the age of the child and the injury. The younger the child the faster the healing capacity and the greater the remodelling capacity.

Vitamin D is essential for calcium homeostasis and thus affects bone development and remodelling. This is considered in more detail in Chapter 23. The practitioner should consider assessing the vitamin D level of children that present with repeat fractures and when considering the possibility of non-accidental injury.

Specific Conditions and Fractures Presenting in Children

Osteogenesis Imperfecta

Osteogenesis imperfecta (OI) is a genetic skeletal dysplasia in which the skeleton is osteoporotic (Cole 2002). It is clinically manifested in tissues in which type I collagen is the principal matrix protein: bone, dentin, sclera and ligaments. It is described as dominant or recessive. In dominant OI there is a protein defect that affects type I collagen formation. Either there is a reduction in the amount of collagen manufactured by the body or there is a reduction in the amount of collagen mixed with some defective collagen (Cole 2002). In recessive OI genetic mutations cause deficiency in the collagen components. Both dominant and recessive forms result in reduced bone mass and strength, making the bone fragile and susceptible to fracture, deformity and growth deficiency (Forlino et al. 2011). The condition is rare, affecting around six per 100 000 of the population (van Dijk et al. 2011). Its clinical presentation ranges from silent forms with osteoporosis to intrauterine death.

Children with OI usually present with a fracture from a low impact injury, multiple or sequential fractures that may be in different stages of union, and a family history of 'easy' fractures and/or bone disease. Fractures often heal with abundant callus. Abnormal reparative bone may give rise to malunion or pseudarthrosis. Children with more severe forms of OI tend to present earlier and with more numerous fractures. Fracture incidence decreases after puberty. Other main musculoskeletal features are short stature, pectus excavatum, kyphoscoliosis and Wormian bone. Kyphoscoliosis occurs in 40–60% of cases and may be progressive after maturity. In Wormian bone small independent areas of primary ossification are seen within membranous bone on X-ray, most often seen on a skull X-ray. Alteration of the tissues containing type I collagen also causes dentinogenesis imperfecta, blue sclera and ligamentous laxity.

OI is classified in to four types:

- The mildest form is type 1. These patients have blue sclera, bone fragility varies from mild to severe and dentinogenesis imperfecta may be present.
- Type 2 is the severest form of OI. It is incompatible with life and usually results in intrauterine death. Babies rarely survive the neonatal period and there is extreme bone fragility with crumpled long bones.
- In type 3 bone fragility is variable, being more severe in infancy; skeletal deformity is progressive with blue sclera.
- In type 4 OI there is bone fragility, normal sclera with variable skeletal deformity and dentin abnormality.

OI is difficult to diagnose; 20.5% of children with OI are initially diagnosed as non-accidental injury (Pandya et al. 2011).

Children with OI should be managed by the multidisciplinary team. Systemic management aims to improve skeletal strength. A group of drugs called bisphosphonates may be prescribed. These decrease osteoclast activity to improve the mineral content of bone (van Dijk et al. 2011) with the intention of decreasing fracture risk. Calcium, vitamins C and D, fluoride and calcitonin are used to try and strengthen the bone with growth hormone used in an attempt to correct short stature.

Management aims to maximise independent mobility by minimising disability that can result from fractures and skeletal deformity. OI is a chronic condition and requires long-term routine therapy. This consists of physiotherapy and hydrotherapy to maintain muscle control and strength. Lightweight orthotics are used to support limbs and prevent deformity, and spinal braces to control kyphoscoliosis. Custom made seating is provided for non-ambulators. Parents and carers need to be taught proper handling and positioning to avoid fractures. It is preferable that fractures are treated conservatively and are immobilised in lightweight casts for short durations to allow for early motion. Prolonged immobilisation results in further osteoporosis, leading to repeat fractures.

Surgery can be used to stabilise skeletal deformity. Options include intramedullary nailing of the long bones, with or without correctional osteotomies, or using telescopic rods that are fixed in the epiphysis and elongate with the bone during growth. Stabilisation aims to improve bone alignment, decrease the risk of refracture and improve rehabilitation. Spinal fusion is recommended for curves over 35°, but surgical fixation is complicated by the poor bone quality and the lack of autogenous bone graft. It is important to remember that patients with OI have a tendency to bleed excessively.

Fractures in Children with Special Needs

Children with special needs are at increased risk of pathological fractures because of low bone mineral density. Many have a decreased weight-bearing status that contributes to osteoporosis (Marreiros et al. 2010), require parenteral nutrition because of poor gastrointestinal absorption that affects their nutritional status, may have epilepsy and need anticonvulsant drugs that have been shown to lower bone mineral density (Gniatkowska-Nowakowska 2010) and/or underlying pathology such as osteomyelitis that affects skeletal strength (Belthur et al. 2012) or neurofibromatosis. Some syndromes (e.g. Turner's syndrome) have a known association with increased fracture risk but the physiology is not yet fully understood (Holroyd et al. 2010).

There is a tripartite approach to caring for the disabled child with a fracture. The main principles of fracture management apply: pain control and limb immobilisation, and conservative or surgical treatment appropriate for the underlying pathology and the child's ability to manage the suggested treatment. Traction may be a preferable treatment. Early mobilisation is preferable, splints and braces may be more appropriate than casts and all need to be lightweight. Many children with special needs are at greater risk of pressure ulcers due immobility, neurological deficit, nutritional issues and fragile skin. This must be considered when prescribing immobilisation devices.

Pathological Fractures

Some fractures are pathological in origin. This means that there is underlying disease or alteration of the biochemistry of the bone that predisposes it to fracture. There can be many causes: malnutrition, neurophysiological disorders that affect the musculoskeletal system, osteomyelitis, skeletal syndromes and dysplasias, bone cysts and tumours. Bone chemistry is altered and bone density is reduced. Pharmacological regimes used to treat other conditions can affect the bone density (e.g. epilepsy drugs and chemotherapy).

To complicate matters, when a child presents with a fracture without clear evidence of injury the practitioner must consider non-accidental injury (NAI) but must also be mindful of pathological causes. Each hospital must have sound child protection procedures/safeguarding in place and designated child protection specialists. The practitioner needs to know and follow the local child protection guidelines if there is any concern about the mechanism of the injury. Sadly, this is especially significant as reported child maltreatment continues to rise (Gilbert et al. 2012). The consequences of not identifying child abuse are severe, with 50% presenting with further injury and 10% dying from abuse. See Chapter 22 for further discussion of safeguarding children.

The first priority when managing a child with a pathological fracture is to diagnose the cause (Saraph and Linhart 2005). Attempting to treat the fracture without understanding the pathological cause is largely futile. If a child has osteomyelitis, then the fracture will not heal until the infection has been appropriately treated. Expediency is also key. A pathological fracture from a bone lesion diagnosed on X-ray may have resulted from a simple bone cyst or an osteosarcoma, which is life threatening. Initial principles of fracture management apply pain control and limb immobilisation, but further management is dependent on the underlying diagnosis (Chapter 15).

Fracture Diagnosis, Classification and Management in Childhood

The principles of diagnosis, classification and management of fractures in the adult are considered in Chapter 17. For the sake of completeness in this chapter an overview of fracture care in children is also considered here with some overlap but the reader may also wish to refer to Chapter 17.

Diagnosis

A fracture is described as a disruption of bone continuity and is most often the result of accidental trauma. On initial presentation the child experiences pain, swelling and loss of function of the affected limb, although in stable undisplaced fractures not all these criteria may be present. It is important to obtain a full medical history, complete a clinical examination and obtain an X-ray to assist with diagnosis. Not all fractures are clearly evident on X-ray, and it may be necessary to use other forms of imaging to clarify the injury, such as magnetic resonance image (MRI) or computerised tomography (CT).

The medical history should identify how the injury happened, the age of the child and the age of the injury. Information about the mechanism of injury will allow for any concerns regarding non-accidental injury to be considered and, hopefully, ruled out. Information about the velocity and impact of injury can give vital information. If a fracture that is normally associated with a high impact injury, for example fractured femur, occurred as a result of low impact then the clinician should be suspicious of a pathological fracture and further investigations are needed. If the child has been involved in major trauma (i.e. road traffic accident) then the clinician must consider the possibility of other injuries (Chapter 16).

Fractures can be diagnosed clinically. The main indices are pain, swelling and loss of function. Palpation over the suspected site of injury will be uncomfortable if there is an underlying fracture. Assessment of the limb must include assessment for neurovascular deficit/compartment syndrome (Wright 2007b). Radiological imaging is used to confirm the diagnosis of a fracture. Initially an X-ray is obtained. It is important to obtain two views: anterior–posterior and lateral. The body is three dimensional and thus one X-ray view may not show evidence of fracture. If an X-ray does not illustrate a fracture but there is a high index of clinical suspicion, then other imaging such as an oblique X-ray view, MRI or CT may be requested. MRIs show the soft tissues and CTs provide better definition of bones. In addition, if the injury is complex, for example a triplane fracture of ankle, which as the name suggests is a three-dimensional injury, then further imaging is requested so that the surgeon can have a full understanding of the injury.

Fracture Classification

Fractures are generally classified as closed or open injuries, by the anatomical location, the direction of fracture line, the level of the fracture within the bone, as a description of the fracture pattern and, if the injury involves the growth plate, using the growth plate classification Salter Harris. There is a detailed and complex fracture classification system for long bones called the AO system of long bone fracture classification (Müller et al. 1990); a further version was created for paediatric long bone fractures by Slongo and Audigé (2007).

In closed fractures, the skin surrounding the fracture is intact. If a fracture is described as open, then the skin has been punctured and the skin integrity has been compromised. In this instance, there is a high risk of infection, especially as debris from the scene of the incident may be embedded inside the bone and surrounding tissues. This is also known as a compound fracture and the bone may be

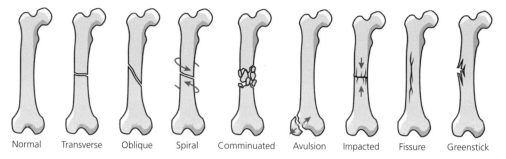

Normal Transverse Oblique Spiral Comminuated Avulsion Impacted Fissure Greenstick

Figure 24.3 Types of fracture. *Source:* Reproduced with permission from ASU Ask a Biologist.

protruding from the skin. Haemorrhage is likely with an open fracture.

Primary fracture description involves identifying the fractured bone, for example fractured left tibia or fractured right metacarpal of index finger. The anatomical reference points are used to describe the level of the fracture, i.e. diaphysis, epiphysis. The Salter Harris classification system is used to describe fractures that involve the physis (Chapter 24). The fracture is then further described by the direction of the fracture line: transverse, linear, oblique or spiral, as demonstrated in Figure 24.3. In a transverse fracture, the fracture line crosses the shaft of the bone at a right angle to the bone's long axis. In a linear fracture, the fracture line is parallel along the bone's long axis. In an oblique fracture, the fracture line is diagonal and in a spiral fracture, the fracture line twists around the long axis of the bone. Other terms used to describe fractures are impacted, comminuted and avulsed. Impacted fractures occur when the bone fragments are driven into each other. In comminuted or multifragment fractures the bone has broken into a number of fragments. With an avulsion fracture, the muscle that attaches to the bone via a tendon has been pulled away by sudden contraction of the muscle. The sudden and forceful muscle contraction results in a fragment of bone being pulled off from the bone. The levels of the fracture site are also used in fracture description: proximal, mid shaft and distal. Figure 24.4 applies these terms to the femur.

The levels of fracture site are also described as the proximal third, middle third or distal third. Terms that describe the fracture pattern are also used. A hairline fracture is a thin, fine fracture where there is no clear evidence of fracture on X-ray, but clinical indices are high. Depressed fractures are inwardly displaced, often caused by a direct blow. Intraarticular fractures involve part of the joint surface. Pathological fracture occurs when the bone is weakened by disease and fractures with minimal force.

Fractures Unique to Childhood

Buckle fractures and greenstick fractures are unique to children. The juvenile skeleton has thicker periosteum, and this partially protects the bone from injury when a high-impact force is sustained, reducing the severity of the fracture. The result is an incomplete 'buckle' or 'greenstick' fracture. The term buckle refers to the buckling of the bone without disturbing the whole bone. This is also known as a torus fracture, from the Latin word *tori* meaning swelling or protuberance. Buckle fractures most commonly occur in the distal radius, typically when a child falls on an outstretched hand. These fractures can be successfully treated using a temporary removable wrist splint (Wright 2011). A greenstick fracture describes a fracture in which one cortex of the bone is broken and the other cortex is intact. These fractures are treated conservatively by immobilising in a cast because angulation can occur at the fracture site due to the asymmetry of the fracture (Chapter 25).

Growth Plate Injuries

Fractures that include the epiphyseal plate are classified using the Salter Harris (SH) classification. This classification describes the physeal injury and appoints a number to each type. The gradient is from one to five; a Salter Harris 5 injury is the severest injury and poses the greatest likelihood of an angulatory deformity or bone length discrepancy. Salter Harris classification and management is further explored in Chapter 25.

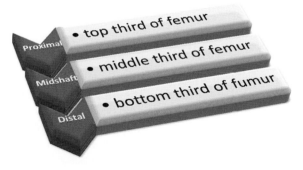

• top third of femur
Proximal
• middle third of femur
Midshaft
• bottom third of fumur
Distal

Figure 24.4 Bone descriptors applied to the femur.

Potential Diagnostic Pitfalls

The altered physiology of the child's skeleton complicates diagnosing children's fractures. The cartilaginous component of the child's skeleton does not show on X-ray and may result in the true extent of the injury not being appreciated. This is particularly true of SH1 and fractures of the lateral condyle of the humerus. An SH1 fracture of long bone presents with the fracture line traversing the physis; a child's physis is cartilage and will therefore not be evident on radiological imaging (Gaston et al. 2012). Similarly, the physis of the lateral condyle of the humerus is the last growth plate in the elbow to fuse, at around 13 years of age, making radiological diagnosis difficult. This is particularly significant because there is a high incidence of non-union (Storm et al. 2006). These injuries are usually treated conservatively (Marcheix et al. 2011) but, due to the risk of non-union, some surgeons prefer to treat them surgically with fracture reduction and K wire fixation. Either way, children with these injuries should be followed up in the outpatient clinic until fracture healing has been confirmed radiologically.

Hairline or stress fractures are not always evident radiologically. These injuries are usually the result of minor trauma or repeated stress (e.g. when participating in sports). Mostly they are stable fractures that will heal well, but the scaphoid is an exception. Scaphoid fractures usually occur in the adolescent (Bhatti et al. 2012) and have a high incidence of painful non-union (Eastley et al. 2012). If there is clinical suspicion of a scaphoid fracture, the limb should be immobilised in a cast. Further imaging by MRI is recommended to aid diagnosis (Yin et al. 2012). Once the cast is removed the child is reviewed in clinic until there is radiological evidence of fracture healing and the patient is symptom free.

Overlooking these injuries can result in deformity and disability. If there is a clinical suspicion of a fracture, even if the injury is not confirmed on X-ray, the limb should be immobilised and further imaging requested to confirm or refute the diagnosis. Furthermore, children's ligaments are stronger than bone, which makes it rare for a child to sustain a 'strain' or 'sprain'. When a child presents with, for example, ankle pain and a history of trauma with no evidence of fracture on X-ray, the practitioner should suspect an SH1 fracture and take appropriate action.

Joint Dislocations

Joint dislocations occur with high-impact events, usually sport related. The two bones that constitute a joint are completely displaced from one another. There is no articulation and the joint cannot function. Subluxation is a variance of this where the two bones are partially dislocated, but some contact is maintained. Dislocation of joints most commonly occurs in the shoulder and the patella. Treatment involves manipulating the bones back into the correct position followed by a period of immobilisation then gradual rehabilitation with physiotherapy to strengthen the musculature that supports the joints.

Fracture Dislocations

Fracture dislocations are a complex group of injuries where a joint is dislocated alongside a fracture. These injuries usually require surgical reduction but can be difficult to reduce and may be unstable. Children with these injuries require close supervision as joint stiffness and avascular necrosis are common complications. An uncommon but unique fracture dislocation in children is the Monteggia fracture. This is a fracture dislocation in which a fracture of the proximal ulna is coupled with dislocation of the radial head (Beutel 2012). While the ulna fracture is usually identified, the radial head dislocation is sometimes initially overlooked (Babb and Carlson 2005). This can cause a valgus deformity of the elbow, restriction of forearm rotation and pain with activity (Bhaskar 2009). With all ulna fractures, the position of the radial head should be confirmed. Surgical reduction of a displaced ulna fracture is needed with which the radial head spontaneously reduces (Ring et al. 1998).

Articular Fractures

If the fracture extends into a joint surface, it is classified as an articular fracture. Two descriptions are used: 'complete' and 'partial'. In a complete articular fracture, the joint line is completely separated. These injuries can also be considered fracture dislocations. In partial articular fractures, also described as intra-articular, part of the joint is separated. The significance of these injuries is that there is usually residual joint stiffness and they can predispose to early osteoarthritis.

Main Principles of Fracture Treatment

The priorities of initial fracture management are to ensure that the neurovascular status of the limb is healthy and that there are no indications of compartment syndrome (Wright 2008a), relieve pain and support the injured limb. The aim of secondary management is to ensure the bone ends are in continuity so that healing can occur without residual deformity and the limb is restored to full normal function. Fractures can be treated conservatively using casts, splintage or traction. If the fracture is displaced, then surgical correction is required; this ranges from manipulation under anaesthetic to open reduction with either internal or external fixation (refer to Chapters 8 and 17).

Casting

Casts made of plaster of Paris (POP) or resin can be used to support and align fractured limbs. PoP casts are easier to mould by the clinician but are heavier and take longer to dry. Resin casts dry within 30 minutes, are available in different colours and are lightweight.

The purpose of casting is:

- to maintain bone alignment for fracture healing
- to maintain surgical correction until healed
- to promote pain relief by resting the affected limb or joint
- to correct deformities by wedging or serial casting.

Casts should always be applied by a suitably qualified practitioner.

There are three layers:

- stockinette to protect the skin
- wool to add padding and further protection
- the casting material.

Each layer should be applied smoothly, to avoid creasing, which may cause pressure sores, and snugly, to support and mould the cast to the limb (Wright 2008b).

After application the plaster will feel warm due to chemical reaction. The wet cast should be handled by the palm of the hand to avoid cast denting, which may cause pressure. The cast should be allowed to dry naturally. Casts can conduct heat and resting a casted limb on a radiator or using a hair drier may cause a burn. The affected limb should be elevated to reduce swelling so the limb should be rested/elevated on pillows covered with a towel to absorb the moisture from the cast. Children in large body casts should be turned 2-hourly to facilitate drying of the cast. The practitioner should observe the cast for dents, cracks or skin rubbing and assess the patient for complaints of pain or discomfort. If any of these are noted, then medical staff should be informed. It may be necessary to modify or remove the cast (Wright 2008b). See Chapter 8 for further information.

When discharged the child and family should be advised to keep the cast dry. It should not be covered with plastic for showering or bathing as steam condenses on the inside of plastic bags and will make the cast wet. The best advice is to cover the cast with a towel to absorb water splashes. Nothing should be put down the cast because of the risk of developing pressure ulcers and nothing should be used to scratch under the cast as the skin may be lacerated and there is a risk of subsequent infection. The family should be advised to avoid beaches and sandpits to prevent sand getting inside the cast as this can rub the skin and cause excoriation (Wright 2007a).

The patient should be advised to observe for the following and to seek medical assistance should any of the following signs and symptoms occur (Lucas and Davis 2005):

- the toes or fingers become blue, swollen and painful to move
- the limb becomes more painful
- pins and needles or numbness are felt in the digits
- if the cast feels uncomfortable or is rubbing
- if an unpleasant smell is noticed from the cast and/or a discharge is seen on the cast.

Orthotic Splints

Orthotic splints are used in the management of fractures to immobilise and rest a limb. They are particularly useful when a child has underlying pathology and traditional treatment such as casting may do more harm than good. Orthotic splints are either dynamic or fixed. A fixed splint is rigid and will support and control the limb and/or correct deformity (Wright 2012), for example removable wrist splints used in the management of buckle fractures (Wright 2011). Dynamic splints support the limb but allow for a controlled range of movement that can help soft tissue development and healing (Wright 2012). The IROM (immobilise range of movement) brace is an example of a dynamic splint; following patellar dislocation it is used to allow controlled knee flexion.

Traction

Traction is a pulling force that is applied to an injured limb using weights and pulleys. This is considered in more detail in Chapter 8 but is considered briefly here for the sake of the completeness of this chapter. It has been used as an orthopaedic treatment since Egyptian times, but is still a valid current treatment option (Choudhry et al. 2020). Traction is applied superficially to the limb, with the force being indirectly exerted on the underlying structures:

- In fixed traction the traction force is exerted against a fixed point (e.g. Thomas splint traction).
- In balanced traction the traction pull is exerted against an opposing force, usually provided by the weight of the body when the foot of the bed is raised.

There are three types of traction: skin, skeletal and manual.

- In skin traction the traction apparatus is applied directly to the patient's skin.

Table 24.1 Traction type and injury

Traction type	Injury
Bucks or Pughs	Hip injury or infection
Gallows	Fractured femur under 2 years of age pre-hip surgery
Halter neck	Torticollis
Dunlop	Supracondylar fracture of humerus (rarely used now)
Thomas splint	Fractured femur over 2 years of age
Tibial (Denham or Steinmann pin)	Fractured femur – adolescent (rarely used now)
Skull/halo	Spinal injuries and deformities (rarely used now)

- In skeletal traction the traction pull is exerted via pins, screws, wires or tongs that have been surgically applied to the skeleton (e.g. Steinman pin through the tibia).
- Manual traction is applied by a person pulling on the affected limb, used during traction application and fracture manipulation.

Traction is used in fracture treatment to restore and maintain fracture alignment and to assist with pain relief by controlling muscle spasm. Different types of traction are used according to the injury (Table 24.1) and are described in more detail in Chapter 8.

Surgical Management

Surgical management falls into four categories:

- closed reduction
- closed reduction with surgical pinning
- open reduction with or without internal fixation
- external fixation.

Closed reduction is achieved by manipulating the fracture while the patient is anaesthetised. With general anaesthetic the muscles are relaxed and the patient is unaware of pain allowing the surgeon to manipulate the fracture ends back to anatomical position. This is used when the fracture is minimally displaced. First manual traction is applied, pulling the limb distally. This corrects limb shortening and often, because the muscles are relaxed from the general anaesthetic, this may be enough to correct the bone alignment. The next step is to push or angulate the bone ends until reduction is achieved. Alignment is radiologically confirmed in theatre and a cast is applied. There has been a recent change of practice with a move towards manipulating distal radial fractures in the emergency department with the use of Entonox and supportive analgesia (Kurien et al. 2016), avoiding the stress and inconvenience of a hospital admission as well as being more cost-effective and efficient.

If the fracture position slips, with intraoperative closed reduction percutaneous Kirschner wires (K wires) are inserted across the fracture site. After confirmation of alignment by X-ray a back slab cast is applied. The K wires loosen in the bone over the next few weeks and are normally removed 4–6 weeks after insertion. There is a best practice debate about whether the K wires should be removed in the outpatient clinic or as a day-case procedure under general anaesthesia. Removing the K wires in a clinic takes a few seconds and is slightly uncomfortable, although the sight of the pliers used to remove the wires can be frightening. To have the wires removed in theatre means having to fast the child and it carries the risks of general anaesthesia. The practitioner should discuss this with the child and family. Generally, if the child is under 8 years of age the K wires should be removed under general anaesthesia and in the clinic if older.

Open Reduction and Internal Fixation

Open reduction is used if satisfactory fracture reduction has not been achieved with closed reduction or the best way to achieve fracture alignment is to expose the fracture to allow reduction under direct vision with or without internal fixation. If the injury is an open fracture, then the site is already exposed and further surgical opening may be needed to fully debride the wound and apply the necessary internal fixation. With open fractures there is the added complication of poor skin integrity. It may not be possible to surgically close the wound and plastic surgery may be needed. Internal fixation secures the anatomical alignment and is beneficial for complex injuries such as intra-articular or fracture dislocation.

A variety of devices can be used for internal fixation: screws, plates, wires, nails and tension sutures. A recent development is absorbable screws and sutures (Yuxi et al. 2019), which avoid the possibility of the child needing to undergo further surgery for removal of metalwork. Internal fixation may be beneficial in major trauma, stabilising the limb injuries and allowing focus on more life-threatening aspects of the patient's care. It also allows for early mobilisation. This may be particularly beneficial to a child with special needs. To internally fix a fracture the surgery is more invasive, with the possibility of infection, and the child will be under general anaesthesia for longer.

External Fixation

External fixation is particularly useful when managing open and/or comminuted fractures. Pins are inserted percutaneously into the bone above and below the fracture site. The pins are then attached to a rigid external frame and the fracture ends can be brought into alignment by manipulation of the frame. When there is severe soft tissue damage, the external fixator allows the fracture to be stabilised whilst the skin can be accessed for wound management. External circular frames such as the Ilizarov and Taylor spatial frame use wires that are thinner than pins and can be placed in individual bone fragments for comminuted fractures. External fixators are visible, there is a risk of pin site infection and the patient needs to be involved in pin site care (see Chapter 8 for further detail).

Factors Complicating Healing

Infection can delay fracture healing. The more interventional the management strategy employed to stabilise the fracture, the greater the risk of infection. Sometimes there is delayed healing that proceeds to non-union. Non-union in otherwise healthy children is rare but can happen if fibrous tissue is within the fracture. Smoking and poor diet can contribute to delayed or non-union. It is known that certain fractures, of the scaphoid for instance, are at risk of non-union due to poor vasculature of the scaphoid bone. Mal union occurs when the fracture ends have united in a suboptimal anatomical position. It is unusual in children and the management depends on the presenting clinical deformity and effect on function.

Further Reading

Benson, M.K.D. (2010). *Children's Orthopaedics and Fractures*, 3rde. London: Churchill Livingstone.

Rang, M., Pring, M., and Wenger, D. (2005). *Rang's Children's Fractures*, 3rde. Philadelphia: Lippincott Williams and Wilkins.

Royal College of Nursing (2021). *RCN Traction: Principles and Application*. London: Royal College of Nursing.

Valerio, G., Gallè, F., Mancusi, C. et al. (2010). Pattern of fractures across pediatric age groups: analysis of individual and lifestyle factors. *BioMedCentral Public Health* 10: 656. http://www.biomedcentral.com/1471-2458/10/656. (accessed 20 March 2013).

References

Aleman, K.B. and Meyers, M.C. (2010). Mountain biking injuries in children and adolescents. *Sports Med.* 40 (1): 77–90.

Babb, A. and Carlson, W.O. (2005). Monteggia fractures: beware! *South Dakota J. Med.* 58 (7): 283–285.

Belthur, M.V., Birchansky, S.B., Verdugo, A.A. et al. (2012). Pathologic fractures in children with acute staphylococcus aureus osteomyelitis. *J. Bone Joint Surg. Am.* 94 (1): 34–42.

Beutel, B.G. (2012). Monteggia fractures in pediatric and adult populations. *Orthopedics* 35 (2): 138–144. https://doi.org/10.3928/01477447-20120123-32.

Bhaskar, A. (2009). Missed Monteggia fracture in children: is annular ligament reconstruction always required? *Indian J. Orthopaedics* 43 (4): 389–395.

Bhatti, A.N., Griffin, S.J., and Wenham, S.J. (2012). Deceptive appearance of a normal variant of scaphoid bone in a teenage patient: a diagnostic challenge. *Orthopedic Rev. (Pavia)* 4 (1): e6. Epub 2 February 2012.

Blatz, A.M., Gillespie, C.W., Katcher, A. et al. (2019). Factors associated with nonaccidental trauma evaluation among patients below 36 months old presenting with femur fractures at a level-1 pediatric trauma center. *J. Pediatr. Orthopaedis* 39 (4): 175–180.

Choudhry, B., Leung, B., Filips, E. et al. (2020). Keeping the traction on in orthopaedics. *Cureus* 12 (8): e10034. https://doi.org/10.7759/cureus.10034.

Clarke, N.M., Shelton, F.R., Taylor, C.C. et al. (2012). The incidence of fractures in children under the age of 24 months in relation to non-accidental injury. *Injury* 43 (6): 762–765. Epub 19 September 2011.

Cole, W. (2002). Bone, cartilage and fibrous tissue disorders. In: *Children's Orthopaedics and Fractures*, 2nde (ed. M. Benson, J. Fixen, M. Macnicol and K. Parsch), 67–92. London: Churchill Livingstone.

van Dijk, F.S., Cobben, J.M., Kariminejad, A. et al. (2011). Osteogenesis imperfecta: a review with clinical examples. *Mol. Syndromol.* 1: 1–20. Epub October 2011.

Doong, J.L. and Lai, C.H. (2012). Risk factors for child and adolescent occupants, bicyclists, and pedestrians in motorized vehicle collisions. *Traffic Inj. Prev.* 13 (3): 249–257.

Dunbar, G. (2012). The relative risk of nearside accidents is high for the youngest and oldest pedestrians. *Accid. Anal. Prev.* 5: 517–521. Epub 25 September 2011.

Eastley, N., Singh, H., Dias, J.J., and Taub, N. (2012). Union rates after proximal scaphoid fractures; meta-analyses and review of available evidence. *J. Hand Surg. (European Volume)*. Epub 26 June 2012.

Forlino, A., Cabral, W.A., Barnes, A.M., and Marini, J.C. (2011). New perspectives on osteogenesis imperfecta. *Nat. Rev. Endocrinol.* 9: 540–557. https://doi.org/10.1038/nrendo.2011.81.

Gaston, M.S., Irwin, G.J., and Huntley, J.S. (2012). Lateral condyle fracture of a child's humerus: the radiographic features may be subtle. *Scottish Med. J.* 57 (3): 182.

Gilbert, R., Fluke, J., O'Donnell, M. et al. (2012). Child maltreatment: variation in trends and policies in six developed countries. *Lancet* 379 (9817): 758–772. Epub 9 December 2011.

Gniatkowska-Nowakowska, A. (2010). Fractures in epilepsy children. *Seizure* 19 (6): 324–325. Epub 20 May 2010.

Holroyd, C.R., Davies, J.H., Taylor, P. et al. (2010). Reduced cortical bone density with normal trabecular bone density in girls with turner syndrome. *Osteoporosis Int.* 21 (12): 2093–2099. Epub 5 February 2010.

Howard, A.W., Macarthur, C., Rothman, L. et al. (2009). School playground surfacing and arm fractures in children: a cluster randomized trial comparing sand to wood chip surfaces. *PLoS Med.* 6 (12): e1000195. Epub 15 December 2009.

Hyman, J.E., Gaffney, J.T., Epps, H.R., and Matsumoto, H. (2011). Impact of fractures on school attendance. *J. Pediatr. Orthopaedics* 31 (2): 113–116.

Jones, I.E., Williams, S.M., Dow, N., and Goelding, A. (2002). How many children remain fracture free during growth? A longitundinal study of children and adolescents participating in the Dunedin multidisciplinary health and development study. *Osteoporosis Int.* 13: 990–995.

Kosuge, D. and Barry, M. (2015). Changing trends in the management of children's fractures. *Bone Joint J.* 97-B: 4. Instructional review: Free Access Published Online: 1 Apr 2015. https://doi.org/10.1302/0301-620X.97B4.34723.

Kurien, T., Price, K.R., Pearson, R.G. et al. (2016). Manipulation and reduction of paediatric fractures of the distal radius and forearm using intranasal diamorphine and 50% oxygen and nitrous oxide in the emergency department a 2.5-year study. *Bone Joint J.* 98-B: 1.

Lucus, B. and Davis, P. (2005). Why restricting movement is important. In: *Orthopaedic and Trauma Nursing* (ed. J. Kneale and P. Davis), 105–139. London: Churchill Livingstone.

Lustenberger, T., Talving, P., Barmparas, G. et al. (2010). Skateboard-related injuries: not to be taken lightly. A National Trauma Databank analysis. *J. Traum. Stress* 69 (4): 924–927.

Majori, S., Ricci, G., Capretta, F. et al. (2009). Epidemiology of domestic injuries. A survey in an emergency department in North-East Italy. *J. Prevent. Med. Hygiene* 50 (3): 164–169.

Marcheix, P.S., Vacquerie, V., Longis, B. et al. (2011). Distal humerus lateral condyle fracture in children: when is the conservative treatment a valid option? *Orthopaedics Traumatol. Surg. Res.* 97 (3): 304–307. Epub 7 April 2011.

Marreiros, H., Monteiro, L., Loff, C., and Calado, E. (2010). Fractures in children and adolescents with spina bifida: the experience of a Portuguese tertiary-care hospital. *Dev. Med. Child Neurol.* 52 (8): 754–759. Epub 19 March 2010.

Mathison, D.J. and Agrawal, D. (2010). An update on the epidemiology of pediatric fractures. *Pediatr. Emerg. Care* 26 (8): 594–603; quiz 604–606.

Milczarek, O., Kuzaj, J., Stanuszek, A. et al. (2021). Characteristics of injuries sustained under the influence of alcohol in a group of adolescents. Is it possible to establish a typical clinical picture of an underage patient who suffered from an injury under the influence of alcohol? *Pediatr. Emergency Care*. Published ahead of print issue. https://doi.org/10.1097/PEC.0000000000002386.

Müller, M.E., Nazarian, S. and Koch, P. (1990) The Comprehensive Classification of Fractures of Long Bones. Springer-Verlag, Berlin.

Mullis, B.H., Gudeman, A.S., Borrelli, J. Jr. et al. (2021). Bone healing: advances in biology and technology. *Orthopaedic Trauma Assoc. Int.* e100. http://dx.doi.org/10.1097/OI9.0000000000000100.

Orton, E., Kendrick, D., West, J., and Tata, L.J. (2012). Independent risk factors for injury in pre-school children: three population-based nested case-control studies using routine primary care data. *PLoS One* 7 (4): e35193. Epub 5 April 2012. http://injuryprevention.bmj.com/content/18/Suppl_1/A231.3.abstract. (accessed 8 April 2014).

Pandya, N.K., Baldwin, K., Kamath, A.F. et al. (2011). Unexplained fractures: child abuse or bone disease? A systematic review. *Clin. Orthopaedics Relat. Res.* 469 (3): 805–812.

Ring, D., Jupiter, J.B., and Waters, P.M. (1998). Monteggia fractures in children and adults. *J. Am. Acad. Orthopaedic Surg.* 6 (4): 215–224.

Ruth, E., Shah, B., and Fales, W. (2009). Evaluating the injury incidence from skate shoes in the United States. *Pediatr. Emerg. Care* 25 (5): 321–324.

Saraph, V. and Linhart, W.E. (2005). Modern treatment of pathological fractures in children. *Injury* 36 (Suppl 1): A64–A74.

Schalamon, J., Dampf, S., Singer, G. et al. (2011). Evaluation of fractures in children and adolescents in a level I trauma center in Austria. *J. Trauma* 71 (2): E19–E25.

Sheng, B., Li, X., Nussler, A.K., and Sheng Zhu, S. (2021). The relationship between healthy lifestyles and bone health. A narrative review. *Medicine* 100: 8. http://dx.doi. org/10.1097/MD.0000000000024684.

Skellern, C.Y., Wood, D.O., Murphy, A., and Crawford, M. (2000). Non-accidental fractures in infants: risk of further abuse. *J. Paediatr. Child Health* 36 (6): 590–592.

Slongo, T.F. and Audigé, L. (2007). AO pediatric classification group. Fracture and dislocation classification compendium for children: the AO pediatric comprehensive classification of long bone fractures (PCCF). *J. Orthopaedic Trauma* 21 (10 Suppl): S135–S160.

Storm, S.W., Williams, D.P., Khoury, J., and Lubahn, J.D. (2006). Elbow deformities after fracture. *Hand Clinics* 22 (1): 121–129.

Valerio, G., Gallè, F., Mancusi, C. et al. (2010). Pattern of fractures across pediatric age groups: analysis of individual and lifestyle factors. *BioMedCentral Publ. Health* 10: 656. http://www.biomedcentral.com/1471-2458/10/656 (accessed 20 March 2013).

Wagner, R., Gosemann, J.H., Sorge, I. et al. (2019). Smartphone-related accidents in children and adolescents a novel mechanism of injury. *Pediatr. Emerg. Care* Publish ahead of print issue. https://doi.org/10.1097/PEC.0000000000001781.

Wang, Q., Wang, X.F., Iuliano-Burns, S. et al. (2010). Rapid growth produces transient cortical weakness: a risk factor for metaphyseal fractures during puberty. *J. Bone Miner. Res.* 25 (7): 1521–1526.

Wright, E. (2007a). Care of Child in a plaster. In: *Oxford Handbook of Children's and Young People's Nursing* (ed. E.A. Glasper, G. McEwing and J. Richards), 510. Oxford: Oxford University Press.

Wright, E. (2007b). Evaluating a paediatric assessment tool. *J. Orthopaedic Nurs.* 11: 20–29.

Wright, E. (2008a). Neurovascular impairment and compartment syndrome: a literature review. *J. Childrens Young Peoples Nurs.* 2 (3): 126–130.

Wright, E. (2008b). Application of plaster and observation for neurovascular deficit. In: *Clinical Skills in Child Health Practice* (ed. J. Kelsey and G. McEwing), 374–378. Churchill Livingstone Elsevier: Edinburgh.

Wright, E. (2011). Treating children's buckle fractures with removable splints. *Nurs. Children Young People* 23 (10): 14–17.

Wright, E. (2012). Musculoskeletal system – splints. In: *Oxford Handbook of Clinical Skills for Children's and Young People's Nursing* (ed. P. Dawson, L. Cook, L.J. Holliday and H. Reddy), 486–489. Oxford: Oxford University Press.

Yin, Z.G., Zhang, J.B., Kan, S.L., and Wang, X.G. (2012). Diagnostic accuracy of imaging modalities for suspected scaphoid fractures: meta-analysis combined with latent class analysis. *J. Bone Joint Surg. (Britain)* 94 (8): 1077–1085.

Yuxi, S., Kai, C., and Jiaqiang, Q. (2019). Retrospective study of open reduction and internal fixation of lateral humeral condyle fractures with absorbable screws and absorbable sutures in children. *Your Journals@OvidMedicine* 98 (44): e17850. AN: 00005792-201911010-00136.

25

Key Fractures Relating to the Infant, Child and Young Person

Thelma Begley[1] and Sonya Clarke[2]

[1] *School of Nursing and Midwifery, University of Dublin Trinity College, Dublin, Ireland*
[2] *Queen's University Belfast, Belfast, UK*

Introduction

Fractures are considered a normal part of an active upbringing (Randsborg 2013; Kitabjian and Ladores 2020), with fractures accounting for up to 25% of all childhood injuries (Rennie et al. 2007). The aim of this chapter is to provide evidence-based guidance for the most common fractures in children and adolescents, the mechanism of injury and the typical management and treatment. As children grow they become more involved in sport, have further freedom and the incidence of fracture increases (Randsborg 2013). A child's musculoskeletal system and the biomechanical composition of children's bones are different to adults, affecting how children's fractures occur and are managed. Differences reduce as a child grows, especially as they reach adolescence (Hart et al. 2006a). Fractures in children tend to heal much more rapidly than in adults as their growth plates/physis are open. This results in shorter periods of immobility and less stiffness. Mal-union and non-union occur rarely as children also have great potential for remodelling and reshaping of bone after a fracture heals (Berg 2005; Randsborg 2013).

The factors that need to be considered when assessing children with fractures include:

- age of the child
- mechanism of injury
- location of fracture
- any potential complications
- possibility of physeal injury
- continuing bone growth
- the possibility of non-accidental injury.

The inclusion of the family in the child's care and awareness of family circumstances also need to be considered.

Physeal Injuries

Physeal (growth plate) injuries are common in children (Jung et al. 2021), with children at risk of them until bone growth is complete. In boys this is age 18 years approximately and for girls it is 2 years after the beginning of puberty (Lipp 1998). Physeal fractures represent between 15% and 18% of all children's fractures (Cepela et al. 2016; Brighton and Vitale 2020). These injuries are common during periods of active growth and more common in boys due to their sporting activities. Injury to the upper limb is more prevalent, with the distal radius most affected (Lipp 1998; Jung et al. 2021) and the distal tibia the second most common area affected (Jung et al. 2021). See Figures 25.1 and 25.2 for examples of growth plate injuries.

The signs of physeal injury are similar to those of a fracture: predominantly pain and swelling located at the ends of bones (Lipp 1998). Diagnosis of the injury is usually by X-ray. Any child presenting with signs and symptoms should be thoroughly assessed as an initial displacement of the epiphysis may occur before returning to a normal position and result in a shearing injury (Lipp 1998). Any injury that involves the physis should be referred to a specialist orthopaedic surgeon for definitive treatment and follow-up as physeal injuries may cause a growth arrest and/or deformity (Cepela et al. 2016). The history of how the injury happened (mechanism) is an essential element of the diagnosis. Injuries are commonly classified using the Salter Harris classification system, which is based on anatomy, pattern of fracture and prognosis (Salter and Harris 1963) (Box 25.1).

Management of the injury and length of immobilisation will depend on the location and extent of injury:

Orthopaedic and Trauma Nursing: An Evidence-based Approach to Musculoskeletal Care, Second Edition. Edited by Sonya Clarke and Mary Drozd.
© 2023 John Wiley & Sons Ltd. Published 2023 by John Wiley & Sons Ltd.

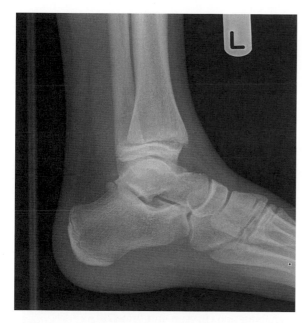

Figure 25.1 Salter Harris type 1 displaced fracture through the inferior tibial growth plate in a 10-year-old girl.

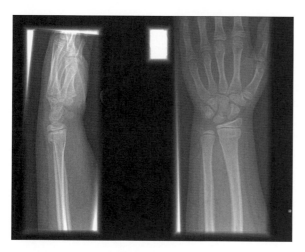

Figure 25.2 Fracture of distal radius Salter Harris type II fracture with slight displacement.

- Salter Harris type I and II are managed by closed reduction and application of a cast.
- Salter Harris type III and IV may require open reduction and internal fixation, and application of a cast (Omeroglu 2018).

A return to mobilisation with full range of motion is the priority following removal of the cast, and may take up to 4 weeks. Disturbance of growth may be associated with this injury but is dependent on the bones involved, the extent of the injury and the age at which injury occurs along with the amount of expected remaining growth (Lipp 1998). Salter Harris type II injuries are the most common type,

> **Box 25.1 Salter Harris Classification of Physeal Injuries**
>
> Salter Harris I: The fracture is across the physis and through the weak zones of growth cartilage.
>
> Salter Harris II: Fractures extend from the physis into the metaphysis.
>
> Salter Harris III: Fracture involves the physis and extends into the epiphysis.
>
> Salter Harris IV: Fractures include the physis and extend into both the epiphysis and metaphysis. There is a great potential for growth disruption with this injury.
>
> Salter Harris V: Fracture represents a crush to the growth plate and death of the reserve zone cells. It is difficult to identify on X-ray as the physis may appear normal or slightly narrowed so there is risk of delayed diagnosis and potential risk for growth disturbance or deformity.

accounting for 74% of physeal injuries, type III and IV are less common but are associated with great risk of complications (Cepela et al. 2016). Complications are uncommon if injuries are managed effectively (Pring and Wenger 2005).

Upper Limb Injuries

Clavicle Fractures

Clavicle (collar bone) fractures are common in children (see Figure 25.3), often accounting for 10–15% of all fractures in children (Bryson and Price 2016) with most occurring due to a fall or trauma directly to the bone. Most clavicle fractures (80–90%) occur in the middle third of the bone (Bryson and Price 2016; Hart et al. 2006b), with some fractures incomplete due to the strong periosteum of the clavicle (Shannon et al. 2009).

Signs of a clavicle fracture are:

- tenderness directly over the fracture site
- bruising

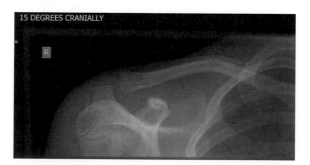

Figure 25.3 Fracture of the mid clavicle with slight angulation in a 2-year-old. The shoulder joint is normal.

- swelling
- crepitus that is easy to palpate as the bone is near the skin surface
- restriction of movement
- holding the arm close to the body and supporting it with the opposite hand.

Neonatal fractures are usually caused by birth trauma, especially in infants with a birth weight greater than 4 kg and following a difficult delivery (Pring and Wenger 2005). Neonatal fractures may be associated with brachial plexus palsy and will require further evaluation (Dunham 2003; Pring and Wenger 2005) as infants may present with a lack of spontaneous movement. Neonatal clavicle fractures usually heal spontaneously and successfully, with the infant starting to move the arm in 2–3 weeks.

With this fracture, neurovascular observation should be performed on the distal extremities to include pulses, motor function, sensation and reflexes (Shannon et al. 2009). A simple sling is recommended for 2–3 weeks until the child is comfortable. Pinning the sleeve to the body or wrapping the arm to the body with bandage may be useful for infants (Pring and Wenger 2005) as it may be difficult to restrict movement in this age group. While most fractures heal uneventfully with the use of a simple sling, some angulation and deformity may occur. Fractures may heal with a visible and palpable bump obvious at the fracture site due to increased callus formation. The child will require follow-up X-rays in 4–6 weeks and contact sports should be avoided for another 2–3 weeks after that (Hart et al. 2006b).

Surgery is rarely indicated but considered if the fracture is open, skin integrity is compromised, the fracture is complicated or comminuted and where there is neurovascular injury (Moonot and Ashwood 2009; O'Neill et al. 2011). Complications from clavicle fractures in children are rare.

Humeral Shaft Fractures

Fractures of the humeral shaft are very rare in children and account for less than 5% of all children's fractures (Bryson and Price 2016; Marengo et al. 2016; Pogorelic et al. 2017). While fractures in neonates are associated with birth trauma, in older infants and toddlers the presence of a fracture in the humeral shaft in a child should raise suspicions that the injury may have occurred from a non-accidental injury (NAI). This is particularly true of spiral fractures of the humeral shaft in infants not yet walking or climbing. Treatment of fractures in infants is usually conservative by immobilising the area in a collar and cuff for approximately 2 weeks. Placing the arm under clothes assists with the immobilisation. From toddlers to adolescents, treatment is

with collar and cuff also, using gravity to apply traction at the site of the fracture. A hanging cast could also be used to achieve the same aim. The treatment duration is determined by the size of the child, their age, how stable the fracture is and how quickly callus develops (Bryson and Price 2016). Problems with nerves can occur with this fracture, so observation of the neurovascular status of the limb is vital. Jerome and Prabu (2021) in a retrospective study of 350 children in one Indian service with humeral shaft fractures found 12 children who had median nerve palsy between 2012 and 2015. Indications of this were absence of thumb flexion, abduction, index finger flexion and sensory loss in the thumb, middle and radial side of the ring finger. Operative treatment, using an intramedullary nail or plate, is indicated when complications are present, namely, open fractures, neurovascular complications, pathological fractures or where there is more than one injury to the child and surgical fixation of the humerus will hasten the child's overall rehabilitation (Bryson and Price 2016).

Elbow Fractures

Elbow fractures are common in children, usually following a fall on an outstretched hand (FOOSH) with elbow in full extension (Siddiq et al. 2020). Care needs to be taken when interpreting X-rays of the elbow and using X-ray as a diagnostic tool; recognition is difficult as the bones of the elbow are poorly developed in childhood and ossify at different rates (Hart et al. 2006b). The location of nerves and vascular structures around the elbow plus the limited ability of the elbow to remodel post fracture means that elbow fractures are commonly subject to open or closed reduction.

The most common fracture in the elbow region in children is a supracondylar fracture of the humerus (Babel et al. 2010; Siddiq et al. 2020), with peak incidence between 5 and 8 years (Siddiq et al. 2020). It has the highest rate of complications of any fracture in children, with a neurological injury or deficit occurring in 20% of cases (Robertson et al. 2012) (Box 25.2).

The most common mechanism of injury is a FOOSH. During the fall the child's arm hyperextends and causes a fracture, with the distal fragment normally being displaced posteriorly (Hart et al. 2006b), which may affect both the vessels and nerves posterior to the fracture (Figures 25.4 and 25.5). Neurovascular assessment of the arm should involve a thorough evaluation of motor, sensory and vascular structures (Box 25.2). The brachial or radial pulse needs to be assessed to ensure that there is no vascular injury. A white or cool hand or absence of pulse usually indicates arterial compromise and need for urgent reduction. Owing to extensive swelling, the arm also needs to be assessed for compartment syndrome (Chapter 9) so neurovascular

Neurological status in paediatric upper limb injuries in the emergency department: current practice (Robertson et al. 2012)

Robertson et al. (2012) retrospectively reviewed the case notes of all children admitted to an emergency department (ED) with upper limb injuries over a 3-month period. Inclusion criteria were that the child had an upper limb injury that required admission and intervention from the orthopaedic team under general anaesthetic. One hundred and twenty-one patients were identified, 61 males and 60 females, and another six who were referred from an ED at another hospital. The age range was from 1 to 12 years. The most common injury was a fractured radius and ulna (39.8%), with a fall the most common mechanism of injury (42.1%). Neurological status was documented in 107 cases (88.4%) using the terms 'NVI', 'CSM', 'sensation' and 'moving'. There was no mention of particular nerves being examined in 114 cases and the anterior interosseous nerve was never mentioned.

In the 3 months, 10 patients had neurological deficits (8.2%), with supracondylar fracture involved in 40% of these. None of these deficits was identified on initial examination in the ED. The authors acknowledge that while some of these may have occurred after ED assessment, this is unclear due to the lack of documentation.

Discussion

Over 90% of patients had no documentation of neurological examination. There were no records of which nerves were assessed or what tests had been performed to assess neurovascular status. This included those who had confirmed neurological injury. The authors concluded that this area of practice was deficient and that there should be documentary evidence that the radial, median, ulnar nerve and anterior interosseous nerve had all been assessed in the ED. Neurovascular assessment of all limb injuries should be standard practice.

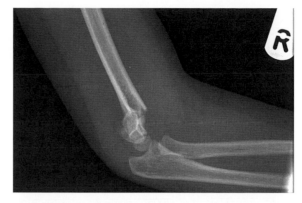

Figure 25.4   Supracondylar fracture of the distal right humerus with significant dorsal angulation of the distal humerus in an 8-year-old.

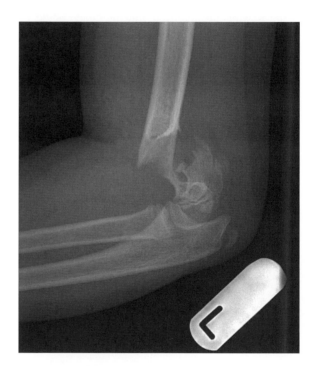

Figure 25.5   Supracondylar fracture of the distal left humerus with gross deformity, displacement and swelling in a 9-year-old.

assessment must be performed regularly and documented accurately (Box 25.2). The fractured bone may also cause puckering of the skin (Platt 2004) with an urgent need for reduction to prevent the overlying skin becoming ischaemic and necrotic. Neurovascular assessment can be difficult as there will be significant swelling and pain, with the child experiencing considerable fear and anxiety. Gaining their cooperation is essential but often difficult because of

the challenges associated with a child's level of understanding and compliance (Robertson et al. 2012). Neurovascular observations are also necessary pre- and post-surgery/treatment alongside elevation of the arm with fingers above the elbow recommended. The anatomy of this region is complex, leading to high complication rates. Damage to the brachial artery, median nerve and/or ulnar nerve may be possible. A complication associated with the fracture is Volkman's ischaemic contracture, a permanent flexion contracture.

The classification that is most widely used based on displacement is Gartland's classification (Gartland 1959)

(Box 25.3). Treatment depends on the grade of fracture. Type 1 is usually placed in an above-elbow cast or sling for 3–4 weeks with the elbow held in 90° of flexion unless swelling impedes this (Hart et al. 2006b). Type 2 and 3 fractures may require surgical intervention with closed or open reduction with pins or Kirschner (K) wires to hold the position after reduction (Bryson and Price 2016). Three weeks after surgery the K wires are removed and the child should be allowed to resume most activities. Children will continue to be monitored for another 2–3 months. If reduction cannot be achieved with closed reduction, open reduction is necessary.

Forearm Fractures

Forearm fractures, particularly radial fractures (Figures 25.6 and 25.7), are common at any age (Schneider et al. 2007; Rimbaldo et al. 2021) but this is an expected fracture in older children with the usual mechanism of injury a

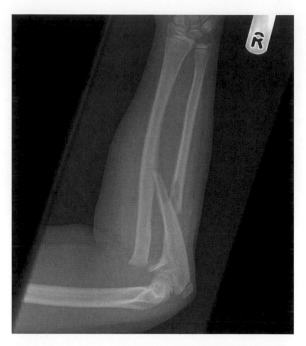

Figure 25.7   Distal radius and ulna buckle fracture without significant deformity and displacement.

FOOSH (Bryson and Price 2016). Increased engagement in sporting activities has increased the incidence of radial fractures (Khosla et al. 2003) and de Putter et al. (2011) report that fractures in the 5–9-years age group are mainly caused by accidents in the home. Those older than 9 years primarily fracture their forearm during sporting activity. Radial fractures can be classified as 'plastic deformation' (bowing), 'buckle' (torus) (Figure 25.7), greenstick, transverse, comminuted or physeal (Hart et al. 2006b). Confirmation of fracture is made by antero-posterior (AP) and lateral X-rays that will also confirm the type of fracture and the bones involved. It is essential in a midforearm fracture that both the wrist and elbow are X-rayed to assess for displacement at the joints above and below.

The management of the fracture will depend on the type and location. Traditionally, this has been managed non-operatively with closed reduction and immobilisation using casting and this continues to be the preferred method (Schneider et al. 2007; Omeroglu 2018; Poutoglidou et al. 2020; Rimbaldo et al. 2021). Simple stable fractures such as the 'buckle' are managed in a short-arm cast for 3–4 weeks, mainly for pain control. After the cast is removed normal activities can resume without restrictions and no review appointment. A splint is an alternative immobilisation option but keeping the splint in place in children can be difficult (Box 25.4).

A thorough examination of the arm must be carried out to identify if ulnar fractures are present as management changes, i.e. application of a long-arm cast and possibly a

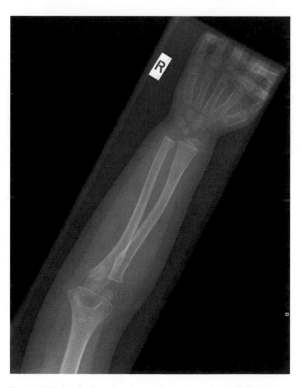

Figure 25.6   Deformity through the proximal radial metaphysis with gross displacement. Displaced and angulated fracture of the proximal ulna shaft.

Box 25.4   Evidence Digest

Cochrane Review: Interventions for treating wrist fractures in children

(Handoll et al. 2018)

This systematic review evaluated the effects of interventions for common distal radial fractures in children, including skeletally immature adults. The best-quality evidence for different treatments for wrist fractures in children was assessed. The Cochrane Bone, Joint and Muscle Trauma Group's Specialised Register, the Cochrane Central Register of Controlled Trials, MEDLINE, Embase, trial registries and associated reference lists were searched up to May 2018. Randomised controlled trials (RCTs) and quasi-RCTs comparing interventions for treating distal radius fractures in children were considered. Data on physical function, treatment failure, adverse events, time taken to return to normal activity, wrist pain and child and parent satisfaction were all assessed. At least two authors performed the study screening, selection, risk of bias assessment and data extraction independently. Data was pooled and GRADE was used to assess the quality of the evidence for each outcome.

Findings

Thirty studies were included, 21 RCTs and seven quasi RCTs. Two did not describe their randomisation method. The studies included 2930 children with reported a mean age of 8–10 years and mostly male children included.

Removable splints and below-elbow casts were compared for buckle fractures in six studies. Various findings were highlighted, including one study showing no difference between the two devices for physical functions at 4 weeks. There was little or no reapplication of either splints or casts needed and there were no refractures. Insufficient evidence was available on pain, time to return to normal activity, minor complications and child or parent satisfaction. Two studies found the splint to be more cost-effective.

Four studies compared a soft or elasticated bandage with a below-elbow cast for buckle fractures. The authors were uncertain regarding the level of disability 4 weeks after bandaging. Three studies reported that few children got their device changed or needed extended immobilisation. No serious adverse events were reported. Again, insufficient evidence was available on recovery time, wrist pain, minor complications and satisfaction. One study reported that children found a bandage more convenient.

Two studies on mainly buckle fractures compared cast removal at home by parents versus clinicians at the hospital fracture clinic. Parents reported greater satisfaction with removal of cast at home (one study) and associated lower healthcare costs for home removal. All children had recovered function at 4 weeks. No serious adverse events or treatment changes were reported. Data were not available on recovery time and number of children with minor complications. It was speculated in one study that there was no difference in pain at 4 weeks.

Four studies compared below-elbow casts and above-elbow cast immobilisation in usually displaced fractures. The results reported were not certain about the difference in children's dependence in below-elbow casts, physical function at 6 months (one study) and whether children in above-elbow casts needed another fracture reduction. No serious adverse events, recovery time or minor complications were reported. Pain at 1 week in below-elbow casts may be less (one study) and healthcare costs were lower for below-elbow casts.

Finally, five studies compared percutaneous wiring and above-elbow cast immobilisation versus above-elbow cast immobilisation alone after closed reduction of displaced fractures. Uncertain data were reported on whether surgery reduces the risk of treatment failure, manipulation for loss of position, fewer adverse events with surgery, recovery time, wrist pain and satisfaction. It is speculated that less physiotherapy is needed after surgery. One study from the USA found treatment costs were similar for both.

Summary

Despite 30 studies available on the management of forearm fractures, limited evidence supports any of the objectives outlined in the studies. The authors report that all of the studies had weaknesses that could affect the reliability of the results and the studies included were deemed to be of low quality, therefore the evidence as to the best way to treat different types of wrist fractures in children is inconclusive. However, findings that suggest a move away from casting in the treatment of wrist fractures are consistent.

longer period of immobilisation. The arm must also be assessed for other fractures caused by a FOOSH, such as a scaphoid or supracondylar fracture (Hart et al. 2006b). Injuries to the radial, median or ulnar nerve can also occur with this fracture. Increased swelling is also a feature, especially if the fracture is displaced, and compartment syndrome can be a complication. The fracture may heal with some displacement but there is no consensus in the literature on how much displacement is acceptable and can be left to normal remodelling (Schneider et al. 2007).

Hand and Finger Fractures

Hand fractures (Figure 25.8) are common in children and young people, with the fifth metacarpal and phalanges the most common bones affected. Treatment is by closed reduction with casting/splinting. It can be difficult to keep a splint on a young child with hand and finger fractures, but they usually heal quite quickly, with casts in place for 3–6 weeks depending on the injury (Hart et al. 2006b).

Different casts are applied depending on the area of the hand involved. Thumb fractures are treated by immobilisation in a thumb spica. Fractures of the index finger are often treated in a radial 'gutter' short-arm cast and those of the long, ring and little fingers with an ulnar gutter short-arm cast (Hart et al. 2006b). Finger fractures must also be assessed for physeal injuries.

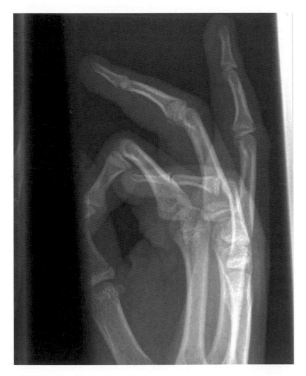

Figure 25.8 Fractures of the palmar aspects of the proximal ends of middle phalanges of the third and fourth fingers.

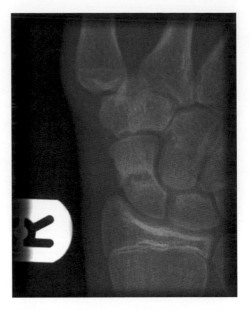

Figure 25.9 An ununited fracture of the mid scaphoid with no evidence of avascular necrosis following an injury 6 months earlier.

Fractures of the scaphoid bone are uncommon in young people (Karir et al. 2020), presenting in isolation or with other injuries of the hand (see Figure 25.9). Diagnosis is made on the basis of patient history, examination and clinical signs plus tenderness of the 'anatomical snuff box' and X-ray. Missed scaphoid fractures can lead to non-union and avascular necrosis, and internal fixation may be necessary to maintain blood supply to fragments if displaced (Karir et al. 2020).

Lower Extremity Fractures

Femoral Shaft Fractures

While fractures of the femoral shaft are less common in children than adults (see Figure 25.10), it is the most typical fracture requiring hospitalisation (Sigrist et al. 2018). Treatment of femoral shaft fractures depend on the site and extent of fracture, the age of the child, weight, socioeconomic and family factors and if open or closed reduction is required (Lindisfarne and Ayodele 2020). While there is no universal classification of femoral shaft fractures they are usually described in terms of open/closed, comminution, fracture pattern and location of fracture (Lindisfarne and Ayodele 2020). Standard treatment is based on age: infants are immobilised in a Pavlik harness (Chapter 23), younger children in traction (Chapter 8), Thomas splint (Chapter 8) or spica cast (Chapter 23), and adolescents are treated with internal fixation with an intramedullary nail. The length of hospitalisation may vary greatly depending on the method of treatment (Table 25.1).

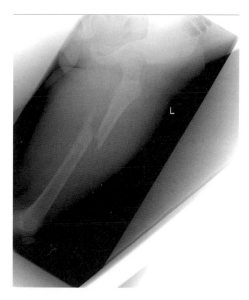

Figure 25.10 Oblique femoral mid-shaft fracture.

Table 25.1 Options for treatment of femoral shaft fractures (Lindisfarne and Ayodele 2020).

Age of child	Fracture pattern	Treatment choices
≤6 months	Shortening >1/2 cm, angulation >30°	Pavlik harness, early spica casting
7 months to 6 years	Shortening <2/3 cm	Early spica casting Traction- spica casting
	Shortening >2/3 cm Multiple or open fractures	(Intramedullary) nailing External fixation
>6–11 years	Transverse or oblique fracture	Traction – spica casting Flexible intramedullary nails
	Comminuted or spiral fracture or very proximal or distal fracture	Submuscular plate or external fixation
>11 years	Length stable Weight <100 lbs (<45 kgs)	Flexible IM nailing
	Length unstable Weight >100 lbs (>45 kgs)	Rigid IM nailing
	Length unstable Very proximal or distal fracture	Submuscular plate External fixation

While age-based algorithms are useful in suggesting treatment methods there are other factors to be considered. The ability to care for a child at home is an important consideration.

Traction still remains a viable option where other treatment options are not suitable. Anglen and Choi (2005) advocate that spica casting in children over 100 lbs (approximately 45 kg) may not be effective or safe and size, weight, activity level and family circumstances will also need to be considered.

Surgical treatment may be considered superior in older or larger children and adolescents. This is especially the case following multiple trauma and with soft tissue injury, obesity or head injury. Adolescents who have reached an acceptable size may be considered for rigid nailing and in younger children flexible nailing may be used (Anglen and Choi 2005). Flexible nailing is well suited to fractures of the central two-thirds of the diaphysis.

Fractures of the femur in children under 5 years usually have further investigation as NAI may be suspected (Anglen and Choi 2005; Pring et al. 2005). However, it must also be noted that this is not the cause in the majority of cases, with a fractured femur also occurring from minimal trauma during play in the young child (Pring et al. 2005). Therefore, this fracture type needs to be managed by experienced professionals in a non-judgmental manner (Chapter 23). Complications associated with fractures of the femur depend on the site of the fracture and the method of treatment. Attention is required in the management to ensure leg length is maintained (Pring et al. 2005), especially as the age of the child increases as there is less time for remodelling.

Tibial Fracture

Tibia fracture is also a common injury in children, with 50% of all tibial fractures occurring in the distal third (Setter and Palomino 2006). The mechanism of injury is usually direct or indirect force. Indirect force is mainly from sports, motor vehicle accidents and falls (Mubarak et al. 2009), with football, skiing and rugby all associated with this type of fracture (Rennie et al. 2007) (Figure 25.11 and Box 25.5).

Fractures of the tibia are usually oblique or spiral (see Figure 25.11), with the younger child requiring less force than in those who are older. Typically, a child with a tibial fracture will present with a history of a traumatic event (either witnessed or unwitnessed), pain, an inability to weight bear, swelling, bruising and deformity (Setter and Palomino 2006). Younger children, especially toddlers, may not have swelling and deformity. In 30% of tibial fractures, a fracture of the fibula will also be present (Hart et al. 2006c). AP and lateral X-ray views that include the knee and ankle are required to confirm the diagnosis.

Simple closed tibial fractures in children can be managed with closed reduction and immobilisation without a need for surgery (Hart et al. 2006c). Surgery may be required if the fracture is open, comminuted and/or irreducible or if casting has been unsuccessful. As always, understanding the

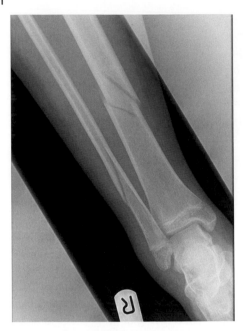

Figure 25.11 An oblique/spiral distal tibial and fibula fracture with minimal deformity.

Box 25.5   Evidence Digest: Buckle Fractures of the Proximal Tibia and Associated Trampoline Use

Saade-Lemus et al. (2019) conducted a retrospective review of charts from one service in Philadelphia from 2010 to 2016. Proximal tibial buckle fractures were found in 145 children. Fractures occurred at a median age of 34 months with 64% of fractures happening in girls.

Around 44% of fractures happened while the child was bouncing and 30% of injuries occurred from falls. In bouncing injuries, 90% of these occurred on a trampoline, 8% on an inflatable bouncer and 2% while jumping on the bed. In 80% of cases, there was more than one person bouncing at a time and 66% occurred when child was bouncing with a larger child and adult. Those injured while bouncing were significantly older compared to those that were injured by non-bouncing mechanisms.

Buckle fractures were associated with a younger age cohort. Concurrent fibula fracture and oblique fractures extending towards the physis were associated with older age. There were no associations identified between fracture patterns or age and gender or side of injury.

The authors concluded that trampoline use was the most common mechanism of injury and weight mismatch is known to cause problems. With the advent of an increased number of trampolines for recreational use, it is important for healthcare professionals to be aware of the patterns of fractures occurring from bouncing, and to be aware that those bouncing with older children and adults are more likely to suffer fractures, particularly of their proximal tibia.

---

mechanism of injury may help in the reduction of the fracture (Mubarak et al. 2009). The length of time in a cast following reduction will depend on type and location of fracture, the treatment and age of the child. The younger the child the less time they spend immobilised, ranging from 3 to 4 weeks for a toddler to 3 to 4 months for a young person/adolescent. A full- or half (short)-leg cast will be applied depending on the fracture location. Mubarak et al. (2009) recommends a long-leg cast to be applied for 4–6 weeks for both non-displaced metaphyseal and physeal fractures. However, a displaced metaphyseal fracture requires a closed or open reduction under general anaesthetic plus a cast for 6–8 weeks. For a displaced physeal fracture, suggested treatment is open reduction with internal fixation, which may need computerised tomography (CT) to help plan for surgery, and a long-leg cast for 4–6 weeks. Finally, extra-articular fractures (through a joint) involving the physis will require either a closed or an open reduction with internal fixation and long-leg cast.

Acute compartment syndrome (ACS) is also a complication of this fracture type. Careful observation of neurovascular status is required regardless of the method of treatment and immobilisation. An acceleration of pain is the predominant symptom of ACS, with presence especially on passive movement, which will require splitting of a cast or padding (Hart et al. 2006c) and a thorough evaluation of the leg, including possible measurement of intracompartmental pressure (Chapter 9). Early recognition of compartment syndrome generally leads to a favourable outcome for the child and the importance of regular neurovascular observations performed accurately cannot be over-emphasised. In fractures with physeal involvement long-term follow-up for evaluation of physeal closure should be advocated (Mubarak et al. 2009).

A 'toddler' fracture is an undisplaced tibial fracture in a child under 3 years of age (Alqarni and Goldman 2018). The child will present with guarding of the limb, a limp or an inability to weight bear (Hart et al. 2006c). Swelling and deformity may not be presenting symptoms. The mechanism of injury varies and occasionally the history is vague, with the injury not noticed until the child is limping. X-rays may be inconclusive, with no fracture visible and follow-up not necessary. It will also be necessary to rule out other causes of a limp such as irritable hip or Perthes disease. Usual management is application of a cast for comfort, with the child allowed to walk, and the site of the fracture determining what kind of cast is applied.

A Cozen's fracture is a fracture of the proximal metaphyseal tibia in children mainly between ages 3 and 6 years. A typical mechanism of injury is trampoline jumping, where often one child gets injured because there are several jumping (Mubarak et al. 2009). Treatment of a non-displaced fracture is with a long-leg cast for 6 weeks with the knee flexed to 10° and a varus mould (Setter and Palomino 2006). A displaced fracture will require reduction under general anaesthetic and a long-leg cast applied for 6–8 weeks. It is an uncommon fracture but clinically important as development of post-fracture progressive valgus deformity can occur. It is reported that this valgus deformity occurs in approximately 50% of fractures in this area (Setter and Palomino 2006). Treatment of valgus deformity in younger children is primarily conservative, monitoring the leg until after puberty as it is possible that some remodelling may take place. The importance of regular follow-up must be stressed to the family. Surgery may be considered if no significant improvement has taken place and the child has reached puberty.

Ankle Fractures

Ankle fractures are also common in children and most fractures happen in the distal third of the tibia and fibula (medial and lateral malleolus) as a result of twisting, falls and direct trauma between the ages of 10 and 15 years. The clinical signs are pain, swelling, deformity and difficulty/inability to weight bear. Initial treatment of ankle fractures is known by the acronym PRICE: protection, rest, ice, compression and elevation (Nicholas and Cooper 2009). Diagnosis is on the basis of both AP and lateral plain X-rays. It is also important to be aware that distal tibial fractures can involve the physis and this is the second most common site of Salter Harris injuries after the radius (Hart et al. 2006c). The grading of injury will affect how the child is managed: closed reduction to grades I and II and open reduction and stabilisation to grades III and IV. All fractures will require casting for 6–8 weeks (Figure 25.12). The majority of fractures in this area have a good prognosis but this depends on the severity of the injury, the skeletal age of the young person, the fracture type and the reduction achieved (Hart et al. 2006c).

Metatarsal Fractures

Fractures of the metatarsal are the most common fracture of the foot in children. See Figure 25.13 for an example. The first and fifth metatarsals are the usual sites. Mechanisms of injury include falling from a low height such as a bed or something heavy falling onto a foot. Physical examination reveals swelling, inability to weight bear, bruising or limp. Diagnosis is determined using anterolateral and oblique X-rays (Hart et al. 2006c), with conservative treatment with application of a short-leg walking cast for 3–4 weeks. Open, displaced or comminuted fractures will require further operative treatment.

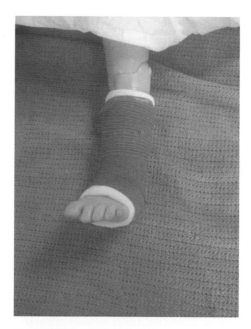

Figure 25.12   Below-knee cast.

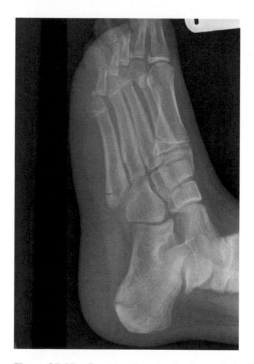

Figure 25.13   Fracture through the base of the fifth metatarsal.

Spinal Cord Injury

Chapter 20 of this book is dedicated to spinal cord injury (SCI). However, it is important to note that spinal injuries in children differ to those of adults in severity, injury patterns, clinical presentation, imaging and treatment (Basu 2012). Only 5% of spinal injuries occur in children (Basu 2012) but the severity is greater. In children under

5 years, the incidence of injury in males and females is equal. However, as they grow older the incidence in males far exceeds that in females. The pattern of injury is related to age and mechanism of injury (Basu 2012). The upper cervical area is injured more often in younger children, whereas the thoracolumbar injures are more common in older children (Puisto et al. 2009; Basu 2012). Worldwide, sports such as diving, soccer, rugby, horseback riding, skiing, wrestling, trampolining and cycling are common causes for spinal injuries. Motor vehicles are the greatest cause and result in more serious injury. Violence is reported as a common cause in adolescents, especially street violence (Mathison et al. 2008). Johnston et al. (2005) retrospectively reviewed the records from 1986 to 2003 of 190 children who had suffered SCI in Pennsylvania and found the most common causes were vehicular ($n = 105$), sports ($n = 25$), gunshot wound ($n = 26$), medical ($n = 16$) and other ($n = 18$). Other reasons included falls, direct trauma to the spine, roller coaster accidents and birth injury.

The diagnosis of SCI in children is comparatively difficult as it is not always obvious on X-rays (Mathison et al. 2008) and many children present with spinal cord injury without radiographic abnormality (SCIWORA). This definition was proposed initially in 1982 (Pang and Wilberger 1982) using plain X-rays but the advent of MRI has advanced the diagnosis of SCIWORA and it is estimated that 30–40% of children with traumatic spinal injury have such a condition (Li et al. 2011). Laxity and elasticity of ligaments in children means that the vertebral column can stretch without disruption (Rush et al. 2013), but the spinal cord can only stretch minimally and so becomes damaged. As children grow this laxity decreases so SCIWORA is most common in children under 8 years of age (Rush et al. 2013). Damage to the spinal cord can be complete or incomplete, with the younger child more at risk of complete injury (Mathison et al. 2008).

Assessment of the child with a spinal injury consists of history, physical examination, X-rays, CT and MRI. While MRI is considered to most advantageous for assessment of spinal injuries, in some children the MRI will be normal in the presence of a spinal injury (Basu 2012). SCIWORA injuries are considered unstable and treatment options are limited, with rest and immobilisation in an age-appropriate orthosis for up to 3 months (Basu 2012) or surgical stabilisation recommended (Mathison et al. 2008; Li et al. 2011). Musculoskeletal complications in children with SCI are scoliosis and hip dysplasia, with a large proportion of those who suffer SCI before puberty developing both and requiring corrective surgery (Vogel et al. 2004). This reduces significantly in those injured after puberty.

The effect of the injury on the child and family is enormous, with changes evident within family dynamics and the team focus must be to ensure both child and family adjust to the injury. The provision of coordinated care by a multidisciplinary team is essential. The goal for all is to maintain active participation at home, school and other activities to ensure the child continues to develop socially. The focus is on promoting independence, rehabilitation and transition from hospital to home (Vogel et al. 2004). The reader should refer to Chapter 20 for further discussion of care following SCI.

Non-accidental Injury

In frequent or multiple fractures in children, the most likely cause is NAI (Jenny 2006). Flaherty et al. (2014) identified metaphyseal, rib, scapular, spinous process or sternal fractures as being the most common fractures caused by non-accidental injury in infants and toddlers. In addition, finger injuries in non-ambulant children, and bilateral and complex skull fractures plus fractures at different stages of healing have been identified as reasons to suspect NAI fractures (Karmazyn et al. 2011).

Children under 2 years and those who arc pre verbal are most at risk (Jenny 2006). Issues for practitioners to consider are:

- fractures are often found in cases of fatal abuse
- fractures of normal bones (non-pathological) require considerable force
- fractures that are sudden and painful: the child does not play normally afterwards
- pain is immediately worse after the fracture
- in late presentation loss of function may be the only symptom
- lack of associated bruising does not exclude NAI
- most abusive fractures are in children under 3 years
- most non-abusive fractures occur in children over 5 years (Selby 2011).

Practitioners also need to remember that several medical conditions may cause multiple fractures in children. These are osteogenesis imperfecta, preterm birth, rickets, osteomyelitis, copper deficiency or bones that are demineralised secondary to paralysis (Flaherty et al. 2014). Many parents whose child has such disorders report they were initially accused of abusing their child and this has severe consequences for both the child and family (Flaherty et al. 2014). Hence, children need a careful assessment if NAI is suspected, including a full history, skeletal survey, bloods for metabolic or bone disease and eye examination

(Jenny 2006). Most units have protocols for assessment and children under 2 years of age will be reviewed by a paediatrician before discharge to ensure that children who may be at risk of future injury are not discharged until review is completed. The reader should review Chapter 22 for further detail regarding NAI.

Obesity and Fractures

The prevalence of obesity has more than doubled in the past few decades in many areas throughout the world, with reports that 1 in 3 children is overweight and 1 in 5 is obese (Nhan et al. 2021). Obesity is recognised as a major medical and physical problem in children. This poses additional complications for those caring for children with fractures who are overweight and obese. Lane et al. (2020) found in a longitudinal cohort study of 466 997 children in Catalonia, Spain that children who were overweight or obese in pre-school had a greater risk of suffering a fracture in childhood. Some studies report increased need for surgical intervention for fractures in overweight and obese children (Nhan et al. 2021). Obese and overweight children in several studies are also reported as having an increased risk of post-operative complications following surgery for a fracture compared with children who are normal weight (Leet et al. 2005; Backstrom et al. 2012; Kim et al. 2016). These complications include increased risk of infection and wound dehiscence, compartment syndrome, nerve injuries and pressure ulcers (Leet et al. 2005). However, other retrospective chart studies have not found this to be the case (Bazelmans et al. 2004; Kwan et al. 2014; Li et al. 2020). Thus, it follows that some additional, larger and more definitive research studies are required on this topic. However, it is still necessary that the care being planned for the child takes body weight into consideration so that safe care is provided to the child and complications are avoided.

Summary

This chapter updates the reader on how best to care for the infant, child and young person presenting with common fractures.

Further Reading

Bryson, D. and Price, K. (2016). Upper limb fractures in children. *Surgery* 35 (1): 18–25.

Waters, P., Skaggs, D., and Flynn, J. (2020). *Rockwood and Wilkins Fractures in Children*, 9e. Philadelphia: Wolters Kluwer.

Wenger, D., Pring, M., Pennock, A., and Mollasani, V. (2018). *Rang's Children's Fractures*, 4e. Philadelphia: Wolters Kluwer.

References

Alqarni, N. and Goldman, R. (2018). Management of toddler's fractures. *Can. Fam. Physician* 64: 740–741.

Anglen, J. and Choi, L. (2005). Treatment options in pediatric femoral shaft fractures. *J. Orthop. Trauma* 19 (10): 724–733.

Babel, J.C., Mehlman, C.T., and Klein, G. (2010). Nerve injuries associated with pediatric supracondylar humeral fractures: a meta- analysis. *J. Pediatr. Orthop.* 30 (3): 253–263.

Backstrom, I.C., MacLennan, P.A., Sawyer, J.R. et al. (2012). Pediatric obesity and traumatic lower-extremity long-bone fracture outcomes. *J. Trauma Acute Care Surg.* 73 (4): 966–971.

Basu, S. (2012). Spinal injuries in children. *Front. Neurol.* 3 (96): 1–8.

Bazelmans, C., Coppieters, Y., Godin, I. et al. (2004). Is obesity associated with injuries among young people. *Eur. J. Epidemiol.* 19: 1037–1042.

Berg, E.E. (2005). Pediatric distal double bone formation fracture remodeling. *Orthop. Nurs.* 24 (1): 55–59.

Brighton, B. and Vitale, M. (2020). Epidemiology of fractures in children. In: *Rockwood and Wilkins Fractures in Children*, 9e (ed. P. Waters, D. Skaggs and J. Flynn). Philadelphia: Wolters Kluwer.

Bryson, D. and Price, K. (2016). Upper limb fractures in children. *Surgery* 35 (1): 18–25.

Cepela, D., Tartaglione, J., Dooley, T., and Patel, P. (2016). Classifications in brief: Salter–Harris classification of pediatric physeal fractures. *Clin. Orthop. Relat. Res.* 474: 2531–2537.

Dunham, E.A. (2003). Obstetrical brachial plexus palsy. *Orthop. Nurs.* 22 (2): 106–116.

Flaherty, E., Perez-Rossello, J., Levine, M. et al. (2014). Evaluating children with fractures for child physical abuse. *Pediatrics* 133 (2): e477–e489.

Gartland, J.J. (1959). Management of supracondylar fractures of the humerus in children. *Surg. Gynecol. Obstet.* 109 (2): 145–154.

Handoll, H., Elliott, J., Iheozor-Ejiofor, Z., and Karantana, A. (2018). Interventions for treating wrist fractures in children (review). *Cochrane Database Syst. Rev.* 12: CD012470. https://doi.org/10.1002/14651858. CD12470.pub2.

Hart, E.S., Albright, M., Gleeson, N.R., and Grottkau, B.E. (2006a). Common pediatric fractures – Part I. *Orthop. Nurs.* 25 (4): 251–256.

Hart, E.S., Grottkau, B.E., Rebello, G.N., and Albright, M.B. (2006b). Broken bones: common pediatric upper extremity fractures – Part II. *Orthop. Nurs.* 25 (5): 311–325.

Hart, E.S., Luther, B., and Grottkau, B.E. (2006c). Broken bones: common lower extremity fractures – Part III. *Orthop. Nurs.* 25 (6): 390–409.

Jenny, C. (2006). Evaluating infants and young children with multiple fractures. *Pediatrics* 118 (3): 1299–1303.

Jerome, J.T. and Prabu, G.R. (2021). Median nerve injuries associated with humerus shaft fractures in children. *Orthop. Surg.* 3 (2021): 17–25.

Johnston, T.E., Greco, M.N., Gaughan, J.P. et al. (2005). Patterns of lower extremity innervation in pediatric spinal cord injury. *Spinal Cord* 43: 476–482.

Jung, H., Park, M., Lee, M. et al. (2021). Growth arrest and its risk factors after physeal injury of the distal tibia in children and adolescents. *Injury* 52: 844–848.

Karir, A., Huynh, M., Carsen, S., et al. (2020). Management and Outcomes of Clinical Scaphoid Fractures in Children. Hand 17(3): 459–464. https://doi.org/10.1177/1558944720930293.

Karmazyn, B., Lewis, M., Jennings, S.G. et al. (2011). The prevalence of uncommon fractures of skeletal surveys performed to evaluate for suspected abuse in 930 children: should practice guidelines change? *Am. J. Roentgenol.* 197 (1): W159–W163.

Khosla, S., Melton, L., Dekutoski, M. et al. (2003). Incidence of childhood distal forearm fractures over 30 years. *J. Am. Med. Assoc.* 290: 1479–1485.

Kim, S., Ahn, J., Kim, H.K., and Kim, J.H. (2016). Obese children experience more extremity fractures than non obese children and are significantly more likely to die from traumatic injuries. *Acta Paediatr.* 105: 1152–1157.

Kitabjian, A. and Ladores, S. (2020). Treatment and management of torus fractures in pediatric patients. *J. Nurse Pract.* 16 (1): 48–56.

Kwan, C., Doan, Q., Oliveria, J.P. et al. (2014). Do obese children experience more severe fractures than non obese children? A cross-sectional study from a paediatric emergency department. *Paediatr. Child Health* 19 (5): 251–255.

Lane, J., Butler, K., Poveda-Marina, J. et al. (2020). Preschool obesity is associated with an increased risk of childhood fracture: a longitudinal cohort study of 466,997 children and up to 11 years of follow up in Catelonia, Spain. *J. Bone Miner. Res.* 35 (6): 1022–1030.

Leet, A., Pichard, C., and Ain, M. (2005). Surgical treatment of femoral fractures in obese children: does excessive body weight increase the rate of complications? *J. Bone Joint Surg. Am.* 87-A (12): 2609–2613.

Li, Y., Glotzbecker, M., Hedequist, D., and Mahan, S. (2011). Pediatric spinal trauma. *Trauma* 14 (1): 82–96.

Li, Y., James, C., Byl, N. et al. (2020). Obese children have different forearm fracture characteristics compared with normal-weight children. *J. Pediatr. Orthop.* 40 (2): e127–e130.

Lindisfarne, E. and Ayodele, O. (2020). Non-accidental injury, femoral shaft and neck fractures in children. *Surgery* 38 (9): 568–580.

Lipp, E.J. (1998). Athletic physeal injury in children and adolescents. *Orthop. Nurs.* 17 (2): 17–22.

Marengo, L., Canavese, F., Cravino, M. et al. (2016). Outcome of displaced fractures of the distal metaphyseal-diaphyseal junction of the humerus in children treated with elastic stable intramedullary nails. *J. Pediatr. Orthop.* 35 (6): 611–616.

Mathison, D., Kadom, N., and Krug, S. (2008). Spinal cord injury in the pediatric patient. *Clin. Pediatr. Emerg. Med.* 9: 106–123.

Moonot, P. and Ashwood, N. (2009). Clavicle fractures. *Trauma* 11: 123–132.

Mubarak, S., Ryul Kim, J., Edmonds, E. et al. (2009). Classification of proximal tibial fractures in children. *J. Child. Orthop.* 3: 191–197.

Nhan, D., Leet, A., and Lee, J. (2021). Associations of childhood overweight and obesity with upper-extremity fracture characteristics. *Medicine (Baltimore)* 100 (18): e25302.

Nicholas, M. and Cooper, L. (2009). Assessment of ankle injuries. *J. Sch. Nurs.* 25 (1): 34–39.

Omeroglu, H. (2018). Basic principles of fracture treatment in children. *Joint Dis. Relat. Surg.* 29 (1): 52–57.

O'Neill, B., Molloy, A., and Curtin, W. (2011). Conservative management of paediatric clavicle fractures. *Int. J. Pediatr.* 2011: ID172571. https://doi.org/10.1155/2011/172571.

Pang, D. and Wilberger, J. (1982). Spinal cord injury without radiographic abnormalities in children. *J. Neurosurg.* 57 (1): 114–129.

Platt, B. (2004). Supracondylar fracture of the humerus. *Emerg. Nurs.* 12 (2): 22–30.

Pogorelic, Z., Kadic, S., Milunovic, K.P. et al. (2017). Flexible intramedullary nailing for treatment of proximal humeral and humeral shaft fractures in children: a retrospective series of 118 cases. *Orthop. Traumatol. Surg. Res.* 103 (2017): 765–770.

Poutoglidou, F., Metaxiotis, D., Kazas, C., and Alvanos, D. (2020). Flexible intramedullary nailing in the treatment of forearm fractures in children and adolescents: A systematic review. *J. Orthop.* 20 (2020): 125–130.

Pring, M. and Wenger, D. (2005). Clavicle. In: *Rang's Children's Fractures*, 3e (ed. M. Rang, M. Pring and D. Wenger), 76–83. Philadelphia: Lippincott Williams and Wilkins.

Pring, M., Newton, P., and Rang, M. (2005). Femoral shaft. In: *Rang's Children's Fractures*, 3e (ed. M. Rang, M. Pring and D. Wenger), 182–200. Philadelphia: Lippincott Williams and Wilkins.

Puisto, V., Kaarainen, S., Impinen, A. et al. (2009). Incidence of spinal and spinal cord injuries and their surgical treatment in children and adolescents. *Spine* 35 (1): 104–107.

de Putter, C.E., van Beeck, E.F., Looman, W. et al. (2011). Trends in wrist fractures in children and adolescents, 1997–2009. *J. Hand Surg.* 236A: 1810–1815.

Randsborg, P.-H. (2013). Fractures in children. *Acta Orthop.* 84 (supp 350): 1–24.

Rennie, L., Court-Brown, C., Mok, J., and Beattie, T. (2007). The epidemiology of fractures in children. *Injury* 38: 913–922.

Rimbaldo, K., Fauteux-Lamarre, E., Babl, F. et al. (2021). Deformed pediatric forearm fractures: predictors of successful reduction by emergency providers. *Am. J. Emerg. Med.* 50 (2021): 59–63.

Robertson, J., Marsh, A., and Huntley, J. (2012). Neurological status in paediatric upper limb injuries in the emergency department – current practice. *BMC Res. Notes* 5: 324. https://doi.org/10.1186/1756-0500-5-324.

Rush, J., Kelly, D., Astur, N. et al. (2013). Associated injuries in children and adolescents with spinal trauma. *J. Pediatr. Orthop.* 33 (4): 393–397.

Saade-Lemus, S., Nguyen, J., Francavilla, M. et al. (2019). Buckle fractures of the proximal tibia in children and frequency of association with trampoline and inflatable bouncer use. *Pediatr. Radiol.* 49 (2019): 1327–1334.

Salter, R.B. and Harris, W.R. (1963). Injuries involving the epiphyseal plate. *J. Bone Joint Surg. Am.* 45-A: 587–623.

Schneider, J., Staubli, G., Kubat, S., and Altermatt, S. (2007). Treating displaced distal forearm fractures in children. *Eur. J. Trauma Emerg. Surg.* 33: 619–625.

Selby, M. (2011). Child protection and safeguarding. *Pract. Nurs.* 41 (4): 32–39.

Setter, K.J. and Palomino, K.E. (2006). Pediatric tibia fractures: current concepts. *Curr. Opin. Pediatr.* 18: 30–35.

Shannon, E., Hart, E., and Grottkau, B. (2009). Clavicle fractures in children: the essentials. *Orthop. Nurs.* 28 (5): 210–216.

Siddiq, K., Mehmood, A., Hamayan, M. et al. (2020). Comparison of outcome with medial versus lateral approach for operative fixation of supracondylar humeral fractures in pediatric patients. *Prof. Med. J.* 27 (10): 2045–2049.

Sigrist, E., George, N., Koder, A. et al. (2018). Treatment of closed femoral fractures in children aged 6 to 10. *J. Pediatr. Orthop.* 39 (5): e355–e359.

Vogel, L., Hickey, K., Klass, S., and Anderson, C. (2004). Unique issues in pediatric spinal cord injury. *Orthop. Nurs.* 23 (5): 300–310.

Index

Orthopaedic and Trauma Nursing: An Evidence-based Approach to Musculoskeletal Care, Second Edition. Edited by Sonya Clarke and Mary Drozd.
© 2023 John Wiley & Sons Ltd. Published 2023 by John Wiley & Sons Ltd.